Artificial Intelligence in Public Health: Current Trends and Future Possibilities

Artificial Intelligence in Public Health: Current Trends and Future Possibilities

Topic Editors

Daniele Giansanti
Giovanni Costantini

MDPI

Basel • Beijing • Wuhan • Barcelona • Belgrade • Novi Sad • Cluj • Manchester

Topic Editors
Daniele Giansanti
Centre Tisp
Istituto Superiore Di Sanita
Rome
Italy

Giovanni Costantini
Department of Electronic
Engineering
University of Rome Tor
Vergata
Rome
Italy

Editorial Office
MDPI AG
Grosspeteranlage 5
4052 Basel, Switzerland

This is a reprint of the Topic, published open access by the journals *Applied Sciences* (ISSN 2076-3417), *Bioengineering* (ISSN 2306-5354), *Healthcare* (ISSN 2227-9032), *International Journal of Environmental Research and Public Health* (ISSN 1660-4601), *Journal of Clinical Medicine* (ISSN 2077-0383) and *AI* (ISSN 2673-2688), freely accessible at: https://www.mdpi.com/topics/C52Z967WA3.

For citation purposes, cite each article independently as indicated on the article page online and as indicated below:

Lastname, A.A.; Lastname, B.B. Article Title. *Journal Name* **Year**, *Volume Number*, Page Range.

ISBN 978-3-7258-5471-4 (Hbk)
ISBN 978-3-7258-5472-1 (PDF)
https://doi.org/10.3390/books978-3-7258-5472-1

Contents

About the Editors

Daniele Giansanti

Daniele Giansanti is a Professor at Sapienza and Catholic University in Rome and a tutor of theses. He is a Board Editor and reviewer for several journals. He has 203 publications indexed on Scopus and more than 200 other contributions, including monographs, book chapters, and conference papers. He received an MD in Electronic Engineering at Sapienza University, Rome, in 1991; a PhD in Telecommunications and Microelectronics Engineering at Tor Vergata University, Rome, in 1997; and an Academic Specialization in Cognitive Psychology and Neural Networks at Sapienza University, Rome, in 1997. He obtained a specialization in Medical Physics at Sapienza University, Rome, in 2005. He was in charge of the Design of VLSI ASICs for DSP in the Civil Field (1991–1997) during his MD and PhD, and he served as a CAE-CAD-CAM system manager and Design Engineer in projects of electronic systems (Boards and VLSI) for the Warfare sector at Elettronica spa (1992–2000), one of the leaders in the military field. More importantly, he has been conducting varied research at ISS (the Italian NIH) since 2000 in the following fields, while also serving as Research Director since 2022: 1) Biomedical engineering and medical physics with the development of wearable and portable devices (three national patents); 2) Telemedicine and e-Health: Technology assessment and the integration of new systems in the fields of telerehabilitation, domiciliary monitoring, digital pathology, and digital radiology; 3) mHealth: Recent interest in the field of integrating smartphones and tablet technology in health care with particular attention to opportunities, risks, abuse, and regulation; 4)Acceptance of and consensus in the use of robots for assistance and rehabilitation; 5) Challenges and acceptance of the use of artificial intelligence in digital radiology and digital pathology; 6) Cybersecurity in the health domain.

Giovanni Costantini

Giovanni Costantini is an Associate Professor at the University of Rome "Tor Vergata," where he has been conducting research since 1995. He earned a degree in Electronic Engineering from "La Sapienza" University of Rome and a Ph.D. in Telecommunications and Microelectronics Engineering from "Tor Vergata." In parallel, he completed his musical studies, graduating in Piano and Electronic Music from the Conservatory of Music, combining technical and artistic expertise in a multidisciplinary path. At the University of Rome "Tor Vergata," Costantini teaches courses in Electrical Engineering, Multimedia Signal Processing, and Electronic Music. He also serves as the Director of the Master's program in Sonic Arts, an advanced program focused on sound technologies, music composition, and sound design for cinema, video games, and other digital media. His main research interests lie at the intersection of electronic engineering, computer science, and neuroscience applied to audio, speech, and biomedical signals. These include artificial intelligence, neural networks, machine learning, and signal processing, with particular emphasis on audio, speech, and biomedical signals. His research focuses on developing methods for analyzing, processing, and generating sound and musical signals, with applications ranging from medicine to multimedia production. His research interests include artificial intelligence, neural networks, machine learning, and signal processing, with a particular emphasis on audio, speech, and biomedical signals. He has authored over 150 publications in scientific journals and international conferences.

Preface

The unprecedented challenges posed by the COVID-19 pandemic have accelerated the transformation of healthcare through artificial intelligence (AI). What was once considered a future possibility has rapidly become an essential component of health systems worldwide. AI has proven crucial in tracking disease outbreaks, optimizing patient care, supporting diagnostics, and managing hospital resources, while also revealing the complexities of integrating such technologies responsibly.

This reprint gathers the research originally published within a comprehensive Topic aimed at exploring AI's multifaceted role in healthcare. In total, the collection includes 26 contributions plus the concluding editorial, encompassing original research, review articles and other contributions. These contributions span scientific and clinical advancements, practical applications, and critical reflections on ethics, equity, and training. The works highlight the diversity of AI applications, ranging from predictive modeling in oncology and emergency medicine to medical imaging, mental health, public health surveillance, and resource management. Reviews further extend the discussion to emerging fields such as mobile radiology, teledermatology, women's health, cardiology, and domestic violence detection, emphasizing both the promise and challenges of AI adoption.

Altogether, these works illustrate how AI and machine learning are reshaping the foundations of healthcare. They underscore AI's transformative potential not only in crisis response but also in building more equitable, efficient, and personalized health systems for the future.

We would like to thank all the authors, reviewers, and contributors whose outstanding work made the reprint of this Topic possible. We also extend our gratitude to the editorial team for their dedication and support and to Editor Pepper Cao for her support and continued guidance. Their combined efforts have been essential in bringing this Topic to fruition.

Daniele Giansanti and Giovanni Costantini
Topic Editors

International Journal of
Environmental Research and Public Health

MDPI

Editorial

Artificial Intelligence in Public Health: Current Trends and Future Possibilities

Daniele Giansanti

Centre Tisp, Istituto Superiore di Sanità, 00161 Rome, Italy; daniele.giansanti@iss.it; Tel.:+39-06-4990-2701

Artificial intelligence (AI) is a discipline that studies whether and how intelligent computer systems that can simulate the capacity and behaviour of human thought can be created.

Specific definitions can be obtained by focusing on applications and by measuring the reliability and effectiveness of behaviour after comparison with human behaviour [1].

What is expected from an AI-based system can be summarized in the following statements [1]:

1. It *must act* in a similar way to human beings: the product of the procedure performed by the artificial intelligent system should be indistinguishable from the one followed by a human being.
2. It *must think* in a similar way to human beings: the sequential activity that leads the intelligent system to face and solve a problem is comparable with the one followed by a human being.
3. It *must behave* (*act* and *think*) in a rational way: the method that leads the intelligent system to solve a problem is a formal structured process following the logic.
4. It *must obtain* the best possible result: the process that leads the intelligent system to solve the problem is the one that allows it to obtain the best-expected outcome based on the provided information.

AI has its roots in and includes scientific disciplines such as computational sciences and neural networks. Starting in the 1980s [2] we began to speak specifically of AI when Deep Blue-type system emerged and were found to be capable of dealing with the human beings in the game of chess and again later on, when NASA used dedicated applications such as Remote Agent to manage the activities of a spacecraft. From these first applications, it was clear that the use of AI has important implications for the user and on the environment; therefore, particular attention must be paid to the ethical, environmental, regulation, and social aspects of AI and to the need to increase transparency and responsibility in the process of use.

In some previous studies focused on AI in digital radiology and digital pathology we have seen this; that is, the real integration of AI in the *health domain* cannot be based on scientific development alone and cannot ignore ethical, regulatory, and social aspects, such as the acceptance of citizens and professionals [3–6].

In 2017, following a conference of world artificial intelligence experts promoted by the Future of Life Institute, a vademecum with 23 principles was drawn up, with broad consensus to address the ethical, social, cultural, and military issues of AI. The document was immediately signed by over 800 experts and later by thousands more [7].

In the *health domain*, when dealing with the health of the individual, all of this is particularly felt. This Special Issue, "Artificial Intelligence in Public Health: Current Trends and Future Possibilities" [8], aims to act as a collector among scholars on issues related to both the development and integration of AI in the health domain. This is addressed both with reference to current trends and by trying to grasp future developments.

This represents a new and hot research topic, as verified through a search on Pubmed, a reference database on issues related to biomedicine and the health domain.

If we search [9]:

(Artificial Intelligence [Title/Abstract]) AND (current trends [Title/Abstract]) Sort by: Publication Date "artificial intelligence" [Title/Abstract] AND "current trends" [Title/Abstract]

We can find 72 articles, 70 of which were published between 2018 and 2022.

Among these, we note a particular development of reviews, 46, all of which are recent (63.9%).

If we search [10]:

(Artificial Intelligence [Title/Abstract]) AND (future possibilities [Title/Abstract]) Sort by: Publication Date "artificial intelligence" [Title/Abstract] AND "future possibilities" [Title/Abstract]

We find 22 articles, all of which were published between 2018 and 2022.

Among these, we note a particular development of reviews, with 15 being found (68.2%).

The high percentage of reviews around these issues certainly denotes a great interest in the cultural and scientific mediation actions dedicated to the intensification of research in this area aimed both at the development and present and future integration of AI on the part of scholars. This is comforting and corroborates the idea of developing a Special Issue dedicated to this [8].

Much is expected of AI both today and tomorrow, both from a development point of view and via integration with the *health domain*, which must also pass regulations, ethical scrutiny, social acceptance.

Research in this area is strategic for the development of health systems and is inextricably linked to the development of digital health, both in regard to this collection, monitoring, and management of information and in regard to the management of hospital and connected government information systems. Think, for example, of the opportunities presented by wearable monitoring, big data, robotic assistance, rehabilitation, and surgery. The applications of artificial intelligence have received growing interest in many sectors, such as in those related to organ, functional tissue, and cell diagnostics [3–6]; care robotics, which assist in interventions, rehabilitation, and supporting the communication and assistance of disabled people [11–14]; the biomedicine sector, where it is implemented in applications from genetics to modelling [15–18]; and precision and personalized biomedicine [19–24]. The consolidation of technologies based on artificial intelligence in the *health domain* is intended to bring benefits to everyone, from the stakeholder to the patient, in the form of equity of care.

In the future, artificial intelligence is expected to have a strong impact on:

- The prevention of the onset of diseases in the individual and in society
- The provision of personal care and assistance.
- Society trends regarding diseases and the impact of biological and behavioural factors.
- The organization of hospital activities with regard to treatment, diagnostics, and decision-making processes.

Thanks to artificial intelligence, on the one hand, big data [25,26] will help us to predict diseases on an individual and collective basis and to identify and correct population behaviours; on the other hand, wearable technologies will allow us to monitor and collect individual medical information and to calibrate the care process. The integration of artificial intelligence with virtual reality and augmented reality [27,28] will allow us to create both virtual medicine services that citizens can access in a simple and direct way as well as robotic surgery applications that are increasingly effective and safe.

Many professionals will be involved in the process of developing and integrating AI into the *health domain* in the present as well as in the future. The sectors of research, diagnosis, and clinical therapy will be called upon to offer ideas and experts in this area. The government, educational, and political sectors will also be called upon to make important decisions. Therefore, stakeholders will have to take on important responsibilities.

The research sector, to which this editorial is addressed, will have a leading role since it is from this sector that not only algorithms and proposals for AI solutions but also concrete ideas of transfer to the *health domain* for a stable use in clinical/biomedical practice will emerge, accompanied by the actions of the regulators acting at all envisaged levels. This key role will also be assumed by the disciplines responsible for the certification of medical devices with artificial intelligence content, which will have to be harmonized and consolidated, particularly at the international level.

It is hoped that this Special Issue [8] will be useful for this purpose and that it will be capable of making important contributions in the levels of intervention related to these issues.

Funding: This study was supported and funded by the Italian Ministry of Health-Ricerca Corrente.

Conflicts of Interest: The author declares no conflict of interest.

References

1. Lieto, A. *Cognitive Design for Artificial Minds*; Routledge, Taylor & Francis: London, UK, 2021; ISBN 978-1-138-20792-9.
2. Heßler, M. The Triumph of "Stupidity": Deep Blue's Victory over Garri Kasparov. The Controversy about its Impact on Artficial Intelligence Research. *NTM* **2017**, *25*, 1–33. [CrossRef] [PubMed]
3. Giansanti, D.; Di Basilio, F. The Artificial Intelligence in Digital Radiology: Part 1: The Challenges, Acceptance and Consensus. *Healthcare* **2022**, *10*, 509. [CrossRef] [PubMed]
4. Di Basilio, F.; Esposisto, G.; Monoscalco, L.; Giansanti, D. The Artificial Intelligence in Digital Radiology: Part 2: Towards an Investigation of acceptance and consensus on the Insiders. *Healthcare* **2022**, *10*, 153. [CrossRef]
5. Giovagnoli, M.R.; Giansanti, D. Artificial Intelligence in Digital Pathology: What Is the Future? Part 1: From the Digital Slide Onwards. *Healthcare* **2021**, *9*, 858. [CrossRef]
6. Giovagnoli, M.R.; Ciucciarelli, S.; Castrichella, L.; Giansanti, D. Artificial Intelligence in Digital Pathology: What Is the Future? Part 2: An Investigation on the Insiders. *Healthcare* **2021**, *9*, 1347. [CrossRef] [PubMed]
7. Available online: https://futureoflife.org/2017/08/11/ai-principles/?cn-reloaded=1 (accessed on 20 September 2022).
8. Available online: https://www.mdpi.com/journal/ijerph/special_issues/C52Z967WA3 (accessed on 20 September 2022).
9. Available online: https://pubmed.ncbi.nlm.nih.gov/?term=%28Artificial+Intelligence%5BTitle%2FAbstract%5D%29+AND+%28current+trends%5BTitle%2FAbstract%5D%29&sort=pubdate&size=100 (accessed on 20 September 2022).
10. Available online: https://pubmed.ncbi.nlm.nih.gov/?term=%28artificial+intelligence%5BTitle%2FAbstract%5D%29+AND+%28future+possibilities%5BTitle%2FAbstract%5D%29&sort=pubdate&size=100 (accessed on 20 September 2022).
11. Bozkurt, E.; Sijberden, J.P.; Hilal, M.A. What Is the Current Role and What Are the Prospects of the Robotic Approach in Liver Surgery? *Cancers* **2022**, *14*, 4268. [CrossRef]
12. Guo, C.; Li, H. Application of 5G network combined with AI robots in personalized nursing in China: A literature review. *Front. Public Health* **2022**, *10*, 948303. [CrossRef]
13. Gu, Y.; Xu, Y.; Shen, Y.; Huang, H.; Liu, T.; Jin, L.; Ren, H.; Wang, J. A Review of Hand Function Rehabilitation Systems Based on Hand Motion Recognition Devices andArtificial Intelligence. *Brain Sci.* **2022**, *12*, 1079. [CrossRef]
14. Benzakour, A.; Altsitzioglou, P.; Lemée, J.M.; Ahmad, A.; Mavrogenis, A.F.; Benzakour, T. Artificial intelligence in spine surgery. *Int. Orthop.* **2022**. [CrossRef]
15. Harris, S.; Bonnici, T.; Keen, T.; Lilaonitkul, W.; White, M.J.; Swanepoel, N. Clinical deployment environments: Five pillars of translational machine learning for health. *Front. Digit. Health* **2022**, *4*, 939292. [CrossRef]
16. Dai, X.; Chen, Y. Computational Biomaterials: Computational Simulations for Biomedicine. *Adv. Mater.* **2022**, e2204798. [CrossRef] [PubMed]
17. Pugliese, R.; Regondi, S. Artificial Intelligence-Empowered 3D and 4D Printing Technologies toward Smarter Biomedical Materials and Approaches. *Polymers* **2022**, *14*, 2794. [CrossRef] [PubMed]
18. Bernstam, E.V.; Shireman, P.K.; Meric-Bernstam, F.; NZozus, M.; Jiang, X.; Brimhall, B.B.; Windham, A.K.; Schmidt, S.; Visweswaran, S.; Ye, Y.; et al. Artificial intelligence in clinical and translational science: Successes, challenges and opportunities. *Clin. Transl. Sci.* **2022**, *15*, 309–321. [CrossRef] [PubMed]
19. Zhou, Y.; Tremmel, R.; Schaeffeler, E.; Schwab, M.; Lauschke, V.M. Challenges and opportunities associated with rare-variant pharmacogenomics. *Trends Pharmacol. Sci.* **2022**, *43*, 852–865. [CrossRef]
20. Acosta, J.N.; Falcone, G.J.; Rajpurkar, P.; Topol, E.J. Multimodal biomedical AI. *Nat. Med.* **2022**. [CrossRef]

21. Al Saiegh, F.; Munoz, A.; Velagapudi, L.; Theofanis, T.; Suryadevara, N.; Patel, P.; Jabre, R.; Chen, C.J.; Shehabeldin, M.; Gooch, M.R.; et al. Patient and procedure selection for mechanical thrombectomy: Toward personalized medicine and the role of artificial intelligence. *J. Neuroimaging* **2022**, *32*, 798–807. [CrossRef]
22. Fountzilas, E.; Tsimberidou, A.M.; Vo, H.H.; Kurzrock, R. Clinical trial design in the era of precision medicine. *Genome Med.* **2022**, *14*, 101. [CrossRef]
23. Thirunavukarasu, R.; Gnanasambandan, R.; Gopikrishnan, M.; Palanisamy, V. Towards computational solutions for precision medicine based big data healthcare system using deep learning models: A review. *Comput. Biol. Med.* **2022**, *149*, 106020. [CrossRef]
24. Zare Harofte, S.; Soltani, M.; Siavashy, S.; Raahemifar, K. Recent Advances of Utilizing Artificial Intelligence in Lab on a Chip for Diagnosis and Treatment. *Small* **2022**, e2203169. [CrossRef]
25. Xu, Y.; Zhang, X.; Li, H.; Zheng, H.; Zhang, J.; Olsen, M.S.; Varshney, R.K.; Prasanna, B.M.; Qian, Q. Smart breeding driven by big data, artificial intelligence and integrated genomic-enviromic prediction. *Mol. Plant.* **2022**. [CrossRef]
26. Jiang, P.; Sinha, S.; Aldape, K.; Hannenhalli, S.; Sahinalp, C.; Ruppin, E. Big data in basic and translational cancer research. *Nat. Rev. Cancer* **2022**, 1–15. [CrossRef] [PubMed]
27. Antel, R.; Abbasgholizadeh-Rahimi, S.; Guadagno, E.; Harley, J.M.; Poenaru, D. The use of artificial intelligence and virtual reality in doctor-patient risk communication: A scoping review. *Patient Educ. Couns.* **2022**, *105*, 3038–3050. [CrossRef] [PubMed]
28. Ma, M.K.I.; Saha, C.; Poon, S.H.L.; Yiu, R.S.W.; Shih, K.C.; Chan, Y.K. Virtual reality and augmented reality- emerging screening and diagnostic techniques in ophthalmology: A systematic review. *Surv. Ophthalmol.* **2022**, *67*, 1516–1530. [CrossRef] [PubMed]

bioengineering

MDPI

Editorial

Artificial Intelligence in Public Health: Bridging Today's Trends with Tomorrow's Possibilities

Daniele Giansanti [1,*] and Giovanni Costantini [2]

1 Centre Tisp, Istituto Superiore Di Sanita, 000161 Rome, Italy
2 Department of Electronic Engineering, University of Rome Tor Vergata, 00133 Rome, Italy; giovanni.costantini@uniroma2.it
* Correspondence: daniele.giansanti@iss.it

Driven by the unprecedented challenges of the COVID-19 pandemic, the healthcare sector has witnessed remarkable—and at times sometimes overwhelming—advancements in the role of artificial intelligence (AI) [1]. The pandemic underscored the urgent need to enhance health systems and better manage healthcare data, prompting a surge in the development and application of AI technologies [2]. From tracking disease outbreaks to optimizing patient care and managing hospital resources, AI has emerged as a critical tool in reshaping health systems, especially in times of crisis [3].

The pandemic has highlighted both the potential and the complexities of integrating AI into healthcare [4]. The rapid shift toward digital health solutions has accelerated the adoption of technologies that were previously seen as futuristic, making them vital to the global response to the health crisis [5]. Innovations such as wearable health monitoring, big data analysis, and robotic surgery have played key roles in addressing the immediate demands of the pandemic [6,7]. The range of AI applications [8] that emerged during this period is broad, including diagnostics for organ and tissue conditions, care robotics for rehabilitation and disability support, biomedicine encompassing genetics and modeling, and precision medicine that tailors treatments to individuals' genetic profiles.

As Henry Ford famously stated, "Real progress happens only when the advantages of a new technology become available to everybody". The COVID-19 pandemic has brought this statement into sharp focus, as the world has recognized the importance of ensuring that the benefits of AI and digital health advancements are accessible to all, regardless of geography or socioeconomic status [9]. AI in healthcare is not merely a technological leap; it represents a critical pathway toward equitable healthcare for all.

The integration of AI in healthcare systems is designed to enhance care quality and promote equity. Its influence will extend far beyond immediate health crises, shaping the future of disease prevention, personal care delivery, and the management of healthcare systems. In particular, AI holds the potential to impact the prevention of diseases at both the individual and societal levels, offering insights into disease prediction, monitoring, and personalized treatment options. The integration of AI with other technologies and solutions [8,9], such as robotics and virtual and augmented reality, could create a new era of accessible virtual healthcare services and further enhance the precision and safety of robotic surgeries.

To address these challenges, a comprehensive Topic [10] was proposed, which included research published in several prominent journals, such as *Healthcare*, *Applied Sciences*, *AI*, Bioengineering, *JCM*, and *IJERPH*. This Topic aims to provide a thorough exploration of AI's role in transforming healthcare systems, spanning from scientific advancements to real-world applications. It also focuses on critical ethical and training considerations,

 https://doi.org/10.3390/bioengineering12060559

encouraging researchers and practitioners to consider how AI can be deployed responsibly and effectively. In this editorial, we will present the results and key findings from the research collected in this Topic, highlighting the significant progress made in AI applications and their implications for the future of public health.

Thanks to the contribution of numerous international research groups, this Topic has reached 26 publications in addition to this concluding editorial. As shown in Figure 1, sixteen articles (AR) [11–26]; seven reviews including two systematic reviews [27–33]; one technical note (TN) [34]; one perspective (P) [35]; and one editorial (ED) [36] presenting the project have been published.

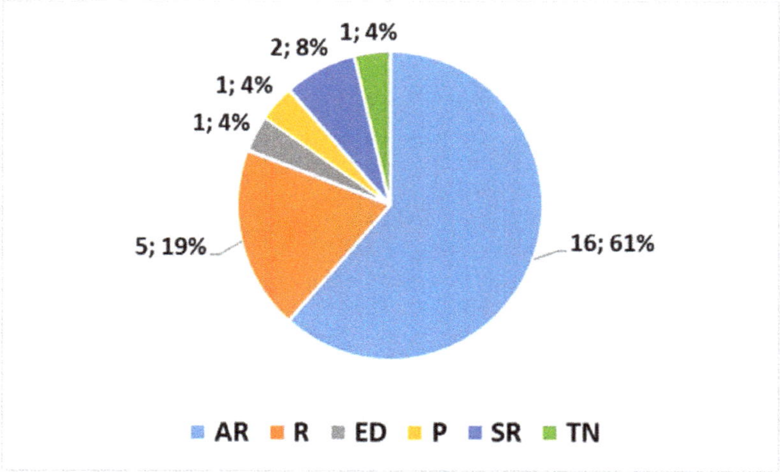

Figure 1. Number and types of publications contributed to the Topic (articles—AR, reviews—R, technical notes—TN, perspectives—P, systematic reviews—SR, editorials—ED).

Contributions of Studies

Table 1 synthesizes the contributions of the studies included in this Topic.

Table 1. Summary of the articles published in this Topic.

Study	Focus	Brief Summary	Contribution
[11]	Indoor transmission of respiratory diseases and real-time contact rate analysis	This study addresses the increasing concern about airborne diseases spreading in indoor spaces, particularly in settings like offices, schools, and hospitals. It introduces an advanced software tool powered by YOLOv8, a state-of-the-art deep learning model, to accurately detect and track individuals from video streams. The tool uses dynamic circular buffer zones and a 2D projective transformation to overlay digital coordinates of the physical environment, visualizing heatmaps of spatial contact patterns and quantifying contact events. This method provides a more precise and automated alternative to traditional manual contact tracing and counting techniques.	This study introduces a transformative shift in public health surveillance by integrating real-time tracking and AI to model disease transmission more accurately and efficiently. The system's ability to offer precise, dynamic tracking within enclosed spaces will significantly enhance epidemiological studies, improve the management of disease outbreaks, and provide public health officials with a robust tool to develop non-pharmaceutical interventions based on real-time, spatially detailed data.

Table 1. *Cont.*

Study	Focus	Brief Summary	Contribution
[12]	Delayed medical treatment behavior in oral cancer patients in Western China and machine learning for prediction	This research investigates the social, economic, and health factors contributing to delays in seeking medical treatment among oral cancer patients in Western China. A combination of logistic regression and machine learning models (such as nearest neighbors, SVM, and random forest) is applied to identify key risk factors and predict the likelihood of delayed treatment. This study compares the behavior of patients before and after the lifting of COVID-19 restrictions, offering insights into the pandemic's impact on medical delays.	This study provides a unique and large-scale analysis of delayed treatment behavior, with a focus on how family dynamics, social support, and external factors like the pandemic influence patients' decision-making. By developing a predictive model, it offers valuable insights into healthcare policies and early intervention strategies, especially in regions with limited healthcare access. It underscores the importance of social support, highlighting the role of family structures in reducing treatment delays and potentially improving outcomes.
[13]	Short- and long-term mortality prediction in emergency department patients using clinical data	This study focuses on creating predictive models for mortality risks in patients admitted to emergency departments (EDs) by using minimal, routine clinical data—specifically, blood biochemistry results from a single admission sample. This study uses datasets from several large Danish hospitals, applying machine learning models to predict patient mortality within 10, 30, 90, and 365 days post-admission. The goal is to enhance patient triage and prioritization, particularly in settings where timely decisions can save lives.	The contribution lies in proving that routine biochemistry tests, often performed at admission, can be leveraged to accurately predict both short-term and long-term mortality. This study proposes a simplified yet highly effective tool for mortality prediction, which could become an integral part of emergency care workflows, helping clinicians make better decisions regarding patient management and resource allocation in EDs.
[14]	AI-assisted mental health evaluation and personalized medical advice generation	This paper proposes an integrated AI system that combines finite state machines, semantic matching algorithms, and medical knowledge graphs to improve mental health assessments. By automating the collection of patient data and conducting preliminary evaluations, the tool optimizes decision-making. It then generates personalized medical advice based on deep learning techniques such as RoBERTa for semantic matching, ensuring accuracy in recommending treatment options.	This study showcases how AI can significantly improve mental healthcare by streamlining the assessment process and providing personalized advice. The integration of AI-driven diagnostics with medical knowledge graphs leads to more accurate recommendations, ensuring efficient use of medical resources. The findings have the potential to reduce the diagnostic burden on mental health professionals and provide a personalized care experience for patients.
[15]	Radiomics and AI in predicting progression-free survival in high-grade glioma patients	This study explores the use of radiomics (the extraction of quantitative features from medical images) combined with AI algorithms to predict progression-free survival (PFS) in patients with high-grade gliomas, a type of brain cancer. The research focuses on preoperative MRI scans, analyzing 109 radiomic features along with clinical factors like age, sex, and tumor location to develop predictive models.	This research contributes to personalized oncology by demonstrating how AI models, when integrated with radiomic features, can provide accurate predictions of progression-free survival in glioma patients. These insights can assist in stratifying patients based on their risk of tumor recurrence, potentially guiding tailored treatment plans. The study emphasizes the importance of early prediction in managing high-grade gliomas and improving patient outcomes through more individualized treatment strategies.

Table 1. *Cont.*

Study	Focus	Brief Summary	Contribution
[16]	Machine learning for predicting length of stay in pediatric intensive care units (PICU)	This study investigates the application of machine learning models to predict the length of stay (LOS) in pediatric intensive care units (PICUs). This research uses data from over 100 North American PICUs, applying algorithms such as support vector machine, Gradient Boosting, and Recurrent Neural Networks (RNNs) to predict patient outcomes at various thresholds (24, 36, 48 h, etc.). The primary goal is to improve resource management and optimize staffing within PICUs.	This study highlights how machine learning can outperform traditional methods of predicting PICU LOS, with models like Gradient Boosting and RNNs achieving higher accuracy and balanced performance. These models provide critical insights that can be used to better allocate resources, optimize staffing, and improve patient care. The findings suggest that further refinement of machine learning models could enhance their applicability in clinical settings, improving operational efficiency in pediatric intensive care units.
[17]	Ensemble machine learning models for injury prediction	This study analyzes the use of ensemble machine learning (ML) models to predict injury codes from the National Electronic Injury Surveillance System (NEISS) dataset. Four ensemble models were tested: random forest (RF) + logistic regression (LR), K-Nearest Neighbor (KNN) + RF, LR + KNN, and a combined LR + RF + KNN approach. The KNN + LR ensemble model achieved 90.47% accuracy for the top injury code, while the combined KNN + LR + RF model excelled with 99.50% accuracy for predicting the top two injury codes.	This study demonstrates how ensemble ML models, particularly the probabilistic framework, can enhance the accuracy of unstructured narrative classification, especially when dealing with imbalanced data. The findings underscore the potential of these models to improve decision-making in public health, especially in injury classification systems.
[18]	Virtual companion for people with dementia in long-term care	This study focuses on developing a virtual companion for people living with dementia (PLWD) in long-term care (LTC). The system, delivered via a head-mounted virtual reality display, initially prompted conversation and reminiscence, and later used advanced AI to allow more nuanced interactions. Testing showed that while the system faced challenges in early stages, the improved AI in later stages led to more meaningful interactions. Despite some issues like speech recognition and display weight, the system was found to be enjoyable for many users.	This research illustrates the application of virtual reality and AI to provide an engaging, socially interactive tool for PLWD in LTC, promoting meaningful conversations and reducing loneliness. It lays the groundwork for future enhancements, emphasizing the need for innovations in both hardware and software to improve user experience.
[19]	Impact of COVID-19 on emergency medical services in Kazakhstan	This retrospective study examines the structure and frequency of ambulance calls in Kazakhstan from 2019 to 2023, focusing on changes during and after the COVID-19 pandemic. The analysis found significant fluctuations in urgency category IV calls, with decreases during the pandemic due to quarantine restrictions and a subsequent increase in the post-pandemic period.	The research provides valuable insights into the dynamics of EMS call volumes in response to the COVID-19 pandemic. It highlights the shifts in healthcare service demand and the long-term impact on emergency medical systems, particularly in less urgent cases. This study offers critical data for improving future emergency healthcare responses during pandemics.
[20]	Comparison of diagnostic accuracy between Google and ChatGPT 3.5 for urological conditions	This study compares the diagnostic accuracy of two freely available platforms, Google and ChatGPT 3.5, for identifying urological pathologies. A sample of 60 clinical cases was used to assess each platform's performance. ChatGPT 3.5 showed superior accuracy, especially for common urological conditions, while Google was less reliable, particularly for rare disorders.	The findings highlight the increasing role of AI platforms in medical diagnosis, showing that ChatGPT 3.5 outperformed Google in providing accurate diagnoses, particularly in common urological conditions. This research sets the stage for exploring the use of AI tools in clinical practice, though further improvements are necessary for rare condition diagnosis.

Table 1. *Cont.*

Study	Focus	Brief Summary	Contribution
[21]	Radiomics and machine learning for predicting survival in NSCLC patients	This retrospective study investigates the use of radiomics and machine learning to predict survival in non-small cell lung cancer (NSCLC) patients using FDG PET/CT imaging. It evaluates a radiomic model, incorporating tumor stage, SUVmax, and selected radiomic features like NGTDM coarseness, and compares it with a traditional survival model based only on tumor stage and SUVmax.	This study demonstrates that integrating radiomic features with traditional clinical data can offer similar predictive power for survival in NSCLC patients. While the radiomic model's accuracy was comparable to traditional methods, the findings suggest a potential for more precise, personalized prognostic models in the future.
[22]	Deep learning for brain tumor detection in MRI scans	This research introduces a novel dual deep convolutional neural network (DCNN) model designed for classifying brain tumor MRI scans. By using two deep learning models (InceptionV3 and DenseNet121) for feature extraction, this study achieves high performance in classifying brain tumors as cancerous or non-cancerous. It compares this dual DCNN approach against other popular deep learning architectures, showing superior performance.	This study presents a highly effective AI model for brain tumor detection, outperforming traditional deep learning methods in terms of accuracy, precision, and recall. This approach highlights the potential for deep learning models to revolutionize early cancer detection through automated analysis of medical images, which could greatly enhance diagnostic efficiency and outcomes.
[23]	Artificial intelligence for early detection of hemorrhage and organ dysfunction during delivery	This study leverages machine learning to establish numerical criteria for identifying organ dysfunction in cases of massive hemorrhage during delivery. The research uses a dataset of 107 deliveries with >2000 mL blood loss from nine national perinatal centers in Japan. By analyzing coagulation factors like fibrinogen and FDP, this study identifies thresholds for predicting hematuria development, which can indicate organ dysfunction. It applies six different machine learning methods, with the support vector machine being the most effective in determining the relevant clinical criteria.	This study presents a novel AI-driven method to detect organ dysfunction in massive hemorrhage cases during delivery. By providing more precise numerical thresholds and combining machine learning with clinical coagulation data, the method could significantly improve the early identification of severe complications in obstetric care, leading to quicker interventions and better patient outcomes.
[24]	Advanced Fuzzy C-Means segmentation for MRI brain tumor detection	This research focuses on improving the Fuzzy C-Means (FCM) segmentation algorithm for MRI images to enhance brain tumor classification. This study integrates feature selection based on tumor shape, texture, and color, which reduces complexity and increases classification accuracy. It then uses the Extreme Learning Machine (ELM) classifier to segment and categorize brain tumors. The performance of this enhanced model is compared with existing methods, and it consistently demonstrates superior accuracy, particularly in detecting gliomas.	The improved FCM-based model delivers better performance for tumor classification in MRI scans, with notable improvements in accuracy, precision, and recall. This algorithm can play a pivotal role in medical imaging for early and accurate brain tumor detection, offering clinicians more reliable tools for diagnosis. Additionally, the model's success in glioma detection has the potential to be a breakthrough in clinical practice for more precise brain tumor identification.
[25]	Exploring AI's role in public health research and scientific authorship	This study explores the potential of GPT-3, an advanced AI model, to support public health research by generating relevant text blocks and summarizing scientific articles. The research specifically tests GPT-3's capacity to provide plausible answers on public health issues. Despite some fabricated content, it demonstrates the potential for AI to assist researchers in compiling and analyzing large amounts of data. It also discusses the implications of using AI as a scientific contributor in research publications while adhering to the principles of scientific integrity.	This study highlights the potential of AI to assist in public health research by summarizing the literature and generating scientific content. However, it also raises critical questions about the credibility of AI-generated information and its appropriate role in authorship. This research emphasizes the importance of establishing guidelines for AI's involvement in scientific research, ensuring that its contributions are valid and adhere to ethical standards.

Table 1. *Cont.*

Study	Focus	Brief Summary	Contribution
[26]	AI-powered COVID-19 CT image diagnosis and lesion segmentation	This study presents a deep learning-based method for accurately segmenting lesions from CT images of COVID-19 patients. The proposed solution, DLShelper, corrects rough initial labels of lesions by analyzing pixel distribution in infected and healthy areas. By improving segmentation accuracy, the system aids in diagnosing COVID-19 and grading the severity of lung lesions. The approach is tested on a public dataset of CT images and has been shown to significantly improve segmentation and diagnosis accuracy, benefiting medical staff with better diagnostic support.	The DLShelper tool offers a promising AI-driven solution for diagnosing COVID-19 through enhanced lesion segmentation and severity grading. It assists clinicians by providing more accurate and detailed diagnostic information, improving decision-making during the diagnosis process. The tool's effectiveness in handling CT images can be adapted for other diagnostic applications, paving the way for more advanced, AI-powered diagnostic systems in healthcare.

The integration of artificial intelligence (AI) and machine learning (ML) has become increasingly important in improving healthcare systems. Studies [11–26] illustrate diverse applications across various domains, from predicting patient outcomes to optimizing diagnostic accuracy and enhancing healthcare management.

One significant area of development is the use of AI for predicting patient outcomes. For example, ref. [12] investigates delayed treatment behavior in oral cancer patients in Western China, using ML models to predict delays and identify risk factors. Similarly, ref. [13] applies ML models to predict mortality risk in emergency department patients based on routine clinical data, aiming to enhance patient triage and prioritization. Both studies demonstrate how AI can support more effective and timely predictions, potentially saving lives by allowing clinicians to intervene earlier. These studies highlight the growing role of AI in supporting medical decision-making and resource allocation.

Medical image analysis also shows promising results, particularly for detecting and classifying diseases. For instance, ref. [15] explores the use of radiomics and AI to predict progression-free survival in high-grade glioma patients, while ref. [22] introduces a dual deep convolutional neural network (DCNN) model to classify brain tumors in MRI scans. By analyzing medical images using AI, clinicians can obtain more precise, personalized treatment plans. Likewise, ref. [24] enhances brain tumor detection through an improved Fuzzy C-Means algorithm, further underscoring AI's potential in improving diagnostic accuracy and early detection. AI-powered diagnostic tools are crucial in improving patient outcomes by enabling earlier intervention and more accurate treatment strategies.

The role of AI in mental health and well-being is another key area that is explored. The authors of [14] propose an AI system to automate mental health evaluations and generate personalized medical advice, highlighting AI's potential in streamlining assessments and offering tailored treatment options. Moreover, ref. [18] investigates the use of a virtual companion for people with dementia in long-term care, which uses AI-driven interactions to reduce loneliness and promote meaningful social engagement. Both studies emphasize AI's ability to provide personalized, patient-centered care in mental health.

AI's impact on public health surveillance is also noteworthy. The authors of [11] explore the use of AI and deep learning models like YOLOv8 for real-time tracking of disease transmission in indoor spaces, improving public health monitoring. This is complemented by [19], which examines the impact of COVID-19 on emergency medical services in Kazakhstan, revealing shifts in healthcare service demand during and after the pandemic. Both studies demonstrate how AI can optimize healthcare responses during health crises and assist in epidemiological monitoring.

Additionally, AI for resource management in healthcare systems is addressed in studies like [16], which uses ML models to predict the length of stay in pediatric intensive care units, and [17], which applies ensemble ML models to predict injuries from the National Electronic Injury Surveillance System dataset. These studies highlight how AI can improve operational efficiency, resource allocation, and decision-making in healthcare settings.

AI's role in improving diagnostic accuracy is examined in [20], which compares the diagnostic accuracy of Google and ChatGPT 3.5 for urological conditions, showing that ChatGPT 3.5 outperforms Google for common conditions. Similarly, ref. [25] discusses AI's role in summarizing scientific research for public health applications, demonstrating its potential in assisting researchers with literature reviews and scientific writing. The authors of [26] present the DLShelper tool, which enhances the segmentation of lesions in CT images, aiding in more accurate COVID-19 diagnoses.

Overall, these studies collectively demonstrate AI's transformative potential across various healthcare domains, from improving diagnostic accuracy and predicting patient outcomes to optimizing resource management. As AI continues to evolve, it offers promising solutions to address challenges in patient care, health management, and public health, providing a foundation for more efficient and personalized healthcare systems.

Contribution of Review Studies

Table 2 presents a summary of the review studies included in this Topic.

Table 2. Summary of the reviews published in this Topic.

Study/Type	Focus	Brief Summary	Contribution
[27]/R	Artificial intelligence in cytopathology	This umbrella review delves into the integration of artificial intelligence (AI) into the field of cytopathology, highlighting its potential to improve diagnostic accuracy and operational efficiency. This study examines 21 review articles to identify key trends, opportunities, challenges, and best practices for AI adoption in cytopathology. It emphasizes the importance of validation processes, integration with existing clinical workflows, and addressing ethical issues such as algorithmic bias and data privacy.	This review contributes by offering an extensive analysis of the current landscape of AI in cytopathology, revealing how AI can automate diagnostic processes, reduce errors, and improve patient outcomes. It highlights critical challenges, such as high implementation costs, the need for empirical data on diagnostic accuracy, and the integration of AI with existing clinical systems. This review also provides a roadmap for future AI development in cytopathology, informed by advancements in related fields like histopathology and radiology.
[28]/SR	Generative Adversarial Networks (GANs) in head and neck surgery	The review explores the application of Generative Adversarial Networks (GANs) in the field of head and neck surgery. GANs are a class of AI algorithms capable of generating new data from existing data. This review examines how GANs are being used in diagnostic imaging and treatment planning in craniofacial surgery, particularly for conditions such as craniosynostosis, chronic sinusitis, and various bone defects. The review assesses 9 studies out of 700, summarizing 8 key applications of GANs in the head and neck region.	This study highlights the emerging role of GANs in improving diagnostic accuracy and treatment outcomes in head and neck surgery. It identifies several practical applications of GANs, including the enhancement of diagnostic imaging, surgical planning, and post-operative prediction. The review emphasizes GANs as a transformative tool in personalized healthcare, providing a more precise and data-driven approach to treating head and neck pathologies, including oncological cases.

Table 2. *Cont.*

Study/Type	Focus	Brief Summary	Contribution
[29]/R	Mobile and domiciliary radiology with AI integration	This review investigates the growing integration of mobile radiology and AI technologies in healthcare, particularly focusing on how these innovations have transformed domiciliary (home-based) radiology services. This study assesses 21 recent publications to analyze the effectiveness of mobile X-ray equipment, AI-enhanced diagnostic tools, and telemedicine applications, with a focus on the post-COVID-19 era. Notably, it explores how mobile mammography units have become essential for breast cancer screening in underserved populations.	The contribution of this review is in examining how AI, mobile radiology, and telemedicine technologies can significantly improve access to diagnostic services in rural and underserved areas. It also discusses the potential of AI in enhancing pediatric radiology and the broader implications for healthcare equity. The review offers insights into the future of domiciliary radiology, suggesting the importance of multi-domain technology assessment and regulatory frameworks for the responsible integration of these technologies.
[30]/SR	AI chatbots in women's health	This systematic review and meta-analysis explores the use of AI-powered chatbots in improving health outcomes for women, specifically focusing on mental health (e.g., anxiety, depression), health behaviors (e.g., cancer self-care), and preconception care. By analyzing 10 studies published between 2019 and 2023, this review assesses the effectiveness of chatbot interventions in various health domains, including reproductive health, eating disorders, and relationship management.	This study underscores the positive impact AI chatbots can have on women's health by providing accessible, digital therapeutic interventions. This review provides evidence that chatbots can improve mental health outcomes and health behaviors among women, offering a cost-effective and scalable solution for addressing issues such as anxiety, depression, and self-care practices. It emphasizes that chatbots could become a critical tool in healthcare interventions, especially for women in remote or underserved areas.
[31]/R	AI and language models in cardiology	This review examines the integration of generative AI, such as ChatGPT-4, and other language models in cardiology. It focuses on how AI can assist in diagnosing heart disease, recommending treatment plans, and improving physician efficiency through administrative task automation. It discusses the challenges associated with AI, such as outdated information, high costs, and the potential loss of human empathy in patient care.	This study explores the role of AI in revolutionizing cardiology by improving diagnostic accuracy, treatment planning, and operational efficiency. It highlights both the benefits of AI tools—such as enhancing physician decision-making and reducing administrative burdens—and the challenges, such as maintaining up-to-date knowledge and ensuring equitable access to these technologies. This review calls for comprehensive training for healthcare professionals and careful integration of AI into medical practices to ensure patient-centered care.
[32]/R	AI in teledermatology	This review discusses the role of AI in advancing teledermatology, particularly in diagnosing skin conditions remotely through telemedicine platforms. It evaluates the integration of AI in eHealth and mHealth for self-care, quality control, and patient management in dermatology. This study also addresses the challenges of app validation, standardization, cybersecurity, and the need for legal and regulatory frameworks.	This study highlights the potential of AI to improve the quality of care in dermatology by facilitating remote diagnosis and patient monitoring. It identifies key benefits such as increased accessibility, reduced healthcare costs, and improved efficiency in diagnosis. However, this review also emphasizes the need for enhanced app design, better cybersecurity measures, and standardized protocols for AI applications in teledermatology. It suggests that regulatory frameworks and position statements from scientific societies are critical to ensuring responsible implementation.

Table 2. *Cont.*

Study/Type	Focus	Brief Summary	Contribution
[33]/R	Machine learning in domestic violence detection	This review explores the use of machine learning (ML) algorithms in detecting and predicting domestic violence (DV) through the analysis of digital data, including social media, surveys, and health records. The study reviews 22 articles and identifies key applications of both supervised and unsupervised ML methods, focusing on their ability to classify, predict, and explore patterns associated with DV.	The contribution of this review lies in demonstrating the potential of machine learning techniques to identify early signs of domestic violence by analyzing digital text data. It provides insights into the algorithms used in this field, such as random forests and support vector machines, and discusses the challenges, including data quality, algorithmic bias, and the need for extensive data preparation. The review encourages further development of ML models specifically designed for DV detection, which could significantly enhance early intervention efforts.

These studies explore a range of AI applications in different healthcare fields, demonstrating the transformative potential of these technologies across diverse medical specialties.

The review on artificial intelligence in cytopathology [27] provides an umbrella review that assesses the integration of AI into cytopathology, focusing on how it can improve diagnostic accuracy and operational efficiency. AI's ability to automate processes, reduce diagnostic errors, and enhance patient outcomes is explored, although challenges such as high implementation costs and algorithmic biases remain.

The systematic review on Generative Adversarial Networks (GANs) in head and neck surgery [28] investigates how GANs, which can generate new data from existing data, are used in craniofacial surgery. It identifies their potential to enhance diagnostic imaging, surgical planning, and post-operative predictions, particularly in treating complex conditions like craniosynostosis and bone defects.

Mobile and domiciliary radiology with AI integration is investigated in the overview reported in [29] that discusses the growing role of mobile radiology and AI in improving healthcare access, especially in rural and underserved areas. AI-powered diagnostic tools and mobile X-ray units, particularly in breast cancer screening, have been transformative in domiciliary radiology, making it an essential service post-COVID-19.

The systematic review on AI chatbots in women's health [30] instigates how AI-powered chatbots are used to improve mental health, health behaviors, and preconception care among women. This study emphasizes the effectiveness of these chatbots in addressing mental health issues such as anxiety and depression, and how they offer a scalable, cost-effective solution for women's health, particularly in remote or underserved areas.

The review on AI and language models in cardiology [31] explores the use of generative AI, such as ChatGPT-4, in cardiology, focusing on how these tools can assist in diagnosing heart disease, recommending treatment plans, and automating administrative tasks. It underscores the benefits of AI in improving efficiency and diagnostic accuracy, but also highlights concerns like outdated data and the loss of human empathy in patient care.

The review on AI in teledermatology [32] examines how AI is enhancing teledermatology, particularly in remote skin condition diagnosis. This review highlights AI's role in increasing accessibility, reducing healthcare costs, and improving diagnosis efficiency. However, it also calls for better app design, cybersecurity, and regulatory frameworks to ensure that AI applications are safely implemented.

The review on machine learning in domestic violence detection [33] explores how machine learning algorithms are being used to detect early signs of domestic violence by analyzing digital data. This review identifies the potential of ML in predicting domestic violence and enhancing early intervention, but it also acknowledges challenges related to data quality and algorithmic biases.

Overall, these studies collectively emphasize how AI and machine learning are revolutionizing various aspects of healthcare, from diagnostics and treatment planning to improving access to care. The common message across all these studies is that AI is becoming a powerful tool in medical fields, enhancing efficiency, improving patient outcomes, and addressing healthcare inequalities. However, challenges such as data privacy, algorithmic bias, and integration with existing systems need to be carefully addressed to fully realize the potential of these technologies.

Contribution of Other Studies

Table 3 presents a summary of other studies published in this Topic.

Table 3. Summary of other studies published in this Topic.

Study/Type	Focus	Brief Summary	Contribution
[34]/TN	Machine learning for effective dose calculation	This study explores the use of machine learning (ML) algorithms to predict organ doses and effective dose conversion coefficients (DCCs) for various anthropomorphic phantoms. Traditionally, Monte Carlo methods are used for these calculations, which are time-consuming and require expertise. By compiling a comprehensive dataset from Monte Carlo studies, the authors train ML models (XGB, GB, and Extra Trees regressor) to predict the effective dose. This study evaluates the ML models' performance using error metrics and compares them with ICRP values.	This study highlights the potential of ML techniques to predict effective doses efficiently, offering a solution to the traditional Monte Carlo method's limitations. The ML models demonstrated good accuracy at mid-range neutron energies, providing a faster alternative for dose prediction, especially in scenarios requiring quick results. Additionally, this study suggests improvements in data representation and the inclusion of larger datasets to enhance model accuracy, thereby contributing to personalized dosimetry in radiation protection.
[35]/P	Neural network models for causal variable analysis in medical and climatic studies	This paper presents a neural network-based method to analyze non-linear systems, focusing on small datasets. The authors propose a strategy to identify the roles (linear, non-linear, or threshold) of causal variables in predicting the behavior of a target variable. They apply this method to climate studies and medical research, particularly cancer studies. The approach allows for predictions about future scenarios based on causal variables.	This paper introduces a complementary approach to deep learning by focusing on understanding causal relationships within datasets. The methodology has applications in medical research, particularly in cancer studies, by helping identify important causal variables and predicting future trends. The approach's utility in small datasets makes it valuable for medical studies with limited data, and its potential to influence research on cancer treatment is a key contribution.

The two studies presented in Table 3 focus on the application of AI in healthcare and environmental research.

Machine learning for effective dose calculation is investigated in a technical note [34], exploring how ML algorithms can predict organ doses and effective dose conversion coefficients (DCCs) for anthropomorphic phantoms. Traditionally, these calculations are performed using Monte Carlo methods, which are time-consuming. By training ML models like XGB, GB, and Extra Trees regressor on Monte Carlo datasets, the authors demonstrate that ML can predict doses efficiently, providing a faster alternative. This approach offers a solution to the time and expertise required for traditional methods, contributing to personalized dosimetry in radiation protection.

Neural network models for causal variable analysis in medical and climatic studies are investigated in a perspective [35], presenting a neural network-based method to analyze non-linear systems with small datasets, focusing on identifying causal variables in medical and climate research. The methodology helps predict future trends, particularly in cancer studies. This approach is valuable for medical research with limited data and provides insights into causal relationships. This study's contribution lies in improving predictions and understanding complex factors, which could influence cancer treatment and other medical applications. Both studies demonstrate the potential of AI to improve efficiency and accuracy in healthcare and research, offering practical solutions and insights for better decision-making and predictions.

Conclusions and message for future work

The studies reviewed here highlight the increasing role of artificial intelligence (AI), and, in particular, machine learning (ML), in advancing healthcare practices, particularly in diagnostic accuracy, treatment planning, and personalized medicine. In various medical fields, such as radiology, cardiology, dermatology, and domestic violence detection, AI and ML are improving the efficiency, accuracy, and accessibility of healthcare services. These innovations not only enhance diagnostic precision but also contribute to reducing operational costs, optimizing workflows, and fostering personalized approaches to care, especially for underserved populations.

A recurring theme across these studies is the importance of integrating AI and ML technologies into existing healthcare frameworks. This involves addressing challenges related to data quality, algorithmic biases, and clinical workflow integration, ensuring that these technologies are both clinically and ethically appropriate. Additionally, the need for rigorous validation, regulatory frameworks, and ongoing assessment remains central to their responsible use in healthcare.

The studies on mobile and domiciliary radiology and AI chatbots for women's health, in particular, highlight the potential of these technologies to bridge gaps in healthcare access. By leveraging mobile devices and telemedicine platforms, AI innovations can improve healthcare access in rural or underserved regions, thereby improving health outcomes and promoting equity.

Despite promising results, significant challenges remain. The adoption of AI and ML tools in healthcare requires careful consideration of technical constraints, such as the need for larger and more diverse datasets, and ethical concerns, including data privacy, security, and bias mitigation. Comprehensive training for healthcare professionals is also essential to ensure they can effectively use AI tools in clinical decision-making.

Future work should focus on the following areas:

- Expanding datasets to improve the accuracy and generalizability of AI/ML models across different healthcare populations and settings.
- Developing interdisciplinary frameworks for better integration of AI solutions into clinical contexts, addressing ethical concerns, and ensuring equity.
- Exploring AI's potential in less-explored areas, such as mental health, long-term disease management, and healthcare logistics.
- Enhancing regulatory frameworks to keep pace with the rapid development of AI/ML technologies, ensuring safe and responsible implementation.
- Promoting the development of user-friendly AI tools that clinicians can adopt without disrupting existing workflows.

In conclusion, while AI and ML have the potential to revolutionize healthcare, their integration must be approached with care, balancing technological innovation with patient safety, ethics, and equity. Future work should focus on overcoming existing barriers and optimizing AI solutions for real-world clinical applications.

Conflicts of Interest: The authors declare no conflict of interest.

References

1. Wang, L.; Zhang, Y.; Wang, D.; Tong, X.; Liu, T.; Zhang, S.; Huang, J.; Zhang, L.; Chen, L.; Fan, H.; et al. Artificial Intelligence for COVID-19: A Systematic Review. *Front. Med.* **2021**, *8*, 704256. [CrossRef] [PubMed] [PubMed Central]
2. Jemioło, P.; Storman, D.; Orzechowski, P. Artificial Intelligence for COVID-19 Detection in Medical Imaging—Diagnostic Measures and Wasting—A Systematic Umbrella Review. *J. Clin. Med.* **2022**, *11*, 2054. [CrossRef] [PubMed]
3. Mohammadi, S.; SeyedAlinaghi, S.; Heydari, M.; Pashaei, Z.; Mirzapour, P.; Karimi, A.; Afsahi, A.M.; Mirghaderi, P.; Mohammadi, P.; Arjmand, G.; et al. Artificial Intelligence in COVID-19 Management: A Systematic Review. *J. Comput. Sci.* **2023**, *19*, 554–568. [CrossRef]
4. Jiang, L.; Wu, Z.; Xu, X.; Zhan, Y.; Jin, X.; Wang, L.; Qiu, Y. Opportunities and challenges of artificial intelligence in the medical field: Current application, emerging problems, and problem-solving strategies. *J. Int. Med. Res.* **2021**, *49*, 3000605211000157. [CrossRef] [PubMed] [PubMed Central]
5. Gawande, M.S.; Zade, N.; Kumar, P.; Gundewar, S.; Weerarathna, I.N.; Verma, P. The role of artificial intelligence in pandemic responses: From epidemiological modeling to vaccine development. *Mol. Biomed.* **2025**, *3*, 1. [CrossRef] [PubMed] [PubMed Central]
6. Channa, A.; Popescu, N.; Skibinska, J.; Burget, R. The Rise of Wearable Devices during the COVID-19 Pandemic: A Systematic Review. *Sensors* **2021**, *21*, 5787. [CrossRef] [PubMed] [PubMed Central]
7. Alsunaidi, S.J.; Almuhaideb, A.M.; Ibrahim, N.M.; Shaikh, F.S.; Alqudaihi, K.S.; Alhaidari, F.A.; Khan, I.U.; Aslam, N.; Alshahrani, M.S. Applications of Big Data Analytics to Control COVID-19 Pandemic. *Sensors* **2021**, *21*, 2282. [CrossRef]
8. Chang, Z.; Zhan, Z.; Zhao, Z.; You, Z.; Liu, Y.; Yan, Z.; Fu, Y.; Liang, W.; Zhao, L. Application of artificial intelligence in COVID-19 medical area: A systematic review. *J. Thorac. Dis.* **2021**, *13*, 7034–7053. [CrossRef] [PubMed] [PubMed Central]
9. Nawaz, F.A.; Khan, A.R.; Boillat, T. AI-enhanced solutions during COVID-19: Current trends and future innovations. *Ann. Med. Surg.* **2022**, *80*, 104158. [CrossRef] [PubMed] [PubMed Central]
10. Artificial Intelligence in Public Health: Current Trends and Future Possibilities. Topic. 2024. Available online: https://www.mdpi.com/topics/C52Z967WA3 (accessed on 20 March 2025).
11. Baligh Jahromi, A.; Attarian, K.; Asgary, A.; Wu, J. Advancing Indoor Epidemiological Surveillance: Integrating Real-Time Object Detection and Spatial Analysis for Precise Contact Rate Analysis and Enhanced Public Health Strategies. *Int. J. Environ. Res. Public. Health* **2024**, *21*, 1502. [CrossRef]
12. Yang, Y.; Ning, H.; Liang, B.; Mai, H.; Zhou, J.; Yang, J.; Huang, J. Exploring Factors Influencing Patient Delay Behavior in Oral Cancer: The Development of a Risk Prediction Model in Western China. *Healthcare* **2024**, *12*, 2252. [CrossRef] [PubMed]
13. Jawad, B.N.; Altintas, I.; Eugen-Olsen, J.; Niazi, S.; Mansouri, A.; Rasmussen, L.J.H.; Schultz, M.; Iversen, K.; Normann Holm, N.; Kallemose, T.; et al. Prospective and External Validation of Machine Learning Models for Short- and Long-Term Mortality in Acutely Admitted Patients Using Blood Tests. *J. Clin. Med.* **2024**, *13*, 6437. [CrossRef] [PubMed]
14. Wu, Y.; Xie, H.; Gu, L.; Chen, R.; Chen, S.; Wang, F.; Liu, Y.; Chen, L.; Tang, J. Advancing Mental Health Care: Intelligent Assessments and Automated Generation of Personalized Advice via M.I.N.I and RoBERTa. *Appl. Sci.* **2024**, *14*, 9447. [CrossRef]
15. Kwiatkowska-Miernik, A.; Wasilewski, P.G.; Mruk, B.; Sklinda, K.; Bujko, M.; Walecki, J. Estimating Progression-Free Survival in Patients with Primary High-Grade Glioma Using Machine Learning. *J. Clin. Med.* **2024**, *13*, 6172. [CrossRef]
16. Ganatra, H.A.; Latifi, S.Q.; Baloglu, O. Pediatric Intensive Care Unit Length of Stay Prediction by Machine Learning. *Bioengineering* **2024**, *11*, 962. [CrossRef]
17. Vichare, S.; Nanda, G.; Sundararajan, R. Probabilistic Ensemble Framework for Injury Narrative Classification. *AI* **2024**, *5*, 1684–1694. [CrossRef]
18. Sheehy, L.; Bouchard, S.; Kakkar, A.; El Hakim, R.; Lhoest, J.; Frank, A. Development and Initial Testing of an Artificial Intelligence-Based Virtual Reality Companion for People Living with Dementia in Long-Term Care. *J. Clin. Med.* **2024**, *13*, 5574. [CrossRef] [PubMed]
19. Messova, A.; Pivina, L.; Ygiyeva, D.; Batenova, G.; Dyussupov, A.; Jamedinova, U.; Syzdykbayev, M.; Adilgozhina, S.; Bayanbaev, A. Lessons of the COVID-19 Pandemic for Ambulance Service in Kazakhstan. *Healthcare* **2024**, *12*, 1568. [CrossRef]
20. Guimaraes, G.R.; Figueiredo, R.G.; Silva, C.S.; Arata, V.; Contreras, J.C.Z.; Gomes, C.M.; Tiraboschi, R.B.; Bessa Junior, J. Diagnosis in Bytes: Comparing the Diagnostic Accuracy of Google and ChatGPT 3.5 as an Educational Support Tool. *Int. J. Environ. Res. Public. Health* **2024**, *21*, 580. [CrossRef]

21. Ciarmiello, A.; Giovannini, E.; Tutino, F.; Yosifov, N.; Milano, A.; Florimonte, L.; Bonatto, E.; Bareggi, C.; Dellavedova, L.; Castello, A.; et al. Does FDG PET-Based Radiomics Have an Added Value for Prediction of Overall Survival in Non-Small Cell Lung Cancer? *J. Clin. Med.* **2024**, *13*, 2613. [CrossRef]
22. Saeed, Z.; Bouhali, O.; Ji, J.X.; Hammoud, R.; Al-Hammadi, N.; Aouadi, S.; Torfeh, T. Cancerous and Non-Cancerous MRI Classification Using Dual DCNN Approach. *Bioengineering* **2024**, *11*, 410. [CrossRef] [PubMed]
23. Miyagi, Y.; Tada, K.; Yasuhi, I.; Tsumura, K.; Maegawa, Y.; Tanaka, N.; Mizunoe, T.; Emoto, I.; Maeda, K.; Kawakami, K.; et al. A Novel Method for Determining Fibrin/Fibrinogen Degradation Products and Fibrinogen Threshold Criteria via Artificial Intelligence in Massive Hemorrhage during Delivery with Hematuria. *J. Clin. Med.* **2024**, *13*, 1826. [CrossRef] [PubMed]
24. Bhimavarapu, U.; Chintalapudi, N.; Battineni, G. Brain Tumor Detection and Categorization with Segmentation of Improved Unsupervised Clustering Approach and Machine Learning Classifier. *Bioengineering* **2024**, *11*, 266. [CrossRef] [PubMed]
25. Jungwirth, D.; Haluza, D. Artificial Intelligence and Public Health: An Exploratory Study. *Int. J. Environ. Res. Public. Health* **2023**, *20*, 4541. [CrossRef] [PubMed]
26. He, T.; Liu, H.; Zhang, Z.; Li, C.; Zhou, Y. Research on the Application of Artificial Intelligence in Public Health Management: Leveraging Artificial Intelligence to Improve COVID-19 CT Image Diagnosis. *Int. J. Environ. Res. Public. Health* **2023**, *20*, 1158. [CrossRef]
27. Giansanti, D. AI in Cytopathology: A Narrative Umbrella Review on Innovations, Challenges, and Future Directions. *J. Clin. Med.* **2024**, *13*, 6745. [CrossRef]
28. Michelutti, L.; Tel, A.; Zeppieri, M.; Ius, T.; Agosti, E.; Sembronio, S.; Robiony, M. Generative Adversarial Networks (GANs) in the Field of Head and Neck Surgery: Current Evidence and Prospects for the Future—A Systematic Review. *J. Clin. Med.* **2024**, *13*, 3556. [CrossRef]
29. Lepri, G.; Oddi, F.; Gulino, R.A.; Giansanti, D. Reimagining Radiology: A Comprehensive Overview of Reviews at the Intersection of Mobile and Domiciliary Radiology over the Last Five Years. *Bioengineering* **2024**, *11*, 216. [CrossRef]
30. Kim, H.-K. The Effects of Artificial Intelligence Chatbots on Women's Health: A Systematic Review and Meta-Analysis. *Healthcare* **2024**, *12*, 534. [CrossRef]
31. Gala, D.; Makaryus, A.N. The Utility of Language Models in Cardiology: A Narrative Review of the Benefits and Concerns of ChatGPT-4. *Int. J. Environ. Res. Public Health* **2023**, *20*, 6438. [CrossRef]
32. Giansanti, D. The Artificial Intelligence in Teledermatology: A Narrative Review on Opportunities, Perspectives, and Bottlenecks. *Int. J. Environ. Res. Public Health* **2023**, *20*, 5810. [CrossRef] [PubMed]
33. Hui, V.; Constantino, R.E.; Lee, Y.J. Harnessing Machine Learning in Tackling Domestic Violence—An Integrative Review. *Int. J. Environ. Res. Public Health* **2023**, *20*, 4984. [CrossRef] [PubMed]
34. Alghamdi, A.A.A. Machine Learning for Predicting Neutron Effective Dose. *Appl. Sci.* **2024**, *14*, 5740. [CrossRef]
35. Pasini, A.; Amendola, S. A Neural Modelling Tool for Non-Linear Influence Analyses and Perspectives of Applications in Medical Research. *Appl. Sci.* **2024**, *14*, 2148. [CrossRef]
36. Giansanti, D. Artificial Intelligence in Public Health: Current Trends and Future Possibilities. *Int. J. Environ. Res. Public Health* **2022**, *19*, 11907. [CrossRef]

applied sciences

MDPI

Article

Advancing Mental Health Care: Intelligent Assessments and Automated Generation of Personalized Advice via M.I.N.I and RoBERTa

Yuezhong Wu [1], Huan Xie [1], Lin Gu [2], Rongrong Chen [3], Shanshan Chen [4], Fanglan Wang [4], Yiwen Liu [5], Lingjiao Chen [1] and Jinsong Tang [4,*]

[1] School of Rail Transit, Hunan University of Technology, Zhuzhou 412007, China; wuyuezhong@hut.edu.cn (Y.W.); m22085400045@stu.hut.edu.cn (H.X.); chenlingjiao@hut.edu.cn (L.C.)
[2] RIKEN AIP (RIKEN Center for Advanced Intelligence Project (AIP)), Rigaku Kenkyujo Kakushin Chino Togo Kenkyu Senta, Tokyo 103-0027, Japan; lin.gu@riken.jp
[3] School of Business, Hunan University of Technology, Zhuzhou 412007, China; chenrongrong@hut.edu.cn
[4] School of Medicine, Zhejiang University, Hangzhou 310020, China; sschen33@zju.edu.cn (S.C.); 12118265@zju.edu.cn (F.W.)
[5] School of Computer Science, Hunan University of Technology, Zhuzhou 412007, China; m23085400026@stu.hut.edu.cn
* Correspondence: tangjinsong@zju.edu.cn

Abstract: As mental health issues become increasingly prominent, we are now facing challenges such as the severe unequal distribution of medical resources and low diagnostic efficiency. This paper integrates finite state machines, retrieval algorithms, semantic-matching models, and medical-knowledge graphs to design an innovative intelligent auxiliary evaluation tool and a personalized medical-advice generation application, aiming to improve the efficiency of mental health assessments and the provision of personalized medical advice. The main contributions include the folowing: (1) Developing an auxiliary diagnostic tool that combines the Mini-International Neuropsychiatric Interview (M.I.N.I.) with finite state machines to systematically collect patient information for preliminary assessments; (2) Enhancing data processing by optimizing retrieval algorithms for efficient filtering and employing a fine-tuned RoBERTa model for deep semantic matching and analysis, ensuring accurate and personalized medical-advice generation; (3) Generating intelligent suggestions using NLP techniques; when semantic matching falls below a specific threshold, integrating medical-knowledge graphs to produce general medical advice. Experimental results show that this application achieves a semantic-matching degree of 0.9 and an accuracy of 0.87, significantly improving assessment accuracy and the ability to generate personalized medical advice. This optimizes the allocation of medical resources, enhances diagnostic efficiency, and provides a reference for advancing mental health care through artificial-intelligence technology.

Keywords: mental health; artificial intelligence; natural language processing; medical-knowledge graph; automatic generation

1. Introduction

With modern life accelerating and societal competition increasing, mental and psychological health issues have become significant global public health challenges. A World Health Organization report indicates that over one billion people globally suffer from various mental health issues [1]. However, many individuals still lack access to proper detection and treatment. These issues not only profoundly affect individuals but also place a substantial burden on families and societies [2]. Globally, there is a severe imbalance in the distribution of mental and psychological healthcare resources across various countries and regions [3]. This imbalance is especially pronounced in developing countries and low-income areas, marked by a lack of professional personnel and medical facilities, complicating access to high-quality medical services. In developed countries, the distribution of mental health services frequently fails to meet population needs, leading to many patients struggling to receive timely and effective treatment.

Current medical practice faces multiple challenges in assessing, diagnosing, and treating mental and psychological disorders [4]. Firstly, the uncertainty of symptoms and subjectivity of patient perception make accurate disease state assessment difficult for doctors in clinical practice. Secondly, the lack of objective indicators means these subjective perceptions often compromise the accuracy of assessment, diagnosis, and treatment. Despite abundant online professional medical knowledge, existing knowledge retrieval systems often provide low-quality information and lack precision. Some specialized platforms provide reliable online consultation services with professional psychiatrists, but these services are typically time-consuming and labor-intensive.

To tackle these challenges, this paper leverages the latest computer technology and artificial-intelligence algorithms. Specifically, we integrate the RoBERTa model, based on BERT [5] (Bidirectional Encoder Representations from Transformers), for effective processing and analysis of medical literature and patient records. Additionally, we use the M.I.N.I tool [6], a validated, simple, and effective diagnostic tool for psychiatric disorders. The combination of these methods aims to improve the accuracy of assessments and medical-advice generation for mental and psychological disorders.

Existing research mainly relies on doctors' clinical experience and traditional diagnostic tools, which are often lacking in flexibility and personalization [7]. The limited understanding of complex and variable mental disorder characteristics constrains the effectiveness and adaptability of medical advice. Therefore, this paper aims to develop a novel auxiliary assessment tool and an application for generating personalized medical advice. The goal is to enhance the accuracy of mental disorder assessments and treatment efficiency through technological innovation. Our approach aims to comprehensively and objectively assess patients' mental states and provide tailored medical advice, improving medical resource allocation and patient quality of life. We believe this innovation will benefit patients directly and offer new perspectives and tools for medical practice.

2. Literature Review

The assessment and diagnosis of mental and psychological disorders are complex and multidimensional processes. Traditionally, this field has relied on physicians' clinical experience and standardized assessment tools, such as DSM-5 [8] and ICD-10 [9], which provide guidelines for diagnosing mental disorders. Chakraborty, N., Ali, A., et al. [10] highlighted the World Health Organization's mhGAP Intervention Guide's effectiveness and practicality in assessing and providing mental health services. However, their practical application is limited by the need for professional knowledge and flexibility in the assessment and diagnostic process. The M.I.N.I questionnaire, popular for its brevity and structured format, allows for quicker assessment of major mental disorders. Arrow, K., Resnik, P., Michel, H., et al. [11] demonstrated these tools' feasibility and effectiveness in assessing mental and psychological symptoms.

In medicine, text-generation technology [12–14] is an emerging research area. Researchers like Hasani, A.M. and Singh, S. [15] have successfully used advanced pre-trained deep-learning models like GPT-4 for generating and standardizing medical reports. However, this method, while flexible, has limitations in content control, and its reliability and safety in medicine are not fully established. A more prudent approach is using information-retrieval technology to find relevant information and extract keywords and key information for generating medical advice.

Most text-retrieval technologies [16,17] rely on full-sentence matching, which is fast but lacks specificity in key information extraction. To address this issue, some researchers have proposed semantic retrieval-based models [18–20]. While these improve knowledge-acquisition precision, their effects vary, and they are computationally intensive. They also do not fully consider the patient's unique situation for personalized medical advice. We propose a keyword-weight [21,22] matching algorithm for preliminary information filtering. In addition, Liu, Y., Ott, M., Goyal, N., et al. [23] confirmed that RoBERTa, a variant of BERT, performed exceptionally well in semantic sentence-matching tasks. Therefore, we adopted a RoBERTa model based on the Cross-Encoder [24,25] network structure to further enhance the accuracy of information retrieval.

This combination lays the foundation for generating personalized medical advice. The introduction of medical-knowledge graphs [26–29] offers a structured way to organize and query medical information, showing great potential in medical-advice generation.

Building on existing literature and technologies, this paper aims to combine finite state machines, the RoBERTa model, and medical-knowledge graphs to improve mental disorder assessment accuracy and the personalization and universality of medical-advice generation. Our method focuses on assessment accuracy and emphasizes medical-advice personalization and specificity, addressing issues like uneven resource distribution and variable service quality. The following sections will elaborate on our research methods, experimental design, and results and discuss how these innovations can enhance the quality and efficiency of mental and psychological health services.

3. Materials and Methods

3.1. Materials

The dataset, named "Huatuo-26M" [30] is one of the largest Chinese medical Q&A datasets currently available, compiled from multiple reliable sources, as detailed in Table 1. It contains over 26 million high-quality medical Q&A pairs, primarily sourced from public medical Q&A forums on the internet. The forums feature responses from certified medical professionals, with verifiable personal and employment details, ensuring data reliability and credibility.

Table 1. Huatuo-26M dataset information.

Source	Data Fields
Online Medical Encyclopedia	Huatuo_encyclopedia_qa
Medical-Knowledge Graph	Huatuo_knowledge_graph_qa
Public Online Medical Q&A Forums	Huatuo_consultation_qa

The dataset includes diverse Q&A pairs, with internet forum data being particularly valuable due to their detailed patient-related information, aligning well with this study's experimental environment. For this paper, data from these forums were meticulously gathered and cleaned to build a preliminary dataset. By applying a set of keywords specific to the mental and psychological domain, high-quality Q&A data were filtered and saved as pairs, with questions containing detailed information such as names, symptoms, medications, and patients' personal information. The answer section consists of expert treatment methods, guidance, and suggestions, totaling approximately 1 million entries.

To date, several studies have utilized the "Huatuo-26M" dataset to construct and evaluate medical question-and-answer systems [31–33], demonstrating its advantages in improving the accuracy and practicality of medical Q&A. The "Huatuo-26M" dataset encompasses a wide range of medical fields, including internal medicine, surgery, pediatrics, and obstetrics and gynecology, among others. The content of the Q&A covers the diagnosis, treatment, and prevention of common diseases, primarily focusing on general medical knowledge. Additionally, it includes a substantial number of Q&A pairs in both the mental and psychological domains, thereby forming a comprehensive medical question-and-answer knowledge base.

Data for constructing the domain-knowledge graph in mental and psychological health were sourced from online medical encyclopedias, medical websites, books, academic papers, and other resources.

The data used to construct the knowledge graph in the field of mental and psychological health were collected from various sources, including online medical encyclopedias, medical information websites, medical books, and academic papers. The entire graph includes 5 types of entities, with a total of 2430 instances; 8 types of attributes; and 9 types of entity relationships, with 5575 instances, as shown in Table 2 below.

Table 2. Knowledge graph data.

Data Category	Category Count	Total Count
Entity	5	2430
Attribute	8	N/A
Public Online	9	5140

3.2. Methods

The methodology proposed in this article consists of three main components: the development and implementation of an auxiliary assessment tool for mental and psychological health, the generation of personalized medical advice, and the application of a medical-knowledge graph. Firstly, patient information is gathered using the auxiliary assessment tool and is then evaluated. This information is then used to generate personalized medical advice. In instances where the data quality is poor or the model matching accuracy falls below a predetermined threshold, making it insufficient for generating personalized advice, the system employs the knowledge graph to produce universally applicable medical advice. The overall architecture is depicted in Figure 1.

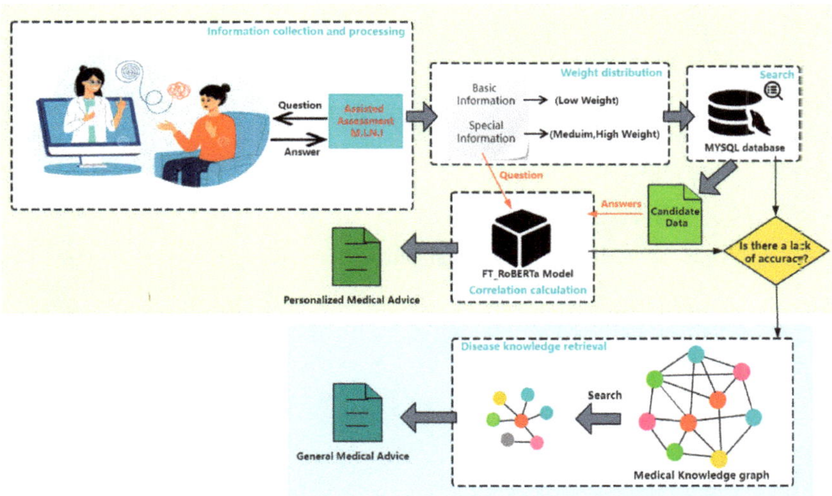

Figure 1. Overall architecture.

3.2.1. Construction and Implementation of the M.I.N.I-Based Diagnostic Tool

With advancements in medical technology and the growth of digitalization, an increasing number of diagnostic tools are utilizing computer technology to boost their efficiency and accuracy. In this study, M.I.N.I version 6.0.0 serves as the basis for the auxiliary assessment of mental and psychological disorders. It is supported by technologies like finite state machines and web interaction for automated and intelligent information support.

1. Overview of M.I.N.I

M.I.N.I is an extensive diagnostic assessment tool, comprising 16 independent modules from A to P. Each module covers a broad range of content and employs intricate logical calculations and judgment mechanisms. Considering the substantial differences in the assessment methods of diagnostic results among these modules, simplifying M.I.N.I into a standard questionnaire is not recommended.

To realize the objectives of automation and intelligence, this paper adopts a specialized modeling approach for each module. By applying the finite-state-machine model, precise logic calculations and logical jumps based on user responses are possible. This approach not only facilitates the flexible collection of multiple indicator information but also enables comprehensive result assessment based on this data. Once information collection is completed in all modules, the system can generate an integrated preliminary assessment report. The use of this method is expected to significantly enhance the precision and efficiency of diagnoses. The implementation effect is illustrated in Figure 2. The picture presents three parts from left to right: an overview of the overall auxiliary diagnosis module, the information collection process, and the evaluation results.

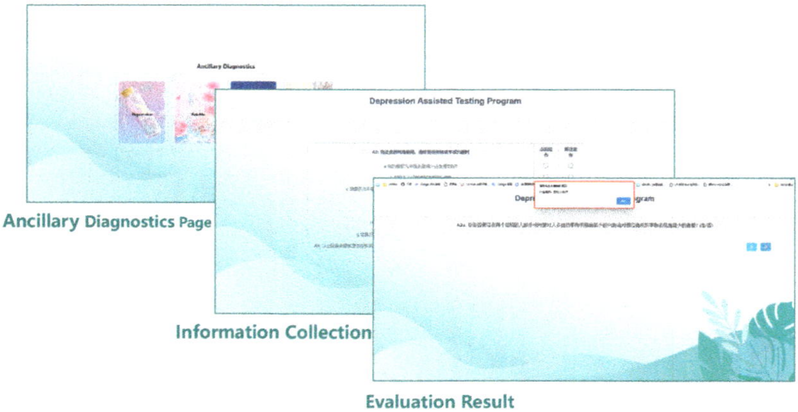

Figure 2. Auxiliary assessment effect.

2. Finite state machine and its application in this study

State machines [34,35] are computational models that describe the behavior or state transitions of objects or systems in response to external events or conditions. In event-driven systems, their behavior or state changes in response to external events or conditions. Table 3 shows the basic components of a state machine. A simple diagram illustrating this concept is shown in Figure 3.

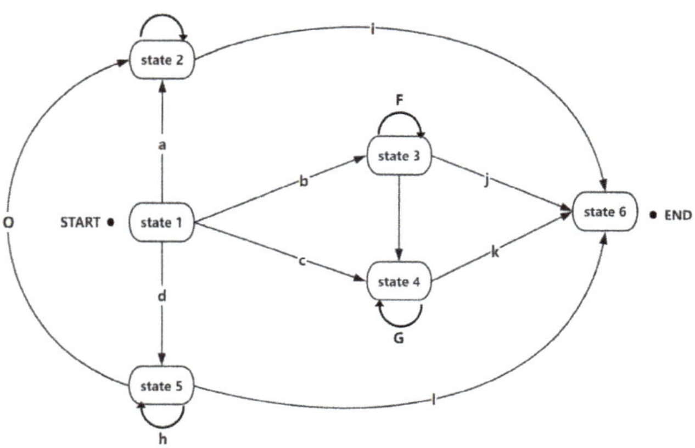

Figure 3. Working principle diagram of finite state machine.

Table 3. State-machine component table.

Component	Category Count
States	Different operational phases of the system, representing specific behaviors or attributes.
Events	External factors that trigger state changes, such as user input or sensor feedback.
Transitions	Rules for transitioning between states, associated with specific events and conditions.
Actions	Specific operations performed during state transitions.

In this study, we utilize the principles of the state-machine model to structure each module of M.I.N.I 6.0.0. Each user's response to a question triggers an event, determining the next question to be asked. This process continues until either the assessment criteria are met or all questions in the module are answered, followed by result evaluation. The flowchart for this process is depicted in Figure 4.

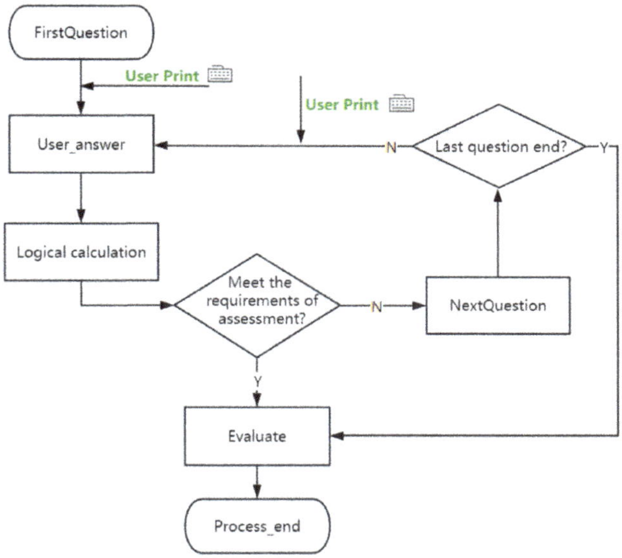

Figure 4. Program flowchart.

3.2.2. Generation of Personalized Medical Advice

In the age of big data, the increasing demand for personalized medical care matches well with the growing volume of medical data. The internet abounds with high-quality medical advice from medical experts, tailored to patients' conditions. By leveraging advanced computer technology, we can effectively gather and share this knowledge, providing robust support for generating personalized medical advice.

1. Information collection

The generation of personalized medical advice primarily depends on two types of information:

Basic Information: Includes gender, age, etc., collected before using the tool.

Special Information: Includes diagnostic results, personal experiences, drug allergy history, concurrent symptoms, etc., gathered during the use of the diagnostic tool.

2. Retrieval matching strategy

The evolution of text-retrieval technology has progressed from the initial Boolean retrieval models [36] to modern deep-learning-based models, such as the Transformer architecture [37]. These technologies have strong information-retrieval capabilities. However, in specific scenarios, particularly with limited data volumes, they may not fully meet precise retrieval requirements.

This study adopts a keyword-weight-matching method. Initially, patient-related information is collected via the M.I.N.I tool, and this is then cleaned and filtered to extract keywords and assign weights. Using these keywords, a preliminary match is performed on a pre-stored high-quality mental and psychological Q&A dataset in MySQL 5.7, forming subsets of question–answer pairs. These subsets are then ranked according to their weight scores, and the top N-ranked data are selected as the candidate set. The advantage of this method is its focus on key information, significantly enhancing the quality of the final data, while also substantially reducing the computational load of subsequent semantic matching. The process schematic is illustrated in Figure 5.

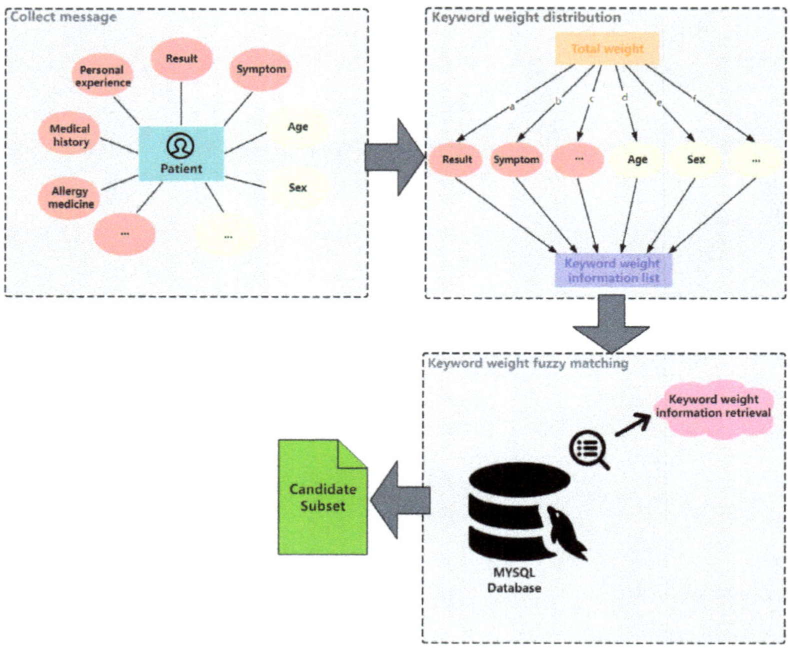

Figure 5. Keyword-weight matching. Letters a–f represent different weight values.

3. Semantic matching model

Semantic matching, the process of measuring textual similarity, has evolved from early neural network-based methods, like Word2Vec [38] and GloVe [39], to Long Short-Term Memory networks (LSTM/BiLSTM) [40]. In 2018, Devlin et al. [5] introduced the BERT model, based on the Transformer architecture, which excels in learning deep language representations from unlabeled text and exhibits remarkable multi-tasking capabilities. Its Cross-Encoder structure, depicted in Figure 6, assesses the relationship between two texts by providing a direct relational score, considering both inputs in their entirety. A variant of BERT, RoBERTa, shows superior performance in tasks like semantic sentence matching.

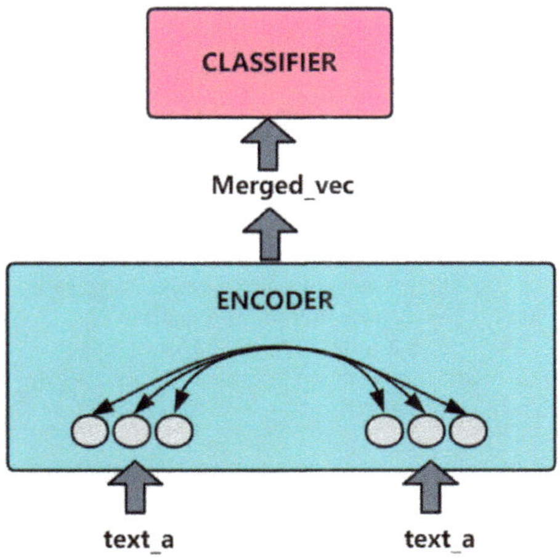

Figure 6. Cross-Encoder structure.

This study employs the RoBERTa model and a Cross-Encoder structure to develop a semantic-matching model, fine-tuned with knowledge in mental and psychological health. It evaluates the relevance between Text_Question (question) and Text_Answer (answer), as shown in Figure 7. Equations (1) and (2) illustrate the ReLU and Sigmoid activation functions, respectively, commonly used in neural networks and deep learning.

$$ReLU(x) = \max(0, x) \quad (1)$$

$$Sigmoid(x) = \frac{1}{1 + e^{-x}} \quad (2)$$

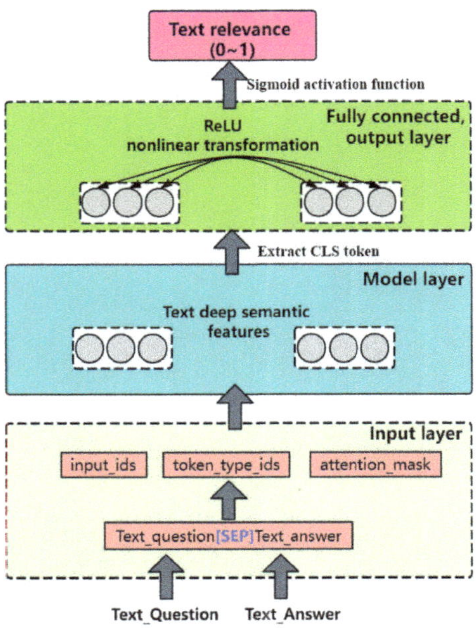

Figure 7. RoBERTa model based on Cross-Encoder.

The model architecture includes the following four main layers, as detailed in Table 4.

Table 4. Model structure.

Layer	Function	Description
Input	Text Preprocessing	Merges text and uses a tokenizer to convert it into the three standard inputs for RoBERTa.
Model	Semantic Extraction	Uses the pre-trained RoBERTa model to extract semantic information from text, outputting token embedding vectors.
Fully Connected	Feature Transformation	Extracts the CLS token vector from RoBERTa's output and performs a nonlinear transformation using Equation (1).
Output	Relevance Scoring	Uses a fully connected layer with the activation function in Equation (2) to map to a relevance score between 0 and 1.

After training and fine-tuning with mental and psychological disorder-related data, the model outputs a relevance score ranging from 0 (unrelated) to 1 (closely related), effectively measuring the connection between Text_Question and Text_Answer. This architecture is designed to deeply understand text content and capture complex relationships.

4. Generate medical advice

We propose an innovative framework for generating personalized medical advice, integrating natural language processing technology with expert medical knowledge. Initially, patient information collected via the M.I.N.I tool is used to form a preliminary subset of candidate advice using a keyword-weight-matching algorithm. This subset is then processed through the semantic-matching model, which scores the advice based on relevance, selecting the top M pieces. The refinement process includes data cleaning and extraction, filtering out various treatment methods, medications, and suggestions, and information filtering and analysis, identifying commonly and uniquely occurring treatment plans, removing duplicates, and retaining unique, relevant advice.

Finally, new templates are designed based on the filtered information to generate personalized medical advice containing core treatment plans. The detailed process of generating medical advice is illustrated in Figure 8.

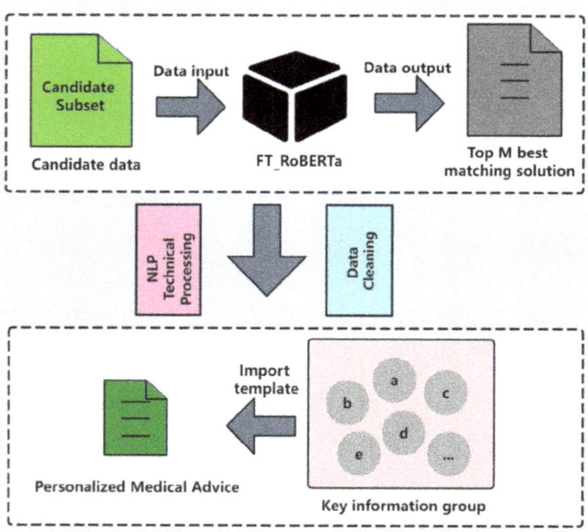

Figure 8. Medical advice generation process flowchart. Letters a–e represent different keywords.

Compared to advice generated solely by text generation technology, this method ensures data reliability and effectiveness, as all medical advice originates from human medical experts and undergoes professional review. It also guarantees the quality of the final medical advice by extracting key information from multiple sources, providing patients with more trustworthy and personalized advice.

3.2.3. Application of Medical-Knowledge Graph

A knowledge graph is a structured management tool for knowledge, with medical-knowledge graphs extensively used to integrate and organize a vast array of medical and health-related information. Leveraging the foundations of artificial intelligence and data science, these graphs aim to provide comprehensive medical knowledge and insights and have broad applications.

1. Knowledge generation

When encountering complex cases with scarce relevant Q&A examples, difficulties arise in matching appropriate medical advice due to a lack of precision. In such instances, the characteristics of medical-knowledge graphs can be utilized to provide universal and structured medical information as a supplement, achieving the goal of generating universally applicable medical advice. The process of knowledge generation is shown in Figure 9.

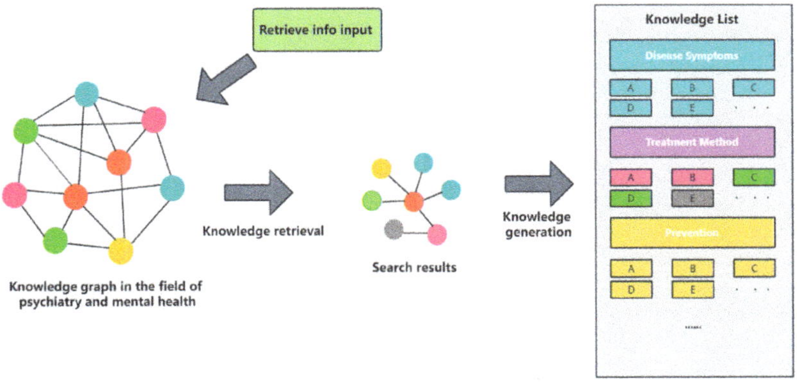

Figure 9. Knowledge generation process in the mental and psychological health domain-knowledge graph. Different colors represent entity categories, and different letters represent subcategories of the same entity.

Initially, the patient's disease assessment results obtained from the M.I.N.I auxiliary assessment tool are used as input. Then, multiple combinational searches are conducted in the mental and psychological health domain-knowledge graph. The search results include information on disease symptoms, treatment methods (including treatment modalities, medications, recommended diets), prevention measures, etc. Finally, after the classification and organization of knowledge, the information is compiled into a knowledge list.

4. Experiment Details

4.1. RoBERTa Model Fine-Tuning

To train an efficiently fine-tuned FT_RoBERTa model for accurately determining the relevance of question–answer pairs, the following steps were employed:

4.1.1. Data Preparation

- Positive Examples: We used original question–answer pairs as highly relevant instances, where each question was paired with its correct answer. These pairs were labeled as positive (e.g., label 1), representing high relevance.

- Negative Examples: To generate low-relevance or irrelevant instances, we deliberately disrupted the original question–answer pairings. This was done by randomly selecting mismatched answers for the questions, creating instances that were unrelated to the specific questions. These mismatched instances were assigned negative labels (e.g., label 0), representing low relevance or irrelevance.

4.1.2. Model Training

The model was fine-tuned using the labeled positive and negative examples, with the optimization guided by the cross-entropy loss function, as shown below:

$$L = -[y \cdot log(p) + (1-y) \cdot log(1-p)] \quad (3)$$

where:

- y represents the true label (0 or 1),
- p is the predicted probability from the model.

To prevent overfitting, we employed an early stopping strategy during training. Additionally, learning rates and batch sizes were adjusted to achieve optimal performance.

4.2. Data Processing in the System

Before introducing the FT_RoBERTa model for relevance calculation, the keyword information collected by the M.I.M.I. assistant evaluation tool was flexibly assigned different weights based on importance. The total weight was normalized to 1. Then, fuzzy keyword matching was applied to the question portion of the dataset stored in the MySQL database, scoring the matches based on the assigned weights. To ensure data reliability, only the top-ranked data with a score greater than 0.7 were selected as the candidate dataset.

After filling the keyword information into a question template to form a complete question, the FT_RoBERTa model was used to compute the relevance between this question and the candidate dataset. Instances with a relevance score greater than 0.85 were selected for the final dataset.

The final dataset underwent data cleaning using NLP techniques. Common and unique treatment methods, medications, and recommendations were extracted from the medical advice within the dataset. The filtered information was then applied to a pre-designed medical recommendation template to generate personalized medical suggestions.

5. Results and Discussion

5.1. Keyword-Weight-Matching Algorithm

By assigning different weights to keywords related to diagnostic results, symptoms, and patient basic information, we can effectively enhance the focus and accuracy of matching. For example, the keyword information group ['depression': 0.4, 'insomnia': 0.2, 'low spirits': 0.1, 'appetite': 0.1, 'motor inhibition': 0.1, 'female': 0.05, '24': 0.05] is weighted as shown in Figure 10, with an average precision score of 7.5.

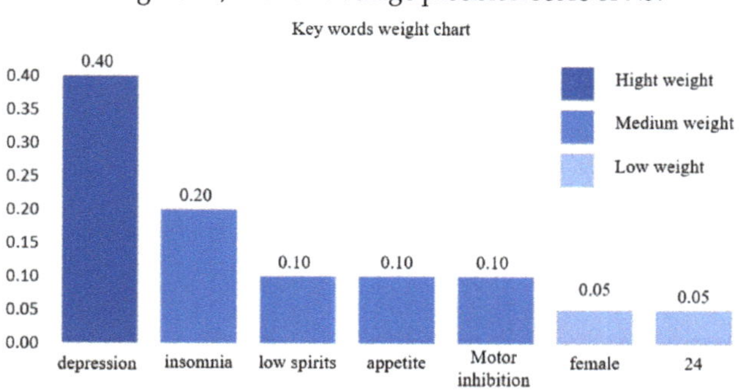

Figure 10. Weight distribution.

Taking 30 different keyword information groups to the MySQL database for fuzzy matching and scoring by weight, the top 15 Q&A pairs averaged 0.7 (out of 1), as shown in Figure 11, indicating rich content and high quality.

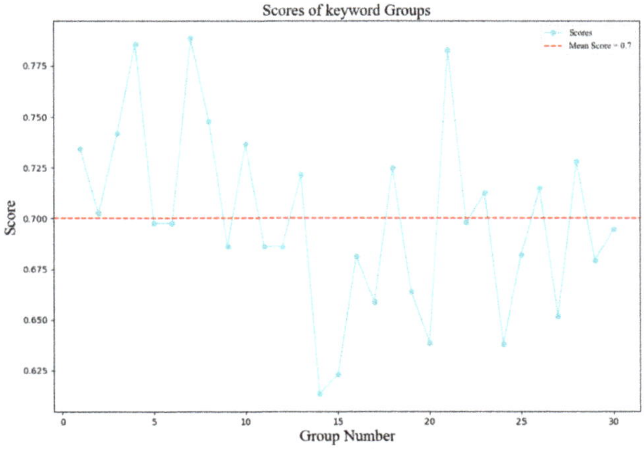

Figure 11. Weight-matching score.

5.2. Semantic-Matching Models

The assessment metrics for this experiment were relevance and precision. We used a pre-trained RoBERTa-based model to generate embeddings for template questions and for each answer. For the template question (Text1) and answers (Text2. . .n) in the dataset, corresponding vector representations v1 and v1. . .n were generated. The relevance between these vectors was measured by calculating the Manhattan Distance, Euclidean Distance, and Cosine Similarity between them. The formulas for these calculations are as follows: (4)–(6), where P and Q represent two points and p_i and q_i are their coordinates on the ith dimension. Manhattan Distance sums the absolute differences in each dimension, reflecting the cumulative difference between two points; the larger the value, the greater the difference. Euclidean Distance calculates the "straight-line" distance between two points, representing the spatial distance; the larger the value, the further apart the points. Cosine Similarity calculates the angle between vectors, with a larger value indicating greater similarity.

$$D_{\text{manhattan}}(P,Q) = \sum_{i=1}^{n} |p_i - q_i| \quad (4)$$

$$D_{\text{euclidean}}(P,Q) = \sqrt{\sum_{i=1}^{n} (p_i - q_i)^2} \quad (5)$$

$$\text{Cosine}(\vec{v_1}, \vec{v_2}) = \frac{\vec{v_1} \cdot \vec{v_2}}{\| \vec{v_1} \| \times \| \vec{v_2} \|} \quad (6)$$

Precision is the ratio of correctly retrieved relevant Q&A pairs ($U1$) to all retrieved Q&A pairs ($U2$). A Q&A pair is defined as correctly retrieved if its cosine similarity with the template question is greater than 0.85, calculated using Formula (7):

$$\text{Accuracy}(U1, U2) = \frac{U1}{U2} \quad (7)$$

The candidate data obtained from the keyword-weight-matching step are further processed using the semantic-matching model, significantly enhancing the precision and quality of answers. For instance, with the template question "[Gender: female, age: 24], suffering from [depression] with symptoms of [insomnia, low spirits, loss of appetite, motor inhibition], what treatment should be taken? What medication? Any suggestions?", we conducted comparative experiments on several advanced models with 15 different template questions and their corresponding candidate answer datasets. The average results are presented in Table 5.

Table 5. Comparative experimental results of different methods.

Model	Manhattan Distance	Euclidean Distance	Cosine Value
BERT	158	7.32	0.84
RoBERTa	52	4.26	0.88
ALBERT [41]	278	6.67	0.73
XLNet [42]	767	69.72	0.87
FT_RoBERTa	50	4.46	0.90

Figures 12–14 illustrate the line graphs showing the scores of various models across 15 sets of data for different metrics. From Figure 14, it is clear that RoBERTa's cosine similarity score (0.88) is the closest to XLNet's (0.87), and both significantly outperform BERT (0.84) and ALBERT (0.73). Figures 12 and 13 show that RoBERTa maintains lower scores for Manhattan distance (52) and Euclidean distance (4.62), while XLNet's scores for Manhattan distance (767) and Euclidean distance (69.72) remain extremely high. Based on these analyses, we conclude that RoBERTa outperforms the other models in terms of both vector similarity and spatial distance when processing our dataset, demonstrating its superior performance. This further indicates that RoBERTa exhibits higher precision and robustness in capturing semantic similarity.

Specifically, RoBERTa's deeper pre-training and more optimized training strategies enable it to better understand and represent complex medical question–answer pairs, leading to higher relevance and accuracy in semantic-matching tasks. Furthermore, the method employed in this study, which incorporates a keyword-weight-matching algorithm, not only significantly reduces computational costs compared to previous semantic retrieval models but also enhances the focus and accuracy of the matching process. This strategy prioritizes highly relevant question–answer pairs during the initial candidate data screening, providing more precise input for subsequent semantic matching. This is one of the key reasons behind the superior overall performance of our approach.

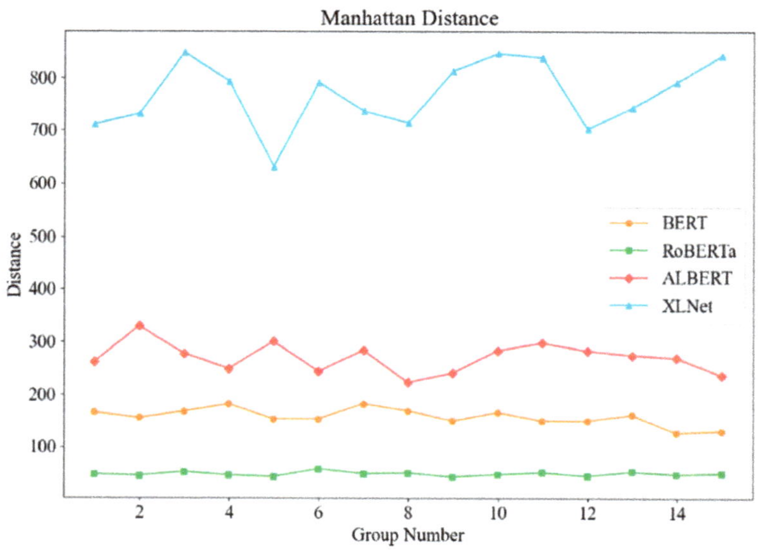

Figure 12. Manhattan distance score.

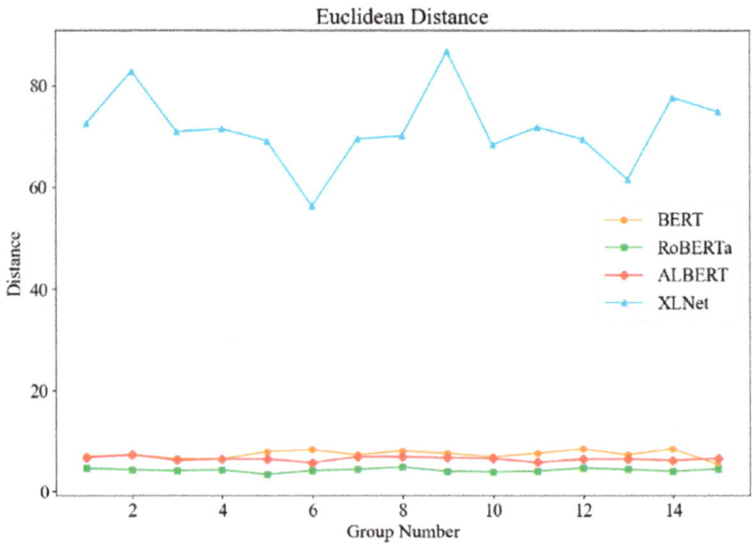

Figure 13. Euclidean distance score.

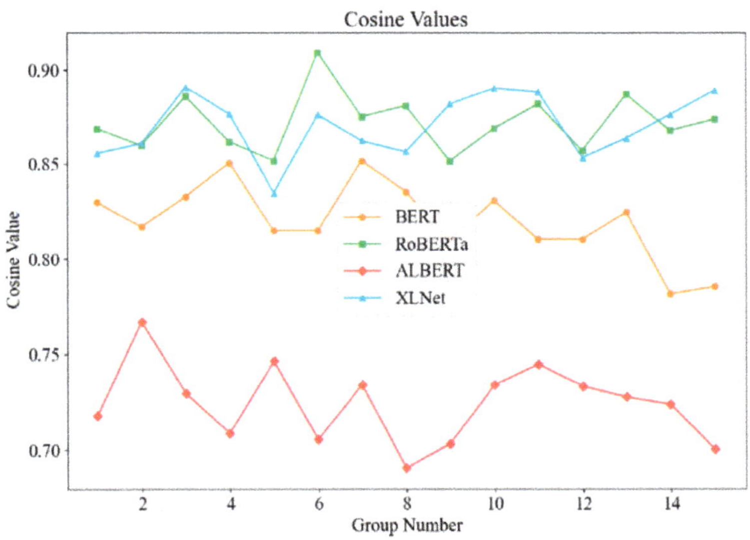

Figure 14. Cosine value score.

Using domain-specific data from the mental health field, we fine-tuned the RoBERTa model to create a new FT_RoBERTa model, which was then tested on the same 15 datasets. As shown in the scatter plot in Figure 15, the fine-tuned FT_RoBERTa model achieved an average cosine similarity score of 0.9 for semantic relevance, an improvement of 0.02 compared to the original RoBERTa model (0.88). According to the calculation in Equation (7), both models achieved a precision score of 0.87, indicating that the fine-tuned FT_RoBERTa model performed well and showed a slight improvement.

Several groups of data selected through the semantic-matching model are combined with advanced natural language processing (NLP) technology to generate personalized medical advice. This advice includes treatment suggestions, recommended medications, lifestyle advice, and mental health guidance, all highly accurate, complete, and consistent, matching the patient's personal circumstances and derived from solutions provided by experts in the relevant medical field.

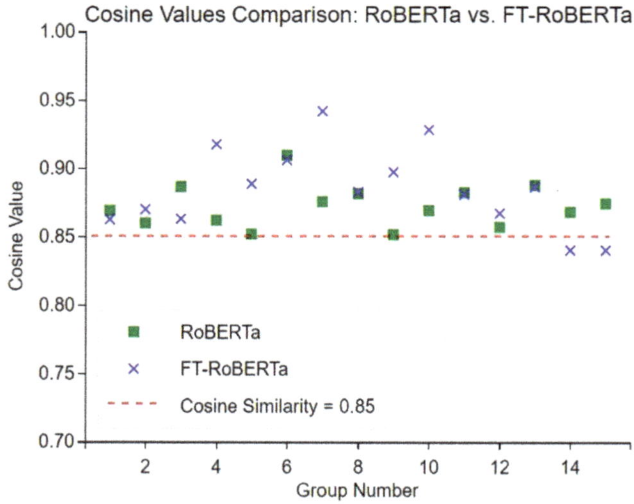

Figure 15. RoBERTa vs. FT-RoBERTa.

5.3. Construction of Medical-Knowledge Graph

To support knowledge retrieval and the generation of universally applicable medical advice in the field of mental and psychological health, we specifically constructed a domain-knowledge graph. The mental and psychological health domain medical-knowledge graph developed in this experiment, as illustrated in Figures 16–19, displays information related to entity categories, entity attributes, and entity relationship types. It includes five entity types with 2430 entities, eight attribute types, and nine relationship types with 5140 relationships, showing a well-developed initial scale.

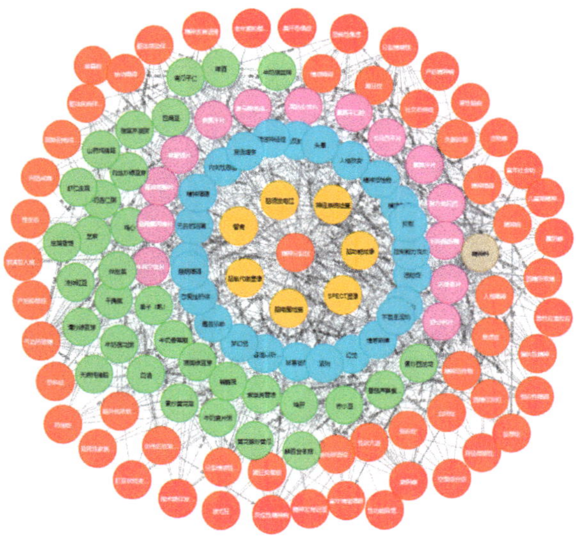

Figure 16. Mental and psychological health domain medical-knowledge graph.

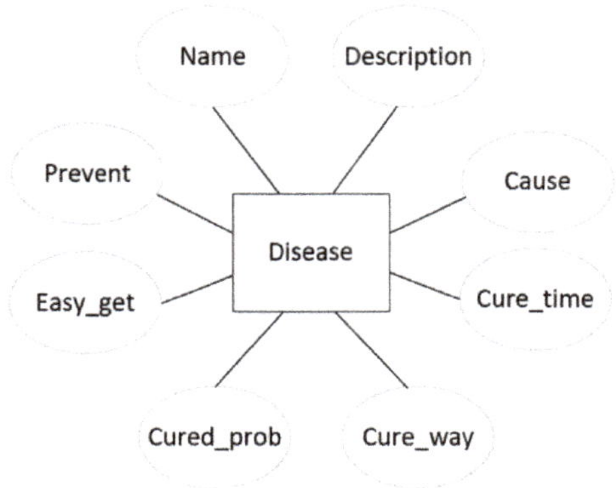

Figure 17. Entity-related info.

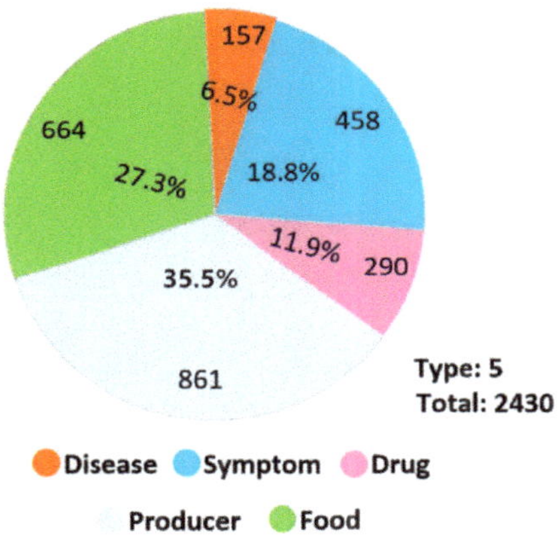

Figure 18. Attribute-related info.

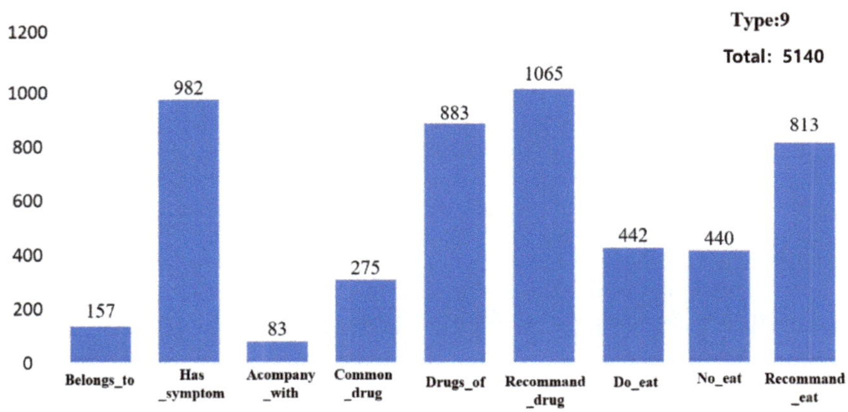

Figure 19. Entity relationship-related Info.

This knowledge graph enables the retrieval of extensive knowledge related to mental and psychological illnesses through specific query templates. For diseases such as depression and mania, the knowledge graph provides detailed information, including symptoms, comorbidities, susceptible populations, treatment duration, cure probabilities, treatment methods, medication use, recommended diets, foods to avoid, and preventive measures.

Figures 20 and 21 show the effectiveness of using query statements to retrieve data from the knowledge graph and filling the results into prepared templates, effectively generating universally applicable medical advice.

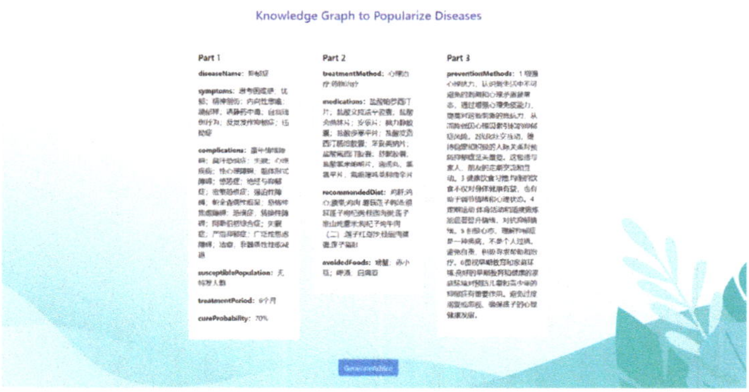

Figure 20. Depression knowledge generation.

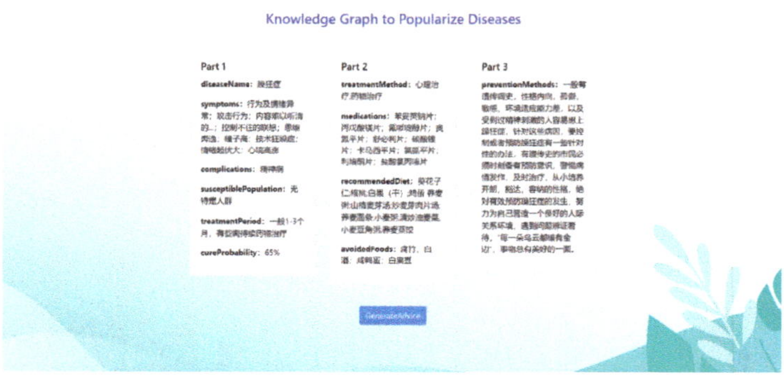

Figure 21. Mania knowledge generation.

5.4. Limitations and Future Work

While our methods have shown promising results on a subset of the Huatuo-26M dataset, several limitations exist. Firstly, although models like BERT and RoBERTa capture deep semantic meanings, they are not specifically tailored for the mental and psychological health domain, potentially limiting precision. Future work includes fine-tuning these models with larger domain-specific datasets to enhance accuracy. Secondly, the use of the Cross-Encoder structure with RoBERTa incurs high computational costs and poses challenges in parallelization. Exploring more efficient network architectures is planned to reduce computational overheads. Thirdly, the dataset and the mental health-knowledge graph used are not comprehensive. Expanding these resources and testing with more diverse datasets are future objectives.

Importantly, our methods have not yet been validated in real clinical settings, which may affect clinician adoption due to concerns about clinical validity. To address this, future work will focus on the following:

- Clinical Validation: Collaborating with mental health professionals to deploy our tools in clinical environments and compare their performance against standard clinical practices.
- Feedback Collection: Gathering insights from clinicians and patients on usability and practical utility.
- Evaluating Key Metrics: Assessing improvements in assessment time, diagnostic accuracy, and patient satisfaction.

By undertaking these steps, we aim to demonstrate the practical applicability of our work, addressing concerns about clinical validity and encouraging adoption in real-world settings.

6. Conclusions

This paper developed a strategy for auxiliary assessment and personalized medical-advice generation in the mental and psychological health domain. Initially, an effective auxiliary assessment tool using M.I.N.I was constructed, enabling the automatic and intelligent collection of patient data and providing preliminary diagnostic results. Subsequently, a keyword-weight-matching retrieval algorithm and an improved semantic-matching model based on RoBERTa were proposed. This approach enhances data quality by focusing on key information through keyword weighting, and the semantic model filters the most relevant data. A medical-advice generation template was then designed, with NLP technology extracting key information from various pieces of advice. After cleaning, calculation, and filtering, this resulted in personalized medical advice. Additionally, a method using a knowledge graph was introduced to generate universally applicable advice in cases of data insufficiency. The proposed algorithms and models were validated on a public benchmark dataset and demonstrated good performance and reliability in generating medical advice. This work aims to alleviate resource distribution issues in mental and psychological health care and enhance diagnostic and treatment efficiency, ultimately improving mental health services' quality and efficiency. Future efforts will focus on optimizing algorithm performance and expanding the knowledge graphs for broader clinical application.

Author Contributions: Conceptualization, Y.W. and J.T.; Methodology, Y.W. and H.X.; Software, H.X.; Validation, H.X.; Formal analysis, R.C.; Investigation, L.G.; Data curation, S.C.; Writing—original draft, Y.W. and H.X.; Writing—review & editing, L.G. and J.T.; Visualization, F.W.; Supervision, Y.L.; Project administration, L.C.; Funding acquisition, J.T. All authors have read and agreed to the published version of the manuscript.

Funding: This work was funded in part by the National Key RD Program of China under Grant no.2022YFE010300; in part by the Natural Science Foundation of Hunan Province under Grant no.2021JJ50050; in part by the Scientific Research Fund of Hunan Provincial Education Department under Grant no.22A0422; in part by the University IUR Innovation Foundation of China under Grant no.2022IT052; National Natural Science Foundation of China (62106074, Research on influence mechanism of research collaboration networks from the network evolution), Ling-Jiao Chen.

Institutional Review Board Statement: Not applicable.

Informed Consent Statement: Not applicable.

Data Availability Statement: Publicly available datasets were analyzed in this study. This data can be found here: https://github.com/FreedomIntelligence/Huatuo-26M.

Conflicts of Interest: The authors declare no conflict of interest.

References

1. World Health Organization. *World Mental Health Report: Transforming Mental Health for All*; World Health Organization: Geneva, Switzerland, 2022. Available online: https://www.who.int/publications/i/item/9789240049338 (accessed on 6 February 2023).
2. Vigo, D.; Thornicroft, G.; Atun, R. Estimating the true global burden of mental illness. *Lancet Psychiatry* **2016**, *3*, 171–178. [CrossRef] [PubMed]
3. World Health Organization. *WHO Report Highlights Global Shortfall in Investment in Mental Health*; World Health Organization: Geneva, Switzerland, 2023. Available online: https://www.who.int/news/item/08-10-2021-who-report-highlights-global-shortfall-in-investment-in-mental-health (accessed on 6 December 2023).
4. Patel, V.; Saxena, S.; Lund, C.; Thornicroft, G.; Baingana, F.; Bolton, P.; Chisholm, D.; Collins, P.Y.; Cooper, J.L.; Eaton, J.; et al. The Lancet Commission on global mental health and sustainable development. *Lancet* **2018**, *392*, 1553–1598. [CrossRef] [PubMed]
5. Devlin, J.; Chang, M.W.; Lee, K.; Toutanova, K. BERT: Pre-training of Deep Bidirectional Transformers for Language Understanding. *arXiv* **2018**, arXiv:1810.04805.

6. Heehan, D.V.; Lecrubier, Y.; Sheehan, K.H.; Amorim, P.; Janavs, J.; Weiller, E.; Hergueta, T.; Baker, R.; Dunbar, G.C. The Mini-International Neuropsychiatric Interview (M.I.N.I.): The development and validation of a structured diagnostic psychiatric interview for DSM-IV and ICD-10. *J. Clin. Psychiatry* **1998**, *59* (Suppl. S20), 22–33; quiz 34–57. [PubMed]
7. Jones, S.R.; Fernyhough, C. A new look at the neural diathesis–stress model of schizophrenia: The primacy of social-evaluative and uncontrollable situations. *Schizophr. Bull.* **2007**, *33*, 1171–1177. [CrossRef]
8. American Psychiatric Association. *Diagnostic and Statistical Manual of Mental Disorders*, 5th ed.; American Psychiatric Publishing, Inc.: Washington, DC, USA, 2013.
9. World Health Organization. *The ICD-10 Classification of Mental and Behavioural Disorders*; World Health Organization: Geneva, Switzerland, 1993.
10. Chakraborty, N.; Ali, A.; Alakpa, C. Diagnostic categories of mental illness in a rural African setting-the mhGAP experience in Edawu (Nigeria). *Int. J. Ment. Health* **2021**, *50*, 91–95. [CrossRef]
11. Arrow, K.; Resnik, P.; Michel, H.; Kitchen, C.; Mo, C.; Chen, S.; Espy-Wilson, C.; Coppersmith, G.A.; Frazier, C.; Kelly, D. Evaluating the Use of Online Self-Report Questionnaires as Clinically Valid Mental Health Monitoring Tools in the Clinical Whitespace. *Psychiatr. Q.* **2023**, *94*, 221–231. [CrossRef]
12. Pan, Y.; Chen, Q.; Peng, W.; Wang, X.; Hu, B.; Liu, X.; Chen, J.; Zhou, W. MedWriter: Knowledge-Aware Medical Text Generation. In Proceedings of the 28th International Conference on Computational Linguistics, Barcelona, Spain, 8–13 December 2020; International Committee on Computational Linguistics: New York, NY, USA, 2020; pp. 2363–2368.
13. Luo, R.; Sun, L.; Xia, Y.; Qin, T.; Zhang, S.; Poon, H.; Liu, T.-Y. BioGPT: Generative pre-trained transformer for biomedical text generation and mining. *Brief. Bioinform.* **2022**, *23*, bbac409. [CrossRef]
14. Kumichev, G.; Blinov, P.; Kuzkina, Y.; Goncharov, V.; Zubkova, G.; Zenovkin, N.; Goncharov, A.; Savchenko, A. MedSyn: LLM-Based Synthetic Medical Text Generation Framework. In *Machine Learning and Knowledge Discovery in Databases*; Applied Data Science Track; ECML PKDD 2024; Lecture Notes in Computer Science; Bifet, A., Krilavičius, T., Miliou, I., Nowaczyk, S., Eds.; Springer: Cham, Switzerland, 2024; Volume 14950. [CrossRef]
15. Hasani, A.M.; Singh, S.; Zahergivar, A.; Ryan, B.; Nethala, D.; Bravomontenegro, G.; Mendhiratta, N.; Ball, M.; Farhadi, F.; Malayeri, A. Evaluating the performance of Generative Pre-trained Transformer-4 (GPT-4) in standardizing radiology reports. *Eur. Radiol.* **2023**, *34*, 3566–3574. [CrossRef]
16. Thakur, N.; Reimers, N.; Rucklé, A.; Srivastava, A.; Gurevych, I. BEIR: A Heterogenous Benchmark for Zero-shot Evaluation of Information Retrieval Models. *arXiv* **2021**, arXiv:2104.08663.
17. Zhu, Y.; Yuan, H.; Wang, S.; Liu, J.; Liu, W.; Deng, C.; Dou, Z.; Wen, J. Large Language Models for Information Retrieval: A Survey. *arXiv* **2023**, arXiv:2308.07107.
18. Tang, X.; Luo, Y.; Xiong, D.; Yang, J.; Li, R.; Peng, D. Short text matching model with multiway semantic interaction based on multi-granularity semantic embedding. *Appl. Intell.* **2022**, *52*, 15632–15642. [CrossRef]
19. Cai, Y.; Fan, Y.; Guo, J.; Sun, F.; Zhang, R.; Cheng, X. Semantic Models for the First-Stage Retrieval: A Comprehensive Review. *ACM Trans. Inf. Syst.* **2021**, *54*, 66.
20. Nigam, S.; Goel, N. Nigam@COLIEE-22: Legal Case Retrieval and Entailment using Cascading of Lexical and Semantic-based models. *arXiv* **2022**, arXiv:2204.07853.
21. Zou, Y.; Liu, H.; Gui, T.; Wang, J.; Zhang, Q.; Tang, M.; Li, H.; Wang, D. Divide and Conquer: Text Semantic Matching with Disentangled Keywords and Intents. *arXiv* **2022**, arXiv:2203.02898.
22. Gupta, S.; Mishra, A. Publisher Side Profit Optimization Using Adaptive Keyword Weighted Sponsored Search Technique. *J. Web Eng.* **2022**, *21*, 1449–1469. [CrossRef]
23. Liu, Y.; Ott, M.; Goyal, N.; Du, J.; Joshi, M.; Chen, D.; Levy, O.; Lewis, M.; Zettlemoyer, L.; Stoyanov, V. RoBERTa: A Robustly Optimized BERT Pretraining Approach. *arXiv* **1907**, arXiv:1907.11692.
24. Reimers, N.; Gurevych, I. Sentence-BERT: Sentence Embeddings using Siamese BERT-Networks. *arXiv* **2019**, arXiv:1908.1008.
25. Li, Z.; Yang, N.; Wang, L.; Wei, F. Learning Diverse Document Representations with Deep Query Interactions for Dense Retrieval. *arXiv* **2022**, arXiv:2208.04232.
26. Zhu, Y.; Li, Y.; Cui, Y.; Zhang, T.; Wang, D.; Zhang, Y.; Feng, S. A Knowledge-Enhanced Hierarchical Reinforcement Learning-Based Dialogue System for Automatic Disease Diagnosis. *Electronics* **2023**, *12*, 4896. [CrossRef]
27. Smith, J.; Johnson, A.B. Medical knowledge graphs: An in-depth review. *Big Data Min. Anal.* **2023**, *6*, 201–217. [CrossRef]
28. Wu, X.; Duan, J.; Pan, Y.; Li, M. Medical Knowledge Graph: Data Sources, Construction, Reasoning, and Applications. *Big Data Min. Anal.* **2023**, *6*, 113–128. [CrossRef]
29. Chandak, P.; Huang, K.; Zitnik, M. Building a knowledge graph to enable precision medicine. *Sci. Data* **2023**, *10*, 67. [CrossRef] [PubMed]
30. Li, J.; Wang, X.; Wu, X.; Zhang, Z.; Xu, X.; Fu, J.; Tiwari, P.; Wan, X.; Wang, B. Huatuo-26m, a large-scale chinese medical qa dataset. *arXiv* **2023**, arXiv:2305.01526, 2023.
31. Li, W.; Yu, L.; Wu, M.; Liu, J.; Hao, M.; Li, Y. DoctorGPT: A Large Language Model with Chinese Medical Question-Answering Capabilities. In Proceedings of the 2023 International Conference on High Performance Big Data and Intelligent Systems (HDIS), Macau, China, 6–8 December 2023; pp. 186–193. [CrossRef]
32. Ye, Q.; Liu, J.; Chong, D.; Zhou, P.; Hua, Y.; Liu, A. Qilin-med: Multi-stage knowledge injection advanced medical large language model. *arXiv* **2023**, arXiv:2310.09089.

33. Yang, S.; Zhao, H.; Zhu, S.; Zhou, G.; Xu, H.; Jia, Y.; Zan, H. Zhongjing: Enhancing the chinese medical capabilities of large language model through expert feedback and real-world multi-turn dialogue. In Proceedings of the AAAI Conference on Artificial Intelligence, Vancouver, BC, Canada, 20–27 February 2024; Volume 38, pp. 19368–19376.
34. Jung, S.; Han, S.-Y.; Kang, B. Design of a Variable-Mode Sync Generator for Implementing Digital Filters in Image Processing. *J. Inst. Korean Electr. Electron. Eng.* **2023**, *27*, 273–279.
35. Islam, K.Z.; Murray, D.; Diepeveen, D.; Jones, M.G.K.; Sohel, F. LoRa-based outdoor localization and tracking using unsupervised symbolization. *Internet Things* **2023**, *25*, 101016. [CrossRef]
36. Steven, W. Boolean operations. In *Information Retrieval Data Structures & Algorithms*; Prentice-Hall, Inc.: Saddle River, NJ, USA, 1992; ISBN 0-13-463837-9.
37. Aswani, A.; Shazeer, N.; Parmar, N.; Uszkoreit, J.; Jones, L.; Gomez, A.N.; Kaiser, L.; Polosukhin, I. Attention Is All You Need. *arXiv* **2017**, arXiv:1706.03762.
38. Mikolov, T.; Chen, K.; Corrado, G.; Dean, J. Efficient Estimation of Word Representations in Vector Space. *arXiv* **2013**, arXiv:1301.3781.
39. Pennington, J.; Socher, R.; Manning, C.D. GloVe: Global Vectors for Word Representation. In Proceedings of the 2014 Conference on Empirical Methods in Natural Language Processing (EMNLP), Doha, Qatar, 25–29 October 2014.
40. Hochreiter, S.; Schmidhuber, J. Long Short-Term Memory. *Neural Comput.* **1997**, *9*, 1735–1780. [CrossRef]
41. Lan, Z.; Chen, M.; Goodman, S.; Gimpel, K.; Sharma, P.; Soricut, R. ALBERT: A Lite BERT for Self-supervised Learning of Language Representations. *arXiv* **2019**, arXiv:1909.11942.
42. Yang, Z.; Dai, Z.; Yang, Y.; Carbonell, J.; Salakhutdinov, R.; Le, Q.V. XLNet: Generalized Autoregressive Pretraining for Language Understanding. In Advances in Neural Information Processing Systems (Vol. 32). *arXiv* **2019**, arXiv:1906.08237.

Journal of
Clinical Medicine

MDPI

Article

Estimating Progression-Free Survival in Patients with Primary High-Grade Glioma Using Machine Learning †

Agnieszka Kwiatkowska-Miernik [1,*], Piotr Gustaw Wasilewski [1], Bartosz Mruk [1], Katarzyna Sklinda [1], Maciej Bujko [2] and Jerzy Walecki [1,*]

[1] Centre of Radiological Diagnostics, National Medical Institute of the Ministry of the Interior and Administration, Wołoska 137, 02-507 Warsaw, Poland

[2] Department of Neurosurgery, National Medical Institute of the Ministry of the Interior and Administration, Wołoska 137, 02-507 Warsaw, Poland

* Correspondence: akwiatkowskamiernik@gmail.com (A.K.-M.); jerzywalecki1@gmail.com (J.W.)

† This article is a revised and expanded version of a paper entitled "Application of artificial intelligence algorithms in estimating progression-free survival in patients with primary high-grade glioma (WHO 4)", which was presented at 1st International Caparica Conference on Prescriptomics and Precision Medicine 2024 11–13 May 2024 | Caparica | Portugal.

Abstract: Background/Objectives: High-grade gliomas are the most common primary malignant brain tumors in adults. These neoplasms remain predominantly incurable due to the genetic diversity within each tumor, leading to varied responses to specific drug therapies. With the advent of new targeted and immune therapies, which have demonstrated promising outcomes in clinical trials, there is a growing need for image-based techniques to enable early prediction of treatment response. This study aimed to evaluate the potential of radiomics and artificial intelligence implementation in predicting progression-free survival (PFS) in patients with highest-grade glioma (CNS WHO 4) undergoing a standard treatment plan. **Methods**: In this retrospective study, prediction models were developed in a cohort of 51 patients with pathologically confirmed highest-grade glioma (CNS WHO 4) from the authors' institution and the repository of the Cancer Imaging Archive (TCIA). Only patients with confirmed recurrence after complete tumor resection with adjuvant radiotherapy and chemotherapy with temozolomide were included. For each patient, 109 radiomic features of the tumor were obtained from a preoperative magnetic resonance imaging (MRI) examination. Four clinical features were added manually—sex, weight, age at the time of diagnosis, and the lobe of the brain where the tumor was located. The data label was the time to recurrence, which was determined based on follow-up MRI scans. Artificial intelligence algorithms were built to predict PFS in the training set (n = 75%) and then validate it in the test set (n = 25%). The performance of each model in both the training and test datasets was assessed using mean absolute percentage error (MAPE). **Results**: In the test set, the random forest model showed the highest predictive performance with 1-MAPE = 92.27% and a C-index of 0.9544. The decision tree, gradient booster, and artificial neural network models showed slightly lower effectiveness with 1-MAPE of 88.31%, 80.21%, and 91.29%, respectively. **Conclusions**: Four of the six models built gave satisfactory results. These results show that artificial intelligence models combined with radiomic features could be useful for predicting the progression-free survival of high-grade glioma patients. This could be beneficial for risk stratification of patients, enhancing the potential for personalized treatment plans and improving overall survival. Further investigation is necessary with an expanded sample size and external multicenter validation.

Keywords: radiomics; glioma; artificial intelligence; recurrence

1. Introduction

Glioma is a brain tumor associated with a high mortality rate [1]. According to the World Health Organization's (WHO) classification of central nervous system (CNS) tumors, grade 4 tumors are the most common primary malignant brain tumors in adults [2]. These neoplasms remain predominantly incurable due to, among others, the genetic diversity within each tumor, leading to varied responses to specific drug therapies [3]. Currently, the most widely used therapy around the world for primary high-grade gliomas is the so-called new Stupp protocol, which consists of maximal surgical resection of the tumor with adjuvant radiotherapy (RT) and chemotherapy (CHTH) with temozolomide (TMZ) [4–6]. The implementation of this therapy is associated with an extension of the mean overall survival to 14.6 months [7]. However, with the emergence of new targeted and immune therapies, which have demonstrated promising results in clinical trials, there is a growing need for image-based methods to predict treatment response.

The answer to this growing demand may lie in the application of artificial intelligence, which is increasingly being used in medicine, especially in radiology. One of the subfields of radiology today is radiomics, which is characterized by the extraction of new data in quantitative form from radiological images. Analysis of such acquired data by artificial intelligence models leads to the discovery of new clinically important information in radiological images. In daily clinical practice, visual analysis of images is based on qualitative descriptors (such as signal intensity, density, heterogeneity, and level of contrast enhancement) or simple quantitative characteristics (for example, dimension, volume, and number of lesions). The sensitivity of such measurements is not high and strongly dependent on the experience of the evaluating radiologist. By automatically extracting the same features from imaging data, computational methods eliminate these disadvantages. These new digital features, which are not intuitively recognizable by humans, are called radiomic features and can be divided into three main groups:

1. Morphological features, which particularly describe the size and shape of the previously segmented region of interest.
2. First-order features, which are based on a histogram of pixel/voxel intensities of the region of interest.
3. Second-order features, which describe the texture of the region of interest. Texture-based features are the most complex and describe the heterogeneity of the image. In radiomics, they are also often the most important due to the more accurate description of the image. Figure 1 shows an example of two images that, when described by radiomic features, would not differ in morphological features and first-order features but differ significantly in texture.

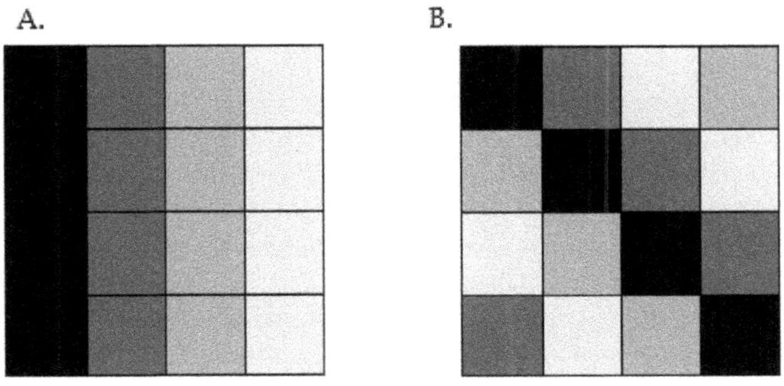

Figure 1. Assuming that each small square represents a pixel, the morphological and first-order features of images (**A**,**B**) would be the same, but the images differ in texture.

Neuro-oncology is one of the specialties in which the advances in radiomics are the most noticeable. Numerous studies have evaluated the use of radiomics models in predicting the presence of mutations in gliomas or the time to recurrence of gliomas after treatment [8]. Ailing He et al. proposed a radiomics model based on MRI images to predict IDH mutation status in low-grade gliomas. The model performed well in validation datasets with an AUC of 0.873 [9]. Jiangwei Lao et al. proposed a radiomics model for the prediction of overall survival in glioblastoma multiforme. The model performed OS prediction with a C-index = 0.710 [10].

However, to the best of the authors' knowledge, there is currently no adequate clinical or image-based predictive model to predict precise PFS (calculated in days) in patients with the highest-grade glioma treated uniformly. Therefore, this study aimed to develop and evaluate an AI model based on radiomic features for prediction of progression-free survival (PFS) in patients with the highest-grade glioma (CNS WHO 4) undergoing a standard treatment plan. The developed machine learning model can help clinicians identify patients who are most likely to benefit from the standard treatment plan and support the implementation of personalized therapy.

2. Materials and Methods

This study carried out a self-evaluation using METRICS, the details of which are provided in Supplementary S1 [11].

The flowchart of the study is shown in Figure 2.

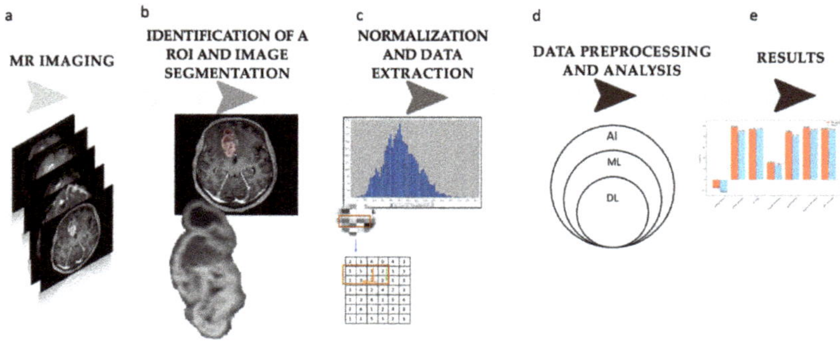

Figure 2. Study flowchart. (**a**) Magnetic resonance (MR) imaging; the study is based on contrast-enhanced T1—w images. (**b**) Identification of a region of interest (ROI) and semi-automatic image segmentation. (**c**) Normalization and radiomic feature extraction from the defined ROI; 109 radiomic features were obtained in the study. (**d**) Data preprocessing and analysis; five different machine learning (ML) models were trained on the received data (AI—artificial intelligence, DL—deep learning). (**e**) Results.

2.1. Study Group

This retrospective study analyzed the medical records of 210 adult patients with pathologically confirmed primary high-grade glioma (CNS WHO 4). As the study included patients hospitalized before 2021, the diagnosis of glioblastoma multiforme fulfilling the World Health Organization's criteria at that time now corresponds to both glioblastoma CNS WHO 4 and astrocytoma CNS WHO 4 [2]. The inclusion criteria were as follows:

- A histopathologic diagnosis of glioma CNS WHO 4;
- Available preoperative MR imaging, including contrast-enhanced T1WI;
- Available follow-up MR imaging with a reported recurrence or imaging follow-up up to two years that showed no features of tumor recurrence.

The exclusion criteria were as follows:

- Artifacts in MR images;
- Treatment program other than complete resection with adjuvant treatment consisting of temozolomide chemotherapy and radiotherapy;
- Inconclusive result of the follow-up MR examination.

A total of 51 patients were ultimately included in the study.

Data were obtained from the authors' institution and the publicly available Cancer Genome Atlas Glioblastoma (TCGA-GBM) clinical database and the associated imaging data from the Cancer Imaging Archive (TCIA) [12,13].

The detailed patient selection process is shown in Figure 3. The main exclusion factor was the standard treatment plan, as some patients from the TCGA-GBM database received bevacizumab, cisplatin, or targeted molecular therapy, among others, as adjuvant chemotherapy instead of temozolomide.

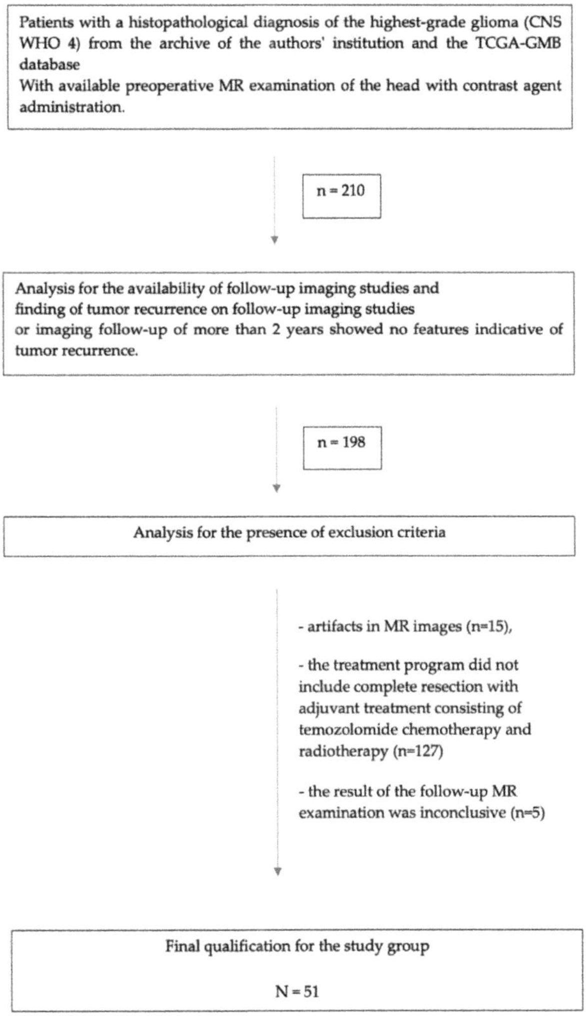

Figure 3. Flowchart of the patient selection process.

2.2. *Identification of a Region of Interest (ROI) and Segmentation*

Preoperative MRIs were analyzed using Syngo.Via VB10, Research Frontier, Siemens Healthineers. Segmentation of the lesion was performed semi-automatically by a single reader (a fourth-year radiology resident). The 2D region of interest (ROI) was marked on the axial view of contrast-enhanced T1-weighted imaging (CE T1WI) on the cross-section in which the tumor had the largest area, and the zone of visible contrast enhancement was identified as the tumor boundary. An example of semi-automated tumor segmentation is shown in Figure 4.

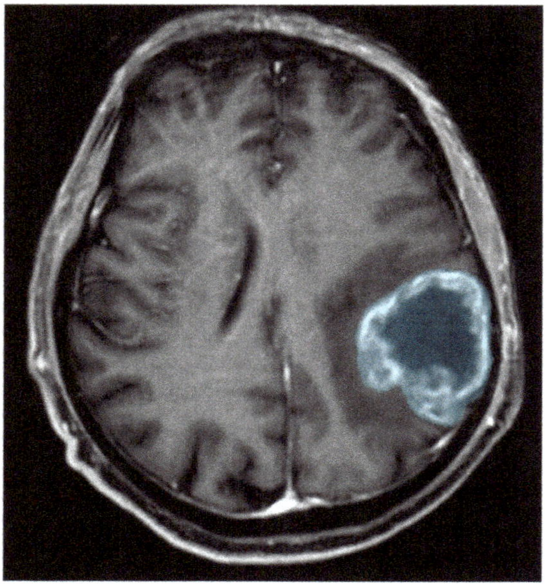

Figure 4. Glioma CNS WHO 4 in the left parietal lobe. T1-weighted image after administration of contrast agent; the blue color was used to mark the tumor segmented by the semi-automated method.

2.3. Normalization and Extraction of the Data

Given that the database included data from multiple sites, there were variations in scanner models, pixel spacing, slice thickness, and contrast within the selected cohort. Normalization was carried out to account for these differences using Syngo.Via VB10, Research Frontier, Siemens Healthineers. All images were resampled to a common voxel resolution of 1 mm^3, and the intensities within each voxel were normalized to a [0, 1] range.

For each patient, 109 radiomic features of the tumor were obtained, and feature groups used in the study are shown in Table 1. Four features were added manually—sex, weight, age at the time of diagnosis, and the lobe of the brain where the tumor was located. The data label was the time to recurrence (calculated in days), which was determined based on follow-up MRI exams evaluated by an experienced radiologist.

Table 1. Groups of radiomic features used in the study.

Feature Group	Number of Features in Each Group
First-order features based on image intensity histogram descriptors	18
Features describing size and shape	16
Features describing the texture extracted from analysis:	75
- Gray-level co-occurrence matrices (GLCM)	24
- Run-length matrix (RLM)	16
- Size-zone matrix (SZM)	16
- Neighboring gray tone difference matrix (NGTDM)	5
- Gray-level run-length matrix (GLRLM)	14

2.4. Data Preprocessing

Reducing the number of features was essential, as the large set of 109 radiomic features could lead to overfitting when predicting progression-free survival (PFS). Additionally, some features might have no variance, be highly correlated with others, or be minimally relevant to PFS prediction. The authors employed methods like locally linear embedding (LLE) and principal component analysis (PCA) to enhance the model's generalizability and obtain higher model performance. Tools for data multiplication of the learning set were used by generating non-repeating data from existing examples while fully considering the underlying patterns and relationships. With the artificial neural network algorithm, a data compression tool based on an encoder–decoder neural network architecture was used.

The dataset was randomly split into training and validation sets in a 75:25 ratio. The training set was utilized to build the predictive model, while the validation set was used for an independent assessment of the model's performance. The details of data preprocessing are shown in Table 2.

Table 2. The details of data preprocessing.

ML Model	Task	Data Multiplication	Dimensionality Reduction
Decision tree (DT)	Classification	×19	Dimensional reduction of up to 11
Random forest (RF)	Classification		
Support vector machine (SVM)	Classification		
Gradient boosting (GBoost)	Classification		
Artificial neural network (ANN)	Classification	×19	Dimensional reduction of up to 66

Among the clinical data, confounding factors were analyzed. None of the added clinical data (gender, age, and weight) individually had a statistically significant effect on PFS ($p < 0.01$); therefore, they were not excluded.

2.5. Development and Validation of Models

Progression-free survival (PFS) was defined as the time from therapy initiation to identification of tumor recurrence on MRI follow-up examination. If the patient was not found to have a tumor recurrence at the last follow-up, the PFS was censored at the time of the last follow-up (at least 2 years).

Due to the diverse properties of artificial intelligence models, we utilized five different machine learning models: decision tree (DT), random forest (RF), support vector machine (SVM), gradient boosting (GBoost), and artificial neural network (ANN).

For statistical analyses, Python Version 3.12 was used. Mean absolute percentage error (MAPE) was used to assess the performance of the models.

3. Results

3.1. Patient Characteristics

A total of 51 patients were included in the study, including 17 women and 34 men. The mean age of the patients included in the study was 56 years, and the median was 59 years. The mean time to recurrence was 352 days, and the median was 215 days. The Kaplan–Meier curve of PFS for patients in the study group is shown in Figure 5.

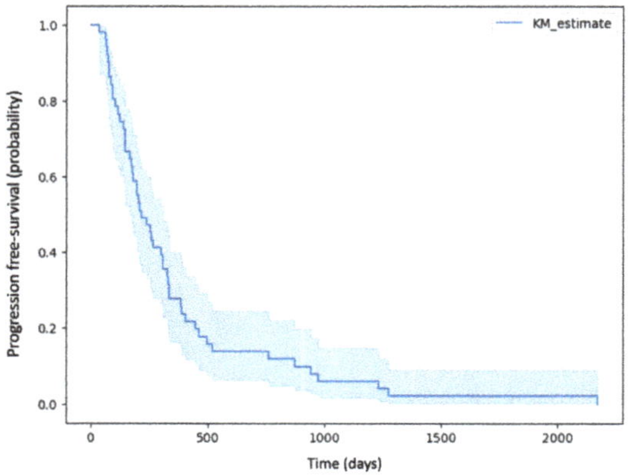

Figure 5. Kaplan–Meier curve of PFS for patients in the study group.

3.2. Model Interpretation

There are several methods to evaluate the performance of a regression model. A common traditional approach is to measure how accurately the predictions match the actual outcomes [14]. This can be carried out using methods like mean absolute error (MAE), mean squared error (MSE), root mean squared error (RMSE), R-squared (R^2), and mean absolute percentage error (MAPE). Another method is the C-index (concordance index). The performance of each model in both the training and test datasets is shown in Tables 3 and 4.

The values of 1-MAPE for each model are shown in Figure 6.

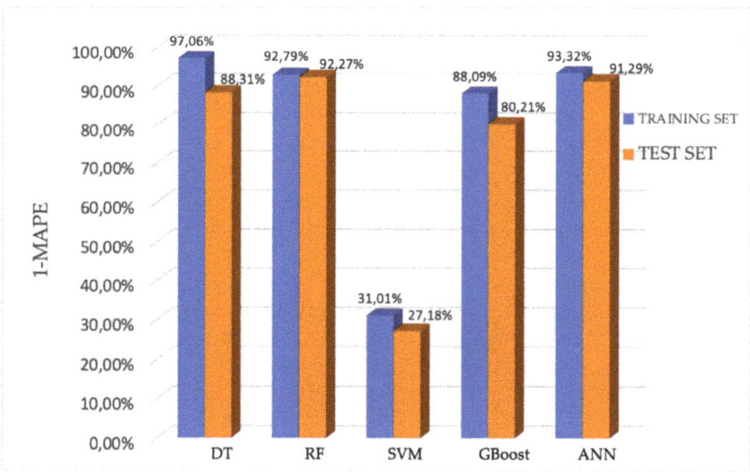

Figure 6. Performance of the five models for predicting the PFS presented using 1-MAPE.

In the training set, the 1-MAPE of the DT, RF, SVM, GBoost, and ANN models were 97.06%, 92.79%, 31.01%, 88.09%, and 93.32%, respectively. Accordingly, in the testing set, the 1-MAPE of these five models were 88.31%, 92.27%, 27.18%, 80.21%, and 91.29%, respectively.

The estimation performance of the DT, RF, GBoost and ANN models reached values above 80% on the test set, which means that these models predict the PFS (calculated in days) with more than 80% accuracy. Among them, the random forest model showed the highest efficiency, predicting PFS on the test set with 92.27% accuracy (C-index: 0.95). The

Kaplan–Meier curve of predicted PFS for the test set by the random forest model is shown in Figure 7 together with the Kaplan–Meier curve of PFS for patients in the study group.

Table 3. Results of each model in the training set presented using mean absolute error, mean squared error, root mean squared error, R^2 score, mean absolute percentage error, and 1-mean absolute percentage error.

	Decision Tree (DT)	Random Forest (RF)	Support Vector Machine (SVM)	Gradient Boosting (GBoost)	Artificial Neural Network (ANN)
Mean absolute error	7.4973	19.1089	180.0376	21.8983	33.9342
Mean squared error	254.1967	3250.7404	92,385.7830	900.2685	8942.9704
Root mean squared error	15.9435	57.0153	303.9503	30.0045	94.5673
R^2 score	0.9969	0.9606	−0.1200	0.9891	0.8799
Mean absolute percentage error	2.9382	7.2073	68.9886	11.9109	6.6754
1-mean absolute percentage error	97.0618	92.7927	31.0114	88.0891	93.3246

Table 4. Results of each model in the test set presented using mean absolute error, mean squared error, root mean squared error, R^2 score, mean absolute percentage error, 1-mean absolute percentage error, C-index.

	Decision Tree (DT)	Random Forest (RF)	Support Vector Machine (SVM)	Gradient Boosting (GBoost)	Artificial Neural Network (ANN)
Mean absolute error	24.8663	25.4891	178.8463	37.3006	45.8352
Mean squared error	4931.2071	4005.8066	79,090.9032	3712.5782	11,766.1994
Root mean squared error	70.2226	63.2914	281.2310	60.9309	108.4721
R^2 score	0.9282	0.9417	−0.1514	0.9460	0.8706
Mean absolute percentage error	11.6877	7.7275	72.8181	19.7899	8.7136
1-mean absolute percentage error	88.3123	92.2725	27.1819	80.2101	91.2964
C-index	0.9413	0.9544	0.5743	0.9254	0.9284

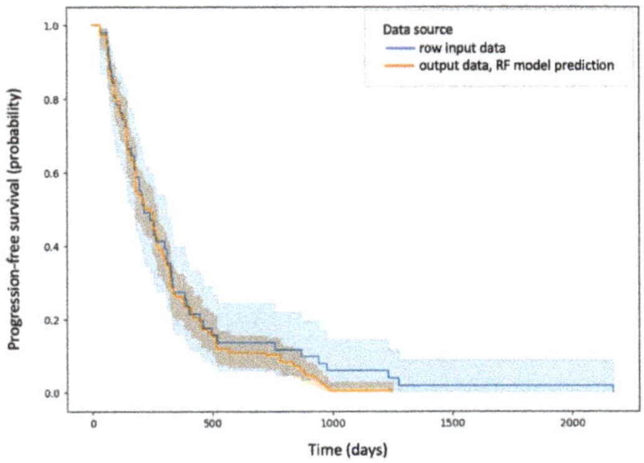

Figure 7. Kaplan–Meier curve of predicted PFS for the test set by the random forest model marked in blue and Kaplan–Meier curve of PFS for patients in the study group marked in orange.

As data multiplication and reduction of dimensionality were used, it was not possible to obtain exact information on which radiomic features made the greatest contribution to the results.

4. Discussion

The results of our study indicate that based on radiomic analysis, which involves extracting texture and morphologic features from numerous medical images in combination with artificial intelligence models, it is possible to build a group of models with a high predictive ability of progression-free survival (PFS). By utilizing advanced computational techniques, these AI-driven models can process vast amounts of radiomic data and identify subtle patterns and correlations, resulting in high prediction performance.

Medical imaging data are predicted to soon represent 30% of global data storage [15]. It is important to use them as efficiently as possible. Machine learning models used to analyze them appear to be key. Therefore, it is important to use several algorithms to analyze the same radiomic data, primarily to expand our knowledge of it. The results of this study show that some of the algorithms have similar accuracy, and the accuracy of the support vector machine (SVM) model is insufficient. However, in a study conducted by Rachel Zhao et al., in which the authors used machine learning models based on clinical data to predict time to recurrence, the accuracy of the SVM model was the highest among the applied models, and the random forest (RF) model had the lowest accuracy (C-index 0.767, 0.771, and 0.57 for Cox proportional hazard (CPH), SVM, and RF models, respectively) [16]. This supports the appropriateness of using several algorithms to analyze the same data.

The implementation of an artificial intelligence (AI) algorithm able to predict recurrence-free time (PFS) with up to 92% accuracy in patients diagnosed with WHO 4 CNS gliomas creates new possibilities in clinical decision-making of these most aggressive brain tumors. One of the main challenges in treating gliomas is their heterogeneity, their ability to infiltrate surrounding brain structures, and, perhaps related to this, their tendency to recur [3]. These features make glioma CNS WHO 4 extremely difficult to treat. Even with a combination of surgical treatment, radiation therapy, and chemotherapy, most patients experience recurrence within a relatively short time. Therefore, a key aspect of improving treatment outcomes is the ability to predict recurrence early. Accurate diagnosis of PFS before treatment could directly influence the choice of treatment options, enhancing the potential for personalized treatment. In addition, it can be a way to find early so-called long-term survivors (LTSs) and extreme long-term survivors (ELTSs). In the glioma CNS WHO 4 patient population, LTSs represent 13% of patients and are characterized by survival of at least 2 years, while ELTSs represent <1% of patients and their survival time is >10 years [17,18]. Identifying this group as early as possible at the beginning of the diagnostic pathway would be extremely significant for clinicians and patients.

Our study has several limitations that should be noted. Firstly, the retrospective nature of the study and the small sample size limit the generalizability of our findings. Despite efforts to mitigate overfitting caused by high dimensionality through techniques such as dimension reduction and data augmentation, the prediction model still requires further validation with a larger dataset. Future research should focus on multicenter studies with larger sample sizes and prospective designs to confirm the model's broader applicability.

Secondly, the process of semi-automatic segmentation of the 2D tumor region of interest (ROI) may impact reproducibility and is a labor-intensive task. Adopting an automatic 3D tumor segmentation algorithm based on deep learning could significantly improve reproducibility and streamline the analysis process, making it more feasible for large-scale data applications.

Thirdly, our study did not incorporate multimodal MRI images, which could potentially enhance the performance and accuracy of the predictive model. Including various imaging modalities in future research could provide more comprehensive data and improve model outcomes.

Lastly, the biological relevance of the radiomic features used in our study is not yet fully understood. Further research is needed to elucidate the connections between radiomics data and tumor biology, which could enhance the interpretability and clinical utility of the predictive models.

5. Conclusions

The results of our study show that artificial intelligence models combined with radiomic features could be useful for predicting the progression-free survival of high-grade glioma patients. This could be beneficial for risk stratification of patients, enhancing the potential for personalized treatment plans and improving overall survival.

Supplementary Materials: The following supporting information can be downloaded at https://www.mdpi.com/article/10.3390/jcm13206172/s1, Supplementary S1. Self-evaluation using METhodological RadiomICs Score (METRICS).

Author Contributions: Conceptualization, J.W., A.K.-M., K.S., B.M. and M.B.; methodology, A.K.-M.; software, B.M. and A.K.-M.; validation, J.W. and K.S.; formal analysis, P.G.W. and A.K.-M.; investigation, A.K.-M.; resources, J.W. and K.S.; data curation, A.K.-M. and B.M.; writing—original draft preparation, A.K.-M.; writing—review and editing, J.W., B.M., P.G.W., K.S. and M.B.; visualization, A.K.-M.; supervision, J.W., B.M. and K.S.; project administration, J.W.; funding acquisition, J.W. All authors have read and agreed to the published version of the manuscript.

Funding: This research was funded by the Centre of Postgraduate Medical Education, grant number 50110283023/24.

Institutional Review Board Statement: The study was conducted in accordance with the Declaration of Helsinki. Ethical review and approval were waived for this study due to the fact that the identity of the human subjects cannot be ascertained directly or through identifiers linked to the subjects, the investigator did not contact the subjects, and the investigator will not re-identify subjects.

Informed Consent Statement: Patient consent was waived due to the retrospective nature of the study.

Data Availability Statement: The results published here are partly based on data generated by the TCGA Research Network: http://cancergenome.nih.gov/ (accessed on 10 January 2024).

Conflicts of Interest: The authors declare no conflicts of interest. The funders had no role in the design of the study; in the collection, analyses, or interpretation of data; in the writing of the manuscript; or in the decision to publish the results.

References

1. Ostrom, Q.T.; Gittleman, H.; Fulop, J.; Liu, M.; Blanda, R.; Kromer, C.; Wolinsky, Y.; Kruchko, C.; Barnholtz-Sloan, J.S. CBTRUS Statistical Report: Primary Brain and Central Nervous System Tumors Diagnosed in the United States in 2008–2012. *Neuro-Oncology* **2015**, *17* (Suppl. S4), iv1–iv62. [CrossRef] [PubMed]
2. Louis, D.N.; Perry, A.; Wesseling, P.; Brat, D.J.; Cree, I.A.; Figarella-Branger, D.; Hawkins, C.; Ng, H.K.; Pfister, S.M.; Reifenberger, G.; et al. The 2021 WHO Classification of Tumors of the Central Nervous System: A summary. *Neuro-Oncol.* **2021**, *23*, 1231–1251. [CrossRef] [PubMed]
3. Wen, P.Y.; Kesari, S. Malignant gliomas in adults. *N. Engl. J. Med.* **2008**, *359*, 492–507, Erratum in *New Engl. J. Med.* **2008**, *359*, 877. [CrossRef] [PubMed]
4. Stupp, R.; Dietrich, P.Y.; Kraljevic, S.O.; Pica, A.; Maillard, I.; Maeder, P.; Meuli, R.; Janzer, R.; Pizzolato, G.; Miralbell, R.; et al. Promising survival for patients with newly diagnosed glioblastoma multiforme treated with concomitant radiation plus temozolomide followed by adjuvant temozolomide. *J. Clin. Oncol.* **2002**, *20*, 1375–1382. [CrossRef] [PubMed]
5. Gilbert, M.R.; Wang, M.; Aldape, K.D.; Stupp, R.; Hegi, M.E.; Jaeckle, K.A.; Armstrong, T.S.; Wefel, J.S.; Won, M.; Blumenthal, D.T.; et al. Dose-dense temozolomide for newly diagnosed glioblastoma: A randomized phase III clinical trial. *J. Clin. Oncol.* **2013**, *31*, 4085–4091. [CrossRef] [PubMed]
6. Fisher, J.P.; Adamson, D.C. Current FDA-Approved Therapies for High-Grade Malignant Gliomas. *Biomedicines* **2021**, *9*, 324. [CrossRef] [PubMed]
7. Stupp, R.; Mason, W.P.; van den Bent, M.J.; Weller, M.; Fisher, B.; Taphoorn, M.J.B.; Belanger, K.; Brandes, A.A.; Marosi, C.; Bogdahn, U.; et al. Radiotherapy plus Concomitant and Adjuvant Temozolomide for Glioblastoma. *N. Engl. J. Med.* **2005**, *352*, 987–996. [CrossRef] [PubMed]

8. Liu, C.; Li, Y.; Xia, X.; Wang, J.; Hu, C. Application of radiomics feature captured from MRI for prediction of recurrence for glioma patients. *J. Cancer* **2022**, *13*, 965–974. [CrossRef]
9. He, A.; Wang, P.; Zhu, A.; Liu, Y.; Chen, J.; Liu, L. Predicting IDH Mutation Status in Low-Grade Gliomas Based on Optimal Radiomic Features Combined with Multi-Sequence Magnetic Resonance Imaging. *Diagnostics* **2022**, *12*, 2995. [CrossRef] [PubMed]
10. Lao, J.; Chen, Y.; Li, Z.C.; Li, Q.; Zhang, J.; Liu, J.; Zhai, G. A Deep Learning-Based Radiomics Model for Prediction of Survival in Glioblastoma Multiforme. *Sci. Rep.* **2017**, *7*, 10353. [CrossRef] [PubMed]
11. Kocak, B.; Akinci D'Antonoli, T.; Mercaldo, N.; Alberich-Bayarri, A.; Baessler, B.; Ambrosini, I.; Andreychenko, A.E.; Bakas, S.; Beets-Tan, R.G.H.; Bressem, K.; et al. METhodological RadiomICs Score (METRICS): A quality scoring tool for radiomics research endorsed by EuSoMII. *Insights Imaging* **2024**, *15*, 8. [CrossRef] [PubMed]
12. Clark, K.; Vendt, B.; Smith, K.; Freymann, J.; Kirby, J.; Koppel, P.; Moore, S.; Phillips, S.; Maffitt, D.; Pringle, M.; et al. The Cancer Imaging Archive (TCIA): Maintaining and Operating a Public Information Repository. *J. Digit. Imaging* **2013**, *26*, 1045–1057. [CrossRef] [PubMed]
13. Scarpace, L.; Mikkelsen, T.; Cha, S.; Rao, S.; Tekchandani, S.; Gutman, D.; Saltz, J.H.; Erickson, B.J.; Pedano, N.; Flanders, A.E.; et al. The Cancer Genome Atlas Glioblastoma Multiforme Collection (TCGA-GBM) (Version 5) [Data Set]. The Cancer Imaging Archive. 2016. Available online: https://www.cancerimagingarchive.net/collection/tcga-gbm/ (accessed on 10 January 2024).
14. Gerds, T.A.; Cai, T.; Schumacher, M. The performance of risk prediction models. *Biom. J.* **2008**, *50*, 457–479. [CrossRef] [PubMed]
15. High-Level Expert Group on Scientific Data (2010) Riding the Wave—How Europe Can Gain from the Rising Tide of Scientific Data. Final Report to the European Commission. pp. 1–40. Available online: https://www.researchgate.net/publication/255181186_Riding_the_wave_How_Europe_can_gain_from_the_rising_tide_of_scientific_data_Final_report_of_the_High_Level_Expert_Group_on_Scientific_Data_A_submission_to_the_European_Commission (accessed on 9 October 2024).
16. Zhao, R.; Zhuge, Y.; Camphausen, K.; Krauze, A.V. Machine learning based survival prediction in Glioma using large-scale registry data. *Health Inform. J.* **2022**, *28*, 14604582221135427. [CrossRef] [PubMed]
17. Gately, L.; McLachlan, S.A.; Philip, J.; Ruben, J.; Dowling, A. Long-term survivors of glioblastoma: A closer look. *J. Neurooncol.* **2018**, *136*, 155–162. [CrossRef] [PubMed]
18. Jovčevska, I. Genetic secrets of long-term glioblastoma survivors. *Bosn. J. Basic Med. Sci.* **2019**, *19*, 116–124. [CrossRef] [PubMed]

Journal of
Clinical Medicine

MDPI

Article

Prospective and External Validation of Machine Learning Models for Short- and Long-Term Mortality in Acutely Admitted Patients Using Blood Tests

Baker Nawfal Jawad [1,2,*], Izzet Altintas [1,2,3], Jesper Eugen-Olsen [1], Siar Niazi [4], Abdullah Mansouri [5], Line Jee Hartmann Rasmussen [1] Martin Schultz [6], Kasper Iversen [2,7,8], Nikolaj Normann Holm [1,9], Thomas Kallemose [1], Ove Andersen [1,2,3] and Jan O. Nehlin [1]

1 Department of Clinical Research, Copenhagen University Hospital Amager and Hvidovre, 2650 Hvidovre, Denmark; jan.nehlin@regionh.dk (J.O.N.)
2 Department of Clinical Medicine, University of Copenhagen, 2200 Copenhagen, Denmark
3 Emergency Department, Copenhagen University Hospital Amager and Hvidovre, 2650 Hvidovre, Denmark
4 Department of Cardiology, North Zealand Hospital, 3400 Hillerød, Denmark
5 Emergency Medical Services, Capital Region, 2750 Ballerup, Denmark
6 Department of Geriatrics, Copenhagen University Hospital Amager and Hvidovre, 2650 Hvidovre, Denmark
7 Department of Emergency Medicine, Copenhagen University Hospital Herlev and Gentofte, 2730 Herlev, Denmark
8 Department of Cardiology, Copenhagen University Hospital Herlev and Gentofte, 2730 Herlev, Denmark
9 Department of Applied Mathematics and Computer Science, Technical University of Denmark, 2800 Kongens Lyngby, Denmark
* Correspondence: baker.jawad@regionh.dk

Abstract: Background: Predicting mortality in emergency departments (EDs) using machine learning models presents challenges, particularly in balancing simplicity with performance. This study aims to develop models that are both simple and effective for predicting short- and long-term mortality in ED patients. Our approach uses a minimal set of variables derived from one single blood sample obtained at admission. **Methods**: Data from three cohorts at two large Danish university hospitals were analyzed, including one retrospective and two prospective cohorts where prognostic models were applied to predict individual mortality risk, spanning the years 2013–2022. Routine biochemistry analyzed in blood samples collected at admission was the primary data source for the prediction models. The outcomes were mortality at 10, 30, 90, and 365 days after admission to the ED. The models were developed using Light Gradient Boosting Machines. The evaluation of mortality predictions involved metrics such as Area Under the Receiver Operating Characteristic Curve (AUC), sensitivity, specificity, negative predictive values, positive predictive values, and Matthews correlation coefficient (MCC). **Results**: A total of 43,648 unique patients with 65,484 admissions were analyzed. The models showed high accuracy, with very good to excellent AUC values between 0.87 and 0.93 across different time intervals. **Conclusions**: This study demonstrates that a single assessment of routine clinical biochemistry upon admission can serve as a powerful predictor for both short-term and long-term mortality in ED admissions.

Keywords: machine learning models; mortality prediction; emergency department; clinical biochemistry; biomarkers; short-term mortality; long-term mortality; explainable artificial intelligence (XAI)

1. Introduction

Effectively identifying patients at low and high risk of adverse outcomes is crucial for optimal resource allocation and treatment prioritization in healthcare systems. With the global population aging [1], the demand on emergency departments (EDs) is expected to rise significantly [2,3]. Consequently, this underlies the urgent need for innovative, personalized care strategies to ensure efficient resource use and patient care. However, in advancing these novel strategies, finding a balance between simplicity and performance becomes critical. High-performance solutions often come with complexity that may limit their practicality in dynamic settings such as EDs. Addressing this challenge is critical to developing effective yet manageable tools that can adapt to the fast-paced nature of emergency care.

In clinical practice, predicting all-cause mortality and assessing risk have consistently been crucial outcomes for clinicians [4–9]. Various scores and indices based on simple linear relationships have been proposed and used to predict mortality; however, their accuracy is only moderate [4,8,10]. In recent years, the application of ML to healthcare data has surpassed these traditional methods, offering enhanced accuracy in predicting outcomes for various patient groups, including those with conditions such as cardiac disease [11], COVID-19 [12], trauma [13], sepsis [14], and those in intensive care units (ICUs) [15]. While ML algorithms offer significant advantages, their integration into clinical practice presents challenges, primarily due to the incorporation of numerous clinical and nonclinical variables. This complexity poses a challenge for clinicians in terms of comprehension and practical application within the fast-paced environment of Eds [16]. Despite advancements in ML for mortality prediction, significant research gaps persist: most models are either designed as triage tools for short-term outcomes or as risk assessment tools for long-term mortality, typically focusing on specific patient cohorts. Additionally, there is a lack of models that address both short- and long-term outcomes simultaneously across a diverse patient population, and few of these models are interpretable. The effectiveness of ML models in clinical settings is closely linked to their transparency and interpretability, highlighting the need for predictive and comprehensible models for clinicians.

Recent developments in deep learning, particularly Transformer-based models, have shown great promise in medical data [17,18]. However, based on the better interpretability [19,20] and superior performance demonstrated in our previous findings [21], we opted to use the LightGBM algorithm. In this study, we aimed to develop and externally validate an easily adaptable prognostic machine learning tool, the short- and long-term mortality models (SLTM), which are designed to predict both short-term and long-term mortality among patients acutely admitted to the ED. These models utilize a single blood sample for routine clinical biochemistry analysis, including biomarkers of vital organs and the immune system. We also aimed to incorporate explainable ML techniques to more clearly explain how the models use input variables to make predictions, thereby assisting clinicians in understanding the ML model's predicted outcomes.

2. Materials and Methods

2.1. Study Design and Settings

In this study, we evaluated data from three study cohorts. First, the retrospective 29K cohort study from the ED at the Copenhagen University Hospital Amager and Hvidovre (AHH), Denmark, was included. The 29K cohort included all patients admitted to the acute medical unit with an available blood sample. The 29K cohort consisted of 51,007 patient records from ED admissions between 18 November 2013 and 17 March 2017. The acute medical unit at the ED receives patients across all specialties, except for children (patients under 18 years), gastroenterological patients, and obstetric patients. Second, a prospective observational cohort, the TRIAGE Study, from the ED at North Zealand University Hospital (NZH), Hilleroed, Denmark, was included [22]. The TRIAGE cohort included all patients admitted to the ED with an available blood sample and consisted of 6383 patient records from ED admissions between 5 September 2013 and 6 December 2013 [22]. Children and obstetric patients were excluded. Third, a prospective observational cohort from the specialized COVID-19 Unit of the ED at AHH was included. This RESPOND-COVID cohort (Respiratory Emergency Surveillance and suPAR Outcome in COVID and Non-COVID Disease) included patients admitted with respiratory symptoms and suspected of having COVID-19. The RESPOND-COVID cohort consisted of 28,210 patient records from admissions between 10 March 2020 and 31 March 2022. The follow-up for vital status data was retrieved from the Central Public Server at Statistics Denmark and the Danish Civil Registration System, which record the status of all Danish residents. Identification was through the Central Personal Registry (CPR) number, unique to each citizen. During the study period, patients who left the country had their last admission data censored.

This study was reported in accordance with the transparent reporting of a multivariable prediction model for individual prognosis or diagnosis (TRIPOD) statement [23]. The research conducted in this study was in strict compliance with both regional and national guidelines and received the necessary approvals from the appropriate Danish authorities. The Danish Data Protection Agency (29K: HVH-2014-018, 02767; TRIAGE: J. 2007-58-0015) and the Danish Health and Medicines Authority (29K: 3-3013-1061/1; TRIAGE: 31-1522-102) approved the studies and analyses. Furthermore, the Legal Office at the Capital Region of Denmark, specifically the Team for patient medical records, issued a permit with reference numbers R-22041261 and R-20064514 for the usage and management of healthcare data within the region. The study adhered to all relevant ethical and legal standards required for research within Denmark.

2.2. Medical Records

Information regarding hospital admissions and discharges for the 29K cohort was extracted from the Danish National Patient Registry (NPR). In the RESPOND-COVID and TRIAGE cohorts, information related to patients' health conditions, vital signs, triage, events in-hospital requiring continued care at the ED, and duration of hospital stay was retrieved from the patient's health records in OPUS Arbejdsplads (version 2.5.0.0 Computer Sciences Corporation [CSC], Falls Church, VA, USA) and "Sundhedsplatformen" (Epic, version 2016, Verona, WI, USA). The TRIAGE study also involved the review of each patient record by two experts in internal or emergency medicine, who evaluated whether each admission was necessary or could have been avoided. An admission was deemed unnecessary only if both specialists agreed on this assessment. These reviewers were blinded to their own roles as either primary or secondary evaluators of each case and to the other reviewer's decisions. An unnecessary admission was defined as one where the patient's condition could have been adequately managed by a general practitioner or in an outpatient setting within 1–2 weeks. For all three cohorts, blood test results were obtained from the LABKA II national database [24]. Using each person's unique personal identification number from the Danish Civil Registration System, we linked the data, encompassing biochemistry, diagnoses, records of hospital admissions, readmissions, and mortality.

2.3. Biomarkers

For all three cohorts, blood samples were collected upon admission to the ED, and routine whole blood counts along with clinical biochemistry were analyzed by AHH's and NZH's respective Departments of Clinical Biochemistry. The results were extracted from the LABKA database. The admission blood tests included C-reactive protein (CRP), soluble urokinase plasminogen activator receptor (suPAR), alanine aminotransferase (ALAT), albumin (ALB), International Normalized Ratio (INR), coagulation factors 2, 7, 10 (KF2710), total bilirubin (BILI), alkaline phosphatase (ALP), creatinine, lactate dehydrogenase (LDH), blood urea nitrogen (BUN), potassium (K), sodium (NA), estimated glomerular filtration rate (eGFR), hemoglobin (HB), and counts of leukocytes, lymphocytes, neutrophils, monocytes, thrombocytes, eosinophils, and basophils. All procedures were executed following the appropriate guidelines and standards.

2.4. Outcomes

In this study, the outcomes were 10-, 30-, 90-, and 365-day mortality after admission at the ED. We define short-term mortality as death within 30 days, intermediate-term mortality as death within 90 days, and long-term mortality as death within 365 days.

2.5. Data Preparation

A standard format was applied to all data. Patient admissions with more than 50% of the data (routine clinical biochemistry results) missing were dropped. The median percentage of missing blood biochemistry results for each study was: 29K: 2.6%; TRIAGE: 3.0%; and RESPOND-COVID: 2.4%, with an overall interquartile range (IQR) ranging from 1.6% to 7.7%.

The 29K cohort was split into training and test sets. To avoid information leakage, as some patients were readmitted multiple times, we ensured that the same patient ID did not appear in both training and test sets. The TRIAGE and RESPOND-COVID datasets were exclusively used as test data.

To handle missing values, we employed iterative imputations from the Python scikit-learn package, version 1.5.2 [25]. This method was chosen due to its ability to impute missing values by modeling each feature as a function of the others iteratively, which can improve the accuracy of the imputation compared to simpler methods such as mean or median imputation. The imputation model used all available features as predictors to minimize data loss. Training and test sets were imputed separately to avoid data leakage. To validate the quality of our imputation process, we conducted a sensitivity analysis comparing models trained on imputed versus non-imputed data. The performance metrics showed minimal differences, suggesting that imputation did not significantly impact the result.

To handle class imbalance in our target outcome, we addressed imbalanced data by exploring several resampling methods, including random undersampling, random oversampling, and SMOTE. We ultimately chose random oversampling technique from the Imbalanced-Learn Package (Python), version 0.12.4 [26] during training. To reduce the impact of magnitude on the variance, we normalized the values of all variables in the data by the z score. This process was applied to the training data. For the test data, normalization was based on the mean and standard deviation estimated from the training data. To achieve a normal distribution approximation for our variables, we employed the Yeo-Johnson transformation [27] on the training data. For the test data, the transformation was based on the estimates derived from the training set. These preprocessing steps significantly enhanced the model's performance on the validation set.

2.6. Model Construction

All the models were crafted using Python (version 3.8.0). We employed the classification module from PyCaret (version 2.2.6) [28] to develop models using four distinct algorithms for predicting 10-, 30-, 90-, and 365-day mortality. PyCaret is a low-code machine learning library that streamlines the entire machine learning process.

For hyperparameter optimization, we used the tune_model() function within PyCaret. The tuning process was configured to perform 100 iterations, optimizing the models based on the AUC metric. We selected Bayesian optimization, a search approach that chooses hyperparameters by learning from previous evaluations to improve future selections, as the search algorithm, leveraging the scikit-optimize library. To enhance computational efficiency, early stopping was implemented using the Asynchronous Successive Halving Algorithm. This approach allows for the early termination of underperforming models during the hyperparameter search process. The parameter choose_better = True was specified to ensure that the best-performing model, according to the AUC metric, was selected.

2.7. Algorithm Selection and Performance Measures

Fifteen machine learning algorithms were trained and evaluated using PyCaret through 10-fold cross-validation (Random Forest (RF), SVM-Radial Kernel (RBFSVM), Extra Trees Classifier (ET), Extreme Gradient Boosting (XGBOOST), Decision Tree Classifier (DT), neural network (MLP), Light Gradient Boosting Machine (LIGHTBM), K Neighbors Classifier (KNN), Gradient Boosting Classifier (GBC), CatBoost Classifier (CATBOOST),

Ada Boost Classifier (ADA), Logistic Regression (LR), Linear Discriminant Analysis (LDA), Quadratic Discriminant Analysis (QDA), and Naive Bayes (NB)) [21].

These models were developed using fifteen biomarkers (ALAT, ALB, ALP, BUN, creatinine, CRP, eosinophils, KF2710, leukocytes, LDH, lymphocytes, neutrophils, platelets, sodium, and suPAR) from a single routine blood test, along with age and sex as additional variables. The feature selection was informed by previous work (Baker et al., 2014). However, in the TRIAGE cohort, mean corpuscular volume (MCV) and mean corpuscular hemoglobin concentration (MCHC) were not available. Therefore, based on the findings from Baker et al., 2024 [21], new models were trained using the top fifteen biomarkers, excluding MCV and MCHC.

The best machine learning algorithm (Light Gradient Boosting Machine [LIGHTGBM]) was fine-tuned and evaluated through a 10-fold cross-validation on the 29K cohort, then tested on an unseen test sample of the same cohort and on TRIAGE and RESPOND-COVID data. Model selection was based on the area under the receiver operating characteristic curve (AUC). Additionally, the sensitivity, specificity, positive predictive value (PPV), negative predictive value (NPV), and Matthew's correlation coefficient (MCC) for the complete data were estimated for the validation and test data and evaluated between them. To evaluate the reliability of our predictive model's performance, we used a bootstrap resampling technique to calculate confidence intervals (CIs) for key metrics, including AUC, sensitivity, specificity, PPV, NPV, and MCC. We performed 1000 bootstraping iterations.

2.8. Calibration

To improve our predictive model's ability to estimate probabilities that accurately reflect actual outcomes, we implemented probability calibration using isotonic regression from the scikit-learn package (version 1.4) in Python [25]. Calibration was performed on unseen test data to prevent overfitting and ensure unbiased adjustments to the predicted probabilities.

To evaluate the model's precision, we employed the Brier score as an accuracy metric, comparing its values before and after the calibration process. We observed that the Brier score improved after calibration, indicating that the calibrated model's probability estimates were more accurate.

As expected, the AUC remained stable after calibration for all outcomes, indicating that the model's ability to discriminate between classes did not change. However, when using the default threshold of 0.50, we observed notable shifts in sensitivity and specificity. Calibration impacted the probability estimates, leading to the default threshold no longer providing an optimal balance between sensitivity and specificity. To optimize the decision threshold for the best balance between sensitivity and specificity, we employed the Youden Index on the calibrated probabilities for all outcomes. This method empirically determines the optimal cutoff point post-calibration to achieve an optimal tradeoff between sensitivity and specificity.

2.9. Explaining Model Predictions

We used TreeExplainer, version 0.45.1 [29], a method based on the approximation of the set of trees to calculate the SHapley Additive exPlanations (SHAP) [30] values, to interpret our machine learning models' predictions, quantifying the impact of each variable on individual predictions. SHAP values were calculated using the SHAP library package in Python, which helped assess variable contributions in terms of magnitude and direction. To visualize these contributions, we employed waterfall plots. These plots illustrated the influence of individual variables on individual model predictions.

2.10. Statistical Analysis

Statistical analyses were performed using R (version 4.1.0) and Python (version 3.8.0). Categorical variables are presented as frequencies (N) and percentages (%), whereas continuous variables are represented by their median values and IQR. To evaluate the differences between datasets, we employed the Student's *t* test, setting our significance level at 5% for continuous variables and the chi-square test for categorical variables.

3. Results

3.1. Description of the Cohorts Used in the Study

In this study, we included a total of 65,484 admissions from the EDs of two different Danish hospitals, the Copenhagen University Hospital Amager and Hvidovre (AHH) and the North Zealand University Hospital (NZH). From AHH we included ED data from both retro and prospective cohorts: 29K (2013–2017) and RESPOND-COVID (2020–2022), respectively, in our analysis. From NZH, we included ED data from a prospective cohort, TRIAGE (2013). The hospital and patient characteristics are summarized in Table 1.

Table 1. Patient baseline characteristics and mortality rates.

Variable	Retrospective	Prospective	Prospective
Cohort	AHH (29K)	NZH (Triage)	AHH (RESPOND-COVID)
Year	2013–2017	2013	2020–2022
N of unique patients	28,671	6124	8451
N of admissions	48,841	6150	10,493
Demographics			
Age	65.6 (48.2–78.5)	63.0 (46.0–76.0)	66.0 (49.1–78.2)
Sex (female) [6]	52.3%	50.5%	51.2%
	Laboratory Biomarkers		
ALAT [1]	21.0 (15.0–33.0)	20.8 (14.8–31.5)	23.0 (16.0–35.0)
Albumin [2]	34.0 (30.0–37.0)	37.2 (33.5–39.8)	34.0 (30.0–37.0)
Alkaline Phosphatase [1]	75.6 (63.0–94.0)	84.2 (69.3–105.9)	79.0 (63.0–103.0)
Bilirubin [3]	7.0 (5.0–10.1)	7.9 (5.7–11.2)	8.0 (5.0–11.0)
BUN [4]	5.1 (3.8–7.2)	5.2 (4.0–7.1)	5.3 (3.9–7.7)
Creatinine [3]	77.0 (62.0–97.0)	71.0 (59.0–88.0)	77.0 (62.0–98.0)
CRP [5]	7.0 (2.0–39.0)	5.2 (2.9–23.2)	12.0 (2.6–54.0)
HB [4]	8.1 (7.2–8.9)	8.4 (7.6–9.0)	8.2 (7.3–9.0)
INR	1.0 (1.0–1.1)	1.0 (0.9–1.1)	1.0 (1.0–1.1)
Potassium [4]	3.9 (3.6–4.2)	4.0 (3.8–4.3)	3.9 (3.6–4.2)
KF2710	0.9 (0.8–1.0)	0.9 (0.8–1.1)	0.8 (0.7–0.9)
LDH [1]	186.0 (169.0–214.0)	182.6 (157.6–217.3)	214.0 (184.0–260.0)
Leukocytes [6]	8.7 (6.9–11.3)	8.2 (6.5–10.6)	8.7 (6.6–11.8)
Lymphocytes [6]	1.7 (1.1–2.3)	1.6 (1.2–2.0)	1.4 (0.9–2.1)
Monocytes [6]	0.7 (0.5–0.9)	0.6 (0.5–0.8)	0.7 (0.5–0.9)
Neutrophils [6]	5.8 (4.1–8.3)	5.7 (4.0–7.9)	6.0 (4.1–8.9)
suPAR (ng/mL)	3.3 (2.3–5.0)	4.5 (3.5–6.4)	4.1 (2.9–5.9)
Thrombocytes [6]	247.0 (201.0–302.0)	238.0 (196.0–288.0)	248.0 (196.0–310.0)
Eosinophils [6]	0.1 (0.0–0.2)	0.2 (0.1–0.4)	0.1 (0.0–0.2)
eGFR (mL/min)	80.0 (60.0–90.0)	86.3 (67.6–90.0)	77.0 (58.0–84.5)
Sodium [4]	139.0 (136.0–141.0)	139.0 (136.9–140.6)	138.0 (135.0–140.0)
Mortality Rates			
Mortality rate 10 days [6]	4.4% (1252)	2.9% (177)	4.0% (341)
Mortality rate 30 days [6]	8.2% (2338)	4.6% (284)	8.4% (712)
Mortality rate 90 days [6]	11.8% (3394)	7.8% (475)	12.4% (1052)
Mortality rate 1 year [6]	16.3% (4677)	11.9% (729)	18.5% (1560)

The results are expressed as median (IQR, interquartile range) for continuous variables. For categorical variables, the results are expressed as the number of participants (percentage). ALAT: alanine-aminotransferase; BUN: blood urea nitrogen; CRP: C-reactive protein; eGFR: estimated glomerular filtration rate; HB: hemoglobin; INR: prothrombin time and international normalized ratio; KF2710: coagulation factors 2, 7, 10; LDH: lactate dehydrogenase; suPAR: soluble urokinase plasminogen activator receptor. 29K: Emergency Department at the Copenhagen University Hospital Amager and Hvidovre (AHH), 2013–2017. TRIAGE: Emergency Department at North Zealand University Hospital (NZH), 2013. RESPOND-COVID: Emergency Department at AHH, 2020–2022. [1]: (U/L); [2]: (g/L); [3]: (μmol/L); [4]: (mmol/L); [5]: (mg/L); [6]: number in (%).

For the 29K dataset, there were 51,007 admissions at the ED of AHH involving 28,683 unique patients during the study period. After excluding 2166 patient records for missing data, the study cohort consisted of 48,841 admissions from 28,671 unique patients (Figure 1). The cohort was herof named 29K. Of these, 34,187 (70%) were allocated as training data, 7327 (15%) as validation data, and 7327 (15%) as internal test data. The median age of the 29K patients at admission was 65.6 years (IQR: 48.2–78.5), with 52.3% being female.

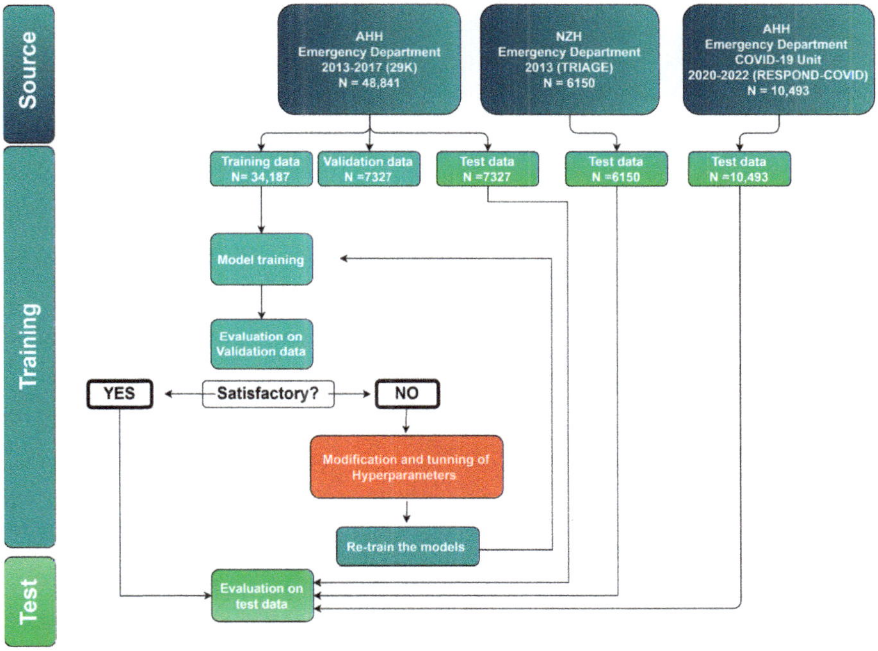

Figure 1. Flowchart of data training, validation, and testing using two ML algorithms. Patient medical records originated from three cohorts at two Danish hospitals: (1) 29K: Emergency Department at the Copenhagen University Hospital Amager and Hvidovre (AHH), 2013–2017, (2) TRIAGE: Emergency Department at North Zealand University Hospital (NZH), 2013, and (3) RESPOND-COVID: Emergency Department at AHH, 2020–2022. N = number of admissions.

The TRIAGE cohort from the NZH included 6383 admissions in the ED, involving 6356 unique patients. After excluding 233 patient records with missing data, the study cohort comprised 6150 admissions involving 6071 unique patients (Figure 1). All the TRIAGE data were used for external data validation. The median age of the TRIAGE patients at admission was 63.0 years (IQR: 46.0–76.0), with 50.6% being female.

The RESPOND-COVID cohort from AHH consisted of 28,210 patient records from 8853 unique patients; however, only 10,493 admissions from 8451 unique patients with a suPAR measurement were included. The median age of the RESPOND-COVID patients at admission was 66.0 years (IQR 49.1–78.2), with 51.2% being female.

Patients from the two AHH cohorts (29K and RESPOND-COVID) were slightly older ($p < 0.0001$), had a higher proportion of females ($p < 0.01$), and exhibited higher mortality rates ($p < 0.0001$), 4.0% and 4.4%, respectively, compared to patients from the NZH cohort, who had a mortality rate of 2.9% (Table 1). In general, the distributions of all the variables were significantly different among the three datasets. Patients excluded based on missing data from the 29K and TRIAGE datasets showed no significant differences compared to those included. However, in the RESPOND-COVID cohort, the excluded patients were predominantly older, mostly female, and had a lower mortality rate at 10 to 365 days.

3.2. Model Performance

Figure 2 illustrates the predictive performance of the LightGBM models, assessed by the AUC, for mortality predictions at 10, 30, 90, and 365 days. Additional performance metrics are detailed in Table 2. ROC curves for each time interval can be found in the Supplementary (Figures S1–S4). For the 29K test dataset, the LightGBM model demonstrated high predictive accuracy, exhibiting an AUC of 0.93 (95% CI: 0.92–0.94) for 10-day mortality predictions and an MCC of 0.30 (95% CI: 0.28–0.32). The model maintained high performance for 30-day mortality predictions with an AUC of 0.92 (95% CI: 0.90–0.92) and an MCC of 0.40 (95% CI: 0.38–0.42). For 90-day mortality, the AUC was 0.91 (95% CI: 0.90–0.92) alongside an MCC of 0.51 (95% CI: 0.49–0.53), and for 365-day mortality, the AUC was 0.91 (95% CI: 0.91–0.91), with an MCC of 0.53 (95% CI: 0.51–0.55).

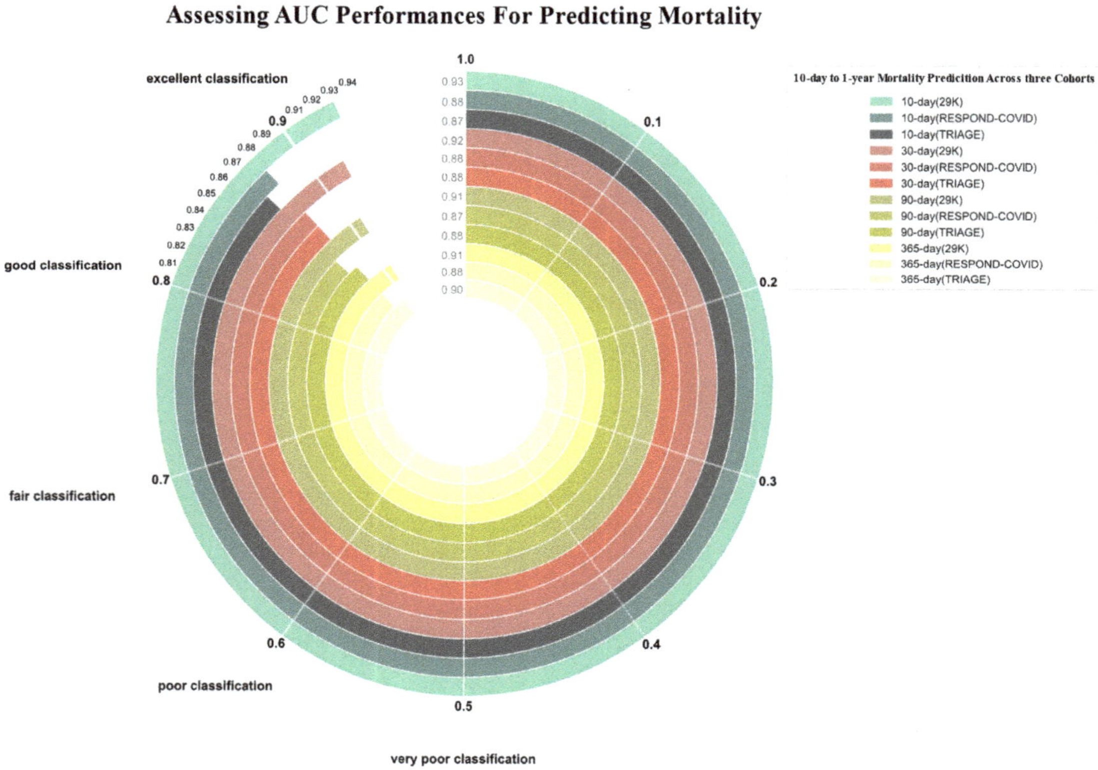

Figure 2. Area under the receiver operating characteristic curve (AUC). Performance for predicting 10-day (green shaded circles), 30-day (peach-shaded circles), 90-day (dark yellow shaded circles), and 365-day (light yellow shaded circles) mortality in each of the three cohorts, 29K, TRIAGE, and RESPOND-COVID, was examined.

Table 2. Results from test data for predicting short- and long-term mortality.

Test Data	N	AUC	Sensitivity	Specificity	PPV	NPV	MCC
10-day Mortality							
29K	7.327 (272)	0.93 (0.92–0.94)	0.90 (0.86–0.93)	0.82 (0.81–0.83)	0.12 (0.11–0.14)	1.0 (1.0–1.0)	0.30 (0.28–0.32)
RESPOND-COVID	10.493 (341)	0.88 (0.86–0.89)	0.88 (0.84–0.91)	0.70 (0.69–0.71)	0.09 (0.08–0.10)	0.99 (0.99–1.0)	0.22 (0.22–0.24)
TRIAGE	6.150 (177)	0.87 (0.85–0.89)	0.72 (0.65–0.79)	0.84 (0.84–0.85)	0.12 (0.10–0.14)	0.99 (0.99–0.99)	0.25 (0.22–0.29)
30-day mortality							
29K	7.327 (537)	0.92 (0.90–0.92)	0.89 (0.86–0.91)	0.83 (0.82–0.83)	0.23 (0.21–0.24)	0.99 (0.99–0.99)	0.40 (0.38–0.42)
RESPOND-COVID	10.493 (712)	0.88 (0.87–0.89)	0.89 (0.86–0.91)	0.68 (0.68–0.69)	0.18 (0.17–0.19)	0.99 (0.98–0.98)	0.32 (0.30–0.33)
TRIAGE	6.150 (284)	0.88 (0.86–0.90)	0.76 (0.71–0.81)	0.84 (0.83–0.85)	0.18 (0.16–0.21)	0.99 (0.98–0.99)	0.34 (0.30–0.37)
90-day Mortality							
29K	7.327 (982)	0.91 (0.90–0.92)	0.84 (0.82–0.86)	0.85 (0.84–0.86)	0.38 (0.36–0.40)	0.98 (0.98–0.98)	0.51 (0.49–0.53)
RESPOND-COVID	10.493 (1052)	0.87 (0.86–0.88)	0.84 (0.82–0.86)	0.73 (0.72–0.74)	0.28 (0.26–0.29)	0.97 (0.97–0.97)	0.38 (0.36–0.40)
TRIAGE	6.150 (475)	0.88 (0.86–0.90)	0.77 (0.73–0.81)	0.84 (0.83–0.85)	0.30 (0.27–0.32)	0.98 (0.97–0.98)	0.40 (0.37–0.43)
365-day mortality							
29K	7.327 (1812)	0.91 (0.91–0.91)	0.87 (0.86–0.88)	0.79 (0.79–0.79)	0.47 (0.46–0.48)	0.97 (0.96–0.97)	0.53 (0.51–0.55)
RESPOND-COVID	10.493 (1569)	0.88 (0.86–0.90)	0.85 (0.83–0.87)	0.78 (0.77–0.79)	0.45 (0.44–0.47)	0.96 (0.96–0.97)	0.43 (0.42–0.45)
TRIAGE	6.150 (729)	0.90 (0.89–0.91)	0.87 (0.84–0.89)	0.75 (0.74–0.76)	0.32 (0.30–0.34)	0.98 (0.97–0.98)	0.43 (0.41–0.45)

N denotes the total number of admissions in the RESPOND-COVID and TRIAGE cohorts and the number of test admissions in the 29K cohort, with the number in parentheses indicating the number of deaths. The results are based on the calibrated models and are presented as the means with 95% confidence intervals. AUC: area under the receiver operating curve based on test data. PPV: positive predictive value; NPV: negative predictive value; MCC: Matthews correlation coefficient.

In the RESPOND-COVID dataset, the AUCs were 0.88 (95% CI: 0.86–0.89) for the 10-day mortality prediction, 0.88 (95% CI: 0.87–0.89) for the 30-day mortality prediction, 0.87 (95% CI: 0.86–0.88) for the 90-day mortality prediction, and 0.88 (95% CI: 0.86–0.90) for the 365-day mortality prediction. The MCC values corresponded to 0.22 (95% CI: 0.20–0.24), 0.32 (95% CI: 0.30–0.33), 0.38 (95% CI: 0.36–0.40), and 0.43 (95% CI: 0.41–0.45), respectively. Lastly, for the TRIAGE dataset, the AUCs were 0.87 (95% CI: 0.85–0.89) for 10-day mortality, 0.88 (95% CI: 0.86–0.90) for 30-day, 0.88 (95% CI: 0.86–0.90) for 90-day, and 0.90 (95% CI: 0.89–0.91) for 365-day mortality. The MCCs were 0.25 (95% CI: 0.23–0.27), 0.34 (95% CI: 0.32–0.36), 0.40 (95% CI: 0.38–0.42), and 0.43 (95% CI: 0.41–0.45), respectively.

The calibrated LightGBM models, showed varying levels of sensitivity and specificity across the datasets for mortality prediction intervals (Table 2). In the 29K dataset, the sensitivity for predicting mortality ranged from 84–90%, while the specificity was between 79–83%. Within the RESPOND-COVID dataset, the model sensitivity was between 84–88%, with a specificity ranging from 70–78%. For the TRIAGE dataset, the sensitivity varied from 72–87%, and the specificity showed a narrow range of 75–84%.

3.3. Machine Learning Prediction Application

From our prospective cohort dataset TRIAGE at NZH, upon which we tested the prediction model, we analyzed a case of an elderly male patient with a history of cardiovascular and neurological conditions (Figure 3a). This patient was brought to the ED with symptoms suggesting an infection in the respiratory system. Upon arrival, the patient was categorized as having moderate urgency based on the triage (Early Warning Score).

Laboratory tests revealed elevated levels of inflammatory markers, indicating a bacterial infection. The patient was treated with standard outpatient antibiotics and discharged the same day. Unfortunately, the patient's condition deteriorated, leading to the patient's passing a few days later. The short-term mortality model, predicting 10-day mortality, estimated a high mortality risk of 97.5% for this patient.

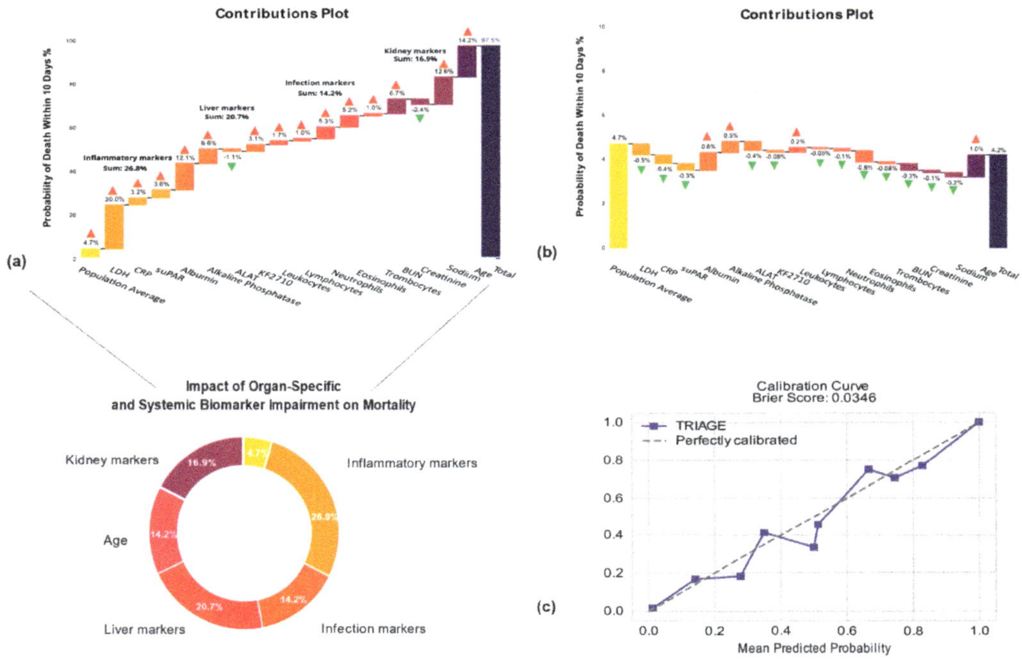

Figure 3. The Light Gradient Boosting Machine (LIGHTBM) model's individualized predictions of 10-day mortality risk for two specific patient cases in the prospective TRIAGE cohort. In this analysis, we utilized explainable artificial intelligence (XAI) techniques, particularly those using estimated SHAP values, to analyze the LGBM model's predictions of 10-day mortality risk for two specific patient cases within the TRIAGE cohort. These plots were based on the calibrated model (**a**). Case 1: a notable case of an elderly male patient who was admitted to the Emergency Department at North Zealand Hospital. *X*-axis: Displays the percentage contribution of biomarkers taken at the ED to the prediction of mortality risk. Below, these biomarkers are categorized by function: inflammatory, infection-related, liver, and kidney markers. (**b**) Case 2: This case involves an elderly female patient who presented at an Emergency Department in TRIAGE with a suspected infection. The model estimated a relatively low 10-day mortality risk of 4.2% for her. In case 1 and 2 variable sex is not shown (value 0.002) (**c**). Calibration plots on the TRIAGE cohort. *X*-axis: Mean Predicted Probability; *Y*-axis: Observed Frequency. The diagonal dash line stretching from the bottom left to the top right represents perfect agreement between the predicted probabilities and actual outcomes. The blue line is the model´s predicted probabilities and actual outcomes.

The contribution plot created using explainable artificial intelligence (XAI), depicted in Figure 3a, provides insights into how the patients impaired organ-specific biomarkers contributed to the model's overall output of mortality risk. In this case, the most important contributors to mortality risk prediction were identified as markers of the inflammatory response to the infection (27%), markers of the immune system (14%), markers of liver function (21%), and kidney function (17%). These insights shed light on the specific factors driving the elevated risk for this patient. With this knowledge, this patient should have been hospitalized. Subsequent independent reviews by two specialists suggested that a hospital admission might have been necessary for this patient.

Moving to a different scenario, in another case, we examined an elderly female patient with a history of cardiovascular conditions and metabolic disease, presenting also with symptoms indicative of an infection in the respiratory system (Figure 3b). The patient was categorized as urgent upon triage. Laboratory tests indicated signs of infection, with elevated inflammatory markers and abnormal blood cell counts. Other notable laboratory results included imbalances in electrolytes and liver enzymes. Despite these findings, the LGBM model, analyzed through XAI, predicted a lower 10-day mortality risk of only 4.3%. The patient was hospitalized and treated with IV antibiotics for three days. However, subsequent reviews by specialists suggested that hospital admission might have been unnecessary.

4. Discussion

In this study, we utilized routine clinical biochemistry data from a single time point upon admission, representing vital organ and immune system function, to predict mortality risk in acutely admitted patients. By incorporating explainable ML methods, we ensured that the model's outputs could be interpreted, thereby aiding clinicians in understanding the predicted ML outcomes. Our results for both short- and long-term mortality models demonstrated very good to excellent performance metrics, achieving high AUC values ranging from 0.87 to 0.93. Although a small decline in AUC values in the TRIAGE and RESPOND-COVID datasets was observed compared to the 29K dataset, this was anticipated due to significant differences in patient characteristics and mortality rates across cohorts. Performance metrics, especially AUC and MCC, showed overlapping confidence intervals for the RESPOND-COVID and TRIAGE datasets. This overlap indicates that the models performed similarly across these datasets. Nonetheless, we observed variability in the models' sensitivity and specificity across the different cohorts.

Overall, the models demonstrated low PPVs ranging from 9% to 47%, indicating a large proportion of false positives, while showing very high NPVs ranging from 96% to 100%. A trend toward increases in PPV and MCC values was observed from short-term to long-term mortality prediction, indicating a higher probability to predict the outcome over the length of time. The low PPV in short-term mortality prediction could be attributed to the low mortality prevalence in the studied patient populations. Additionally, it is possible that the model identifies patients (false positive) as being at high risk of mortality, but upon readmission and/or subsequent treatment after their initial discharge, these patients survive. As regards the high NPV, the results should be interpreted considering the dataset's overall low mortality rate, or conversely, its high survival rate.

In clinical practice, screening tools that offer high sensitivity and high NPV are preferred and well justified [31,32], as these tools align with clinicians' needs for safely excluding individuals at low risk of adverse outcomes in the future. This approach is preferred due to the low pretest probability, and the goal of the diagnostic test will be "ruling out" the condition, emphasizing high sensitivity where a negative result effectively excludes the condition. This is in contrast with diagnostic tools, where a high pretest probability of a condition leads to the goal of "ruling-in" the condition, emphasizing high specificity and PPV, as a positive result effectively confirms the condition. Our ML models embody this clinical principle, providing reliable decision support that matches the preferences of healthcare practitioners. This alignment with clinical practices not only supports the utility of the models but also sets a foundation for their potential development and application in healthcare settings.

Comparing our models with existing ML models, in terms of short-term mortality prediction, our models achieved an AUC of 0.87 to 0.93 for 10-day mortality predictions across the studied cohorts. This performance, when compared to other promising models, seems to be either on par or clearly superior, as explained below. Nevertheless, it is crucial to acknowledge that comparing results from data across diverse populations can be complex, given the multifaceted nature of socioeconomic, health factors, and other variables. Furthermore, mortality rates can be different in each population. Despite these complexities, when reviewing the literature, we find notable results. For instance, Trentino et al. conducted a study analyzing data from three adult tertiary care hospitals in Australia [33]. This study achieved a remarkable AUC of 0.93 for predicting in-hospital mortality among all admitted patients, regardless of whether their cases were medical or surgical. The predictive model used in this study incorporated various variables, including demographics, diagnosis codes, administrative information, and the Charlson comorbidity index. Similarly, an ED triage tool, the Score for Emergency Risk Prediction (SERP), to predict mortality within 2 to 30 days for ED patients was initially applied in a cohort from a Singaporean ED and subsequently underwent external validation in a South Korean ED [34,35]. These studies demonstrated AUCs of 0.81–0.82 for in-hospital mortality and 0.80–0.82 for 30-day mortality prediction. The SERP scores incorporate variables, including age, vital signs, and comorbidities. Additionally, in a study conducted on hospitalized patients in the U.S. by Brajer et al., reported an AUCs between 0.86 and 0.89 based on 57 electronic health record data variables [36]. In contrast, our models performed competitively, achieving comparable or superior results for short-term mortality prediction using just 15 biomarkers measured from a single routine blood sample collected upon arrival in the ED. For 30-day mortality, our models consistently maintained high AUCs (0.88–0.92) in both the internal and external evaluations. Likewise, the long-term mortality models showed near-excellent performance, with AUCs ranging from 0.87 to 0.91 for 90-day mortality prediction and 0.88 to 0.91 for 365-day mortality prediction. The performance of this model is either superior or comparable to similar studies in the field.

The random forest models developed by Sahni et al. achieved an AUC of 0.86 for 1-year mortality prediction [37]. Their model incorporated various variables, including demographic, physiological, biochemical factors, and comorbidities. Similarly, Woodman et al. developed a ML model trained on a patient cohort aged > 65 years. Their model achieved an AUC of 0.76 and incorporated variables including demographic, BMI, anticholinergic risk score, biochemical markers, and a comprehensive geriatric assessment.

In this study, we have adopted a streamlined biomarker approach that aligns with the latest recommendations for AI deployment in healthcare settings, prioritizing consistency and reduced error susceptibility [38]. This approach, which is centered on a single blood sample routinely analyzed for a select set of standard vital organ and immune system biomarkers, presents significant advantages. Unlike existing tools that primarily focus on triage, our models extend their utility to encompass resource allocation, treatment planning, discharge, and potentially preventing overtreatment and ensuring that care aligns with the patient's preferences and recovery potential. Specifically, it provides a stable and chronic disease-oriented perspective, which is crucial for uncovering underlying pathologies that might not be apparent with other data types.

In stark contrast to other models that depend on various inputs—such as continuous vital sign monitoring, administrative variables, medical history, comorbidities, and medication profiles—our model's simplicity integrates more fluidly into clinical workflows and mitigates the 'black box' nature that often accompanies complex AI systems, where the intricacy of ML models and the use of non-clinical features can make it challenging to understand the rationale behind the model output. Our methodology, with its deliberately limited parameters, enhances the models' output transparency and interpretability, thereby building confidence and trust among clinicians in AI-assisted decision-making.

4.1. Limitations

The exclusion of specific patient groups from the cohorts, including children and obstetric patients, limits the trained model applicability of our models to these populations. Furthermore, the retrospective design of our cohort introduces inherent limitations, such as the potential for selection and information biases. These biases can impact the validity of our findings and their applicability to broader, more diverse populations. There are also several limitations to the SHAP values. SHAP values are used for interpreting predictions of ML models, specifically by quantifying the contribution of each feature to a particular prediction. However, they do not provide causal insights. This means that while SHAP values can tell us which variables were important in the model's decision-making process, they do not imply a cause-and-effect relationship between these variables and the prediction. Lastly, the models were primarily validated within the same geographical region and governing clinical jurisdiction. While they were evaluated across different cohorts, this regional focus might constrain the generalizability of our findings.

4.2. Future Research

The present models are only meant as a proof-of-concept study. Refining and validating these models with diverse datasets remains a priority. We also plan to perform further generalizability testing on external datasets from other countries and outpatient populations in future research to ensure applicability across different geographical regions and demographics. Future research should similarly focus on enhancing the PPV and incorporating more comprehensive patient data before implementation in clinical practice.

5. Conclusions

In this study, we have successfully developed and externally validated machine learning models that predict both short-term and long-term mortality in acutely admitted patients based on a single set of routine blood tests. With AUC scores ranging from 0.87 to 0.93, we have demonstrated that a simplified approach can achieve sufficient high predictive accuracy, with the potential to warrant investigation into its applicability as an additional tool in clinical decision-making.

Supplementary Materials: The following supporting information can be downloaded at: https://www.mdpi.com/article/10.3390/jcm13216437/s1. Supplementary Figure S1: ROC curve for 10-day mortality; Figure S2: ROC curve for 30-day mortality; Supplementary Figure S3: ROC curve for 90-day mortality; Supplementary Figure S4: ROC curve for 365-day mortality.

Author Contributions: B.N.J., J.O.N. and O.A. were responsible for the research idea. T.K., O.A., L.J.H.R., J.E.-O., K.I. and M.S. were responsible for the study design. B.N.J., S.N., and T.K. were responsible for the statistical analysis and algorithm training and evaluation. B.N.J., I.A., A.M., T.K., A.M., S.N., N.N.H. and J.O.N. were responsible for the interpretation of the results. All the authors contributed important intellectual content during the manuscript drafting or revision, accepted personal accountability for their own contributions, and agreed to ensure that questions pertaining to the accuracy or integrity of any portion of the work were appropriately investigated and resolved. All authors have read and agreed to the published version of the manuscript.

Funding: This research received no external funding.

Institutional Review Board Statement: The study was conducted in accordance with the Declaration of Helsinki, and the protocol was approved by the Danish Data Protection Agency (29K: HVH-2014-018, 02767; TRIAGE: J. 2007-58-0015), and the Danish Health and Medicines Authority (29K: 3-3013-1061/1; TRIAGE: 31-1522-102) approved the studies and analyses. Furthermore, the Legal Office at the Capital Region of Denmark, specifically the Team for patient medical records, issued a permit with reference numbers R-22041261 and R-20064514 for the usage and management of healthcare data within the region. The study adhered to all relevant ethical and legal standards required for research within Denmark.

Informed Consent Statement: Informed consent was not deemed necessary.

Data Availability Statement: The datasets analyzed during the current study are not publicly available due to privacy considerations (data use agreements) and ethical restrictions. However, they can be made available from the corresponding author upon reasonable request and after obtaining the necessary approvals from the relevant authorities. The underlying code for this study, as well as the training and validation datasets, is not publicly available for proprietary reasons. However, qualified researchers may request access from the corresponding author, and they can be provided upon reasonable request.

Acknowledgments: The authors thank the Department of Clinical Biochemistry at Amager and Hvidovre Hospital and at North Zealand University Hospital for all analyses used in this study. We thank the contribution from Anders Stockmarr for valuable input.

Conflicts of Interest: J.E.O. is a cofounder, shareholder, and Chief Scientific Officer of ViroGates A/S. J.E.O., and O.A. are named inventors on patents covering suPAR owned by Copenhagen University Hospital Amager and Hvidovre, Hvidovre, Denmark and licensed to ViroGates A/S. All remaining authors declare no financial or non-financial competing interests.

References

1. ONU. *World Population, Ageing*; ST/ESA/SER.A/390; Department of Economic and Social Affairs, Population Division: New York, NY, USA, 2015.
2. Veser, A.; Sieber, F.; Groß, S.; Prückner, S. The demographic impact on the demand for emergency medical services in the urban and rural regions of bavaria, 2012–2032. *J. Public Health* **2015**, *23*, 181–188. [CrossRef] [PubMed]
3. Businger, A.P.; Kaderli, R.; Burghardt, L.R.; Osinga, R.; Liesch, M.; Furrer, M. Demographic Changes and Their Implications in a Nonacademic Emergency Department in Switzerland: An 11-Year Trend Analysis (2000–2010) of 104,510 Patients. *ISRN Emerg. Med.* **2012**, *2012*, 1–6. [CrossRef]
4. Lemeshow, S.; Gehlbach, S.H.; Klar, J.; Avrunin, J.S.; Teres, D.; Rapoport, J. Mortality Probability Models (MPM II) Based on an International Cohort of Intensive Care Unit Patients. *JAMA J. Am. Med. Assoc.* **1993**, *270*, 2478–2486. [CrossRef]
5. Toma, T.; Abu-Hanna, A.; Bosman, R.J. Discovery and inclusion of SOFA score episodes in mortality prediction. *J. Biomed. Inform.* **2007**, *40*, 649–660. [CrossRef]
6. Burch, V.C.; Tarr, G.; Morroni, C. Modified early warning score predicts the need for hospital admission and inhospital mortality. *Emerg. Med. J.* **2008**, *25*, 674–678. [CrossRef] [PubMed]
7. HKlausen, H.H.; Petersen, J.; Bandholm, T.; Juul-Larsen, H.G.; Tavenier, J.; Eugen-Olsen, J.; Andersen, O. Association between routine laboratory tests and long-term mortality among acutely admitted older medical patients: A cohort study. *BMC Geriatr.* **2017**, *17*, 62. [CrossRef]
8. Phungoen, P.; Khemtong, S.; Apiratwarakul, K.; Ienghong, K.; Kotruchin, P. Emergency Severity Index as a predictor of in-hospital mortality in suspected sepsis patients in the emergency department. *Am. J. Emerg. Med.* **2020**, *38*, 1854–1859. [CrossRef]
9. Mahmoodpoor, A.; Sanaie, S.; Saghaleini, S.H.; Ostadi, Z.; Hosseini, M.-S.; Sheshgelani, N.; Vahedian-Azimi, A.; Samim, A.; Rahimi-Bashar, F. Prognostic value of National Early Warning Score and Modified Early Warning Score on intensive care unit readmission and mortality: A prospective observational study. *Front. Med.* **2022**, *9*, 938005. [CrossRef] [PubMed]
10. Knaus, W.A. APACHE 1978-2001: The development of a quality assurance system based on prognosis: Milestones and personal reflections. *Arch. Surg.* **2002**, *137*, 37–41. [CrossRef]
11. Sherazi, S.W.A.; Jeong, Y.J.; Jae, M.H.; Bae, J.-W.; Lee, J.Y. A machine learning-based 1-year mortality prediction model after hospital discharge for clinical patients with acute coronary syndrome. *Health Inform. J.* **2020**, *26*, 1289–1304. [CrossRef]
12. Yadaw, A.S.; Li, Y.-C.; Bose, S.; Iyengar, R.; Bunyavanich, S.; Pandey, G. Clinical features of COVID-19 mortality: Development and validation of a clinical prediction model. *Lancet Digit. Health* **2020**, *2*, e516–e525. [CrossRef] [PubMed]
13. Bonde, A.; Bonde, M.; Troelsen, A.; Sillesen, M. Assessing the utility of a sliding-windows deep neural network approach for risk prediction of trauma patients. *Sci. Rep.* **2023**, *13*, 5176. [CrossRef] [PubMed]
14. Kijpaisalratana, N.; Sanglertsinlapachai, D.; Techaratsami, S.; Musikatavorn, K.; Saoraya, J. Machine learning algorithms for early sepsis detection in the emergency department: A retrospective study. *Int. J. Med. Inform.* **2022**, *160*, 104689. [CrossRef]
15. HThorsen-Meyer, H.-C.; Nielsen, A.B.; Kaas-Hansen, B.S.; Toft, P.; Schierbeck, J.; Strøm, T.; Chmura, P.J.; Heimann, M.; Dybdahl, L.; Spangsege, L.; et al. Dynamic and explainable machine learning prediction of mortality in patients in the intensive care unit: A retrospective study of high-frequency data in electronic patient records. *Lancet Digit. Health* **2020**, *2*, e179–e191. [CrossRef]
16. Kirk, J.W.; Nilsen, P. Implementing evidence-based practices in an emergency department: Contradictions exposed when prioritising a flow culture. *J. Clin. Nurs.* **2016**, *25*, 555–565. [CrossRef] [PubMed]
17. Huang, P.; Li, C.; He, P.; Xiao, H.; Ping, Y.; Feng, P.; Tian, S.; Chen, H.; Mercaldo, F.; Santone, A.; et al. MamlFormer: Priori-experience guiding transformer network via manifold adversarial multi-modal learning for laryngeal histopathological grading. *Inf. Fusion* **2024**, *108*, 102333. [CrossRef]
18. Huang, P.; Xiao, H.; He, P.; Li, C.; Guo, X.; Tian, S.; Feng, P.; Chen, H.; Sun, Y.; Mercaldo, F.; et al. LA-ViT: A Network With Transformers Constrained by Learned-Parameter-Free Attention for Interpretable Grading in a New Laryngeal Histopathology Image Dataset. *IEEE J. Biomed. Health Inform.* **2024**, *28*, 3557–3570. [CrossRef]
19. Singh, P.; Chahat, R.K.; Kr, S.; Anup, M.; Yadav, L.; Singla, S. Comparative Analysis of Tree-Based Models and Deep Learning Architectures for Tabular Data: Performance Disparities and Underlying Factors. In Proceedings of the 2023 International Conference on Advanced Computing & Communication Technologies (ICACCTech), Banur, India, 23–24 December 2023; pp. 224–231. Available online: https://api.semanticscholar.org/CorpusID:268045915 (accessed on 28 August 2024).
20. Frasca, M.; La Torre, D.; Pravettoni, G.; Cutica, I. Explainable and interpretable artificial intelligence in medicine: A systematic bibliometric review. *Discov. Artif. Intell.* **2024**, *4*, 15. [CrossRef]

21. Jawad, B.N.; Shaker, S.M.; Altintas, I.; Eugen-Olsen, J.; Nehlin, J.O.; Andersen, O.; Kallemose, T. Development and validation of prognostic machine learning models for short- and long-term mortality among acutely admitted patients based on blood tests. *Sci. Rep.* **2024**, *14*, 5942. [CrossRef]
22. Plesner, L.L.; Iversen, A.K.S.; Langkjær, S.; Nielsen, T.L.; Østervig, R.; Warming, P.E.; Salam, I.A.; Kristensen, M.; Schou, M.; Eugen-Olsen, J.; et al. The formation and design of the TRIAGE study—Baseline data on 6005 consecutive patients admitted to hospital from the emergency department. *Scand. J. Trauma. Resusc. Emerg. Med.* **2015**, *23*, 106. [CrossRef]
23. Collins, G.S.; Reitsma, J.B.; Altman, D.G.; Moons, K.G.M. Transparent reporting of a multivariable prediction model for individual prognosis or diagnosis (TRIPOD): The TRIPOD Statement. *Eur. Urol.* **2015**, *67*, 1142–1151. [CrossRef] [PubMed]
24. Arendt, J.F.H.; Hansen, A.T.; Ladefoged, S.A.; Sørensen, H.T.; Pedersen, L.; Adelborg, K. Existing data sources in clinical epidemiology: Laboratory information system databases in Denmark. *Clin. Epidemiol.* **2020**, *12*, 469–475. [CrossRef] [PubMed]
25. Pedregosa, F.; Varoquaux, G.; Gramfort, A.; Michel, V.; Thirion, B.; Grisel, O.; Blondel, M.; Prettenhofer, P.; Weiss, R.; Dubourg, V.; et al. Scikit-learn: Machine learning in Python. *J. Mach. Learn. Res.* **2011**, *12*, 2825–2830.
26. Lemaître, G.; Nogueira, F.; Aridas, C.K. Imbalanced-learn: A python toolbox to tackle the curse of imbalanced datasets in machine learning. *J. Mach. Learn. Res.* **2017**, *18*, 1–5.
27. Yeo, I.; Johnson, R.A. A new family of power transformations to improve normality or symmetry. *Biometrika* **2000**, *87*, 954–959. [CrossRef]
28. Moez, A. PyCaret: An Open Source, Low-Code Machine Learning Library in Python. 2020. Available online: https://www.pycaret.org (accessed on 8 March 2023).
29. Lundberg, S.M.; Erion, G.; Chen, H.; DeGrave, A.; Prutkin, J.M.; Nair, B.; Katz, R.; Himmelfarb, J.; Bansal, N.; Lee, S.-I. From local explanations to global understanding with explainable AI for trees. *Nat. Mach. Intell.* **2020**, *2*, 56–67. [CrossRef]
30. Lundberg, S.M.; Lee, S.-I. A Unified Approach to Interpreting Model Predictions. In Proceedings of the 31st International Conference on Neural Information Processing Systems, Long Beach, CA, USA, 4–9 December 2017; pp. 4768–4777.
31. Bartol, T. Thoughtful use of diagnostic testing: Making practical sense of sensitivity, specificity, and predictive value. *Nurse Pract.* **2015**, *40*, 10–12. [CrossRef]
32. Galvin, R.; Gilleit, Y.; Wallace, E.; Cousins, G.; Bolmer, M.; Rainer, T.; Smith, S.M.; Fahey, T. Adverse outcomes in older adults attending emergency departments: A systematic review and meta-analysis of the Identification of Seniors At Risk (ISAR) screening tool. *Age Ageing* **2017**, *46*, 179–186. [CrossRef]
33. Trentino, K.M.; Schwarzbauer, K.M.; Mitterecker, A.M.; Hofmann, A.D.R.M.; Lloyd, A.M.; Leahy, M.F.M.; Tschoellitsch, T.; Böck, C.M.; Hochreiter, S.; Meier, J. Machine Learning-Based Mortality Prediction of Patients at Risk During Hospital Admission. *J. Patient Saf.* **2022**, *18*, 494–498. [CrossRef]
34. Xie, F.; Ong, M.E.H.; Liew, J.N.M.H.; Tan, K.B.K.; Ho, A.F.W.; Nadarajan, G.D.; Low, L.L.; Kwan, Y.H.; Goldstein, B.A.; Matchar, D.B.; et al. Development and Assessment of an Interpretable Machine Learning Triage Tool for Estimating Mortality after Emergency Admissions. *JAMA Netw. Open* **2021**, *4*, e2118467. [CrossRef]
35. Yu, J.Y.; Xie, F.; Nan, L.; Yoon, S.; Ong, M.E.H.; Ng, Y.Y.; Cha, W.C. An external validation study of the Score for Emergency Risk Prediction (SERP), an interpretable machine learning-based triage score for the emergency department. *Sci. Rep.* **2022**, *12*, 1–8. [CrossRef] [PubMed]
36. Brajer, N.; Cozzi, B.; Gao, M.; Nichols, M.; Revoir, M.; Balu, S.; Futoma, J.; Bae, J.; Setji, N.; Hernandez, A.; et al. Prospective and External Evaluation of a Machine Learning Model to Predict In-Hospital Mortality of Adults at Time of Admission. *JAMA Netw. Open* **2020**, *3*, e1920733. [CrossRef] [PubMed]
37. Sahni, N.; Simon, G.; Arora, R. Development and Validation of Machine Learning Models for Prediction of 1-Year Mortality Utilizing Electronic Medical Record Data Available at the End of Hospitalization in Multicondition Patients: A Proof-of-Concept Study. *J. Gen. Intern. Med.* **2018**, *33*, 921–928. [CrossRef] [PubMed]
38. Kristiansen, T.B.; Kristensen, K.; Uffelmann, J.; Brandslund, I. Erroneous data: The Achilles' heel of AI and personalized medicine. *Front. Digit. Health* **2022**, *4*, 862095. [CrossRef]

bioengineering

MDPI

Article

Pediatric Intensive Care Unit Length of Stay Prediction by Machine Learning

Hammad A. Ganatra [1,*], Samir Q. Latifi [1,2] and Orkun Baloglu [1,2]

[1] Division of Pediatric Critical Care, Cleveland Clinic Children's, Cleveland, OH 44195, USA; latifis@ccf.org (S.Q.L.); baloglo@ccf.org (O.B.)
[2] Division of Cardiology and Cardiovascular Medicine, Cleveland Clinic Children's, Cleveland, OH 44195, USA
* Correspondence: ganatrh@ccf.org

Abstract: Purpose: To develop and validate machine learning models for predicting the length of stay (LOS) in the Pediatric Intensive Care Unit (PICU) using data from the Virtual Pediatric Systems (VPS) database. **Methods**: A retrospective study was conducted utilizing machine learning (ML) algorithms to analyze and predict PICU LOS based on historical patient data from the VPS database. The study included data from over 100 North American PICUs spanning the years 2015–2020. After excluding entries with missing variables and those indicating recovery from cardiac surgery, the dataset comprised 123,354 patient encounters. Various ML models, including Support Vector Machine, Stochastic Gradient Descent Classifier, K-Nearest Neighbors, Decision Tree, Gradient Boosting, CatBoost, and Recurrent Neural Networks (RNNs), were evaluated for their accuracy in predicting PICU LOS at thresholds of 24 h, 36 h, 48 h, 72 h, 5 days, and 7 days. **Results**: Gradient Boosting, CatBoost, and RNN models demonstrated the highest accuracy, particularly at the 36 h and 48 h thresholds, with accuracy rates between 70 and 73%. These results far outperform traditional statistical and existing prediction methods that report accuracy of only around 50%, which is effectively unusable in the practical setting. These models also exhibited balanced performance between sensitivity (up to 74%) and specificity (up to 82%) at these thresholds. **Conclusions**: ML models, particularly Gradient Boosting, CatBoost, and RNNs, show moderate effectiveness in predicting PICU LOS with accuracy slightly over 70%, outperforming previously reported human predictions. This suggests potential utility in enhancing resource and staffing management in PICUs. However, further improvements through training on specialized databases can potentially achieve better accuracy and clinical applicability.

Keywords: length of stay; machine learning; artificial intelligence; intensive care units; pediatric; deep learning

1. Introduction

Machine learning (ML) and artificial intelligence (AI) are revolutionizing healthcare, with potential to transform patient care [1], enhance diagnostic accuracy [2], and optimize treatment pathways [3]. From assisting in interpreting radiological studies [4,5] to personalizing oncology therapy plans [2], these technologies offer significant potential across various healthcare fields. Analyzing electronic health records (EHRs) and large databases using ML and AI has also shown promise in improving patient outcomes and operational efficiency [6], particularly in critical care settings.

Pediatric intensive care units (PICUs) are resource-intensive environments within healthcare, necessitating specialized staffing and advanced medical equipment to cater to the complex needs of critically ill children. The nature of care in these units is compounded by the variability in patient ages, underlying conditions, and the critical interventions required. Consequently, PICUs face significant challenges in resource allocation, including the need for precise staffing levels and the availability of specialized equipment.

In this context, predicting the length of stay (LOS) in PICUs holds significant potential for improving resource allocation and staff scheduling. Accurate LOS predictions can lead to more efficient bed management, staffing decisions, and equipment planning, ultimately enhancing patient care and operational efficiency within the unit. Additionally, it can help better prepare patients and their families for the duration of their stay. Applying ML to predict LOS in PICUs presents a novel approach to these challenges. By utilizing the vast amounts of data generated in PICUs, ML models can identify patterns and predictors of LOS that might not be evident through traditional analytical methods.

To this end, the objective of this study is to use the Virtual Pediatric Systems (VPS, LLC http://www.myvps.org/ accessed on 23 September 2024) database, a comprehensive repository of pediatric critical care data, to develop and validate a machine learning model for predicting LOS in the PICU. The VPS database compiles clinical and administrative data on pediatric critical care admissions from over 100 North American PICUs and provides a readily available dataset for exploring the application of ML in this context.

2. Materials and Methods

2.1. Data Acquisition and Preprocessing

The study was reviewed by the Cleveland Clinic Institutional Review Board and approved as IRB-exempt research. It was not registered, and formal protocol was not prepared. We sourced our dataset by exporting the VPS database in CSV file format. The data extracted spans from the year 2015 to 2020, encompassing a broad temporal range to ensure development of a comprehensive ML model. We utilized Jupyter Notebooks version 7.2.2 as our integrated development environment (IDE), offering the ability to execute code blocks incrementally for data exploration. Additionally, its support for inline documentation and visualization makes it an ideal tool for collaborative data science projects, facilitating clear communication of methodologies and findings [7].

We employed Pandas version 2.2.3 [8] for preliminary data cleanup and analysis and removed patient records with essential missing variables. We consolidated certain variables (e.g., age groups, patient origin) to create more discrete and useful classes, such as recoding 28 categories of patient origin into 4: Emergency Department, Operating Room or Procedure Room, Lower Level of Care, and Another ICU. This processing made it easier to correlate patient demographics, initial care settings, and LOS in the PICU. Additionally, we simplified model development by focusing only on the primary organ system involved, streamlining the dataset for further processing and ensuring the quality and reliability of our predictive models. The above tasks were assisted by PandasAI version 2.2.15, a Python library that adds generative AI capabilities to Pandas, allowing analysis through natural language queries.

2.2. Data Transformation and Scaling

The LOS variable, originally continuous, was recoded into binary variables for different model thresholds. These binary variables represented whether LOS was less than or more than specific cutoffs: 24 h, 36 h, 48 h, 72 h, 96 h, 5 days, and 7 days, all clinically relevant thresholds for resource planning in PICUs. We utilized Scikit Learn's (SKL version 1.6.0) OrdinalEncoder [9] to transform non-numeric categorical data into integers, ensuring that all features, regardless of their original format, were included in the predictive model. We preferred ordinal encoding for our categorical data since the main categories (e.g., LOS) have an inherent order that we wanted to preserve by converting them into integer values. This is important for models like gradient boosting and SVM, which benefit from maintaining the rank without assuming exact numeric distances. Unlike one-hot encoding, which loses ordinal information, and target encoding, which risks bias or leakage, OrdinalEncoder keeps the ordinal structure intact, aligning with model assumptions and capturing relationships more accurately. For other models such as KNN or RNN, ordinal encoding may not always provide a distinct advantage because these models may not inherently leverage the order of categories in the same way. However, it does not offer a disadvantage either.

We created input and output vectors for the ML models, with the output vector representing binary recoded LOS and the input vector including patient demographics, physiological, and diagnostic variables (listed in Figure 1). Data normalization was performed using the MinMaxScaler from SKL [9], scaling values to 0–1, which is essential for effective ML model training and consistent performance.

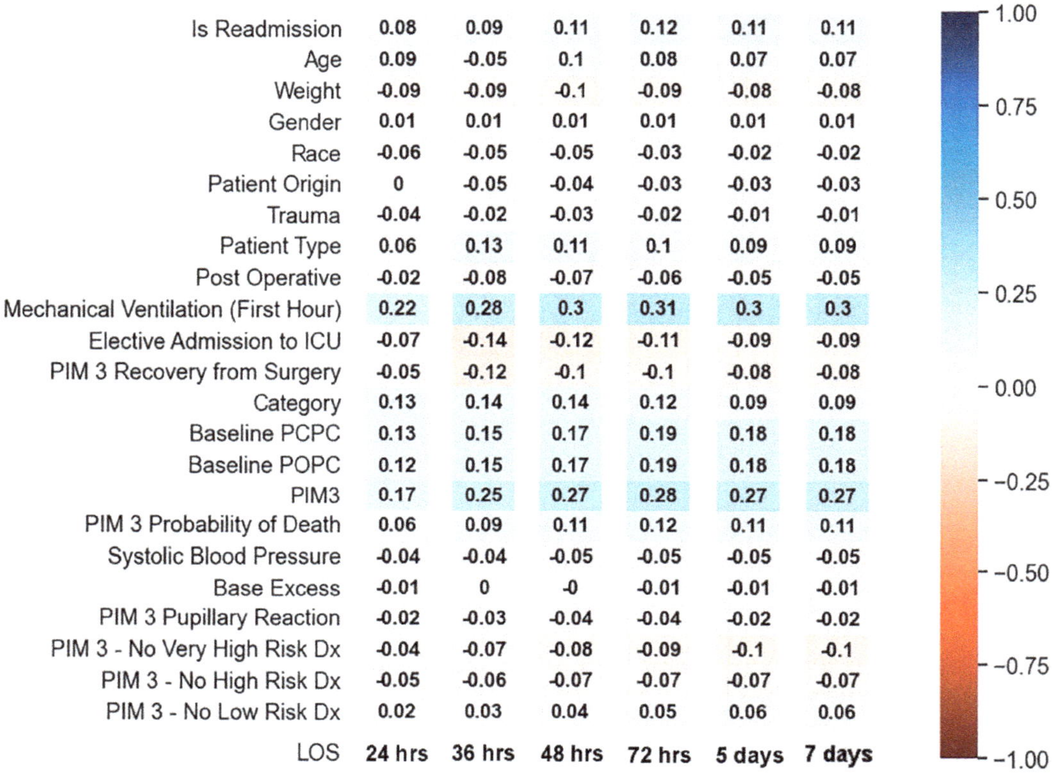

Figure 1. Input variables and their Pearson correlation heatmaps at each LOS threshold.

2.3. Model Development and Evaluation

For each LOS cutoff iteration, we generated heatmaps using the Pearson coefficient to visualize variable correlations with LOS. These heatmaps provided a comprehensive, color-coded view of potential predictors, showing the complex and multifactorial nature of LOS determinants. This process is useful when initiating a ML project like ours, highlighting the limitations of using a single variable to predict LOS due to patient variability and the dynamic nature of critical care. The moderate to weak correlations observed for individual variables underscore the need for a multivariate approach in developing predictive ML models.

For each LOS cutoff, we trained and tested multiple well-established shallow learning algorithms: Support Vector Machine (SVM), Stochastic Gradient Descent Classifier (SGDC), K nearest neighbor (KNN), Decision Tree classifier, Gradient Boost, and Cat Boost. Each algorithm has specific strengths, and we wanted to explore which best served our healthcare dataset complexities. SVM is suited for high-dimensional spaces, robust against overfitting, and ideal for datasets rich in patient metrics. SGDC offers efficiency in linear classification and is beneficial for large-scale and sparse data that can be typical in healthcare datasets. KNN adapts well to new data, using a similarity vote among nearest neighbors, while Decision Tree Classifier provides easy-to-understand visualizations, crucial for explaining predictions in medical settings. Gradient Boosting effectively minimizes errors and improves accuracy by sequentially learning from past mistakes. Finally, Cat Boost is optimized for categorical variables that are common in healthcare and requires minimal data preprocessing.

We excluded other algorithms because they were not as well suited to the characteristics of our dataset or the goals of our analysis. For example, Naive Bayes assumes conditional independence between features, which is unrealistic in complex healthcare datasets where patient metrics are often correlated. Random Forest, while useful, tends to be less effective than Gradient Boosting or CatBoost in reducing bias and handling categorical variables in high-dimensional data. We also did not select Logistic Regression because it is too simplistic for multi-class healthcare data and does not capture non-linear relationships as effectively as decision trees or boosting methods. Lastly, AdaBoost, while similar to Gradient Boosting, can struggle with noisy data and is sensitive to outliers, making it less robust for our dataset. By choosing SVM, SGDC, KNN, Decision Trees, Gradient Boost, and CatBoost, we focused on models that offer a balance between performance, interpretability, and efficiency, making them better suited for addressing the complexities of healthcare data.

All shallow algorithms were imported from the SKL open access library [9]. The data were randomly split 80:20, with 80% for training and 20% for testing each algorithm's LOS predictive performance. Additionally, we developed and tested a recurrent neural network (RNN) model using Keras version 3.5.0 [10] and Tensorflow 2.16.1 [11] framework developed by Google™. For this model, the data were split 60:20:20 for training, validation, and testing, facilitating the tuning and evaluation of the RNN's performance [10].

We evaluated these models using various metrics: accuracy, sensitivity (true positive rate), specificity (true negative rate), negative predictive value (NPV), positive predictive value (PPV, also known as "precision" in ML parlance), and the area under the receiver operating characteristic curve (AUC-ROC). The model's accuracy was the outcome of primary interest, but it was put into perspective by the AUC-ROC, which weighs the true positive against the false positive rate. These metrics provided insights into the models' classification accuracy, balance between true and false positives, and overall diagnostic ability in predicting LOS outcomes.

The Jupyter Notebook file with complete Python code and markdown is available as Supplementary Data in PDF (read-only) format.

3. Results

Our study analyzed data from 608,512 ICU patient encounters, treating repeat PICU admissions during the same hospitalization as separate encounters. After rigorous data processing, we retained 123,485 encounters, excluding those with missing variables like the Pediatric Overall Performance Category (POPC) and Pediatric Cerebral Performance Category (PCPC) scores. Further refinement removed encounters involving cardiac surgery recovery based on the Pediatric Index of Mortality 3 (PIM3) score, culminating in a final dataset comprising 123,354 encounters (Figure 2). Salient patient characteristics are detailed in Table 1.

Table 1. Demographic characteristics of sample utilized for ML modeling.

Characteristic	Values	Count	Percentage (%)
Age	0–2 years	39,018	31.63%
	Child 2 years to <6 years	23,923	19.40%
	Child 6 years to <12 years	22,927	18.59%
	12 years and up	37,486	30.38%
Gender	Male	67,785	54.96%
	Female	55,567	45.05%
	Ambiguous	2	0.002%

Table 1. *Cont.*

Characteristic	Values	Count	Percentage (%)
Race	White	57,002	46.22%
	Hispanic or Latino	25,688	20.83%
	Black or African American	21,539	17.46%
	Other/Mixed	7686	6.23%
	Unspecified	5569	4.51%
	Asian	2487	2.02%
	Asian/Indian/Pacific Islander	2367	1.92%
	American Indian or Alaska Native	669	0.54%
	Native Hawaiian or Other Pacific Islander	347	0.28%
Patient Origin	Emergency Department	69,441	56.30%
	OR/Procedure	28,013	22.71%
	Lower level of care	23,736	19.25%
	Another ICU	2164	1.75%
Readmission	No	86,939	70.48%
	Yes	36,415	29.52%
Trauma	No	111,927	90.75%
	Yes	11,427	9.25%
Patient Type	Unscheduled	100,194	81.22%
	Scheduled (>12 h in Advance)	23,160	18.78%
Post Operative	No	91,546	74.23%
	Yes	31,808	25.77%
Mechanical Ventilation (First Hour)	No	92,863	75.28%
	Yes	30,491	24.72%

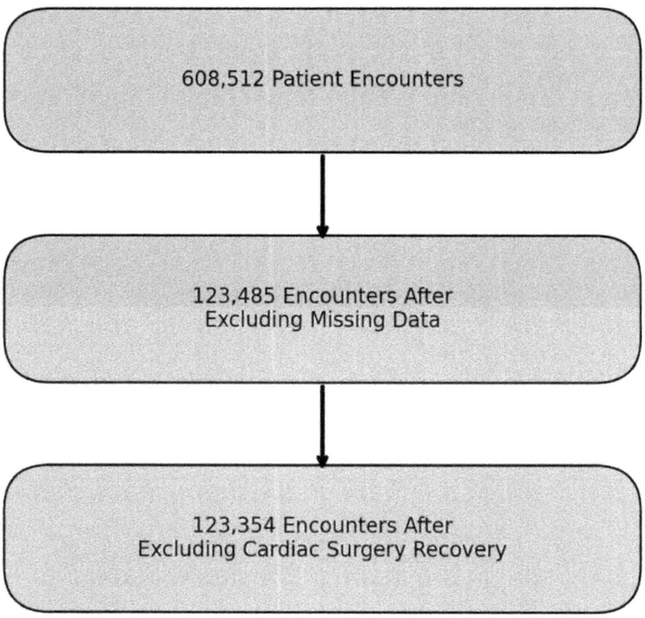

Figure 2. Flowchart depicting the sequential filtering process of patient encounters for inclusion in the machine learning models.

In evaluating the efficacy of various machine learning models to predict the LOS for PICU patients, this study systematically compared the performance across multiple LOS duration cutoffs: 24 h, 36 h, 48 h, 72 h, 5 days, and 7 days. The percentages of samples exceeding these durations were 68%, 52%, 40%, 28%, 16%, and 11%, respectively (Figure 3).

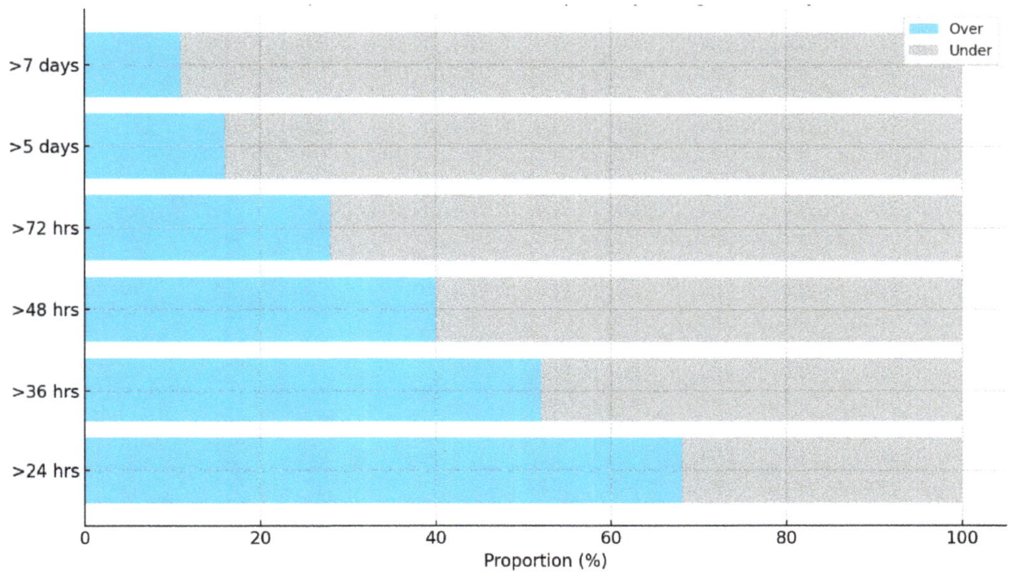

Figure 3. Proportion of patient samples by length of stay.

The Pearson coefficient heatmaps generated at each LOS cutoff are displayed in Figure 1. Correlations approaching +1 or −1 indicate strong positive or strong negative correlations; however, we found that no single input variable had a strong or even moderate correlation with LOS. Mechanical ventilation during the first hour and the PIM3 score were the only variables that showed weak correlation for predicting LOS at most time cutoffs (Pearson coefficient 0.2–0.3).

At the 24 h LOS threshold, Gradient boost and CatBoost demonstrated highest accuracy at 73%, followed by RNN with 72% and KNN with 70% accuracy (Table 2). Most models demonstrated high sensitivity in predicting LOS greater than 24 h (74% to 100%) but very low specificity (6–46%). Similarly, PPVs for LOS greater than 24 h were generally higher, reaching 75% for most models, but the NPVs remained low (45–62%). Finally, AUC-ROC for all ML models was persistently low (0.5–0.63) when attempting to predict LOS less than or greater than 24 h.

Running the models with a 36 h LOS cutoff yielded the best results. Gradient Boosting, CatBoost, and RNN showed robust performance, with accuracy rates of 70–72%, AUC-ROC of 0.70–0.72, and balanced sensitivity (71–74%) and specificity (69–70%), NPV (68–70%) and PPV (72–73%). At the 48 h cutoff, these models had similar accuracy (71–73%) and AUC-ROC (0.70–0.71), but higher specificity (79–82%) and NPV (75–76%), and lower sensitivity (59–62%) and PPV (65–68%).

When predicting longer LOS timeframes (72 h, 5 days, 7 days), all models demonstrated increasing accuracy, up to 89% (Supplemental Table S1). However, this was also associated with significantly increasing bias towards high specificity (84–99%) and high NPV (80–91%), and very low sensitivity (5–47%) and PPV (27–65%). Accordingly, the AUC-ROC scores were as low as 0.50.

Table 2. Summary of evaluation metrics for ML models at selected LOS cutoffs.

ML Model	Accuracy	Sensitivity	Specificity	NPV	PPV	AUC
			24 h			
SVM	68.60%	97%	6%	52%	69%	0.52
SGDC	68.40%	100%	0%	0%	68%	0.50
KNN	70.60%	86%	37%	55%	75%	0.62
Decision Tree	65%	74%	46%	45%	75%	0.60
Gradient boost	73%	90%	36%	62%	75%	0.63
Cat boost	73%	91%	32%	62%	74%	0.62
RNN	72%	90%	33%	60%	74%	0.61
			36 h			
SVM	66%	62%	70%	63%	69%	0.66
SGDC	65%	54%	77%	60%	72%	0.65
KNN	68%	71%	65%	67%	69%	0.68
Decision Tree	63%	65%	62%	61%	65%	0.63
Gradient boost	72%	74%	69%	71%	73%	0.72
Cat boost	71%	73%	69%	70%	72%	0.71
RNN	70%	71%	70%	68%	72%	0.70
			48 h			
SVM	68%	45%	85%	70%	66%	0.65
SGDC	68%	41%	86%	69%	66%	0.63
KNN	69%	56%	79%	73%	64%	0.67
Decision Tree	64%	55%	70%	70%	55%	0.63
Gradient boost	73%	62%	81%	76%	68%	0.71
Cat boost	73%	59%	82%	75%	68%	0.70
RNN	71%	61%	79%	75%	65%	0.70
			72 h			
SVM	75%	30%	93%	78%	60%	0.61
SGDC	74%	46%	84%	80%	53%	0.65
KNN	75%	37%	90%	79%	58%	0.63
Decision Tree	69%	47%	78%	79%	45%	0.63
Gradient boost	78%	42%	91%	81%	65%	0.67
Cat boost	77%	39%	92%	80%	65%	0.65
RNN	76%	43%	89%	80%	61%	0.66

SVM: Support Vector Machine, SGDC: Stochastic Gradient Descent Classifier, KNN: K-Nearest Neighbor, RNN: Recurrent Neural network, NPV: negative predictive value, PPV: positive predictive value, AUC: area under the curve.

4. Discussion

Our findings indicate that several ML models (particularly CatBoost, Gradient Boost, and RNNs) can achieve significant success in predicting PICU LOS, particularly for thresholds of 36 and 48 h (70–73% accuracy, with precision approaching 73%). While an accuracy of 73% may not seem very impressive at first glance, a review of the literature would suggest otherwise. Data show that ICU physicians are not successful at predicting LOS, approaching only 53% accuracy [12]. Similarly, emergency department physicians achieve 46% accuracy when predicting inpatient LOS [13], and intensivists and anesthesiologists successfully predicted ICU LOS after cardiac surgery in roughly 50% cases [14]. Given the perspective where human prediction is tantamount to a coin toss, we would argue that the 70–73% accuracy accomplished by our ML models is a significant improvement.

We believe our findings represent a successful initial exploration, and one of the first documented attempts to utilize AI/ML for LOS prediction in the PICU environment. The high costs of pediatric intensive care underscore the need for accurate predictions of staffing and resource allocation [15], allowing for cost-effective resource use and reduced wastage, which is essential in today's financially constrained healthcare environment. Additionally, the COVID-19 pandemic has intensified staffing challenges for nurses and respiratory therapists [16–18], heightening the importance of reliable LOS predictions that allow healthcare administrators to better optimize staffing. Accurately forecasting LOS through ML models, therefore, addresses both economic and staffing challenges, enhancing patient care and resource management in PICUs.

Our ML models predict LOS more accurately at the 36 h and 48 h thresholds (vs. longer timeframes) due to a more balanced distribution of LOS at these points. As shown in Figure 3, our study sample has a near 50:50 split for LOS under or over 36 h and a 60:40 split for under or over 48 h. Other thresholds have skewed distributions, potentially resulting in ML models adopting a more computationally efficient strategy to "learn" the most common outcome. While this appears to increase accuracy, it tends to reduce precision (PPV) and sensitivity. For instance, predicting LOS greater/less than 7 days yields up to 89% accuracy but only 5% sensitivity and 27% PPV, rendering the prediction essentially unusable. This aligns with studies showing ML classifiers perform better with balanced datasets and tend to favor frequent outcomes in imbalanced data [19]. Such computational efficiency can be beneficial in certain contexts, but also highlights ML limitations in complex environments like the PICU.

Interestingly, in our iterative process we ended up using the PIM3-ROM and PIM3 score, as well as its constituent variables to formulate our best model. Although this may seem counterintuitive initially, it is recognized that inclusion of composite variables in a ML model can enhance its performance by integrating multiple dimensions, reducing noise, and encapsulating interaction effects [20,21]. Also, the PIM3 score was originally designed to predict risk of mortality and is calculated using a formula that assigns fixed coefficients to the component variables. It can be theorized that by including its constituent variables within the model, the model was able to learn and assign different coefficients and weightage to these variables to predict LOS.

A literature review reveals scarce data on using ML to predict LOS, but our results align with a recent Taiwanese investigation using "TabNet" to predict inpatient LOS from a single center's emergency room admissions [22]. Despite their different patient population, their results were similar, with 71% accuracy and 78% precision. Another study using shallow ML models (logistic regression, random forest, and XGBoost) reported 66–77% accuracy for emergency department LOS predictions [23], paralleling our optimal ML model. The consistency across these studies and ours, highlights AI and ML's potential in critical care predictions.

In our study, we explored both deep and shallow learning algorithms to predict the LOS. Shallow learning algorithms like decision trees, linear regression, and support vector machines, with limited layers, suit problems with less complex input–output relationships. Deep learning, with multiple layers, processes large data hierarchically, capturing complex patterns useful in tasks like image and speech recognition [24]. Interestingly, our best results were achieved equally by shallow (Gradient Boost and CatBoost) and deep learning (RNN) models. This suggests that shallow learning algorithms can perform effectively despite the potential of deep learning, emphasizing the need to choose the right approach based on the data and problem characteristics rather than defaulting to more complex models that may be computationally wasteful.

Our moderately effective ML models were trained on the VPS database, which is exceptionally large, encompassing over 600,000 unique encounters. This allowed us to liberally exclude patient encounters lacking complete information, while still retaining more than 120,000 patient encounters for model development and testing. Had we started with a smaller dataset, we would have been forced to handle missing data through less-than-ideal methods like imputation or limit ourselves to only using machine learning algorithms capable of dealing with incomplete data. Of note, in earlier iterations of this project (not published) we utilized statistical imputation to utilize all 600,000 patient encounters. However, this approach resulted in very low accuracy, and we therefore chose to forego imputation and used the best quality data for our modeling. While it may be disconcerting that we excluded almost 80% of the available VPS database, our approach is supported by Kariluoto et al., who have emphasized that the significance of ML models lies in the quality of data rather than the quantity [25].

We would like to emphasize that VPS was not originally designed for predicting LOS, and it has limitations when used in this setting. Although it is comprehensive, it includes optional data elements (e.g., disability scores) that some sites do not collect, or data that might be missing for logistical reasons (e.g., base excess in PIM3 scoring if no arterial or capillary blood gas was taken). Furthermore, clinicians looking to predict LOS might use variables that are not present in VPS. For example, while VPS includes systolic blood pressure (SBP) at admission, it lacks other early vital signs, creating a gap between available data and clinical insights needed for accurate LOS prediction. The first hours of admission offer crucial information affecting a patient's trajectory, and the absence of this data likely limited our model's prediction accuracy.

Moreover, it could be argued that certain variables within VPS are coded in ways that render them less suitable for machine learning modeling. For instance, VPS uses ICD codes or proprietary STAR codes for diagnoses. While these codes standardize diagnoses, they can lack the specificity needed for precise LOS predictions. For instance, septic shock in an immunocompromised oncologic patient differs significantly from that in an immunocompetent child, leading to different clinical courses and PICU LOS. Additionally, the VPS database contains 1533 unique STAR codes, and this large number of classes can weaken model predictive capability. To mitigate some of these challenges, we chose not to rely on specific ICD or STAR diagnoses, and instead categorized by the primary organ system involved (as documented in VPS), thereby reducing the classes from 1533 to just 25.

While traditional statistical methods have been used to identify factors that may be associated with PICU LOS or to produce benchmarks for PICU LOS, these methods are limited to population inferences and lack the ability to make personalized predictions [26]. Machine learning approaches such as ours are practical and implementable from an operational standpoint and can make predictions for an individual patient's LOS by utilizing variables that are easily obtained within an hour of PICU admission. Our findings emphasize the need for databases tailored to support predictive analyses for LOS and similar outcomes. These databases should include a broader range of detailed clinical variables to enhance machine learning models' accuracy, bolstering the case for AI and ML in clinical decisions, and we encourage the pediatric critical care medicine organizations such as SCCM and ESPNIC to facilitate such efforts. Despite challenges, our study shows the feasibility of using ML models to predict LOS in the PICU, which is crucial amid nursing and staffing shortages. By improving census prediction accuracy, our work suggests a path toward more efficient staffing and resource allocation in PICUs. Once adequately developed with more refined datasets, such models can be deployed within the electronic medical record to automatically extract data from a patient's chart within the first few hours of admission. Automatic notifications can be sent to PICU managers about the predicted LOS for all patients in the PICU, and plans can then be updated to adjust nurse staffing and material resources such as ventilators.

5. Conclusions

Our study investigates machine learning models for predicting PICU LOS, marking an early effort in this area. CatBoost, Gradient Boost, and Recurrent Neural Networks showed moderate effectiveness, with accuracy slightly over 70%. Despite the limitations of the VPS database, our research highlights ML's potential in healthcare and the need for specialized databases to improve model accuracy and utility. While not suitable as standalone AI agents yet, we believe future models trained with specialized datasets hold promise as tools for resource and staffing management in PICUs, addressing financial and staffing issues.

Supplementary Materials: The following supporting information can be downloaded at: https://www.mdpi.com/article/10.3390/bioengineering11100962/s1. The source code and extended results are included within the Supplementary Data file.

Author Contributions: All authors were involved in the planning and execution of the research. H.A.G. and O.B. conceived the idea and handled the machine learning aspects of the study. O.B. and S.Q.L. provided continuous feedback for clinical relevance of the developing machine learning models. S.Q.L. provided critical evaluation of the study from an administrative perspective to ensure relevance and applicability to clinical operations and resource management. H.A.G. wrote the first draft of the manuscript, and O.B. and S.Q.L. provided critical review and revisions. All authors have read and agreed to the published version of the manuscript.

Funding: This research received no external funding.

Institutional Review Board Statement: The study was conducted in accordance with the Declaration of Helsinki and approved as IRB exempt research by the Cleveland Clinic Institutional Review Board.

Informed Consent Statement: Study was conducted using an anonymized database and did not recruit individual human subjects; therefore, consent was not applicable.

Data Availability Statement: The database can be obtained through VPS, LLC. The machine learning source code is included in Supplementary Data.

Conflicts of Interest: The authors declare no conflicts of interest.

References

1. Chavva, I.R.; Crawford, A.L.; Mazurek, M.H.; Yuen, M.M.; Prabhat, A.M.; Payabvash, S.; Sze, G.; Falcone, G.J.; Matouk, C.C.; de Havenon, A.; et al. Deep Learning Applications for Acute Stroke Management. *Ann. Neurol.* **2022**, *92*, 574–587. [CrossRef] [PubMed]
2. Varlamova, E.V.; Butakova, M.A.; Semyonova, V.V.; Soldatov, S.A.; Poltavskiy, A.V.; Kit, O.I.; Soldatov, A.V. Machine Learning Meets Cancer. *Cancers* **2024**, *16*, 1100. [CrossRef] [PubMed]
3. Gomez-Cabello, C.A.; Borna, S.; Pressman, S.; Haider, S.A.; Haider, C.R.; Forte, A.J. Artificial-Intelligence-Based Clinical Decision Support Systems in Primary Care: A Scoping Review of Current Clinical Implementations. *Eur. J. Investig. Health Psychol. Educ.* **2024**, *14*, 685–698. [CrossRef] [PubMed]
4. Irmici, G.; Cè, M.; Della Pepa, G.; D'Ascoli, E.; De Berardinis, C.; Giambersio, E.; Rabiolo, L.; La Rocca, L.; Carriero, S.; Depretto, C.; et al. Exploring the Potential of Artificial Intelligence in Breast Ultrasound. *Crit. Rev. Oncog.* **2024**, *29*, 15–28. [CrossRef] [PubMed]
5. Onnis, C.; van Assen, M.; Muscogiuri, E.; Muscogiuri, G.; Gershon, G.; Saba, L.; De Cecco, C.N. The Role of Artificial Intelligence in Cardiac Imaging. *Radiol. Clin. N. Am.* **2024**, *62*, 473–488. [CrossRef]
6. Ridgway, J.P.; Lee, A.; Devlin, S.; Kerman, J.; Mayampurath, A. Machine Learning and Clinical Informatics for Improving HIV Care Continuum Outcomes. *Curr. HIV/AIDS Rep.* **2021**, *18*, 229–236. [CrossRef]
7. Beg, M.; Taka, J.; Kluyver, T.; Konovalov, A.; Ragan-Kelley, M.; Thiéry, N.M.; Fangohr, H. Using Jupyter for Reproducible Scientific Workflows. *Comput. Sci. Eng.* **2021**, *23*, 36–46. [CrossRef]
8. McKinney, W. *Python for Data Analysis: Data Wrangling with Pandas, NumPy, and IPython*, 3rd ed.; O'Reilly Media, Inc.: Sebastapol, CA, USA, 2022.
9. Pedregosa, F.; Varoquaux, G.; Gramfort, A.; Michel, V.; Thirion, B.; Grisel, O.; Blondel, M.; Prettenhofer, P.; Weiss, R.; Dubourg, V.; et al. Scikit-learn: Machine Learning in Python. *J. Mach. Learn. Res.* **2011**, *12*, 2825–2830.
10. Chollet, F. *Deep Learning with Python*, 2nd ed.; Manning Publications Co.: Shelter Island, NY, USA, 2021.
11. Abadi, M.; Agarwal, A.; Barham, P.; Brevdo, E.; Chen, Z.; Citro, C.; Corrado, G.S.; Davis, A.; Dean, J.; Devin, M.; et al. TensorFlow: Large-Scale Machine Learning on Heterogeneous Distributed Systems. *arXiv* **2016**, arXiv:1603.04467.
12. Nassar, A.P., Jr.; Caruso, P. ICU physicians are unable to accurately predict length of stay at admission: A prospective study. *Int. J. Qual. Health Care* **2016**, *28*, 99–103. [CrossRef]
13. Dent, A.W.; Weiland, T.J.; Vallender, L.; Oettel, N.E. Can medical admission and length of stay be accurately predicted by emergency staff, patients or relatives? *Aust. Health Rev.* **2007**, *31*, 633–641. [CrossRef] [PubMed]
14. Tu, J.V.; Mazer, C.D. Can clinicians predict ICU length of stay following cardiac surgery? *Can. J. Anaesth.* **1996**, *43*, 789–794. [CrossRef] [PubMed]
15. Killien, E.Y.; Keller, M.R.; Watson, R.S.; Hartman, M.E. Epidemiology of Intensive Care Admissions for Children in the US From 2001 to 2019. *JAMA Pediatr.* **2023**, *177*, 506–515. [CrossRef]
16. Boston-Leary, K.; Yakusheva, O. It's Time! The Path for Nursing Reimbursement Reform. *Creat. Nurs.* **2024**, *30*, 37–40. [CrossRef]
17. Peters, M. Time to solve persistent, pernicious and widespread nursing workforce shortages. *Int. Nurs. Rev.* **2023**, *70*, 247–253. [CrossRef]
18. Sanford, K. Nursing 2023: A New Emphasis on Nursing Strategy. *Nurs. Adm. Q.* **2023**, *47*, 289–295. [CrossRef]
19. Wei, Q.; Dunbrack, R.L. The role of balanced training and testing data sets for binary classifiers in bioinformatics. *PLoS ONE* **2013**, *8*, e67863. [CrossRef]

20. Kuhn, M.; Johnson, K. *Feature Engineering and Selection: A Practical Approach for Predictive Models*; Chapman and Hall/CRC: Boca Raton, FL, USA, 2019.
21. Zheng, A.; Casari, A. *Feature Engineering for Machine Learning: Principles and Techniques for Data Scientists*; O'Reilly Media, Inc.: Sebastopol, CA, USA, 2018.
22. Lin, Y.T.; Deng, Y.X.; Tsai, C.L.; Huang, C.H.; Fu, L.C. Interpretable Deep Learning System for Identifying Critical Patients through the Prediction of Triage Level, Hospitalization, and Length of Stay: Prospective Study. *JMIR Med. Inform.* **2024**, *12*, e48862. [CrossRef] [PubMed]
23. Canellas, M.M.; Kotkowski, K.A.; Pachamanova, D.A.; Perakis, G.; Reznek, M.A.; Lami, O.S.; Tsiourvas, A. A Granular View of Emergency Department Length of Stay: Improving Predictive Power and Extracting Real-Time, Actionable Insights. *Ann. Emerg. Med.* **2024**, *84*, 386–398. [CrossRef]
24. Baloglu, O.; Latifi, S.Q.; Nazha, A. What is machine learning? *Arch. Dis. Child Educ. Pract. Ed.* **2022**, *107*, 386–388. [CrossRef]
25. Kariluoto, A.; Kultanen, J.; Soininen, J.; Pärnänen, A.; Abrahamsson, P. Quality of Data in Machine Learning. In Proceedings of the IEEE 21st International Conference on Software Quality, Reliability and Security Companion (QRS-C), Hainan, China, 6–10 December 2021; pp. 216–221. [CrossRef]
26. Bzdok, D.; Altman, N.; Krzywinski, M. Statistics versus machine learning. *Nat. Methods* **2018**, *15*, 233–234. [CrossRef] [PubMed]

healthcare

MDPI

Article

Exploring Factors Influencing Patient Delay Behavior in Oral Cancer: The Development of a Risk Prediction Model in Western China

Yuanyuan Yang [1,2,†], Huan Ning [2,†], Bohui Liang [3,†], Huaming Mai [1], Jie Zhou [2], Jing Yang [2] and Jiegang Huang [2,4,*]

1 Hospital of Stomatology, Guangxi Medical University, Nanning 530021, China; yuanyang0122@outlook.com (Y.Y.); huamingmai@outlook.com (H.M.)
2 School of Public Health, Guangxi Medical University, Nanning 530021, China; a15277099623@hotmail.com (H.N.); zhoujie2121@outlook.com (J.Z.); jingyang202220919@outlook.com (J.Y.)
3 School of Computer, Electronics and Information, Guangxi University, Nanning 530004, China; hliangcs@foxmail.com
4 Guangxi Colleges and Universities Key Laboratory of Prevention and Control of Highly Prevalent Diseases, Guangxi Medical University, Nanning 530021, China
* Correspondence: jieganghuang@gxmu.edu.cn; Tel.: +86-7715334215
† These authors contributed equally to this work.

Abstract: Background and Aims: To study the unknown influencing factors of delayed medical treatment behavior in oral cancer patients in western China and to develop a prediction model on the risk of delayed medical treatment in oral cancer patients. Method: We investigated oral cancer patients attending a tertiary Grade A dental hospital in western China from June 2022 to July 2023. The logistic regression and four machine learning models (nearest neighbors, the RBF SVM, random forest, and QDA) were used to identify risk factors and establish a risk prediction model. We used the established model to predict the data before and after the COVID-19 pandemic and test whether the prediction effect can still remain stable and accurate under the interference of COVID-19. Result: Out of the 495 patients included in the study, 122 patients (58.65%) delayed seeking medical treatment before the lifting of the restrictions of the pandemic, while 153 patients (53.13%) did so after the lifting of restrictions. The logistic regression model revealed that living with adult children was a protective factor for patients in delaying seeking medical attention, regardless of the implementation of pandemic control measures. After comparing each model, it was found that the statistical indicators of the random forest algorithm such as the AUC score (0.8380) and specificity (0.8077) ranked first, with the best prediction performance and stable performance. Conclusions: This study systematically elucidates the critical factors influencing patient delay behavior in oral cancer diagnosis and treatment, employing a comprehensive risk prediction model that accurately identifies individuals at an elevated risk of delay. It represents a pioneering large-scale investigation conducted in western China, focusing explicitly on the multifaceted factors affecting the delayed medical treatment behavior of oral cancer patients. The findings underscore the imperative of implementing early intervention strategies tailored to mitigate these delays. Furthermore, this study emphasizes the pivotal role of robust social support systems and positive family dynamics in facilitating timely access to healthcare services for oral cancer patients, thereby potentially improving outcomes and survival rates.

Keywords: oral cancer patients; patient delay; influencing factors; prediction model; Guangxi Province; China's western region; spatial accessibility; machine learning

1. Introduction

Oral cancer is the general term for malignant tumors occurring in the mouth, which are one of the common malignant tumors in the head and neck. Head and neck cancer (HNC)

is considered the sixth most common malignant tumor in the world. The incidence and prevalence of oral cancer have significant geographical differences, and their distribution varies greatly around the world. Reports show that Asia has the highest proportion of confirmed cases of oral cancer (64.2%) and mortality (73.3%) [1,2]. Patient delay is defined as the period between the initial recognition of symptoms by the patient and their first consultation with healthcare professionals regarding those symptoms. For tumor diseases, disease staging serves as a crucial prognostic indicator for predicting patient survival. Allison and colleagues discovered that delays exceeding 3 months could elevate the risk of the disease progressing to an advanced stage [3]. Owing to the lack of public awareness regarding oral cancer and inadequate attention to disease symptoms, patients with oral cancer generally experience delays in seeking treatment, which can impact subsequent treatment and recovery outcomes. Currently, research on the delay in seeking medical attention among oral cancer patients in China is scarce, and numerous potential risk factors affecting the medical behavior of these patients remain undiscovered. Public service accessibility is an important research object in urban and rural planning and urban geography abroad. Reachability methods have proposed standards and methods for identifying areas with shortages of public services. It is an important indicator for measuring the level of equalization of urban and rural public services and provides scientific references for the planning and layout of public services [4]. The low level of accessibility to medical and health services leads to patients having to delay seeking medical treatment. Consequently, this study employs the shortest time distance, grounded in GIS (geographic information systems), to delineate the level of accessibility to medical and health services. This approach facilitates a comparison of the disparities in accessibility to medical and health services between the residences of patients who experienced delays in seeking medical treatment and those who did not.

The machine learning predictive model is a tool that utilizes computer algorithms to learn model parameters from training data, which are then used to predict and analyze unknown data. These models are capable of predicting a continuous outcome or classification label based on the input data features. The construction of predictive models typically involves selecting appropriate machine learning algorithms adjusting the model parameters through a training dataset to achieve an optimal predictive performance. The performance of the model is usually evaluated using metrics such as accuracy, precision, and recall to ensure that the model has good generalization ability and stability. For example, Zhang Yuying and others used machine learning algorithms to build a medical delay risk prediction model for imported malaria cases in Jiangsu Province, thereby discovering new risk prediction factors with good predictive efficacy, which can provide a reference for the health management of imported malaria patients. The factors causing delayed medical treatment in oral cancer patients are complex. If machine learning methods can be used to build a risk prediction model for delayed medical treatment in oral cancer, it will fully tap into data information, handle complex interactions between variables, and process various data formats in dynamic, large-capacity, and complex data environments. Thus, it may identify data trends and patterns that could be overlooked in the risk factors of delayed medical treatment for oral cancer, providing guidance for the prevention of the occurrence and development of oral cancer diseases. However, there have been no reports on machine learning prediction models for delayed medical treatment in oral cancer patients in China.

Public service accessibility is an important research object in foreign urban and rural planning and urban geography. The accessibility method proposes standards and methods for identifying public service shortage areas. It is an important indicator for measuring the level of equalization of public services in urban and rural areas and provides a scientific reference for the planning and layout of public services. The low level of accessibility to medical and health services leads to patients having to delay seeking medical treatment. Therefore, this study is based on a geographic information system (GIS) and uses the shortest time distance to represent the level of accessibility to medical and health services, thereby comparing the differences in the accessibility levels of medical and health services between the residences of patients with delayed medical treatment and those without delayed medical treatment.

The western region of China is an economically underdeveloped region with multiple ethnic groups living together. It has its uniqueness in geography, economy, culture, and medical and health resources. In a recent review [5], researchers included studies on the diagnosis delay of oral cancer conducted in multiple countries from 1994 to 2020. Among them, two studies in China were conducted in Beijing and Jilin (a province in northeast China), with sample sizes of 102 and 128, respectively. Large-sample studies on the western region of China have not yet been reported.

The significance of this study lies in that this study is the first large-sample research on the risk factors of delayed medical-seeking behavior among oral cancer patients in western China. In order to explore new factors related to the delayed medical treatment behavior of oral cancer patients, we investigated various aspects, including the patients' demographic information, their social support status, the site of onset, the impact of the COVID-19, personal health literacy, and the accessibility level of medical and health services in the patients' place of residence. We also established a new predictive model that can avoid the interference of the pandemic and accurately predict the risk factors for delayed medical treatment in oral cancer patients. This model can be applied to guide the formulation of public health policies, improve the medical treatment behavior of oral cancer patients, and enhance patient survival rates.

2. Materials and Methods

2.1. Subject Criteria

A continuous inclusion method was used to investigate eligible oral cancer patients who visited the Department of Oral and Maxillofacial Surgery in the Affiliated Stomatological Hospital of Guangxi Medical University from June 2022 to July 2023. This study was conducted at the Affiliated Stomatological Hospital of Guangxi Medical University, which is the only Grade III Class A stomatological specialty hospital in Guangxi, and its oral cancer case data have a certain representativeness. The inclusion criteria: ① suffering from malignant tumors in the oral region, including cancers in the tongue, lips, cheeks, gums, floor of the mouth (oral floor), hard palate, soft palate, and salivary glands; ② pathologically diagnosed with squamous cell carcinoma; ③ age $\geq$ 18 years old; ④ willing to participate in this study; ⑤ having a certain level of understanding and language expression ability and able to cooperate with the investigation. The exclusion criteria: ① non-permanent residents of Guangxi; ② incomplete medical records. A total of 495 patients met the criteria.

2.2. Research Methods

In this study, the delay in seeking medical treatment for oral cancer was defined as the time from the onset of symptoms to the first visit > 3 months. The main form of investigation was face-to-face interviews or telephone follow-ups to conduct questionnaires. The research variables included the patient's gender, ethnicity, occupation, age, education level, average monthly income, marital status, and inhabiting status, as well as whether they had medical staff as relatives or friends, their type of medical insurance, their systemic disease status, the oral site of symptoms, the initial visit medical institution, self-medication, the impact of the COVID-19 pandemic on visits, smoking and drinking habits, whether they ate betel nuts, personal health literacy (HL), the cognition of the disease, oral health behavior, etc. Furthermore, based on the distribution of medical and health service institutions surrounding the patient's residence and the type of the nearest road, the level of accessibility to medical and health services was ascertained. The above 21 data types were used as independent variables. Electronic medical records were analyzed, and patient histories were collected. According to the patient's delay in seeking medical treatment ($\leq$3 months and >3 months), it was used as the dependent variable. Questionnaire information was double-entered using the software EpiData 3.1 and difference tests were performed. Difference samples were rechecked against the original survey data and re-entered.

This paper uses GIS network analysis to calculate the shortest time distance from the patient's residence to the surrounding primary hospitals, secondary hospitals, tertiary hospitals, dental clinics, and stomatological hospitals, using the shortest time distance to characterize the level of medical and health service accessibility. POI data sources are Gaode Map data from December 2022, including county towns, townships, streets, villages, and urban and rural public service facilities. The road network data is sourced from the OpenStreetMap website, and the traffic network data includes national highways, provincial highways, county roads, township roads, urban arterial roads, secondary arterial roads, and residential area roads. Under the mode of car travel, the speed limits for these roads are 65, 50, 40, 30, 65, 40, and 30 km/h, respectively. The data source for the medical institutions is the Guangxi Medical Insurance Public Service website. The accessibility of medical and health services is divided into four levels, 10~15, 10~20, 20~30, and more than 30 min, which are set as very good, good, poor, and very poor, respectively.

2.3. Statistical Analysis Methods

2.3.1. Impact Factor Analysis

Statistical analysis is performed using SPSS 23.0 software. The chi-square test is used for inter-group count data difference analysis, and continuity corrections or Fisher's exact probability method is used if necessary. After passing the single sample Kolmogorov–Smirnov test, two independent samples' t-tests are used for comparison between groups for measurement data that conforms to a normal distribution. Non-parametric tests are used for comparisons of inter-group differences in non-normally distributed measurement data. $p < 0.05$ indicates a statistically significant difference.

2.3.2. Prediction Model Establishment

Before and after the lifting of the restrictions of the pandemic, patients were randomly assigned to training and test sets in an 8:2 ratio. Python 3.8 software was applied to screen candidate factors in the training sets of the two groups before and after the lifting of the restrictions of the pandemic through the recursive feature elimination (RFE) algorithm. The importance of each feature was obtained by returning the coefficient attribute or feature importance attribute of the learner. RFE was proposed by Guyon et al. [6], based on support vector machines. This method uses a base model for multiple rounds of training. After each round of training, several features with certain weight coefficients are eliminated, and the next round of training is performed based on the new feature set. The implementation steps of RFE in this paper can be summarized as follows: Train a machine learning base model, which is logistic regression in this study. Calculate the importance of different factors in patient delay, eliminate factors with low importance, and repeatedly recurse this step on the feature set until the desired number of features is reached. The most important factors are selected separately in the two groups. A Venn diagram is used to analyze unique or shared factors before and after the lifting of the restrictions of the pandemic.

The above common factors are incorporated into the model to build the overall model. All research subjects are randomly assigned to training sets and test sets in an 8:2 ratio. Risk prediction models are constructed based on four machine learning algorithms: nearest neighbors, the RBF SVM, random forest, and QDA. Ten-fold cross-validation (Figure 1) is used to determine the optimal hyperparameters of the model, which is independently validated on the test set to obtain the model with the highest AUC. The built model is used to predict data before and after the pandemic to test whether the prediction effect is stable and accurate. This process is shown in Figure 2.

The Hospital of Stomatology, Guangxi Medical University, Institutional Review Board provided ethics approval (ethics approval number: 2023006). Written informed consent was obtained from all study participants at the time of initial enrolment. All methods were performed in accordance with the relevant guidelines and regulations.

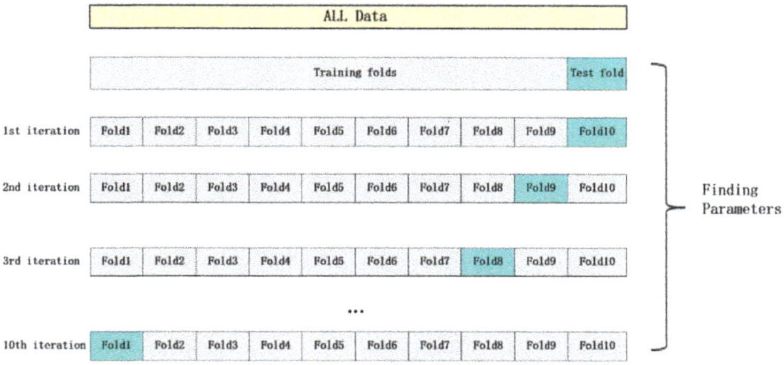

Figure 1. Flowchart of 10-fold cross-validation.

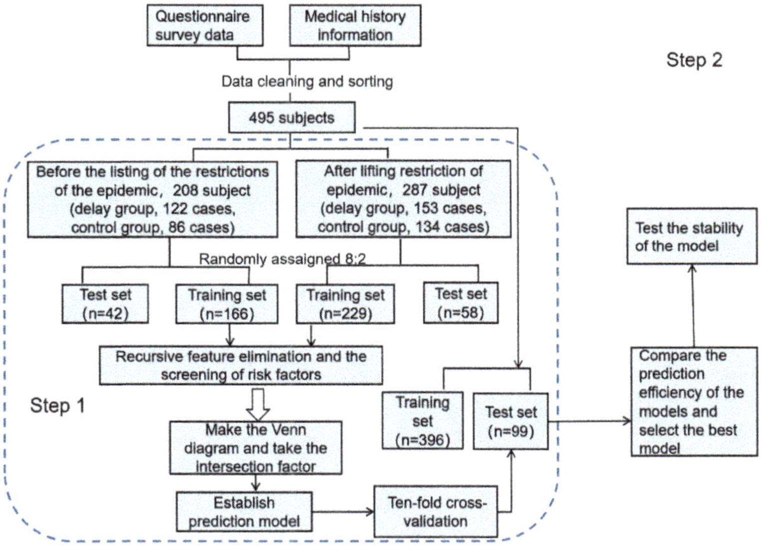

Figure 2. An overview of the model building process and the deep learning model architecture.

3. Results

3.1. Baseline Data Analysis

In this survey, a total of 495 cases of oral cancer in Guangxi were included. The tumor type the participants suffered from, the TNM staging, and whether there were systemic diseases are shown in Table 1. Before the lifting of the pandemic restrictions, there were 208 patients, of whom 122 (58.65%) had delayed seeking medical attention. After the lifting of the pandemic restrictions, there were 287 patients, of whom 153 (53.13%) had delayed seeking medical attention. The demographic characteristics are shown in Table 2. It was found that there were differences in occupation and marital status before and after the relaxation of the pandemic prevention and control. The proportion of workers and farmers decreased after the relaxation, while the proportion of single people increased (Table 2).

The univariate analysis found that before the lifting of the pandemic restrictions, the factors with statistical differences between patients with delayed medical attention and non-delay patients were as follows: sites inside the mouth, heath literacy level, and ways to access knowledge about oral cancer. After the lifting of the restrictions of the pandemic, statistically significant factors associated with patient delay in seeking medical treatment compared to non-delayed patients were having or not having medical as staff friends/relatives and the habit of chewing hard objects (Supplementary File Table S1).

Table 1. Tumor type, TNM staging, and whether there were systemic diseases.

Tumor Type	**Quantity**
Lip/Parotid/Floor of Mouth/Pharynx	61
Cheek	84
Tongue	239
Gum Cancer	84
Palatal Cancer	27
TNM Stage	
Stage 1	71
Stage 2	154
Stage 3	77
Stage 4	193
Presence of Systemic Diseases	
Yes	291
No	204
Systemic Disease Classification	
None	206
Circulatory System Diseases	133
Endocrine System Diseases	35
Others	121

Table 2. Demographic characteristics of patients with oral cancer.

Demographic Data		**During Strict Travel Restrictions**		**Lifted Restrictions**		***p***
Gender	Male	130	62.50%	188	65.50%	0.491
	Female	78	37.50%	99	34.50%	
Nation	Han ethnicity	119	57.20%	173	60.30%	0.518
	Ethnic minorities	89	42.80%	114	39.70%	
Occupation	Workers	41	19.70%	85	29.60%	**0.032 ***
	Farmers	88	42.30%	98	34.10%	
	Professionals and others	79	38.00%	104	36.20%	
Age	<40	17	8.20%	41	14.30%	0.113
	40–59	99	47.60%	127	44.30%	
	>60	92	44.20%	119	41.50%	
Residency	Rural	104	50.00%	149	51.90%	0.674
	Urban	104	50.00%	138	48.10%	
Educational level	Below primary education	11	5.30%	29	10.10%	0.341
	Primary school	43	20.70%	64	22.30%	
	Middle school	65	31.30%	86	30.00%	
	High school	50	24.00%	62	21.60%	
	≥College	39	18.80%	46	16.00%	
Monthly income	<1500 RMB	49	23.60%	99	34.50%	0.112
	1500–3000 RMB	57	27.40%	63	22.00%	
	3001–5000 RMB	62	29.80%	81	28.20%	
	5001–8000 RMB	31	14.90%	34	11.80%	
	>8000 RMB	9	4.30%	10	3.50%	
Marital status	Single	9	4.30%	30	10.50%	**0.007 ***
	Married	184	88.50%	220	76.70%	

* Statistically signifcant.

Regardless of whether it was before or after the lifting of the restrictions of the pandemic, statistically significant differences were observed between patients who delayed seeking medical treatment and those who did not in terms of inhabiting status, urban or rural residence, the impact of the COVID-19 pandemic, the personal health literacy scale, regular oral examination habits, the frequency of tooth brushing, the distance to the nearest medical institution, and the mode of transportation used for medical visits ($p < 0.05$).

The binary logistics regression model indicated that living with adult children was a protective factor in both the periods before and after the lifting of the restrictions of the pandemic. Walking to seek medical care was a risk factor. Before the lifting of the restrictions of the pandemic, being affected by COVID-19, not having regular dental check-up habits, and acquiring knowledge from the internet or other sources were risk factors for patient delay. After the lifting of the restrictions of the pandemic, the habit of biting hard objects with the teeth was a risk factor for affected patients' medical behavior. Patients living within 2–10 km of the nearest medical institution were at a higher risk of patient delay (Table 3).

Table 3. Multivariate analysis of delayed medical treatment in patients with oral cancer.

Parameter	Restrictions Multivariate Analysis		Lifted Restrictions Multivariate Analysis	
	OR (95%CI)	*p*	OR (95%CI)	*p*
Person lived with (Adult children vs. Spouse)	41.99 (10.71~164.56)	**<0.001** *	24.72 (10.11~60.45)	**<0.001** *
Person lived with (Adult children vs. No one or others)	9.09 (1.29~63.84)	**0.026** *	5.77 (2.15~15.53)	**0.001** *
Vehicle (On foot vs. Electric bicycle)	5.65 (1.33~23.99)	**0.028** *	3.09 (1.08~8.84)	**0.035** *
Impact of COVID-19 (Yes vs. No)	8.66 (2.28~32.82)	**0.002** *	-	-
Access to knowledge (Network and others vs. Relatives and friends)	14.83 (1.83~120.55)	**0.012** *	-	-
Checking mouth regularly (No vs. Yes)	26.35 (2.86~242.80)	**0.004** *	-	-
Distance to nearest medical facility (<2 km vs. 2–5 km)	-	-	2.94 (1.04~8.34)	**0.043** *
Distance to nearest medical facility (<2 km vs. 6–10 km)	-	-	4.32 (1.03~18.09)	**0.045** *
Chewing hard objects	-	-	2.15 (1.05~4.38)	**0.035** *

* Statistically signifcant.

3.2. Spatial Accessibility Analysis of Medical and Health Services for Oral Cancer Patients in Guangxi

Oral cancer patients seeking medical care are distributed across various cities in Guangxi, radiating from Nanning City as the center (Figure 3A). The proportion is higher in the southeastern part and lower in the northwestern part. This is related to the location of our hospital in Nanning, which is in the central–southern part of Guangxi, and the relatively distant distance from Nanning to the northwestern region of Guangxi, indicating that spatial distance has a certain impact on patients' medical behavior.

Based on GIS, the shortest time distance was used to represent the accessibility level of medical and health services. Under the mode of automobile travel, the accessibility level of primary hospitals is the highest (Figure 3B): the proportion of patients arriving at first-level institutions within 10 min and 20 min reaches 79.5% and 92.3%, respectively. This indicates that under the background of urban–rural transportation integration, the network of primary medical and health institutions in Guangxi has covered rural areas, making it more convenient for urban and rural residents in Guangxi to seek medical care.

The accessibility level of second-level medical institutions is relatively good (Figure 3C), with the proportion of patients arriving at secondary hospitals within 10 min and 20 min being 55.7% and 71.3%, respectively. The accessibility level of tertiary hospitals is relatively poor (Figure 3D), with only 36.5% and 45.3% of patients able to reach these institutions within 10 min and 20 min, respectively. The regions with better accessibility are mostly urban areas, which may be related to the fact that tertiary medical institutions are mostly built in densely populated urban areas.

The accessibility level of stomatological hospitals is the worst (Figure 3E), with only 17.4% of patients able to arrive within 20 min. There are only two stomatological hospitals in Guangxi, one in Nanning and the other in Guilin, reflecting that residents in Nanning and Guilin enjoy better medical resources. Fortunately, even though the distribution of stomatological hospitals is scarce, oral cancer patients can first go to the stomatology department of general hospitals or dental clinics for screening. The accessibility level of dental clinics is average (Figure 3F). The proportions of patients who can reach a dental clinic within 10 min and 20 min are 46.0% and 55.6%, respectively. However, dental clinics are mostly located in densely populated urban areas and rarely in remote rural areas.

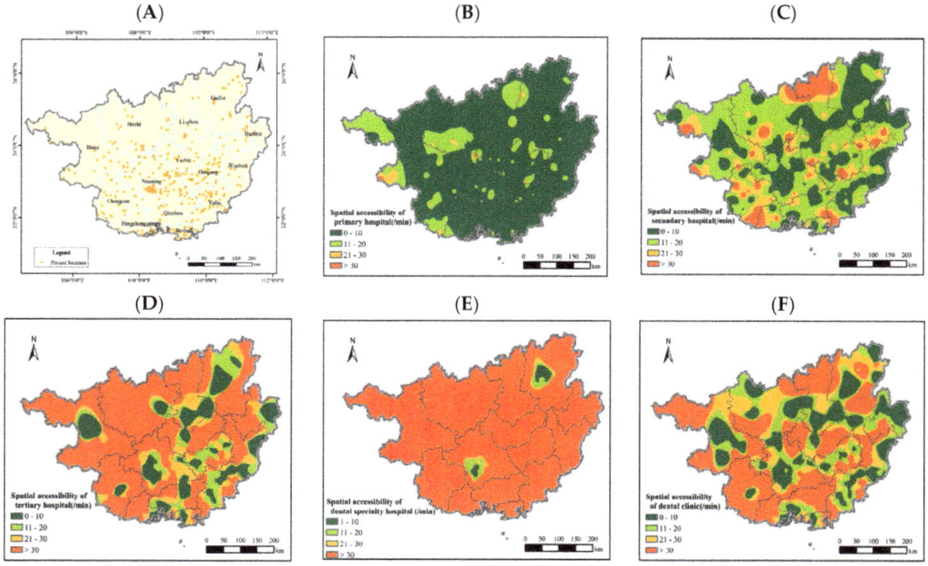

Figure 3. Analysis of the accessibility of medical and health services for oral cancer patients in Guangxi under the mode of automobile travel. ((**A**): Spatial distribution of residence of oral cancer patients in Guangxi; (**B–F**): accessibility of health services to primary, secondary, and tertiary hospitals, dental specialty hospitals, and oral clinics under the automobile travel mode).

3.3. Overall Model Establishment

Feature selection was performed using machine learning methods to remove irrelevant and redundant features and retain representative informative features. In this study, a feature selection method based on the recursive feature elimination (RFE) of logistic regression was used to select factors in the data before and after the lifting of the restrictions of the pandemic (Figure 4). Ten factors were selected before the relaxation: marital status, living with others, the person lived with, the follow-up status of systemic disease, the impact of COVID-19, HL2, HL3, access to knowledge, checking the mouth regularly, and the nearest medical facility. Eighteen factors were selected after the relaxation: living with others, the person lived with, medical staff as friends/relatives, medical insurance type, the type of self-medication, the impact of COVID-19, smoking dosage, second-hand smoking, the consumption of areca nuts, HL1, HL2, HL3, HL score, heath literacy level, presumed cause, checking the mouth regularly, brushing frequency, and the accessibility of secondary care facilities.

Venn diagrams were used to analyze unique or shared factors before and after the lifting of the restrictions of the pandemic. As shown in Figure 5, six shared factors were identified: checking the mouth regularly, HL2, HL3, the impact of COVID-19, living with others, and the person who lives with them. These six factors were included in all the study subjects, and four models were constructed. The hyperparameters of the four machine learning models were adjusted through ten-fold cross-validation, and the optimal hyperparameter combination was determined from each model with the best predictive performance (Figure 6). The ROC curve AUC values of the models were ranked from high to low using random forest (0.838), the RBF SVM (0.809), nearest neighbors (0.787) and QDA (0.776). DeLong's test was used to compare the ROC curve AUC values of random forest with the other three models (the bottom right of Figure 7). The results showed that there was no statistically significant difference in the AUC values between the random forest and nearest neighbors, RBF SVM, and QDA ($p > 0.05$). However, random forest had the highest AUC score (0.8380) and specificity (0.8077) on the test set, and its accuracy (0.7071), precision (0.7115), sensitivity (0.7071), and f1-score (0.7032) were all above 0.70, indicating excellent performance (Table 4).

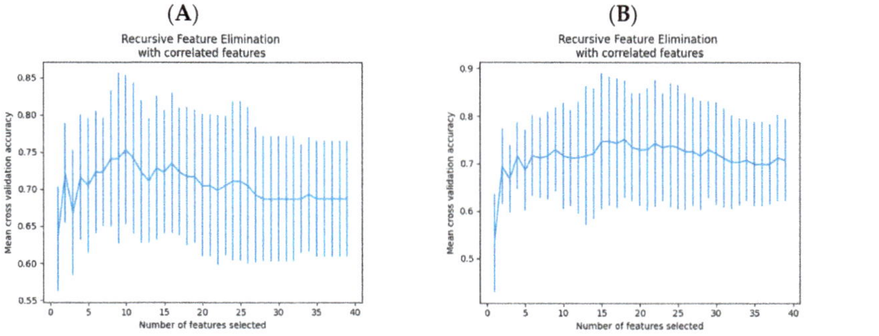

Figure 4. Recursive feature elimination with correlated features ((**A**): features that were screened before the lifting of pandemic restrictions; (**B**): features that were screened after the lifting of pandemic restrictions).

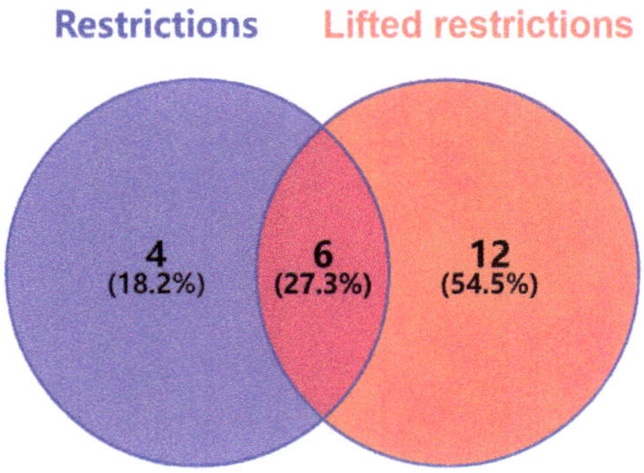

Figure 5. Venn diagram for analysis of common influencing factors before and after lifting of restrictions of pandemic.

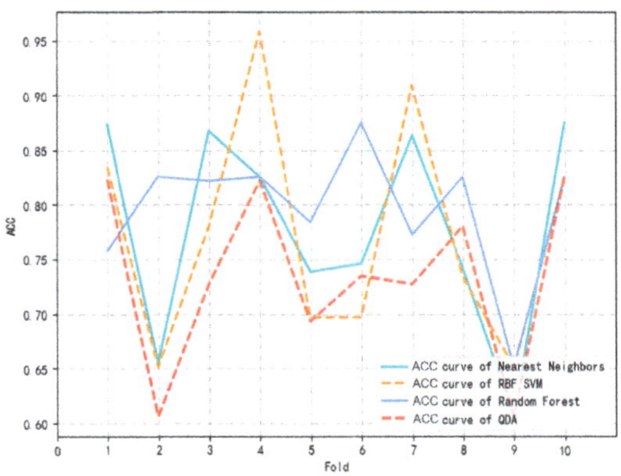

Figure 6. 10-fold ross-validation ACC change chart.

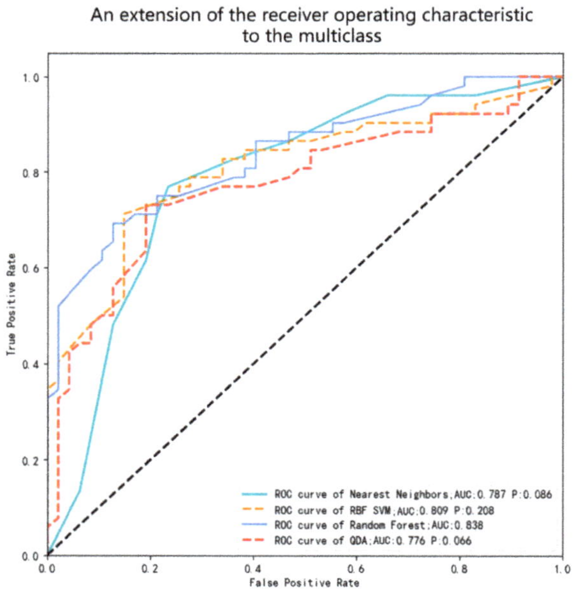

Figure 7. ROC curve of the prediction effectiveness of four models (nearest neighbors, the RBF SVM, random forest, and QDA) on the risk of patient delay behavior for oral cancer in Guangxi.

Table 4. Comparison of comprehensive performance of machine learning prediction models.

	Random Forest	Nearest Neighbors	RBF SVM	QDA
test set				
accuracy	0.7071	0.7677	0.7273	0.6566
AUC score	**0.8380** *	0.7866	0.8089	0.7762
sensitivity	0.7071	0.7677	0.7273	0.6566
specificity	**0.8077** *	0.7692	0.7885	0.8077
precision	0.7115	0.768	0.7282	0.6651
f1-score	0.7032	0.7678	0.7259	0.6469

* Statistically signifcant.

In summary, the overall model built with the random forest algorithm had the best predictive performance. The two sets of data before and after the lifting of the restrictions of the pandemic were, respectively, input into the model, with AUC values of 0.76 and 0.81, showing stable performance (Figure 8).

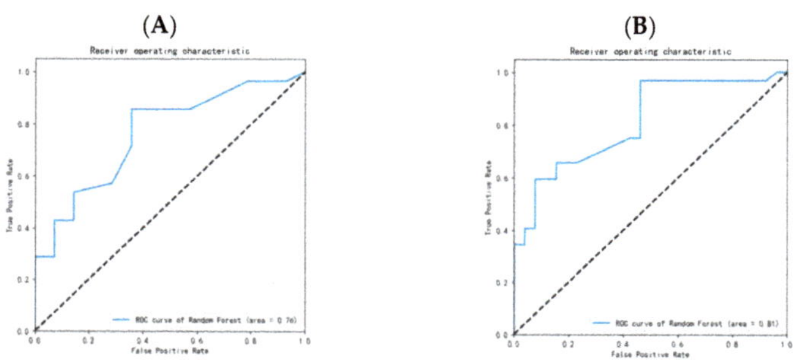

Figure 8. ROC curve of prediction efficiency of random forest model for delayed risk of oral cancer in Guangxi ((**A**): ROC curve before lifting of restrictions of pandemic; (**B**): ROC curve after lifting of restrictions of pandemic).

3.4. Model Stability Assessment

To test the stability of the established overall model's predictive effect, the two sets of data before and after the lifting of the restrictions of the pandemic were each randomly divided into three groups, and the overall and group data were input into the model to test the stability of the indicators of its predictive effectiveness. Since the data did not meet the normal distribution in the normality test ($p < 0.05$), non-parametric tests were used. The results indicated that there were no significant differences in the data indicators across each group ($p > 0.05$), confirming that the model remains stable regardless of whether it is applied to data before or after the lifting of pandemic restrictions, meaning it is not impacted by changes in pandemic prevention and control measures (Table 5).

Table 5. Comparison of comprehensive performance stability of prediction models.

	Group A	Group A (1)	Group A (2)	Group A (3)	Data B	Group B (1)	Group B (2)	Group B (3)	Z	*p*
n	208	69	69	70	287	96	96	95		
test set accuracy	0.7619	0.7857	0.7857	0.7143	0.7071	0.6500	0.6500	0.7368	−2.045	0.057
AUC score	0.7628	0.7708	0.7917	0.9271	0.8125	0.6700	0.6700	0.7670	−1 1620	0.3140
sensitivity	0.7619	0.7857	0.7857	0.7143	0.7414	0.6500	0.6500	0.7368	−1 7530	0.1140
specificity	0.8214	0.8750	0.8333	0.6250	0.6562	0.7000	0.6667	0.7500	−1.155	0.343
precision	0.7619	0.7873	0.7959	0.7440	0.7623	0.6515	0.7188	0.7439	−1 7320	0.1140

(Group A: data before lifting of restrictions of pandemic; Group B: data after lifting of restrictions of pandemic).

3.5. Model Explainability Analysis

The SHAP graph importance results based on the RF model are shown in Figure 9. In the variable SHAP graph, each sample is represented by one point. The horizontal axis represents the SHAP value of the feature, which indicates the impact distribution of each feature on the model's output. The color represents the feature value, with high values represented by red and low values represented by blue. The vertical axis reflects the feature importance ranking. The factors that have a greater impact on the delay in seeking medical treatment for oral cancer patients are as follows: the person lived with >the impact of COVID-19 > the difficulty level of seeking help from others for misunderstood hospital materials (HL2) > the difficulty level of understanding one's health condition through written information (HL3) > checking the mouth regularly > living with others or not.

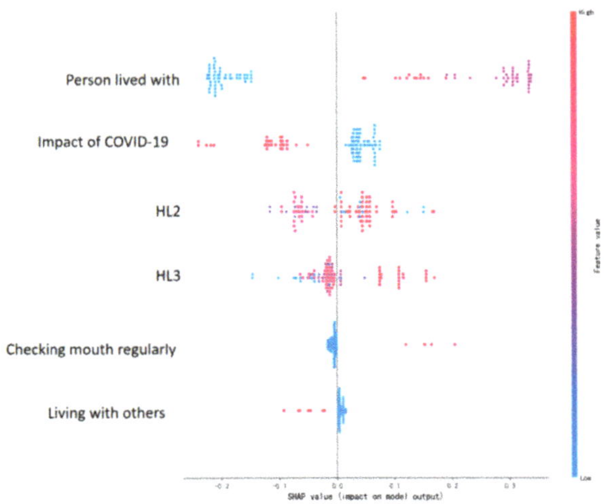

Figure 9. SHAP diagram of risk prediction characteristics of delayed medical treatment for oral cancer patients in Guangxi based on random forest model.

4. Discussion

In 1938, the concept of delay in seeking medical treatment came into being [7]. Scott SE and others summarized the results of eight similar studies and found that the occult nature of oral lesions and diagnostic delays were considered to be the cause of the high incidence of advanced oral cancer [8]. Delays in treatment before the onset of oral cancer can lead to disease progression to advanced disease, resulting in decreased survival rates [9]. Conversely, the early treatment of oral cancer has less damage and a better prognosis, with higher survival rates and quality of life for patients [10]. Fortunately, due to the discovery of a large number of risk factors, a long natural history, and the possibility of the visual inspection of lesions, the prevention of oral cancer is highly feasible [11]. This study is the first large-sample study of factors affecting the delay in seeking medical attention among oral cancer patients in western China, with high research value.

Inhabiting status has a significant impact on patient delay in seeking medical treatment. Previous research results have shown that there are significant differences in the disease burden of oral cancer by age [12], and the incidence and mortality of oral cancer gradually increase with age. Elderly people are a high-risk group for oral cancer. In this study, 42.6% of patients were over 60 years old. Population aging is a serious problem facing China, and it is expected that, by 2050, China will have 400 million elderly people over 65 years old, of which 150 million will be over 80 years old [13]. On the contrary, the number of people in the adult labor force is insufficient, which is related to the one-child policy introduced in 1980 and abolished in 2016. The way Chinese people take care of elderly people is generally dominated by children taking care of elderly people. In this study, the proportion of patients with adult children living with them who experienced delays in seeking medical attention was significantly lower than that of patients without adult children living with them, indicating a statistically significant difference. Adult children have received certain education, have good care ability and mobility, and can detect symptoms early and send patients to the hospital in time. Cohabitants are an important factor affecting patient medical behavior, which is also reflected in the SHAP graph of the risk prediction model.

With the development of urbanization, a large number of adult laborers in rural areas migrate to cities, and the population of "empty nest" elderly people in rural areas increases significantly. Elderly people lack the care and financial support of adult children [14]. These elderly people usually have more chronic diseases (two or more), and over time, they have become accustomed to and adapted to them, so they often ignore chronic symptoms and underestimate the conditions [15]. A large amount of elderly people even have to take care of the left-behind children, leaving elderly people in rural areas no time to take care of their health [16].

In response to the lack of care for "empty nest" elderly people, we suggest gradually addressing the issues of high medical costs and the insufficient coverage of medical insurance for these elderly individuals. It is essential to vigorously develop primary medical services and encourage general practitioners to serve at the grassroots level, providing them with economic and policy subsidies. Additionally, it is important to establish health records for permanent residents in the jurisdiction area and create chronic disease cards. In an oral cancer screening project conducted in Thailand, participants expressed a preference for home visits over going to the hospital themselves [17], which may be related to the older age of the patients and their relative distance from qualified hospitals. Therefore, we believe that home visit services should be fully implemented. Home visits are a supplement to outpatient services and can provide on-site examinations and treatments for elderly and physically challenged patients. The advantages of home visits also include the ability to understand and assess the patient's social support situation on-site, allowing for targeted treatment plans [18].

The place of residence and the accessibility of medical and health services have an effect on the behavior of patients with oral cancer seeking medical treatment. Geographical location and socio-economic inequalities have a significant impact on the occurrence of oral cancer [19,20]. High-incidence areas of oral cancer are mostly located in developing countries in Asia. China is a developing country in Asia, and Guangxi is an economically underdeveloped region in the western part of China, as well as an autonomous region inhabited by many ethnic groups. It has its uniqueness in geography, economy, culture, and medical and health resources. In this study, the difference in the impact of the accessibility of medical and health services on patients' delay in seeking medical attention was not statistically significant, which may be related to the fact that the sample was sourced from a single center. From Figure 3, we can understand the accessibility of Guangxi oral cancer patients to various levels of medical and health institutions.

In China, hospitals are divided into three levels and ten grades based on indicators such as hospital size, medical hardware equipment, talent, and technical strength. The primary institutions include community health service centers, township health centers, and village clinics. In recent years, China has made great efforts to improve the level of medical security in rural areas and reform and improve the operation mechanism of the rural medical and health system [21]. Primary medical and health service institutions have basically been popularized, and the results of this study also reflect this trend; under the mode of car travel, the accessibility level of first-level medical institutions is the highest, and urban and rural residents in Guangxi can conveniently reach primary medical and health institutions for medical treatment. However, the level of medical services provided by primary medical institutions is not optimal. In a study in Sichuan Province, the diagnostic accuracy of primary doctors in rural areas for unstable angina and type 2 diabetes was evaluated using standardized patient methods. A total of 172 rural primary doctors were included in the study, and 186 standardized patient visits were completed. The results showed that the correct diagnosis rate was only 48.39% [22]. In another survey on the cognitive level of primary doctors' knowledge of COPD, 229 rural doctors in Zigong City, Sichuan Province, had a cognitive level of COPD knowledge of only 14.4% [23]. In addition, 73 representative rural primary medical institutions were selected in Hubei, Guangxi, and Jiangxi to investigate the use rate of antibiotics in prescriptions, and it was found that all these institutions had the problem of antibiotic abuse [24]. This study also found that doctors in primary medical institutions tend to prescribe antibiotics for initial patients with "ulcers" or swellings in the mouth rather than referring them to higher-level institutions, which may delay the diagnosis of patient's condition [25].

Tertiary hospitals can provide high-level specialized medical and health services to several regions, and their locations are mostly in densely populated urban areas. However, oral cancer patients mostly live in remote rural areas with scarce medical resources, so their accessibility to tertiary medical institutions is poor. Oral specialty hospitals have the highest level of the diagnosis and treatment of oral cancer, but their accessibility is the worst. At present, Guangxi only has two oral specialty hospitals, located in Nanning and Guilin, the two major cities in Guangxi with relatively complete medical resources. Primary care physicians and dentists play an important role in referring oral cancer cases to specialist services. A study in Canada found that dentists are more likely than primary care physicians to detect asymptomatic cases [26]. Patients with oral cancer can first go to the oral department of a general hospital or an oral clinic for screening. The accessibility level of oral clinics is generally good, they are mostly located in densely populated urban areas and rarely in remote rural areas.

The uneven distribution of medical resources and the low level of the diagnosis and treatment of primary medical service institutions greatly affect the seeking behavior of oral cancer patients in Guangxi. To solve these problems, the government has implemented a medical consortium model, trying to promote communication and exchanges between local tertiary hospitals, secondary hospitals, and primary hospitals and accelerate the construction of primary medical information and the establishment of primary clinical pathways to improve the initial diagnosis ability of primary doctors for common diseases. Guangxi is also accelerating the construction of transportation infrastructure to improve people's convenience in accessing corresponding medical institutions.

The impact of the COVID-19 remains after the lifting of epidemic restrictions. As this study spans before and after the lifting of the restrictions of the epidemic, there was a decline in the utilization of medical services in hospitals during this period, with most people choosing to delay seeking medical care, even in urgent situations. Reports show that the number of emergency department visits decreased during the COVID-19 pandemic [27]; 41% of Americans delayed or avoided going to the hospital for urgent or non-urgent medical care due to COVID-19 [28], and in England, the delay in diagnosis caused by COVID-19 led to a significant increase in preventable cancer mortality [29]. In this study, COVID-19 was a significant factor in the delay in seeking medical care for oral cancer patients.

Six months after China lifted the restrictions of the pandemic, in May 2023, the Director-General of the World Health Organization, Tedros Adhanom Ghebreyesus, announced that the COVID-19 pandemic is now an established and ongoing health issue and no longer constitutes a public health emergency of international concern. However, even after lifting the restrictions of the pandemic, the behavior of oral cancer patients in seeking medical care is still affected, possibly because the aftermath of the pandemic has not yet dissipated. Since the lifting of the restrictions of the pandemic, the risk of contracting COVID-19 has greatly increased, especially for high-risk groups (elderly people, those with underlying diseases, etc.), who are more likely to develop severe symptoms. There is ample evidence that, after "recovery" from COVID-19, a considerable proportion of people experience sequelae in the immune, blood, respiratory, cardiovascular, digestive, and other systems [30]. One study included 443,588 participants with a primary infection, 40,947 with two or more infections, and 5,334,729 uninfected participants [31]. The researchers found that, compared to those with only one infection, individuals with repeated infections had a 2.17 times higher risk of all-cause mortality and a 3.32 times higher risk of hospitalization. Therefore, even if oral cancer patients notice their oral health issues, they may still choose to delay seeking medical care out of fear of contracting COVID-19; another scenario is that patients who have already contracted COVID-19 may choose to go to the hospital to address more urgent symptoms (such as respiratory symptoms, cardiovascular symptoms, etc.) rather than prioritizing oral health issues. However, how long the impact of the COVID-19 pandemic will last remains to be studied in the future.

Health literacy (HL) refers to the cognitive and social skills that determine an individual's motivation to seek, understand, and use information to promote and maintain good health [32]. This study uses the Brief Health Literacy Screen (BHLS) scale, which consists of three questions: (1) How confident are you filling out medical forms by yourself? (2) How often do you have someone (like a family member, friend, hospital/clinic worker, or caregiver) help you read hospital materials? (3) How often do you have problems learning about your medical condition or health because of difficulty understanding written information? The questionnaire uses a Likert five-point scale, where 1 represents very difficult and 5 represents no difficulty at all, with a total score of 15 points; a higher score indicates a higher level of HL. A total score of $\leq$9 indicates insufficient HL [33]. The advantages of this scale are its convenience and speed, and the questions are unlikely to cause patients to feel shame, sensitivity, or anxiety [34]. The scores of the three questions for patients who delay seeking medical care are lower than those of non-delayed patients. The SHAP graph of the risk prediction model shows that the difficult degree of seeking help from others for incomprehensible health information (HL2) and the difficult degree of learning about one's medical condition through reading hospital materials (HL3) are significant factors. Among patients with insufficient health literacy, 53% are over 60 years old. There are many reasons for insufficient health literacy, including low literacy levels, visual impairments, inability to write, and lack of young family members to assist, which make it difficult for patients to obtain health information through their own efforts or support from others, making it challenging to truly understand their medical conditions, directly affecting their behavior in seeking medical care. Having good health literacy is extremely important, as it allows patients to pay attention to oral health issues and even learn self-examination, thus allowing the early detection of oral diseases, timely medical care, and timely and effective treatment.

To improve patients' health literacy, it is essential first to popularize knowledge about oral cancer. In recent years, the government has proposed the Healthy China initiative; one of its major actions is the Health Knowledge Popularization Action, aimed at improving everyone's health literacy, encouraging medical staff to participate in health promotion and education work, and establishing a health science popularization platform using new media. In addition, we suggest that community workers deeply communicate with families and regularly provide one-on-one health guidance for elderly people with low cultural knowledge and mobility issues, increasing their attention to diseases, early detection, and timely medical care.

This study found that, among patients who delay seeking medical attention, the proportion of those with regular oral check-up habits and those who brush their teeth more than twice a day is lower than that of non-delayed patients. People who regularly see dentists are a group that regularly undergo oral cancer screening, which undoubtedly protects high-risk groups. A study in the UK found that oral cancers detected during "routine checks" are more likely to be in the early stages (stage 1 or 2) than those detected after symptoms appear [25]. A large randomized controlled trial on oral cancer screening conducted over 15 years in India showed that oral cancer screening reduced the mortality rate of high-risk groups by 24% [35]. Patients with regular oral check-up habits pay more attention to oral problems, can detect oral diseases in time, and are more willing to seek treatment for oral cancer in hospitals. In a study by the International Head and Neck Cancer Epidemiology Consortium (INHANCE) on the role of oral hygiene in head and neck cancer, they observed a negative correlation between the occurrence of head and neck cancer (HNC) and regular tooth brushing every day [36]. Oral hygiene habits are one of the factors affecting the incidence of oral cancer and also affect patients' behavior in seeking medical attention for oral cancer. Therefore, it is necessary to improve patients' oral hygiene habits and behaviors for the tertiary prevention of oral cancer.

The establishment of the random forest model has predictive significance. In this study, a risk prediction model for delayed medical attention was constructed based on machine learning algorithms, and the predictive effects of four prediction models, nearest neighbors, the RBF SVM, random forest, and QDA, on the delay in seeking medical treatment for oral cancer patients in Guangxi Province were compared and analyzed. This study found that the random forest (RF) model has the best predictive performance and is stable both before and after the lifting of the pandemic restrictions. RF randomly samples the original dataset to form different sample datasets, then builds different decision tree models based on these datasets, and finally obtains the final result based on the average value (for regression models) or voting (for classification models) of these decision tree models. To ensure the generalization ability of the model, random forests usually follow two basic principles when building each tree: data randomness and feature randomness. Its advantages include high classification accuracy, the ability to identify variable importance, and the ability to perform various types of data analysis. Currently, RF is a common ensemble learning method used for classification, regression, and other tasks [37]. In addition, the SHAP diagram ranks the six factors selected according to their importance and directly explains their impact on the medical behavior of oral cancer patients, providing evidence for public health policymakers and healthcare providers to early identify high-risk groups of oral cancer and take corresponding measures.

Since December 2019, the COVID-19 pandemic has swept across the world, and pandemic prevention and control work face serious challenges at present. Due to the particularity of oral diagnosis and treatment, patients cannot wear masks during oral diagnosis and treatment, and close face-to-face contact between doctors and patients greatly increases the risk of infection. Therefore, before the lifting of the restrictions of the pandemic, oral clinics adopted a relatively strict triage system [38]. For suspected or confirmed COVID-19 or close contacts of COVID-19, treatments were postponed as much as possible until after the infection period or the end of self-isolation, which undoubtedly affected the visiting behavior of oral cancer patients. On 7 December, the state announced the "Notice on Further Optimizing and Implementing COVID-19 Prevention and Control Measures," and after three years of COVID-19 prevention and control in China, the novel coronavirus infection returned from initial Class A management to Class B management. This study included patients who visited the hospital from June 2022 to July 2023, which was a transition period from the strict control to the gradual orderly opening of the COVID-19 pandemic, so the impact of the pandemic should be fully considered. We conducted a stability assessment of the established model and found that it has stability whether applied to data before or after the relaxation of pandemic prevention and control measures, meaning it is not affected by changes in COVID-19 pandemic prevention and control.

5. Limitations

This study has some limitations. The sample comes from a single-center convenience sample, making it difficult to directly verify the impact of the level of accessibility of medical and health services on the delayed medical behavior of oral cancer patients. In addition, the constructed model has not been externally validated. Future research will consider multi-center studies, and subsequent research should pay more attention to the practical application value, optimize variable settings, emphasize external validation to further optimize the model, and demonstrate the external adaptability of the model.

6. Conclusions

In summary, factors such as cohabitation status, being affected by the COVID-19 pandemic, the mode of transportation used to seek medical treatment, patients' health literacy, oral examination habits, ways to obtain oral knowledge, oral hygiene habits, the distance between residence and medical institutions, etc., are factors affecting patients' delay in seeking medical treatment. The random forest model constructed based on the data of the delayed medical treatment of oral cancer patients in this study has a good predictive performance and can be used to predict the risk of delayed medical treatment for oral cancer patients in Guangxi Province, providing a reference for public health policymakers and healthcare providers in western China to early identify high-risk groups of oral cancer and take corresponding measures.

Supplementary Materials: The following supporting information can be downloaded at: https://www.mdpi.com/article/10.3390/healthcare12222252/s1, Table S1: Single factor analysis.

Author Contributions: Conceptualisation, Y.Y. and J.H.; data curation, Y.Y. and H.N.; formal analysis, H.N. and J.Y.; methodology, J.Z. and J.Y.; supervision, J.H.; validation, Y.Y. and H.M.; visualization, B.L. and Y.Y.; writing—original draft, Y.Y. and H.N.; writing—review and editing, J.H. and J.Z. All authors have read and agreed to the published version of the manuscript.

Funding: This research was supported by funding from the National Natural Science Foundation of China (Grant/Award Number: 82260586).

Institutional Review Board Statement: This research was approved by the Stomatology Hospital Affiliated to Guangxi Medical University (the ethical code: 2023006; the date of approval: 7 February 2023).

Informed Consent Statement: Written informed consent has been obtained from the patients to publish this paper.

Data Availability Statement: The data that support the findings of this study are available from the Hospital of Stomatology, Guangxi Medical University, but restrictions apply to the availability of these data, which were used under license for the current research, and so are not publicly available. Data are however available from the authors upon reasonable request and with the permission of the Hospital of Stomatology, Guangxi Medical University. The datasets generated during and/or analyzed during the current study are available from the corresponding author on reasonable request.

Conflicts of Interest: The authors declare no competing interests.

References

1. Sarode, G.; Maniyar, N.; Sarode, S.C.; Jafer, M.; Patil, S.; Awan, K.H. Epidemiologic aspects of oral cancer. *Dis.-a-Mon.* **2020**, *66*, 100988. [CrossRef] [PubMed]
2. Macpherson, L.M.D. Raising awareness of oral cancer from a public and health professional perspective. *Br. Dent. J.* **2018**, *225*, 809–814. [CrossRef]
3. Allison, P.; Franco, E.; Feine, J. Predictors of professional diagnostic delays for upper aerodigestive tract carcinoma. *Oral Oncol.* **1998**, *34*, 127–132. [CrossRef] [PubMed]
4. Shen, Y.; Shi, Y.; Wang, H.; Sun, B. The impacts of medical facility accessibility on patients' medical treatment space: A case study in shanghai. *Urban Dev. Stud.* **2019**, *26*, 46–52.
5. da Cunha Lima, A.M.; Meira, I.A.; Soares, M.S.M.; Bonan, P.R.F.; Mélo, C.B.; Dalle Piagge, C.S.L. Delay in diagnosis of oral cancer: A systematic review. *Med. Oral Patol. Oral Y Cirugia Bucal* **2021**, *26*, e815. [CrossRef]
6. Guyon, I.; Weston, J.; Barnhill, S.; Vapnik, V. Gene Selection for Cancer Classification using Support Vector Machines. *Mach. Learn.* **2002**, *46*, 389–422. [CrossRef]
7. Torti, R.A.; Winship, T. Culpability for delay in the treatment of breast cancer. *Med. Ann. Dist. Columbia* **1963**, *32*, 132–133. [PubMed]
8. Scott, S.E.; Grunfeld, E.A.; McGurk, M. The idiosyncratic relationship between diagnostic delay and stage of oral squamous cell carcinoma. *Oral Oncol.* **2005**, *41*, 396–403. [CrossRef]
9. Atula, M.; Aro, K.; Irjala, H.; Halme, E.; Jouppila-Mättö, A.; Koivunen, P.; Wilkman, T.; Blomster, H.; Mäkitie, A.; Atula, T. Patient and health care delays in large (class T3–T4) oral, oropharyngeal, and laryngeal carcinomas. *Head Neck* **2023**, *45*, 1215–1225. [CrossRef]
10. Ford, P.J.; Farah, C.S. Early detection and diagnosis of oral cancer: Strategies for improvement. *J. Cancer Policy* **2013**, *1*, e2–e7. [CrossRef]
11. Elango, K.J.; Anandkrishnan, N.; Suresh, A.; Iyer, S.K.; Ramaiyer, S.K.; Kuriakose, M.A. Mouth self-examination to improve oral cancer awareness and early detection in a high-risk population. *Oral Oncol.* **2011**, *47*, 620–624. [CrossRef] [PubMed]
12. Du, M.; Nair, R.; Jamieson, L.; Liu, Z.; Bi, P. Incidence Trends of Lip, Oral Cavity, and Pharyngeal Cancers: Global Burden of Disease 1990–2017. *J. Dent. Res.* **2020**, *99*, 143–151. [CrossRef]
13. Fang, E.F.; Scheibye-Knudsen, M.; Jahn, H.J.; Li, J.; Ling, L.; Guo, H.; Zhu, X.; Preedy, V.; Lu, H.; Bohr, V.A.; et al. A research agenda for aging in China in the 21st century. *Ageing Res. Rev.* **2015**, *24*, 197–205. [CrossRef] [PubMed]
14. Wu, Y.; Zhang, Q.; Huang, Y.; Qiu, S. Seeking medical services among rural empty-nest elderly in China: A qualitative study. *BMC Geriatr.* **2022**, *22*, 202. [CrossRef]
15. Leung, J.T.Y. Perceived parental sacrifice, filial piety and hopelessness among Chinese adolescents: A cross-lagged panel study. *J. Adolesc.* **2020**, *81*, 39–51. [CrossRef]
16. Zhou, R.Y.; Wang, J.J.; Ma, B.X. The mental and psychological problems in left-behind children in China. *Pediatr. Res.* **2020**, *87*, 802–803. [CrossRef] [PubMed]
17. Klongnoi, B.; Sresumatchai, V.; Clypuing, H.; Wisutthajaree, A.; Pankam, J.; Srimaneekarn, N.; Shrestha, B.; Khovidhunkit, S.P. Histopathological and risk factor analyses of oral potentially malignant disorders and oral cancer in a proactive screening in northeastern Thailand. *BMC Oral Health* **2022**, *22*, 613. [CrossRef]
18. Kaiwen, Y.; Yue, J.; Fuying, Z. Implementation Effect of Home Care: A Case Report and Exploratory Home Follow-up Study. *Chin. Gen. Pract.* **2021**, *24*, 2880–2884. [CrossRef]
19. Dourado Martins, J.; Oliveira Mascarenhas Andrade, J.; Souza Freitas, V.; de Araújo, T.M. Social determinants of health and the occurrence of oral cancer: A systematic literature review. *Rev. Salud Publica (Bogota Colomb.)* **2014**, *16*, 786–798. [CrossRef]
20. Conway, D.I.; Petticrew, M.; Marlborough, H.; Berthiller, J.; Hashibe, M.; Macpherson, L.M. Socioeconomic inequalities and oral cancer risk: A systematic review and meta-analysis of case-control studies. *Int. J. Cancer* **2008**, *122*, 2811–2819. [CrossRef]
21. Sandager, M.T.; Rossen, S.; Hofland, D.T.; Nielsen, C.V.; Maribo, T. Health-related quality of life, needs, and concerns among cancer survivors referred to rehabilitation in primary healthcare setting. *Acta Oncol.* **2024**, *63*, 76–82. [CrossRef] [PubMed]
22. Zhou, Y.S.; Du, Y.; Wu, Y.J.; Ye, R.X.; Wang, Q.Z.; Sun, C.; Zheng, Q.M.; Zhou, H. Evaluation of Accuracy and Influencing Factors for Diagnosis of Two Chronic Diseases by Primary Healthcare Providers in Sichuan Rural Areas Based on Standardized Patients. *Zhongguo Yi Xue Ke Xue Yuan Xue Bao. Acta Acad. Med. Sin.* **2022**, *44*, 213–220. [CrossRef]
23. Liu, J.; Zheng, H.; Pan, H.; Ye, L.; Li, C. Perceptions of Chronic Obstructive Pulmonary Disease among Chronic Disease Managers in Primary Care in Rural Areas. *Chin. Gen. Pract.* **2023**, *26*, 877–885. [CrossRef]
24. Wang, W.j.; Xiao, L.Q.; Li, C. The utilization of essential medicines in rural primary medical institutions in poor or remote areas of three provinces (autonomous regions) in central and western China. *Chin. Health Resour.* **2017**, *20*, 490–494. [CrossRef]
25. Langton, S.; Cousin, G.C.S.; Plüddemann, A.; Bankhead, C.R. Comparison of primary care doctors and dentists in the referral of oral cancer: A systematic review. *Br. J. Oral Maxillofac. Surg.* **2020**, *58*, 898–917. [CrossRef]
26. Groome, P.A.; Rohland, S.L.; Hall, S.F.; Irish, J.; Mackillop, W.J.; O'Sullivan, B. A population-based study of factors associated with early versus late stage oral cavity cancer diagnoses. *Oral Oncol.* **2011**, *47*, 642–647. [CrossRef] [PubMed]
27. Schwarz, V.; Mahfoud, F.; Lauder, L.; Reith, W.; Behnke, S.; Smola, S.; Rissland, J.; Pfuhl, T.; Scheller, B.; Böhm, M.; et al. Decline of emergency admissions for cardiovascular and cerebrovascular events after the outbreak of COVID-19. *Clin. Res. Cardiol. Off. J. Ger. Card. Soc.* **2020**, *109*, 1500–1506. [CrossRef]

28. Czeisler, M.; Marynak, K.; Clarke, K.E.N.; Salah, Z.; Shakya, I.; Thierry, J.M.; Ali, N.; McMillan, H.; Wiley, J.F.; Weaver, M.D.; et al. Delay or Avoidance of Medical Care Because of COVID-19-Related Concerns—United States, June 2020. *MMWR Morb. Mortal. Wkly. Rep.* **2020**, *69*, 1250–1257. [CrossRef] [PubMed]
29. Maringe, C.; Spicer, J.; Morris, M.; Purushotham, A.; Nolte, E.; Sullivan, R.; Rachet, B.; Aggarwal, A. The impact of the COVID-19 pandemic on cancer deaths due to delays in diagnosis in England, UK: A national, population-based, modelling study. *Lancet Oncol.* **2020**, *21*, 1023–1034. [CrossRef]
30. Soriano, J.B.; Murthy, S.; Marshall, J.C.; Relan, P.; Diaz, J.V. A clinical case definition of post-COVID-19 condition by a Delphi consensus. *Lancet Infect. Dis.* **2022**, *22*, e102–e107. [CrossRef]
31. Bowe, B.; Xie, Y.; Al-Aly, Z. Acute and postacute sequelae associated with SARS-CoV-2 reinfection. *Nat. Med.* **2022**, *28*, 2398–2405. [CrossRef] [PubMed]
32. Mirzaie, A.A.; Hanson, N.C.; Neal, D.; Berceli, S.A.; Back, M.R.; Scali, S.T.; Huber, T.S.; Upchurch, G.R., Jr.; Shah, S.K. Limited health literacy is common among vascular surgery patients. *Surgery* **2024**, *175*, 1600–1605. [CrossRef] [PubMed]
33. Sand-Jecklin, K.; Coyle, S. Efficiently assessing patient health literacy: The BHLS instrument. *Clin. Nurs. Res.* **2014**, *23*, 581–600. [CrossRef] [PubMed]
34. Fan, Z.Y.; Yang, Y.; Yin, R.Y.; Tang, L.; Zhang, F. Effect of Health Literacy on Decision Delay in Patients with Acute Myocardial Infarction. *Front. Cardiovasc. Med.* **2021**, *8*, 754321. [CrossRef]
35. Sankaranarayanan, R.; Ramadas, K.; Thomas, G.; Muwonge, R.; Thara, S.; Mathew, B.; Rajan, B. Effect of screening on oral cancer mortality in Kerala, India: A cluster-randomised controlled trial. *Lancet* **2005**, *365*, 1927–1933. [CrossRef]
36. Hashim, D.; Sartori, S.; Brennan, P.; Curado, M.P.; Wünsch-Filho, V.; Divaris, K.; Olshan, A.F.; Zevallos, J.P.; Winn, D.M.; Franceschi, S.; et al. The role of oral hygiene in head and neck cancer: Results from International Head and Neck Cancer Epidemiology (INHANCE) consortium. *Ann. Oncol. Off. J. Eur. Soc. Med. Oncol.* **2016**, *27*, 1619–1625. [CrossRef]
37. Cutler, D.R.; Edwards, T.C., Jr.; Beard, K.H.; Cutler, A.; Hess, K.T.; Gibson, J.; Lawler, J.J. Random forests for classification in ecology. *Ecology* **2007**, *88*, 2783–2792. [CrossRef]
38. Zeng, X.J.; Qu, X.; Zhou, X.D. Routine Epidemic Prevention and Control and Treatment Process Reengineering of Outpatient Dental Care. *Sichuan Da Xue Xue Bao. Yi Xue Ban = J. Sichuan Univ. Med. Sci. Ed.* **2021**, *52*, 485–488. [CrossRef]

Journal of
Clinical Medicine

MDPI

Article

Development and Initial Testing of an Artificial Intelligence-Based Virtual Reality Companion for People Living with Dementia in Long-Term Care

Lisa Sheehy [1], Stéphane Bouchard [2,*], Anupriya Kakkar [1], Rama El Hakim [1], Justine Lhoest [2,3] and Andrew Frank [1]

1 Bruyère Research Institute, 43 Bruyère St., Ottawa, ON K1N 5C8, Canada; lsheehy@bruyere.org (L.S.); afrank@bruyere.org (A.F.)
2 Cyberpsychology Lab of UQO, Université du Québec en Outaouais, Gatineau, QC J8X 3X7, Canada
3 HEC Liège—École de Gestion, Université de Liège, 4000 Liège, Belgium
* Correspondence: stephane.bouchard@uqo.ca; Tel.: +1-819-595-3900 (ext. 2360)

Abstract: Background/Objectives: Feelings of loneliness are common in people living with dementia (PLWD) in long-term care (LTC). The goals of this study were to describe the development of a novel virtual companion for PLWD living in LTC and assess its feasibility and acceptability. **Methods**: The computer-generated virtual companion, presented using a head-mounted virtual reality display, was developed in two stages. In Stage 1, the virtual companion asked questions designed to encourage conversation and reminiscence. In Stage 2, more powerful artificial intelligence tools allowed the virtual companion to engage users in nuanced discussions on any topic. PLWD in LTC tested the application at each stage to assess feasibility and acceptability. **Results**: Ten PLWD living in LTC participated in Stage 1 (4 men and 6 women; average 82 years old) and Stage 2 (2 men and 8 women; average 87 years old). Session lengths ranged from 0:00 to 5:30 min in Stage 1 and 0:00 to 53:50 min in Stage 2. Speech recognition issues and a limited repertoire of questions limited acceptance in Stage 1. Enhanced conversational ability in Stage 2 led to intimate and meaningful conversations with many participants. Many users found the head-mounted display heavy. There were no complaints of simulator sickness. The virtual companion was best suited to PLWD who could engage in reciprocal conversation. After Stage 2, response latency was identified as an opportunity for improvement in future versions. **Conclusions**: Virtual reality and artificial intelligence can be used to create a virtual companion that is acceptable and enjoyable to some PLWD living in LTC. Ongoing innovations in hardware and software will allow future iterations to provide more natural conversational interaction and an enhanced social experience.

Keywords: virtual reality; long-term care; dementia; artificial intelligence; large language models; compassion; reminiscence; elderly; cognitive decline; cognitive impairment

1. Introduction

Dementia is a collection of signs and symptoms that affect memory, executive function, language, and problem-solving to a degree which impacts daily life [1]. In Canada, the number of people living with dementia is expected to double from approximately 500,000 to over 900,000 between 2022 and 2030 [2]. Different but still dramatic estimates are in place for OECD countries (dementia increasing by 50% between 2021 and 2040, from 21 million to 32 million people), and for the entire world (increasing by 166% between 2019 and 2050, from 57.4 million to 152.8 million people) [3,4]. Twenty-five percent of adults over 85 years old have dementia [5], many of whom will require extensive support. As of 2016, in Canada, 69% of the residents living in long-term care (LTC) were living with dementia [6].

Feelings of social isolation are common in residents living in LTC due to factors such as communication difficulties, cognitive impairment, physical limitations, a lack of visitors, and low staffing levels [7]. Loneliness and isolation are associated with depression and reduced quality of life in older adults [8]. People living with dementia (PLWD) are at a much higher risk of depression, with depression presenting in 20–45% of those with dementia compared to 3.0–4.5% of all adults aged 65 and older [9]. Therefore, depression is very common in LTC residents (up to 44% of LTC residents in Canada), and is associated with deteriorating function, decreased quality of life, aggression, conflict with staff, and withdrawal [10].

Increasing LTC residents' opportunities to interact socially contributes to improved mood and quality of life [11]. In one large study, person-centered care training for staff which promoted personalized activities and social interactions significantly improved the quality of life of LTC residents living with dementia [12].

Personalized activities, such as reminiscence therapy and storytelling, can be facilitated by photos, meaningful items (e.g., clothing or toys), music, or life stories (i.e., recorded oral histories), and can be used to improve communication, reinforce relationships between residents and caregivers, and strengthen family interactions [13]. Such therapy may reduce depression and improve the quality of life in LTC residents living with dementia [14]. Residents living with dementia can also interact with dolls, robotic pets, and social robots [15–18]. Robotic pets can respond to voice commands or touch while social robots can play simple video games, sing songs, or facilitate video calls. These innovations have been shown to improve communication, activity participation, mood, social interaction, and quality of life for older adults, residents living in LTC, and PLWD living in the community [15–18].

A novel approach to reducing the feelings of isolation and loneliness in PLWD living in LTC is through conversation with a computer-generated "virtual companion" presented while immersed in virtual reality (VR) using a head-mounted display. VR technology allows participants to become immersed in a computer-generated environment and interact via sensorimotor channels [19]. Furthermore, recent developments in large language model generative artificial intelligence (AI) now permit the interpretation of spoken inputs from a user, and the generation of emotionally appropriate responses [20]. By combining the technological potential of both VR (e.g., ref. [21]) and AI (e.g., ref. [22]), clinical benefits may be achieved.

PLWD living in LTC have been shown to react positively to VR technology [23,24]. Two studies of PLWD living in LTC reported no negative side-effects such as dizziness, nausea, or disorientation in VR sessions lasting up to an average of 8–10 min [25,26]. VR immersion in virtual nature, tourist locations, or relaxation scenarios has the potential to produce pleasure, well-being, improved mood, and alertness in PLWD, including those living in LTC [25–28]. LTC staff also believe that VR experiences can be beneficial to residents [29].

A virtual companion able to utilize aspects of immersive VR and AI may create an outlet for social interaction and conversation for PLWD living in LTC. In contrast to current AI applications dedicated to answering user queries, a virtual companion can actively engage the user to reminisce, potentially reducing loneliness and isolation, and improving quality of life [21]. Being immersed in VR and interacting with a conversational agent may also allow PLWD living in LTC to feel as though they are no longer in their LTC facility, a phenomenon called presence [30,31].

The goals of this study were to accomplish the following: (a) develop a novel virtual companion, presented using a head-mounted VR display, incorporating AI tools to allow conversational abilities, and (b) assess the feasibility and acceptability of this companion in PLWD living in LTC. Feasibility and acceptability assessments included the determination of the ease of use of the hardware and software for PLWD, the enjoyment and acceptability of the virtual companion, and the duration and quality of interactions between PLWD and the virtual companion [32].

2. Materials and Methods

The companion was developed in an iterative process followed by empirical data collection in a two-stage multi-method study design as defined by Elbanna [33], with each stage representing a different version of the virtual companion. At each stage, the development of the virtual companion is described, and the quantitative and subjective results of feasibility are reported to determine whether the intervention should be recommended for efficacy testing [32]. Research ethics approval was obtained from the Bruyère Research Ethics Board (Ottawa, ON, Canada; M16-21-032). The study conformed to the principles laid out in the Declaration of Helsinki and the Tri-Council Policy Statement: Ethical Conduct for Research Involving Humans in Canada.

2.1. Stage 1

2.1.1. Hardware

The virtual companion was run on an Omen desktop gaming computer (Hewlett-Packard: Mississauga, Canada) and was presented using the Meta Quest 2 VR head-mounted display (Meta: Menlo Park, CA, USA) connected to the computer via a Quest Link cable (Meta: Menlo Park, CA, USA). The Meta Quest 2 is equipped with integrated audio microphone and speakers. The optional Elite Strap (Meta: Menlo Park, CA, USA) was available for the improved support of the head-mounted display. Users wore a disposable eye mask for hygienic purposes.

The head-mounted display and controllers were cleaned before and after each use with Accel INTERVention hospital-grade sanitizing wipes (Diversey: Fort Mill, SC, USA) and disinfected with a CX1 UVC LED decontamination unit (Cleanbox Technology: Nashville, TN, USA).

2.1.2. Virtual Environment

The virtual environment and companion were developed by our team, which includes a cognitive neurologist with extensive experience assessing and treating PLWD, a clinical psychologist with extensive experience developing and deploying immersive VR for clinical applications, and a physiotherapist with a PhD in Rehabilitation Science having extensive clinical and research experience working with PLWD and older adults. More than ten clinicians and volunteers with experience working with PLWD, and a technical team with artistic and technical experience in VR and AI [34], were included. Every aspect of the development was created with the end-users (PLWD and their caregivers) in mind.

A virtual companion character, a young woman named "Kiera", was presented sitting on a couch in a living room, with the user immersed in VR seated across the room (Figure 1). The appearance of the virtual companion was determined following discussions among the research team, artistic impressions, and social psychology studies suggesting that people are more likely to feel comfortable talking to and confiding in women [35].

The virtual environment was developed using 3D StudioMax version 2021 (Autodesk: San Francisco, CA, USA), Unity Store Assets version 2021 (Unity Technologies, San Francisco, CA, USA), and Character Creator version 3.4 (Reallusion: Atlanta, GA, USA). The animations of the virtual companion were created using Deepmotion version 2 (San Francisco, CA, USA), UMotions version 2021 (Soxware Interactive: Böhlerwerk, Austria), and Salsa version 2020 (Crazy Minnow Studio: Clear Lake, IA, USA). The virtual environment was rendered in stereoscopy using the Unity 3D engine version 2021 (Unity Technologies: San Francisco, CA, USA).

In Stage 1, the virtual companion interacted with the user using three AI modules: (a) speech-to-text (Recognissimo version 2021 from bluezzzy: San Francisco, CA, USA), (b) interpreting the intent of the text message and selecting pre-scripted replies (Neural-intents Library version 2021 from NeuralNine: Neuberg an der Mürz, Austria, and Flask Library version 1.1.1 in Python: Vienna, Austria), and (c) text-to-speech (using pre-scripted sentences with Speechelo 2021 from Videly Marketing: Dumbravita, Romania). The implemented solution required an operator to start the application, after which the virtual companion introduced herself and then spoke one of eight questions intended to encourage conversation and foster reminiscence, such as "Tell me something about your childhood". After the user replied, the virtual companion could recognize 14 different intentions in the user's sentence, and automatically reply with one of five responses inviting the user to continue the discussion, such as "Tell me more about that". If the application did not detect a response, the operator could manually trigger the companion to provide her own anecdote in order to give the user topics about which to converse. The virtual companion was able to recognize two questions: "Where am I?" and "Who are you?" and automatically respond appropriately. The operator could manually repeat questions, and adjust the volume. At the end of the conversation, the virtual companion concluded with "It was a pleasure chatting with you today". (See Lhoest, 2022 [34] for more technical details).

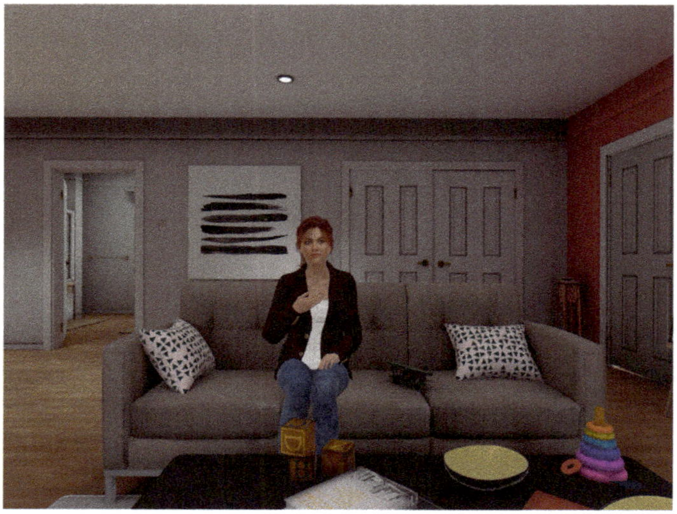

Figure 1. Screenshot of the virtual companion, "Kiera", as seen by the person immersed in virtual reality.

2.1.3. Participants

PLWD living in two LTC residences in Ottawa, Canada were recruited. PLWD were eligible for inclusion if they were diagnosed with dementia of any cause and severity, were not on quarantine measures due to COVID-19, and were able to understand and speak English. Participants were excluded from the study if they had any contraindications to immersive VR (such as hypersensitivity to motion sickness, uncontrolled mood disorder, or seizure disorder), were medically unstable, actively lightheaded or vertiginous, had neck pain or headache, or had an active infection of the face or eyes. Free and informed consent was obtained from the participants' substitute decision makers (the same person who would provide consent for medical decisions). While the participants were not deemed able to provide full consent for research, they could understand the general methods of the proposed study and what impact it may have on them. Interest in participating was obtained from the potential participants before contacting their substitute decision maker. Once consent was obtained, the participants provided verbal assent to the study at each contact point with the research team.

Demographic data were collected to describe the participant sample: age, gender, and Cognitive Performance Scale score indicating the level of dementia [scored from 0 (intact) to 6 (very severe impairment)] [36].

The LTC staff who worked directly with the participants provided free and informed consent to provide feedback on their observations of the participants' interactions with the virtual companion.

2.1.4. Feasibility and Acceptability Measures

The number of sessions per participant and the duration of each session with the virtual companion were recorded. The ease of use, comfort level, interaction and verbal communication with the virtual companion, apparent enjoyment, and interest to use the virtual companion again were collected from the PLWD, LTC staff, and the research team.

At the end of each participant's interaction with the virtual companion, the PLWD and LTC staff were asked questions in a semi-structured format (see Supplementary Files S1 and S2) to explore their interpretation of the experience. Suggestions for improvement were captured to aid in the ongoing iterative development of the virtual companion.

2.1.5. Procedure

A research team member was trained to plug the head-mounted display into the computer, open the application, and run the virtual companion in the VR environment using the operator interface. The participants were seated comfortably and provided with a disposable eye mask. The head-mounted display was adjusted so that the participant was comfortable and could see the VR environment. The participants then conversed with the virtual companion with minimal interruption. Support was provided for the participants after their experience if they expressed distress.

2.1.6. Subjective Analysis

The analysis of comments and semi-structured interviews were performed using a method similar to the framework coding method combining inductive and deductive components [37] using Excel 2019 spreadsheets. The coding and subsequent categorization included the following initial categories: hardware and software set-up, user experience, ease of conversation, and technology comments. As new feedback was collected, information was coded and previous codes and categories were adjusted. Disputes were discussed with a third researcher until consensus was obtained, and thematic relationships were established to analyze the data.

Demographic and user data were presented for each participant. Subjective data were categorized and summarized relative to each feasibility objective.

2.2. *Stage 2*

2.2.1. Hardware

The hardware in Stage 2 was identical to that used in Stage 1. The disposable eye masks were cumbersome for PLWD using the head-mounted display, so their use was discontinued.

2.2.2. Virtual Environment

The appearance of the virtual environment and companion remained the same as in Stage 1, except for small improvements to the animations of facial and non-verbal expressions, making the virtual companion appear friendlier. For example, the virtual companion smiled more and leaned forward at times to suggest active listening and interest in the conversation.

Significant modifications were included given the development of more powerful AI solutions for all three integrated AI modules. The speech-to-text module utilized Whisper version 2 (OpenAI: San Francisco, CA, USA). Importantly, the interpretation of the user's intent and generation of replies was performed by the AI Generative Pre-trained Transformer (GPT) 3.5 large language model application programming interface (API) (OpenAI: San Francisco, CA, USA). Within the GPT 3.5 API settings, the companion's persona was defined as a friendly nurse working with PLWD, who asks questions specifically to inspire reminiscence. Settings were created to automatically detect when the user stopped talking (i.e., a combination of minimal volume threshold to define a silence and duration of the silence), thereby removing the need for an operator to manually trigger responses. Text-to-speech of responses generated by GPT 3.5 was performed by ElevenLabs version 1 (ElevenLabs: New York, NY, USA) using a voice model selected from their library.

2.2.3. Participants

In Stage 2, LTC residents living in one LTC residence in Ottawa, Canada were recruited. Only residents with mild cognitive impairment or mild-to-moderate dementia were considered, as they were more able to carry on a fluent conversation. LTC staff members were not recruited in Stage 2. The same procedures as in Stage 1 were applied in obtaining free and informed consent.

2.2.4. Feasibility and Acceptability Measures

The outcome measures were identical to those used in Stage 1, with the exception that LTC staff members were not included.

2.2.5. Procedure

The procedure was identical to that used in Stage 1. If participants were willing and available, they were invited to engage with the virtual companion a second and third time. Up to three sessions with the virtual companion were offered to each participant, spread out over several weeks.

2.2.6. Subjective Analysis

The analysis was identical to that used in Stage 1.

3. Results

3.1. Stage 1

Ten PLWD living in LTC participated in Stage 1. The descriptive data and interactions with the virtual companion are reported in Table 1. The time spent interacting with the virtual companion ranged from 0:00 to 5:30 min, with an average of 2:48 min.

Table 1. Descriptive data and virtual companion interaction data for the Stage 1 research sample. All the participants participated in one session with the virtual companion. M—man; W—woman.

Participant Number	Gender	Age	Cognitive Performance Score	Length of Session (min:s)	Subjective Reports
2022-1	M	68	3	3:00	The participant had a natural conversation with reminiscence on topics they had not thought about for a long time.
2022-2	W	85	3	1:00	The participant did not speak to the virtual companion.
2022-3	M	81	3	0:00	The participant did not want to wear the head-mounted display.
2022-4	W	93	4	4:30	The participant engaged in some conversation, but used semi-coherent sentences. There was minimal reminiscing.
2022-5	W	74	5	2:00	There was minimal interaction. The participant was happy to be asked questions, and responded with a smile.
2022-6	M	85	3	3:30	The participant engaged with the virtual companion and seemed pleased to answer the questions.
2022-7	W	82	5	4:00	The participant did not interact verbally, but was happy to wear the head-mounted display.
2022-8	W	80	3	2:30	The participant did not seem to understand the virtual companion, and was not interested in interacting.
2022-9	M	84	3	2:00	There was a short interaction. The participant expressed enjoyment and thought that the virtual companion was "friendly".
2022-10	W	87	5	5:30	The participant responded to some questions but not others. There was some laughter.
Frequency or mean (standard deviation)	4 M 6 W	82 (6.9)	3.7 (0.9)	2:48 (1:42)	

3.1.1. Hardware and Software

Setting up the computer, monitor, cables, and head-mounted display was reported to be fairly simple for the trained research staff, and took less than 15 min. Six out of the ten PLWD and most LTC staff felt that the head-mounted display was comfortable, easy to wear, and well-fitted. However, for two out of the ten PLWD, the head-mounted display felt heavy, and for another two out of the ten, the head-mounted display shifted over their eyes easily, obscuring their view of the virtual environment. The Elite Strap was preferred by most users as it provided more support and allowed the head-mounted display to remain in place. The disposable eye masks frequently shifted and were difficult to place accurately over the eyes.

Several software challenges were experienced when setting up the Stage 1 version of the virtual companion. For example, the room with the virtual companion was sometimes seen to be tilted. This could be corrected with the operator interface. The sessions were brief given the limited options provided by the response generation module, which limited reciprocal conversation and deep exploration of any topic.

Prior to the conversation, there were occasions in which the virtual companion would not emit sound and had to be reloaded, or the software unexpectedly reverted to the loading screen. Frequently, the virtual companion experienced speech recognition issues due to a combination of software limitations and different patterns of speech often used by PLWD. The participants often mumbled, spoke few words at a time, or spoke in a quiet voice. The limited ability of the system to recognize speech or when the user was finished talking created both long pauses (if the participant spoke only a short phrase) and interruptions (if the participant talked more at length).

3.1.2. Feasibility and Acceptability, and Subjective Reports

The conversation with the virtual companion flowed relatively naturally for some, and many PLWD, especially those with milder dementia, engaged well. Participant 2022-9 commented that the virtual companion was "friendly, (and) questions were good". The LTC staff also observed that the virtual companion "is a friendly companion and asks interesting questions. Her few responses are well-done, and the anecdotes she gives are just the right length. Conversing with her is pleasant". Indeed, according to both PLWD and LTC staff, the personal anecdotes provided by the virtual companion were helpful to the overall interaction, inducing reminiscence, inviting positive memories, and increasing engagement. Another frequent comment was that the length of the conversation was too short, and that pauses between the questions were not sufficiently long enough to provide a response. The limited number of questions asked by the virtual companion limited reciprocal conversation. One PLWD was confused by the virtual companion and four PLWD did not converse at all. The reasons included an unwillingness to try on the head-mounted display, attempts to remove it as it was being positioned, or being unable or unwilling to speak to the virtual companion.

Because of the severity of their dementia, not all PLWD were able to answer the interview questions regarding their experience with the virtual companion. Participants 2022-4 and 2022-5 mentioned that it was "nice to speak to someone". A majority of the observed interactions involved good memories and social connection, and the LTC staff observed one participant engaging in what they felt was "a good chat". Three PLWD specifically noted that visiting with the virtual companion improved their day and that they would interact with her again.

Further, an LTC staff noted that the virtual companion "is a friendly companion and asks interesting questions. She has a good tone and it is not difficult to suspend disbelief when speaking to her. She imitates a human's behavior to a reasonable degree and the environment is welcoming". However, another LTC staff mentioned that the virtual companion "seems somewhat realistic but lacks nonverbal cues, and can sometimes come off as blunt and robotic".

There were no complaints of simulator sickness in Stage 1.

3.2. *Stage 2*

Ten new LTC residents living with cognitive impairment participated in Stage 2. The descriptive data and interactions with the virtual companion are reported in Table 2. The time spent interacting with the virtual companion ranged from 00:32 to 29:00 min for the first session (average 11:42 min), from 0:00 to 34:48 min for the second session (average 18:07 min), and from 1:07 to 53:50 min for the third session (average 29:39 min).

Table 2. Descriptive data and virtual companion interaction data for the Stage 2 research sample. M—man; W—woman.

Participant Number	Gender	Age	Cognitive Performance Score	Number of Sessions	Length of Session(s) (min:s)	Subjective Reports
2023-1	W	83	1	3	7:32 3:39 2:07	Session 1—The participant's voice was mistaken by the software for a language other than English. Session 2—There was an engaging conversation about the participant's children. The participant enjoyed how immersive the conversation was. Session 3 –The participant gave one-word answers, so the virtual companion kept asking new questions.
2023-2	W	87	1	3	25:00 25:00 53:50	The participant had stimulating, deep, and personal conversations about traveling, teaching, poetry, and death. The participant did not believe that the virtual companion was a real person.
2023-3	W	87	3	3	20:23 29:00 32:53	The participant was very engaged, and did not understand that the virtual companion was not a real person. The participant had deep and intimate conversations about their family.
2023-4	M	93	3	3	22:39 33:53 30:46	Session 1—The participant was engaged but the conversation was "all over the place". Session 2—The participant was very engaged, and talked about their farm. Session 3—This was primarily a question-and-answer conversation (with questions from the virtual companion), but the participant was engaged.
2023-5	W	92	3	1	0:32	The participant asked to take the head-mounted display off as they found it too heavy.
2023-6	W	93	1	2	29:00 34:48	The participant had very positive, lengthy conversations about their pet (Session 1) and cuisine/food (Session 2).
2023-7	W	96	2	2	2:23 9:10	Session 1—The conversation was dry, and the participant thought that the questions were "stupid". Session 2—The participant gave one-word answers so the software was not able to engage and respond appropriately.
2023-8	M	86	4	1	5:50	The participant answered questions but felt overwhelmed.
2023-9	W	86	2	2	0:52 0:00	Session 1—The participant had a hard time understanding the virtual companion but was willing to try a second time. Session 2—The participant immediately asked to remove the headset.
2023-10	W	67	3	2	2:49 9:29	Session 1—The participant took the head-mounted display off but was willing to try a second time. Session 2—The software had difficulty understanding the participant's speech (due to stuttering) but the participant appeared to enjoy the experience.
Frequency or mean (standard deviation)	2 M 8 W	87 (8.1)	2.3 (1.1)	2.2 (0.8)	Session 1: 11:42 (11:13) Session 2: 18:07 (14:04) Session 3: 29:54 (21:15)	

3.2.1. Hardware and Software

Nine out of the ten participants found that the head-mounted display was heavy, especially after a long time. However, six out of the ten also reported that it was "comfortable". For the participants with a reduced ability to hold their heads up, the Elite Strap was used for improved support. The head-mounted display did not fit well over eyeglasses.

Software challenges, such as error codes and freezing, tended to occur 25–30 min into the conversation. At times, the virtual companion unexpectedly started to speak words that were not English. At other times, the virtual companion interrupted the participants while they were talking. However, this did not necessarily create a negative experience according to the participants. The participants who had quiet and raspy voices, or spoke using single words or short phrases, were not able to trigger the microphone threshold to activate the listening mode of the AI speech-to-text module. When the participants provided long answers, the software processing time created long pauses in the conversation.

3.2.2. Feasibility and Acceptability, and Subjective Reports

Half of the participants enjoyed conversing with the Stage 2 version of the virtual companion and provided positive comments. Participant 2023-3 mentioned that "She really knows her stuff", and Participant 2023-2 observed that the virtual companion asked "... great questions, they seem to be written by a human and the questions were very stimulating and made me think". On the other hand, two participants found the interactions overwhelming. Participant 2023-9 stated that "She doesn't understand me and I don't understand her". Participant 2023-4 did not appreciate the virtual companion's many questions, stating that "Yes, I liked, but too fast, can't think, too many things".

The conversation topics varied widely. Many intimate and mentally stimulating conversations took place, such as reminiscing about loved ones, sharing personal experiences and interests, and recalling recent interactions with grandchildren. In many instances, the questions generated by the virtual companion showed great emotional intelligence. However, in one case, the participant was discussing her husband's death, and the virtual companion completely dismissed this, which seemed uncaring. While the conversations occasionally switched suddenly to other topics, most participants did not seem to notice. At the end of their session, one participant stated "Thank you so much, I usually don't talk this much".

There were varied opinions on the appearance and tone of the virtual companion. When asked if they liked the virtual companion and thought that they could trust her, Participant 2023-2 commented that the virtual companion appeared "too fake", "artificial", and "saw it was a robot". Participant 2023-1 stated that they "thought she was a real person at first and then realized she wasn't". However, according to Participant 2023-3, "She talks the way I feel. I like her. She is very friendly. It is like I have known her for years. I like that we feel the same".

Participant 2024-2 mentioned that the virtual companion's hand motions and facial expressions were "stiff" and "she doesn't imitate people". On the other hand, many participants found the companion to be very knowledgeable and interesting. Participant 2023-4 "liked her as a person to do business with, very nice, beautiful and very professional responses ... good at expressing words". Participant 2023-3 commented that "she sounds trustworthy to me. She tells a story like she has been there, makes me feel close to her".

Some participants felt that the experience improved their mood for the moment, though some did not find much value in it. Participant 2023-2 stated "it was fun, made me rethink. I would rather a real person, but it is better than nothing in an area with less people". Participant 2023-6 stated how the companion "... made me happy to see there is a person like this around", while Participant 2023-3 stated "I feel very comfortable, not shy". On the other hand, Participant 2023-7 felt "I think that she is alright, (but) I did not see any point in the conversation". Six out of ten participants agreed that they would be interested in spending time with the virtual companion again.

There were no complaints of simulator sickness in Stage 2.

4. Discussion

This project documents the iterative development of an AI-based "virtual companion", designed for PLWD, through two stages of development. Stage 1, while using a rudimentary version of the companion and AI tools, showed that some PLWD could tolerate wearing a VR head-mounted display and interact with the virtual companion for a few minutes. The software was limited in the questions the companion could pose, and there were delays and some difficulties with voice recognition. It was also recognized that not all PLWD would accept wearing the head-mounted display, or speaking to a stranger about personal topics. Nevertheless, the results supported proceeding to Stage 2.

Conversing with a virtual companion was more feasible for people with milder dementia who were much more verbal and likely to reminisce and tell stories. For this reason, the inclusion criteria were revised in Stage 2 to focus on participants with mild cognitive impairment or mild-to-moderate dementia.

During Stage 2, the virtual companion benefited from recent (as of the autumn of 2023) advances in AI technology to converse much more effectively on a broader range of topics. In particular, generative AI was used for the response module, and an AI solution able to generate natural speech in real time was employed for the text-to-speech module. Software limitations continued to cause conversation delays and interruptions. Because AI systems do not comprehend what the user is saying (for more on how large language models operate and reproduce human-like interactions, see [38]), it is difficult for AI systems to determine exactly when the user is finished expressing their thought. Indeed, a moment of silence when the user is speaking may represent a pause in the ongoing expression of an idea, mumbling, stuttering, a raspy voice, or in fact that the user is finished talking. The available speech-to-text module automatically processed audio information in one batch when the user was considered to be done talking, sometimes leading to noticeable delays while the system was processing all the information at once. At other times, there were interruptions by the virtual companion when users were still talking. However, the substantial increase in conversation length and positive feedback from several participants provided support for yet further development.

VR head-mounted display units are becoming more commonplace, and have been generally well tolerated by residents living in LTC, as well as their care staff [23,24,29]. In our study, a consistent complaint was that the headset was heavy. While the size and weight of VR head-mounted displays may decrease in the future, weight should be considered when choosing a particular display unit for use in this population. Some participants complained of itchiness and irritation, potentially caused by the silicone portion of the headset that contacted the skin, or the cleanser used to sanitize the unit. Furthermore, the head-mounted display did not fit comfortably over many styles and sizes of eyeglasses. Future versions of the virtual companion should be compatible with a variety of different head-mounted displays.

As noted, the availability of generative AI solutions enabled the virtual companion to converse in detail on topics of the user's choosing, for up to almost one hour. The use of more advanced AI technology will help to remove some of the conversation delays and interruptions, which will make interactions with the virtual companion smoother and more realistic. Tailoring the generative AI system to PLWD was very helpful, resulting in a seemingly emotionally intelligent companion able to inspire reminiscence. The focus on engaging the user to reminisce sets this application of AI apart from common applications which focus on decision-making support, assisting therapists, and counselling [39].

Findings from Stage 2 have led to yet further improvements to the virtual companion. Recent (as of the summer of 2024) AI solutions integrating speech, text, and response generation can circumvent many interruptions and delays associated with defining when the user has stopped talking. A new user interface allows choice among the different large language models (from GPT 3.5 to GPT 4o), AI text-to-speech models, and AI voices provided by OpenAI. Animations while the virtual companion is speaking have been improved. The experience can now take place in a virtual apartment or a virtual park (see Figure 2) providing more options to induce a positive mood [40] in people living in LTC.

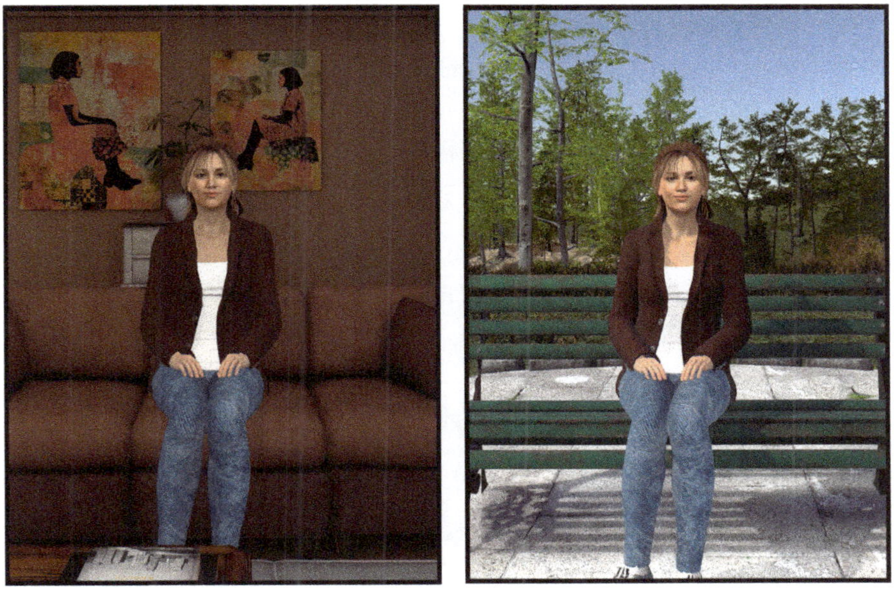

Figure 2. Screenshots of the improved virtual environments for the virtual companion in an apartment (**left**) or in a park (**right**).

The virtual companion was presented in an immersive VR environment using a head-mounted display. The advantage of immersive VR lies in the feeling of presence [30,31], which is the feeling of being somewhere else, rather than, for example, an LTC residence (i.e., the place illusion); the feeling that what is happening in VR is real (i.e., the plausibility illusion); and the feeling of engaging with a real person (i.e., social presence). Some participants made comments suggesting that they indeed experienced presence. Presence has been found to play a significant role in perceived social support [41], the motivation to use conversational agents in human–AI interactions [42], and anthropomorphism, the attribution of human characteristics to a non-human object [43]. The use of immersive VR platforms has led to improved cognitive and motor rehabilitation in PLWD [44]. One recent study [45] determined that the use of immersion during cognitive training provided greater benefits for global cognition than more conventional methods (such as paper-and-pencil or computer tasks) in people living with mild cognitive impairment. However, they found that lower levels of immersion provided more benefit than full immersion, possibly because older adults are less comfortable with full immersion technologies. Therefore, further study is necessary to investigate the role of immersiveness. Importantly, there were no complaints of simulator sickness in our PLWD participant sample, supporting the assertion that immersive VR is well tolerated by PLWD [25,26].

We used an animated computer-generated character instead of a photo-realistic image for the visual representation of the virtual companion. Complex real-time social interactions with photo-realistic images or 360-degree video recordings represent a technical challenge [46]. The impact of small imperfections in a photo-realistic image or in animations can create a sense of "eeriness", while a less life-like image may be more relatable. This tendency has been shown to be even greater in immersive VR [47,48]. Feedback from some participants was that the companion appeared blunt, robotic, stiff, or fake. However, others described her as friendly. Future iterations of the virtual companion will improve the animations of facial expressions and non-verbal behavior. Further studies should assess the impact of virtual companion characteristics (e.g., gender, ethnicity, appearance, and voice) and virtual contexts (e.g., locations relevant to users' life history). The impact of imperfections in verbal and non-verbal behaviors and interruptions must be assessed. Contrary to expectation, a lack of realism has been shown to be trivial among people with anxiety disorders [49] or substance use disorders [50] when the right stimuli were presented in the virtual environment to trigger emotional reactions.

Encouraging PLWD to engage with a virtual companion raises ethical considerations. PLWD may believe that the virtual companion is an actual person, and some participants did mention this. The use of generative AI in Stage 2 of our study increasingly produced human-like conversation, compounding this effect. It has been argued that a robot (or perhaps an AI conversational agent) that acts as if it cares for others can connect with older adults as well or better than human beings who may avoid emotional attachment [51]. So long as the use of a virtual companion does not negatively impact care by healthcare providers, and does not cause distress or become excessive, the benefits of a pleasant recreational activity meet the principles of respect for persons, beneficence, non-maleficence, and justice (for more on the ethics of using chatbots and conversational agents see [52,53]). Large language models have been known to be occasionally inaccurate or produce false claims that have been anthropomorphized by the term hallucination [38]. Although false statements or factual errors generated by AI may pose a risk to vulnerable populations, this is unlikely in an application which is designed to be empathetic and favor reminiscence. The virtual companion is designed to avoid engaging in discussions on delicate topics or providing advice, and to ask questions to the user instead of generating new ideas or explanations about factual events. Our application promotes and supports *reminiscence of a user's own personal history*, which limits the potential risk for people with mental or cognitive disorders of being exposed to inaccuracies, disinformation, or dangerous advice (for more on this topic, see [54]). Future applications should use AI models that are more interpretable and transparent in their internal processing, reasoning, and decision-making patterns than mainstream large language models, and they should use generative AI models specifically developed for empathy and the detection of emotional reactions (e.g., refs. [55–57]).

One limitation of this study is that the feasibility of caregivers or LTC staff directly operating the virtual companion was not tested. This will be assessed in future studies to determine if staff or other caregivers feel that using the virtual companion is both feasible and worthwhile. Reminiscence therapy [14,27] and virtual social interactions [17,18] can be quite beneficial for people living in LTC; therefore, testing the impact of AI-based VR companions on mood, quality of life, and responsive behaviors in PLWD via randomized controlled trials is necessary.

5. Conclusions

A virtual companion was created using multiple AI-based components to rapidly transform speech into text, generate complex and human-like responses, and rapidly engage in conversations using a naturalistic human voice. The virtual companion was presented to PLWD using a VR head-mounted display providing a virtual environment that differed significantly from their LTC facility. Twenty PLWD living in LTC interacted with the virtual companion, some through meaningful and prolonged conversations, providing proof-of-concept that this technology may be beneficial in this population. Ongoing innovations in hardware and software will allow virtual companions to provide more natural conversational abilities and an enhanced social experience.

Supplementary Materials: The following supporting information can be downloaded at: https://www.mdpi.com/article/10.3390/jcm13185574/s1, File S1: Semi-structured interview questions for people living with dementia, File S2: Semi-structured interview questions for long-term care staff.

Author Contributions: Conceptualization, A.F., L.S. and S.B.; methodology, A.F., L.S. and S.B.; software, S.B. and J.L.; validation, R.E.H., A.K. and L.S.; formal analysis, L.S., A.K., R.E.H., A.F. and S.B.; investigation, R.E.H., A.K. and L.S.; resources, S.B. and A.F.; data curation, R.E.H., A.K. and L.S.; writing—original draft preparation, L.S., A.K. and R.E.H.; writing—review and editing, L.S., S.B., A.F., A.K. and R.E.H.; visualization, L.S., S.B., A.F., A.K., R.E.H. and J.L.; supervision, L.S., A.F. and S.B.; project administration, L.S.; funding acquisition, A.F., S.B. and L.S.; accountable for all aspects of the work, A.F, L.S., S.B., A.K., R.E.H. and J.L. All authors have read and agreed to the published version of the manuscript.

Funding: This research was funded by Bruyère Academic Medical Organization (Incentive grant, no grant number), Centre for Aging + Brain Health Innovation (grant number SPARK-6-00449), BioTalent Canada (contract numbers 18750, 81450), The Canada Research Chairs (grant number 231039), and generous donations from the Burnside family to the Bruyère Research Institute.

Institutional Review Board Statement: The study was conducted according to the guidelines of the Declaration of Helsinki and the Canadian Tri-Council Policy Statement: Ethical Conduct for Research Involving Humans—TCPS 2, and approved by the Research Ethics Board of Bruyère Research Institute (M16-21-032; 31 August 2021).

Informed Consent Statement: Informed consent was obtained from all the participants' substitute decision makers and also from all the participants involved in the study.

Data Availability Statement: The dataset is not publicly available due to privacy and ethical restrictions. The data for this study is available upon request addressed directly to the Research Ethics Boards of the Bruyère Research Institute (REB@bruyere.org), which must first approve the request. If the request is approved, anonymized data supporting the conclusions of this manuscript will be made available by the corresponding author.

Acknowledgments: The authors would like to acknowledge all of the participants; the long-term care staff at Bruyère Continuing Care; and Marie-Christine Rivard, Simon Tremblay, and Rezza Amini for their work on the software.

Conflicts of Interest: LS owns a share in Engram Innovations and has received a research grant from AMS Healthcare. She is an AMS Healthcare Fellow. AF owns a share in Engram Innovations. SB is president and owner of Clinique et Development In Virtuo. He also owns a share in Engram Innovations. The terms and arrangements with theses spinoffs have been reviewed and approved by the Université du Québec en Outaouais in accordance with its Conflict of Interest policies. He also receives honoraria from conferences, workshops, and books.

References

1. Alzheimer's Association. (n.d.). *What Is Dementia? Alzheimer's Association*. Available online: https://www.alz.org/alzheimers-dementia/what-is-dementia (accessed on 5 September 2024).
2. Leaver, C.; Moroz, A. *There's Still Time: Paving a Path for Value-Based Dementia Care in Canada*; The Conference Board of Canada: Ottawa, ON, USA, 2022.
3. OECD. *Health at a Glance 2023: OECD Indicators*; OECD Publishing: Paris, France, 2023; pp. 216–217. [CrossRef]
4. Nichols, E.; GBD 2019 Dementia Forecasting Collaborators. Estimation of the global prevalence of dementia in 2019 and forecasted prevalence in 2050: An analysis for the Global Burden of Disease Study 2019. *Lancet Public Health* **2022**, *7*, e105–e125. [CrossRef] [PubMed]
5. Canadian Institute for Health Information (CIHI). (n.d.). *Dementia in* Canada: Summary; CIHI. Available online: https://www.cihi.ca/en/dementia-in-canada/dementia-in-canada-summary (accessed on 4 August 2022).
6. Canadian Institute for Health Information (CIHI). (n.d.). *Dementia in Long-Term Care*; CIHI. Available online: https://www.cihi.ca/en/dementia-in-canada/dementia-care-across-the-health-system/dementia-in-long-term-care (accessed on 9 August 2022).
7. Boamah, S.A.; Weldrick, R.; Lee, T.-S.J.; Taylor, N. Social isolation among older adults in long-term care: A scoping review. *J. Aging Health* **2021**, *33*, 618–632. [CrossRef]
8. Mushtaq, R.; Shoib, S.; Shah, T.; Mushtaq, S. Relationship between loneliness, psychiatric disorders and physical health? A review on the psychological aspects of loneliness. *J. Clin. Diagn. Res.* **2014**, *8*, WE01. [CrossRef] [PubMed]
9. Valkanova, V.; Ebmeier, K.P.; Allan, C.L. Depression is linked to dementia in older adults. *Practitioner* **2017**, *261*, 11–15. [PubMed]
10. Canadian Institute for Health Information (CIHI). *Analysis in Brief: Depression among Seniors in Residential Care*; CIHI: North York, ON, USA, 2010. Available online: https://secure.cihi.ca/free_products/ccrs_depression_among_seniors_e.pdf (accessed on 9 August 2022).

11. Beerens, H.C.; Zwakhalen, S.M.G.; Verbeek, H.; Tan, F.E.S.; Jolani, S.; Downs, M.; de Boer, B.; Ruwaard, D.; Hamers, J.P.H. The relation between mood, activity, and interaction in long-term dementia care. *Aging Ment. Health* **2018**, *22*, 26–32. [CrossRef]
12. Ballard, C.; Corbett, A.; Orrell, M.; Williams, G.; Moniz-Cook, E.; Romeo, R.; Woods, B.; Garrod, L.; Testad, I.; Woodward-Carlton, B.; et al. Impact of person-centred care training and person-centred activities on quality of life, agitation, and antipsychotic use in people with dementia living in nursing homes: A cluster-randomised controlled trial. *PLoS Med.* **2018**, *15*, e1002500. [CrossRef]
13. Park, K.; Lee, S.; Yang, J.; Song, T.; Hong, G.-R.S. A systematic review and meta-analysis on the effect of reminiscence therapy for people with dementia. *Int. Psychogeriatr.* **2019**, *31*, 1581–1597. [CrossRef] [PubMed]
14. Thomas, J.M.; Sezgin, D. Effectiveness of reminiscence therapy in reducing agitation and depression and improving quality of life and cognition in long-term care residents with dementia: A systematic review and meta-analysis. *Geriatr. Nurs.* **2021**, *42*, 1497–1506. [CrossRef]
15. Abbott, R.; Orr, N.; McGill, P.; Whear, R.; Bethel, A.; Garside, R.; Stein, K.; Thompson-Coon, J. How do "robopets" impact the health and well-being of residents in care homes? A systematic review of qualitative and quantitative evidence. *Int. J. Older People Nurs.* **2019**, *14*, e12239. [CrossRef]
16. Koh, W.Q.; Ang, F.X.H.; Casey, D. Impacts of low-cost robotic pets for older adults and people with dementia: A scoping review. *JMIR Rehabil. Assist. Technol.* **2021**, *8*, e25340. [CrossRef]
17. Martin-Garcia, A.; Corregidor-Sanchez, A.I.; Fernandez-Moreno, V.; Alcantara-Porcuna, V.; Criado-Alvarez, J.J. Effect of doll therapy in behavioral and psychological symptoms of dementia: A systematic review. *Healthcare* **2022**, *10*, 421. [CrossRef] [PubMed]
18. Yu, C.; Sommerlad, A.; Sakure, L.; Livingstone, G. Socially assistive robots for people with dementia: Systematic review and meta-analysis of feasibility, acceptability and the effect on cognition, neuropsychiatric symptoms and quality of life. *Ageing Res. Rev.* **2022**, *78*, 101633. [CrossRef] [PubMed]
19. Baus, O.; Bouchard, S. Moving from virtual reality exposure-based therapy to augmented reality exposure-based therapy: A review. *Front. Hum. Neurosci.* **2014**, *8*, 112. [CrossRef] [PubMed]
20. Colombatto, C.; Fleming, S.M. Folk psychological attributions of consciousness to large language models. *Neurosci. Conscious.* **2024**, *2024*, niae013. [CrossRef] [PubMed]
21. Ng, W.H.D.; Ang, W.H.D.; Fukahori, H.; Goh, Y.S.; Lim, W.S.; Siah, C.J.R.; Seah, B.; Liaw, S.Y. Virtual reality-based reminiscence therapy for older adults to improve psychological well-being and cognition: A systematic review. *J. Clin. Nurs.* **2024**, 1–16. [CrossRef]
22. Haque, M.D.R.; Rubya, S. An overview of chatbot-based mobile mental health apps: Insights from app description and user reviews. *JMIR Mhealth Uhealth* **2023**, *11*, e44838. [CrossRef]
23. Hosseini, M.; Thomas, R.; Pilutti, L.; Fallavollita, P.; Jutai, J.W. Assessing virtual reality acceptance in long-term care facilities: A quantitative study with older adults. *Disabil. Rehabil. Assist. Technol.* **2023**, 1–12. [CrossRef]
24. Rmadi, H.; Maillot, P.; Artico, R.; Baudouin, E.; Hanneton, S.; Dietrich, G.; Duron, E. Tolerance of immersive head-mounted virtual reality among older nursing home residents. *Front. Public Health* **2023**, *11*, 1163484. [CrossRef]
25. Appel, L.; Appel, E.; Bogler, O.; Wiseman, M.; Cohen, L.; Ein, N.; Abrams, H.B.; Campos, J.L. Older adults with cognitive and/or physical impairments can benefit from immersive virtual reality experiences: A feasibility study. *Front. Med.* **2020**, *6*, 329. [CrossRef]
26. Pardini, S.; Gabrielli, S.; Gios, L.; Dianti, M.; Mayora-Ibarra, O.; Appel, L.; Olivetto, S.; Torres, A.; Rigati, P.; Trentini, E.; et al. Customized virtual reality naturalistic scenarios promoting engagement and relaxation in patients with cognitive impairment: A proof-of-concept mixed-methods study. *Sci. Rep.* **2023**, *13*, 20516. [CrossRef]
27. Moyle, W.; Jones, D.; Dwan, T.; Petrovich, T. Effectiveness of a virtual reality forest on people with dementia: A mixed methods pilot study. *Gerontologist* **2018**, *58*, 478–487. [CrossRef] [PubMed]
28. Lin, C.X.; Lee, C.; Lally, D.; Coughlin, J.F. Impact of virtual reality (VR) experience on older adults' well-being. In *Human Aspects of IT for the Aged Population: Applications in Health, Assistance, and Entertainment*; Zhou, J., Salvendy, G., Eds.; Springer: Cham, Switzerland, 2018; pp. 129–140. [CrossRef]
29. Moore, R.C.; Hancock, J.T.; Bailenson, J.N. From 65 to 103, older adults experience virtual reality differently depending on their age: Evidence from a large-scale field study in nursing homes and assisted living facilities. *Cyberpsychol. Behav. Soc. Netw.* **2023**, *26*, 886–895. [CrossRef] [PubMed]
30. Berthiaume, M.; Corno, G.; Nolet, K.; Bouchard, S. A novel integrated information processing model of presence. *Presence* **2021**, *27*, 378–399. [CrossRef]
31. Slater, M. Place illusion and plausibility can lead to realistic behaviour in immersive virtual environments. *Philos. Trans. R. Soc. B Biol. Sci.* **2009**, *364*, 3549–3557. [CrossRef]
32. Bowen, D.J.; Kreuter, M.; Spring, B.; Cofta-Woerpel, L.; Linnan, L.; Weiner, D.; Bakken, S.; Kaplan, C.P.; Squiers, L.; Fabrizio, C.; et al. How we design feasibility studies. *Am. J. Prev. Med.* **2009**, *36*, 452–457. [CrossRef]
33. Elbanna, S. *The Role of the Two-Stage Multimethod Design: Developing Relevant Strategy Measures for New Settings*; Sage Research Methods Cases Part 1; SAGE Publications Ltd.: Thousand Oaks, CA, USA, 2020. [CrossRef]
34. Lhoest, J. Développement d'un Agent Conversationnel Dans un Environnement de Réalité Virtuelle au Service des Personnes Atteintes de la Maladie d'Alzheime. Master's Thesis, École de Gestion de l'Université de Liège, Liège, Belgium, 2022.
35. Dindia, K.; Allen, M. Sex differences in self-disclosure: A meta-analysis. *Commun. Res.* **1992**, *19*, 462–482. [CrossRef]
36. Morris, J.N.; Fries, B.E.; Mehr, D.R.; Hawes, C.; Phillips, C.; Mor, V.; Lipsitz, L.A. MDS Cognitive Performance Scale. *J. Gerontol.* **1994**, *49*, M174–M182. [CrossRef]

37. Gale, N.K.; Heath, G.; Cameron, E.; Rashid, S.; Redwood, S. Using the framework method for the analysis of qualitative data in multi-disciplinary health research. *BMC Med. Res. Methodol.* **2013**, *13*, 117. [CrossRef]
38. Hicks, M.T.; Humphries, J.; Slater, J. ChatGPT is bullshit. *Ethics Inf. Technol.* **2024**, *26*, 38. [CrossRef]
39. Arbanas, G. ChatGPT and other chatbots in psychiatry. *Arch. Psychiatry Res.* **2024**, *60*, 137–142. [CrossRef]
40. Di Pompeo, I.; D'Aurizio, G.; Burattini, C.; Bisegna, F.; Curcio, G. Positive mood induction to promote well-being and health: A systematic review from real settings to virtual reality. *J. Environ. Psychol.* **2023**, *91*, 102095. [CrossRef]
41. van Brakel, V.; Barreda-Angeles, M.; Hartmann, T. Feelings of presence and perceived social support in social virtual reality platforms. *Comput. Hum. Behav.* **2023**, *139*, 107523. [CrossRef]
42. Jin, S.V.; Youn, S. Social presence and imagery processing as predictors of chatbot continuance intention in human-AI-interaction. *Int. J. Hum.–Comput. Interact.* **2022**, *39*, 1874–1886. [CrossRef]
43. Konya-Baumbach, A.; Biller, M.; von Janda, S. Someone out there? A study on the social presence of anthropomorphized chatbots. *Comput. Hum. Behav.* **2023**, *139*, 107513. [CrossRef]
44. Ren, Y.; Wang, Q.; Liu, H.; Wang, G.; Lu, A. Effects of immersive and non-immersive virtual reality-based rehabilitation training on cognition, motor function, and daily functioning in patients with mild cognitive impairment or dementia: A systematic review and meta-analysis. *Clin. Rehabil.* **2024**, *38*, 305–332. [CrossRef]
45. Papaioannou, T.; Voinescu, A.; Petrini, K.; Stanton Fraser, A. Efficacy and moderators of virtual reality for cognitive training in people with dementia and mild cognitive impairment: A systematic review and meta-Analysis. *J. Alzheimer's Dis.* **2022**, *88*, 1341–1370. [CrossRef] [PubMed]
46. Restout, J.; Bernache-Assollant, I.; Morizio, C.; Boujut, A.; Angelini, L.; Tchalla, A.; Perrochon, A. Fully immersive virtual reality using 360 videos to manage well-being in older adults: A scoping review. *J. Am. Med. Dir. Assoc.* **2023**, *24*, 564–572. [CrossRef]
47. Hepperle, D.; Ödell, H.; Wölfel, M. Differences in the uncanny valley between head-mounted displays and monitors. In Proceedings of the 2020 International Conference on Cyberworlds (CW), Caen, France, 29 September–1 October 2020. [CrossRef]
48. Hepperle, D.; Purps, C.F.; Deuchler, J.; Wölfel, M. Aspects of visual avatar appearance: Self-representation, display type, and uncanny valley. *Vis. Comput.* **2022**, *38*, 1227–1244. [CrossRef]
49. Robillard, G.; Bouchard, S.; Fournier, T.; Renaud, P. Anxiety and presence during VR immersion: A comparative study of the reactions of phobic and non-phobic participants in therapeutic virtual environments derived from computer games. *Cyberpsychol. Behav.* **2003**, *6*, 467–476. [CrossRef]
50. Simon, J.; Etienne, A.M.; Bouchard, S.; Quertemont, E. Alcohol craving in heavy and occasional alcohol drinkers after cue exposure in a virtual environment: The role of the sense of presence. *Front. Hum. Neurosci.* **2020**, *14*, 124. [CrossRef]
51. Waschmuth, I. Robots like me: Challenges and ethical issues in aged care. *Front. Psychol.* **2018**, *9*, 432. [CrossRef]
52. Beauchamp, T.L. The 'Four Principles Approach' to health care ethics. In *Principles of Health Care Ethics*; Ashcroft, R.E., Dawson, A., Draper, H., McMillan, J., Eds.; John Wiley Sons: Hoboken, NJ, USA, 2007; pp. 3–11.
53. Portacolone, E.; Feddoes, D.E. Should artificial intelligence play a role in cultivating social connections among older adults? *Am. Med. Assoc. J. Ethics* **2020**, *25*, E818–E824. [CrossRef]
54. Monteith, S.; Glenn, T.; Geddes, J.R.; Whybrow, P.C.; Achtyes, A.; Bauer, M. Artificial intelligence and increasing misinformation. *Br. J. Psychiatry* **2024**, *224*, 33–35. [CrossRef]
55. Joudeh, I.O.; Cretu, A.-M.; Bouchard, S. Predicting the arousal and valence values of emotional states using learned, predesigned, and deep visual features. *Sensors* **2024**, *24*, 4398. [CrossRef] [PubMed]
56. Gomez-Zaragozá, L.; Marín-Morales, J.; Parra Vargas, E.; Alice Chicchi Giglioli, I.; Alcaniz Raya, M. An Online Attachment Style Recognition System Based on Voice and Machine Learning. *IEEE J. Biomed. Health Inform.* **2023**, *27*, 5576–5587. [CrossRef]
57. Parra, E.; Chicchi Giglioli, I.A.; Philip, J.; Carrasco-Ribelles, L.A.; Marín-Morales, J.; Alcañiz Raya, M. Combining Virtual Reality and Organizational Neuroscience for Leadership Assessment. *Appl. Sci.* **2021**, *11*, 5956. [CrossRef]

AI

MDPI

Article

Probabilistic Ensemble Framework for Injury Narrative Classification

Srushti Vichare, Gaurav Nanda and Raji Sundararajan *

School of Engineering Technology, Purdue University, West Lafayette, IN 47907, USA; svichar@purdue.edu (S.V.); gnanda@purdue.edu (G.N.)
* Correspondence: raji@purdue.edu

Abstract: In this research, we analyzed narratives from the National Electronic Injury Surveillance System (NEISS) dataset to predict the top two injury codes using a comparative study of ensemble machine learning (ML) models. Four ensemble models were evaluated: Random Forest (RF) combined with Logistic Regression (LR), K-Nearest Neighbor (KNN) paired with RF, LR combined with KNN, and a model integrating LR, RF, and KNN, all utilizing a probabilistic likelihood-based approach to improve decision-making across different classifiers. The combined KNN + LR ensemble achieved an accuracy of 90.47% for the top one prediction, while the KNN + RF + LR model excelled in predicting the top two injury codes with a very high accuracy of 99.50%. These results demonstrate the significant potential of ensemble models to enhance unstructured narrative classification accuracy, particularly in addressing underrepresented cases, and the potential of the proposed probabilistic ensemble framework ML models in improving decision-making in public health and safety, providing a foundation for future research in automated clinical narrative classification and predictive modeling, especially in scenarios with imbalanced data.

Keywords: injury classification; injury narratives; machine learning models; ensemble models

1. Introduction

Injury classification categorizes injuries by location, severity, cause, and type, which is an essential part of tracking public health and safety by understanding the underlying causes and circumstances of injuries and, thus, preventing them and minimizing harm. It also helps in achieving better diagnosis and treatment of injuries [1]. Multiple public health agencies and organizations are involved in the collection and classification of injury narratives from hospital emergency rooms (ERs). The narratives collected at ERs are analyzed by these agencies by assigning different types of diagnostic injury codes, such as their nature, cause, and severity. In the US, the Consumer Product Safety Commission (CPSC) maintains the National Electronic Injury Surveillance System (NEISS), which collects comprehensive narratives outlining the circumstances leading to accidents caused by consumer products [2]. The narratives collected at ERs are crucial for understanding causes and concerns with product safety. The narratives allow public health experts to study and track injury patterns, spot new hazards, and create focused preventive measures. After the narratives are categorized into a structured form by assigning injury diagnostic codes, the statistical analysis of classified injury narratives provides insightful information about the common causes and conditions that lead to injuries. However, the manual approach to categorizing these narratives into injury codes is time-consuming and prone to errors. Previous studies have used machine learning (ML)-based approaches for classifying injury narratives, but the accuracy has been observed to be limited for individual ML models due to the large number of prediction categories and noisy nature of narratives [3–7].

This motivated us to study the prediction performance of three state-of-the-art ML models and different ensemble models, based on their probabilistic likelihood of correctness, in classifying product-related injury narratives.

2. Literature Review

Researchers studied the use of narrative analysis for describing the mechanisms of injury and comparing patterns of work-related fatalities in New Zealand, Australia, and the United States [3]. The study underscored the potential of narrative analysis to bridge these gaps by offering a consistent framework for comparing work-related fatalities across countries. The research revealed the narrative analysis's need in examining work-related deaths by offering an innovative perspective alongside conventional coding methods. The analysis improved the knowledge of job safety and aids in creating more focused preventive measures for different countries and sectors. The narrative analysis minimized misclassification by enabling researchers to use narrators' own words, fixing coding inaccuracies in complex cases [4]. While narrative analysis has its merits, it also presents obstacles that necessitate a structured coding process. Thus, ML techniques are seen to be a substitute for the tedious, manual coding of narratives, offering a faster and efficient classification process.

Fuzzy Bayesian models and automated techniques demonstrated promising results in the past, precisely classifying cause-of-injury codes from narratives and in the capacity to separate out cases for human evaluation [5,6]. Classifying injury narratives from large administrative databases has been made easier with a semi-automated method utilizing Naïve Bayesian algorithms. The method yielded an overall accuracy of 87% and has significantly reduced the requirement for manual review [7]. The rapid development of ML and natural language processing (NLP) technology has provided a viable path towards automating classification, improving precision, and facilitating continuous surveillance [8].

In another study, an NLP framework was deployed to identify e-scooter-related injuries from over 36 million clinical notes [9]. This NLP approach involved refining regular expression techniques previously developed to identify emergency room (ER) visits related to e-scooter injuries. The framework was trained and tested using a three-stage process on ER visit notes. The training data included notes containing keywords, such as "scooter" and specific e-scooter brand names. The NLP model incorporated an ensemble random multi-model deep learning (RMDL) technique that combined convolutional neural networks (CNNs) and deep neural networks (DNNs) to enhance accuracy. The model used global vectors for word representation (GloVe) and term frequency–inverse document frequency (TF-IDF) to process the text, translating it into a series of vectors that convey semantic meaning and context. The combined scores from the CNN and DNN models were averaged through soft voting to determine the probability of an e-scooter injury. The algorithm indicated an overall accuracy of 92%, correctly classifying the majority of notes in the testing set [9].

In [10], researchers used a comprehensive methodology to predict injury severity using proactive and reactive data from a steel manufacturing plant in India. The dataset was merged to build a mixed dataset, which underwent several preprocessing steps to ensure data quality and manage complexities. The study addressed class imbalance by employing four state-of-the-art oversampling techniques: Synthetic Minority Over-sampling Technique (SMOTE), Borderline SMOTE (BLSMOTE), Majority Weighted Minority Oversampling Technique (MWMOTE), and k-means SMOTE (KMSMOTE). Six classification algorithms were used for injury severity prediction, with KMSMOTE being the most effective in balancing datasets and achieving a higher prediction accuracy. The Random Forest algorithm showed superior performance in terms of accuracy and robustness. The study demonstrated that by integrating proactive and reactive data, and effectively handling class imbalance, advanced ML models significantly improved injury severity prediction, offering valuable implications for safety management and preventive measures.

Van Eetvelde et al. [11] highlighted the growing use of ML in injury prediction and prevention. The researchers reviewed ML techniques, such as tree-based ensemble methods, SVM, and ANN, showcasing that ML models can identify high-risk factors. However, the review called for improved methodological rigor and data analysis and inclusion for optimal performance. These studies did not analyze the performance of the likelihood-based ensemble approach using combinations of simple and advanced ML models to classify product injury data; hence, in this study, the classification performance of the likelihood-based ensemble ML approach using three well-established ML models, K-Nearest Neighbor, Random Forest, and Logistic Regression, to classify product injury data was evaluated.

3. Methodology

3.1. Data Description

Injury narratives from the National Electronic Surveillance System (NEISS) [2], leveraging their concise and unstructured format, were utilized. The NEISS is an informative dataset managed by the U.S. Consumer Product Safety Commission (CPSC). The system collects data from over 100 hospitals across various healthcare settings, ensuring data representation and an accurate scale to reflect nationwide trends. NEISS is a critical tool for acquiring and assessing information about injuries, including those brought on by defective consumer goods, adverse drug events, and acts of violence. Preventive initiatives, product recalls, and public safety regulations have benefited from the use of NEISS data. The nationally representative hospitals in the United States and its territories feed the data into NEISS. Every ER visit associated with a consumer product or a kid under five years old's poisoning is reported by each member of the NEISS facility [2]. This dataset holds crucial data elements essential for understanding consumer product-related injury dynamics. It offers a demographic profile of those most affected by specific injuries, detailing the age, sex, race, and ethnicity of the injured. The data include detailed injury information, such as descriptions, affected body areas, diagnoses, and outcomes (treated and released or hospitalized), alongside product data highlighting potential risks and identifying involved consumer products. The data used for this research included detailed injury information, such as descriptions, affected body areas, diagnoses, and outcomes, alongside product data highlighting potential risks and identifying involved consumer products.

The NEISS data collection involved the following steps:

(1) User Affiliation: Affiliation was declared by selecting the category "researcher". This classification affects access and offers context for data usage.
(2) NEISS Data Highlights: Access to summary reports of data was granted through this section, with the selection of "Overview-All Products".
(3) Archived Annual NEISS Data: An Excel file was used for storing the raw data acquired for 2022.
(4) NEISS Estimates Query Builder: The NEISS Estimates Query Builder was utilized for specialized data gathering, enabling comprehension of injury codes with few samples (less than 100). Two files, "neiss2022.xlsx" and "DataDictionary042022.xlsx" were retrieved from the NEISS database from their website [2]. The "neiss2022.xlsx" file, which contains three distinct worksheets, namely, "NEISS_2022", "NEISS_FMT", and "Code Details", was utilized. Figure 1 shows a sample record, where the "Narrative_1" column was used as independent variable (X), and the "Diagnosis" column as the dependent variable (Y). The NEISS dataset's injury codes were decoded using the file "DataDictionary042022.xlsx". The document provided the meaning behind each digit in the injury code, including the kind of injury, body part, gender, and product type. Since the dataset was already processed, it did not contain any missing records.

There were a total of 323,344 data points, encompassing 30 unique codes. Table 1 lists the number of injury cases and description for each injury code in the NEISS data used for this research.

Age	Gender	Race	Body Part	Diagnosis	Product	Narrative_1
34	2	1	82	59	478	34YOF WAS WASHING A GLASS THAT BROKE. DX: LACERATION TO RIGHT HAND
11	2	1	82	53	3286	11YOF INVOLVED IN FOUR WHEELER TURNO-VER. DX: CONTUSION WITH ABRASION LEFT HAND.
12	2	1	30	53	3286	12YOF WITH MVA, WAS PASSENGER ON A FOUR WHEELER. DX: CONTUSION SHOULDER, CONTU-SION RIGHT KNEE.
38	2	1	75	62	698	38YOF, FELL X 4 DAYS GETTING OUT OF HOT TUB, SLIPPED HIT RT SIDE OF HEAD, + LOC DX; FALL, HEADACHE, CLOSED HEAD INJURY, RT KNEE CONTUSION, LT HAND CONTUSION

Figure 1. Sample records in NEISS data files.

Table 1. Data description of different diagnosis codes.

Sr. No	Diagnosis Code	Cause	Data Samples
1	41	Ingestion	3884
2	42	Aspiration	327
3	46	Burns, Electrical	79
4	47	Burns, Not Specified	94
5	48	Burns, Scald	2280
6	49	Burns, Chemical	455
7	50	Amputation	643
8	51	Burns, Thermal	2495
9	52	Concussions	6438
10	53	Contusions, Abrasions	34,775
11	54	Crushing	668
12	55	Dislocation	5113
13	56	Foreign Body	7028
14	57	Fracture	53,849
15	58	Hematoma	4453
16	59	Laceration	50,991
17	60	Dental Injury	1759
18	61	Nerve Damage	1414
19	62	Internal Organ Injury	42,451
20	63	Puncture	2467
21	64	Strain, Sprain	28,840
22	65	Anoxia	940
23	66	Hemorrhage	731
24	67	Electric Shock	192
25	68	Poisoning	4541
26	69	Submersion	380
27	71	Other/Not Stated	61,220

Table 1. *Cont.*

Sr. No	Diagnosis Code	Cause	Data Samples
28	72	Avulsion	2487
29	73	Burns, Radiation	135
30	74	Dermatitis, Conjunctivitis	2214

3.2. *Text Preprocessing*

The classification of injury narratives requires text preprocessing that converts unstructured text data into a more uniform and analytical structure. Text preprocessing involves steps that are necessary to enhance the interpretability of the text by ML models. The following preprocessing steps were carried out:

3.2.1. Tokenization

Narratives were divided into smaller units, such as words, phrases, and symbols. Analyzing and comprehending the structure and meaning of the text required this distinction. The algorithm took into consideration a number of linguistic quirks and norms, such as how contractions and multi-word sentences were handled.

3.2.2. Cleaning

Characters like punctuation, special symbols, and numerals that do not contribute to the meaning of the text were eliminated. This kind of text cleaning reduced the text's complexity and made it useful for the analysis to concentrate on its important aspects.

3.2.3. Normalization and Stop Words Removal

In order to reduce data dimensionality and the influence of lexical diversity, the text was standardized by changing its case to lowercase. The corpus was restructured by eliminating high-frequency stop words to allow for a more focused analysis on more significant words.

3.3. *Training and Test Data*

The preprocessed text was split into training and test datasets, following an 80/20 rule to ensure effective training and generalizability. With the allocation of 80% of the data to training, the model learned comprehensively and identified underlying patterns. The remaining 20% was used for testing that assessed the model's ability to generalize to new data. This strategic division facilitated the detection of overfitting and underfitting, enabling tuning to model complexity and training strategy. This approach optimized the ML model's performance across various injury codes and narrative contexts, enhancing its real-world application potential.

3.4. *Vectorization*

The preprocessed data were transformed into numerical vectors using Count Vectorizer (CV) and Term Frequency Inverse Document Frequency (TF-IDF) Transformer. Count Vectorizer tokenized text narratives by assigning unique features to each word across the corpus. This process enabled ML algorithms to understand the text's content with greater nuance. TF-IDF Transformer refined the textual data representation by calculating token importance based on term frequency within a document and inverse document frequency across the corpus [12]. The integration of CV and TF-IDF transformer accounted for the frequency and uniqueness of words, enhancing document disparity and classification based on thematic relevance [13].

3.5. Machine Learning Models

Three well-established ML models, K-Nearest Neighbor, Random Forest, and Logistic Regression that provided the output in form of prediction and associated likelihood of correctness of prediction, were used.

K-Nearest Neighbor (KNN), a versatile ML model, was utilized for classification tasks. It operates on the principle of instance-based learning, deferring its learning phase until a prediction is required. The core principle of KNN involves predicting the label of a new data point by assessing the "k" nearest labeled data points in the feature space. The "closeness" is determined using a Euclidean distance metric. For this research, KNN was chosen due to its effectiveness in big data analysis, owing to its simplicity and efficiency in handling massive datasets [14]. For each narrative, KNN was utilized to predict both the top 1 and top 2 injury classifications. This approach was adopted to provide a comprehensive understanding of the potential injuries associated with each narrative.

The Random Forest algorithm is an ensemble learning strategy used for classification, which enhances the decision tree method. RF integrates multiple trees to boost prediction accuracy and model stability [15]. The RF model for multiclass classification trains each tree in the forest to predict multiple classes. The training procedure creates bootstrap samples from the original dataset, and each sample is utilized to build a decision tree. RF addresses class imbalance by assigning class weights that effectively prioritize rarer classes. The approach ensures that the less frequented categories are accurately represented in the model's decision-making process.

Logistic Regression effectively extends to multiclass text classification, modeling the text sample's likelihood for predefined categories, and efficiently using the high-dimensional nature of textual data. The "multinomial" method was used to apply LR to injury classification. The approach directly modeled the likelihoods of categories. The model predicted that a given narrative belongs to each code using the SoftMax function, extending the logistic function to multiple categories [16]. This was achieved by computing a set of coefficients for each code that involved maximizing the likelihood of the observed data under the model. These coefficients then determined the influence of each feature on the likelihood of belonging to each category. The sign and magnitude of coefficients indicated the direction and strength of the relationship between features and the log-odds of category elements.

These models were implemented using scikit-learn, a Python library, with default parameters; no hyperparameter tuning was performed.

3.6. Ensemble Modeling

Different ensemble models that integrated the predictive capabilities of the LR, KNN, and RF [17] were developed. The ensemble approach combined the advantageous properties of classifiers into a framework to enhance prediction precision and reliability. The four ensemble models developed were as follows: the KNN + LR model, the KNN + RF model, the RF + LR model, and the KNN + LR + RF model. Combining KNN with LR, we leveraged KNN's ability to capture the nuances of local data structures and LR's powerful probabilistic classification ability. Similarly, making use of RF's strength to handle complex data interconnections and high dimensionality, with KNN's locality-based insights, the number of misclassifications by the individual models were minimized [18].

The third model along with LR used RF, known for its classification efficacy by aggregating multiple decision trees to minimize overfitting while retaining accuracy. The experimental setup and subsequent performance evaluation led to the development of the fourth model [18]. The comprehensive approach integrated the strengths of the KNN, LR, and RF models as depicted in Figure 2. By averaging the likelihood of each category, this model effectively harnessed the combined strengths of the individual models for a more accurate prediction of injury codes from narrative texts. This model enhanced the understanding of injury codes even with limited data points. Unlike conventional strategies that assign a single code to each narrative, these models are intended to predict two potential injury codes, reflecting the complex and diverse character of accidents, which often involve more than one type of injury. The classifier analyzed narratives for probable injury codes that targeted the top 1 (Top1) and top 2 (Top2) potential codes for each narrative. These Top1 and 2 codes were selected based on the likelihood/probability of correctness of prediction, provided as output by the model.

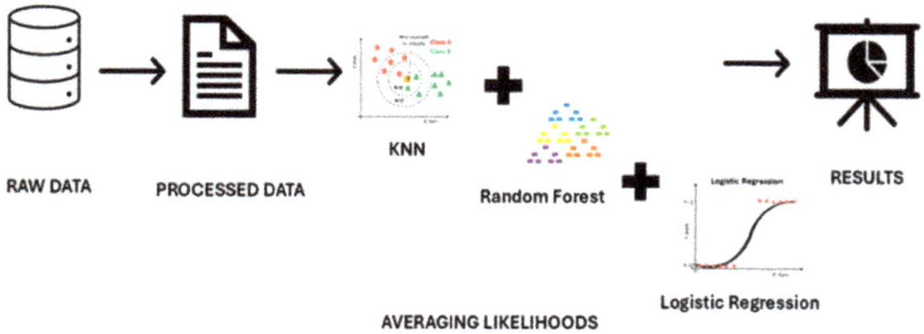

Figure 2. Schematic diagram of ensemble model.

4. Results and Discussion

The performance of these models was quantified using three well-established performance metrics used for machine learning: accuracy, precision, and recall, and the results were reported for both the top 1 (Top1) and top 2 (Top2) predictions. In this context, the Top1 accuracy represents the model's ability to correctly predict the primary injury code, while the Top2 accuracy extends this to include the model's second guess, increasing the chances of a correct prediction. Table 2 presents the performance evaluation metrics for individual ML models of KNN, RF, and LR in predicting the top 1 and 2 injury codes. KNN showed lower performance, particularly in precision and recall for the top 1 predictions, which can be attributed to its sensitivity to noise and reliance on distance measures. In contrast, RF and LR demonstrated superior accuracy in handling high-dimensional data, particularly for the top 2 predictions. LR surpassed RF in precision and recall, benefiting from its strength in binary outcomes and clear decision boundaries.

Table 2. Evaluation metrics of single machine learning models.

Performance Metrics (%)	KNN		RF		LR	
	Top1	**Top2**	**Top1**	**Top2**	**Top1**	**Top2**
Accuracy	71.3	83.6	90.2	97.5	92.2	98.6
Precision	78.2	51.5	89.0	55.5	91.6	55.2
Recall	65.4	77.1	64.9	81.2	77.9	89.7

The RF model showed superior performance in the Top1 predictions across all metrics, particularly in accuracy (90.19%) and precision (89.02%), indicating its effectiveness in correctly identifying the primary injury code with high reliability. The LR model, however, showed remarkable results in the Top2 accuracy (98.63%), suggesting its strength in providing a broader set of potential injury codes that likely include the correct one. Table 2 underscores the variability in model performance based on the metric considered, highlighting the need to balance precision (the model's ability to return relevant results) and recall (the model's ability to find all relevant instances) based on the application's requirements.

The detailed performance of the LR model for each category is shown as a confusion matrix in Figure 3. It depicts the LR model's performance in multi-class variation, highlighting the model's challenges in correctly classifying complex data due to high prediction errors and misclassifications. The results indicate that using a single model, such as LR, is ineffective for handling complex datasets, thus necessitating the need for ensemble models, which combine the strengths and capabilities of multiple algorithms to improve prediction accuracy and reduce errors.

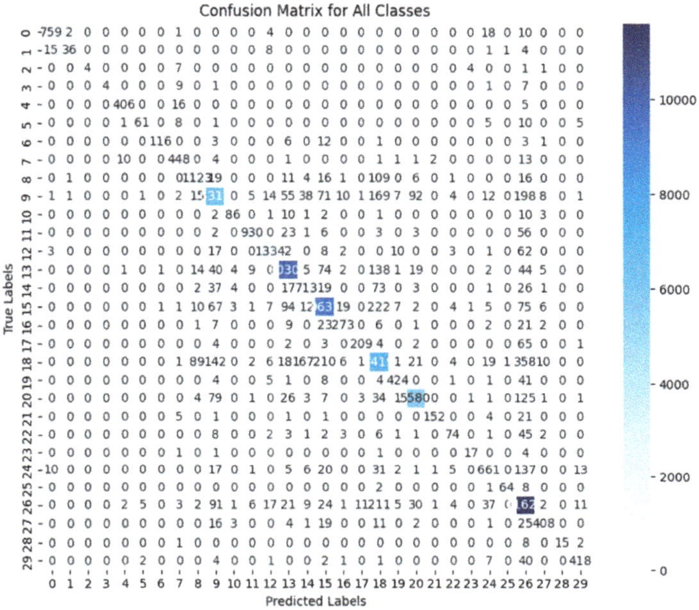

Figure 3. Confusion matrix of top-1 predictions of LR model.

Tables 3 and 4 indicate the analysis of ensemble models, which combine predictions from multiple ML techniques to improve overall prediction accuracy. Table 3 indicates the Top1 prediction performance of ensemble models made from different combinations of KNN, RF, and LR. The RF + LR ensemble showed the highest accuracy (92.27%) and precision (92.01%), suggesting that this combination is particularly effective at identifying the primary injury code accurately. The combination of all three models (KNN + RF + LR) proved to be the most accurate, demonstrating a significant improvement in predictive modeling. The differences in precision and recall among various combinations (e.g., KNN + LR, RF + LR) highlighted the unique advantages of each ensemble, owing to their strategic integration of base model capabilities. Compared to Table 2, showing that individual models had distinct performance limitations, the shift to ensemble methods was an effective strategy to overcome these challenges. While Table 2 presents the highest accuracy of 92.19% (LR for top 1) and 98.63% (LR for top 2), the peak ensemble accuracy in Table 3 is 97.36%. This improvement of up to 5.17% in the top 1 prediction confirms the effectiveness of combining different modeling techniques to address complex prediction tasks.

Table 3. Evaluation metrics of ensemble models—Top one prediction

Performance Metrics (%)	Ensemble Models			
	KNN + LR	**KNN + RF**	**RF + LR**	**KNN + RF + LR**
Accuracy	90.47	83.88	92.27	97.36
Precision	89.66	86.54	92.01	89.08
Recall	77.50	70.14	75.99	76.99

Table 4. Evaluation metrics of ensemble models—Top two predictions.

Performance Metrics (%)	Ensemble Models			
	KNN + LR	KNN + RF	RF + LR	KNN + RF + LR
Accuracy	97.12	95.16	98.50	99.50
Precision	53.04	53.30	59.50	60.23
Recall	88.54	83.58	88.04	88.03

Table 4 depicts the effectiveness of ensemble models in predicting the top two injury codes, representing a trend of improved accuracy and precision compared to single-model predictions. It shows that the ensemble methods address the limitations observed in single models within complex scenarios, as highlighted in Table 2. The KNN + RF + LR ensemble model excelled in accuracy, demonstrating its ability to integrate a broader range of relevant features for more precise predictions. The ensemble model had a drop in precision, from a peak of 91.51% (LR in Table 2 for top 1) to 60.23%. Despite this, the high recall rate compensated for the precision decline, indicating that while the ensemble predicted more than one code, it reliably identified the correct ones due to its comprehensive approach. By integrating the diverse strengths of KNN, RF, and LR, the ensemble model effectively navigated the complexities of the data, ensuring that relevant predictions were not missed.

Figure 4 shows the confusion matrix, illustrating the performance of the ensemble model with KNN, RF, and LR. The values along the diagonal are closer to zero, indicating more accurate predictions compared to the LR model alone. Misclassifications, represented by off-diagonal values, are reduced, suggesting that the ensemble model handles the data efficiently, overall, improving the accuracy and reducing extreme prediction errors.

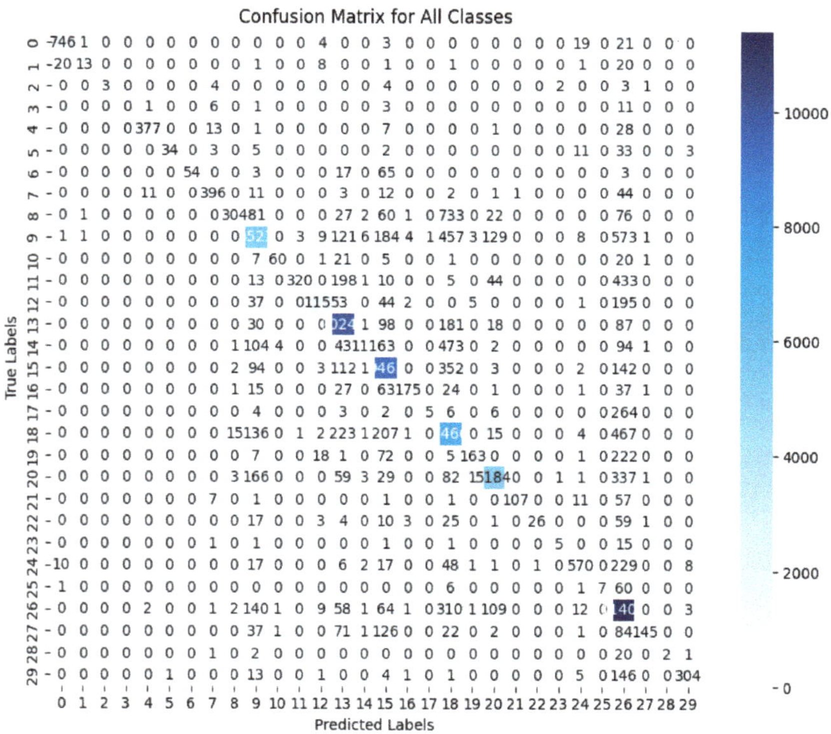

Figure 4. Confusion matrix for top-1 predictions of ensemble model KNN + RF + LR.

5. Conclusions

We developed ensemble models that enhanced the predictive performance across a number of criteria by combining three of the most popular ML models: K-Nearest Neighbor, Random Forest, and Logistic Regression. Our results indicate that ensemble models, especially the KNN +RF + LR combination, are highly effective for injury code prediction using NEISS data, providing a robust tool for accurately identifying injury types from narrative reports. The inclusion of both the Top1 and Top2 prediction evaluations offers a comprehensive view of each model's performance, emphasizing the trade-offs between capturing the most likely injury code and ensuring broader coverage to include possible alternatives.

The combined KNN, LR, and RF model indicated an accuracy of as high as 99.50% for the top two injury predictions, while the KNN + LR ensemble model showcased a robust predictive power with a high accuracy of 90.47%. Our results demonstrate that ensemble machine learning is a useful tool for enhancing clinical accident narrative classification, particularly when individual ML models do not yield a very high accuracy. Future research in clinical narrative analysis can utilize the presented ensemble ML models framework for decision support in injury surveillance and prevention.

The proposed ensemble models' ability to make multiple predictions enhanced reliability and also ensured that cases with fewer samples were considered, which might be overlooked by a conventional (single) prediction model due to underfitting. In real-world applications, this is particularly valuable because certain injury types or scenarios may be underrepresented in the data, making it challenging for a single model to make accurate predictions. The ensemble models address this issue by combining the strengths of multiple algorithms, ensuring that even rare or less common cases are captured in predictions. The ensemble model approach can, thus, aid in emergency response by accurately predicting and prioritizing critical injuries that are not frequently reported, ensuring appropriate resources are allocated in real-world applications.

Our findings demonstrate the potential of ensemble models to mitigate data scarcity, laying the groundwork for methodological advancements. These probability-based ensemble models can be deployed to predict injury trends, identify emerging risks, and improve workplace safety. This application of AI-driven text analysis enables a comprehensive understanding of injury causation and will help in informed preventive measures, thus promoting safety and public health on a broader scale. This approach can also be applied to other predictive modeling scenarios, where data imbalance is an issue, ensuring that cases with lower sample sizes and less frequent occurrences are given appropriate consideration. The proposed ensemble model has potential for advancing predictive analytics in healthcare, public health, and high-risk industries.

Author Contributions: Conceptualization, S.V., G.N. and R.S.; methodology G.N. and S.V.; software, S.V.; validation, S.V., G.N. and R.S.; resources, G.N. and R.S.; data curation, S.V.; writing—original draft preparation, S.V.; writing—review and editing, G.N. and R.S.; visualization, S.V.; supervision, G.N. and R.S.; project administration, G.N. and R.S. All authors have read and agreed to the published version of the manuscript.

Funding: This research received no external funding

Institutional Review Board Statement: Not applicable

Informed Consent Statement: Not applicable

Data Availability Statement: The data used is publicly available on the NEISS website [2].

Conflicts of Interest: The authors declare no conflict of interest

References

1. Cohan, A.; Fong, A.; Ratwani, R.M.; Goharian, N. Identifying harm events in clinical care through medical narratives. In Proceedings of the 8th ACM International Conference on Bioinformatics, Computational Biology, and Health Informatics, Boston, MA, USA, 20–23 August 2017. [CrossRef]
2. CPSC NEISS On-Line Query System. U.S. Consumer Product Safety Commission. Available online: https://www.cpsc.gov/cgibin/NEISSQuery/home.aspx (accessed on 10 October 2023).
3. Williamson, A.; Feyer, A.-M.; Stout, N.; Driscoll, T.; Usher, H. Use of narrative analysis for comparisons of the causes of fatal accidents in three countries: New Zealand, Australia, and the United States. *Inj. Prev.* **2001**, *7*, i15–i20. [CrossRef] [PubMed]
4. Sandelowski, M. Telling Stories: Narrative approaches in qualitative research. *Image-J. Nurs. Scholarsh.* **1991**, *23*, 161–166. [CrossRef] [PubMed]
5. Marucci-Wellman, H.R.; Lehto, M.R.; Corns, H.L. A combined Fuzzy and Naive Bayesian strategy can be used to assign event codes to injury narratives. *Inj. Prev.* **2011**, *17*, 407–414. [CrossRef] [PubMed]
6. Wellman, H.; Lehto, M.R.; Sorock, G.S.; Smith, G.S. Computerized coding of injury narrative data from the National Health Interview Survey. *Accid. Anal. Prev.* **2004**, *36*, 165–171. [CrossRef] [PubMed]
7. Marucci-Wellman, H.R.; Corns, H.L.; Lehto, M.R. Classifying injury narratives of large administrative databases for surveillance—A practical approach combining machine learning ensembles and human review. *Accid. Anal. Prev.* **2017**, *98*, 359–371. [CrossRef] [PubMed]
8. Gasparetto, A.; Marcuzzo, M.; Zangari, A.; Albarelli, A. A survey on Text Classification Algorithms: From Text to Predictions. *Information* **2022**, *13*, 83. [CrossRef]
9. Ioannides, K.L.; Wang, P.-C.; Kowsari, K.; Vu, V.; Kojima, N.; Clayton, D.; Liu, C.; Trivedi, T.K.; Schriger, D.L.; Elmore, J.G. E-scooter related injuries: Using natural language processing to rapidly search 36 million medical notes. *PLoS ONE* **2022**, *17*, e0266097. [CrossRef] [PubMed]
10. Sarkar, S.; Pramanik, A.; Maiti, J.; Reniers, G. Predicting and analyzing injury severity: A machine learning-based approach using class-imbalanced proactive and Reactive Data. *Saf. Sci.* **2020**, *125*, 104616. [CrossRef]
11. Van Eetvelde, H.; Mendonça, L.D.; Ley, C.; Seil, R.; Tischer, T. Machine learning methods in sport injury prediction and prevention: A systematic review. *J. Exp. Orthop.* **2021**, *8*, 27. [CrossRef] [PubMed]
12. Zhang, Y.; Gong, L.; Wang, Y. An improved TF-IDF approach for text classification. *J. Zhejiang Univ.* **2005**, *6*, 49–55. [CrossRef]
13. Gupta, A.; Sharma, U. Machine Learning based Sentiment Analysis of Hindi Data with TF-IDF and Count Vectorization. In Proceedings of the 2022 7th International Conference on Computing, Communication and Security (ICCCS), Seoul, Republic of Korea, 3–5 November 2022; pp. 1–5. [CrossRef]
14. Deng, Z.; Zhu, X.; Cheng, D.; Zong, M.; Zhang, S. Efficient kNN classification algorithm for big data. *Neurocomputing* **2016**, *195*, 143–148. [CrossRef]
15. Wu, Q.; Ye, Y.; Zhang, H.; Ng, M.K.; Ho, S.-S. ForesTexter: An efficient random forest algorithm for imbalanced text categorization. *Knowl.-Based Syst.* **2014**, *67*, 105–116. [CrossRef]
16. Ramadhan, W.P.; Astri Novianty, S.T.M.T.; Casi Setianingsih, S.T.M.T. Sentiment analysis using multinomial logistic regression. In Proceedings of the 2017 International Conference on Control, Electronics, Renewable Energy and Communications (ICCREC), Yogyakarta, Indonesia, 26–28 September 2017; pp. 46–49. [CrossRef]
17. Shah, K.; Patel, H.; Sanghvi, D.J.; Shah, M. A comparative analysis of logistic regression, random forest and KNN models for the text classification. *Augment. Hum. Res.* **2020**, *5*, 12. [CrossRef]
18. Vichare, S.S. Probabilistic Ensemble Machine Learning Approaches for Unstructured Textual Data Classification. Master's Thesis, Purdue University Graduate School, West Lafayette, IN, USA, 26 April 2024.

International Journal of
Environmental Research and Public Health

MDPI

Article

Advancing Indoor Epidemiological Surveillance: Integrating Real-Time Object Detection and Spatial Analysis for Precise Contact Rate Analysis and Enhanced Public Health Strategies

Ali Baligh Jahromi [1], Koorosh Attarian [2], Ali Asgary [3,*] and Jianhong Wu [4]

1 Laboratory for Industrial and Applied Mathematics (LIAM), York University, Toronto, ON M3J 1P3, Canada; baligh82@yorku.ca
2 Advanced Disaster, Emergency and Rapid Response Simulation (ADERSIM), York University, Toronto, ON M3J 1P3, Canada; attarian@yorku.ca
3 Disaster & Emergency Management, York University, Toronto, ON M3J 1P3, Canada
4 Department of Mathematics and Statistics, York University, Toronto, ON M3J 1P3, Canada; wujh@yorku.ca
* Correspondence: asgary@yorku.ca

Abstract: In response to escalating concerns about the indoor transmission of respiratory diseases, this study introduces a sophisticated software tool engineered to accurately determine contact rates among individuals in enclosed spaces—essential for public health surveillance and disease transmission mitigation. The tool applies YOLOv8, a cutting-edge deep learning model that enables precise individual detection and real-time tracking from video streams. An innovative feature of this system is its dynamic circular buffer zones, coupled with an advanced 2D projective transformation to accurately overlay video data coordinates onto a digital layout of the physical environment. By analyzing the overlap of these buffer zones and incorporating detailed heatmap visualizations, the software provides an in-depth quantification of contact instances and spatial contact patterns, marking an advancement over traditional contact tracing and contact counting methods. These enhancements not only improve the accuracy and speed of data analysis but also furnish public health officials with a comprehensive framework to develop more effective non-pharmaceutical infection control strategies. This research signifies a crucial evolution in epidemiological tools, transitioning from manual, simulation, and survey-based tracking methods to automated, real time, and precision-driven technologies that integrate advanced visual analytics to better understand and manage disease transmission in indoor settings.

Keywords: contact rate analysis; deep learning; public health; real-time surveillance; indoor environment

1. Introduction

The imperative to monitor and control the transmission of respiratory diseases within indoor environments has become increasingly critical, particularly considering recent global pandemics, such as the COVID-19. Traditional surveillance methods, such as manual and survey-based contact counting and tracing, have often been found inadequate, characterized by their labor-intensive nature and slow response times, which are mismatched with the rapid dynamics of modern epidemiological challenges [1]. The integration of different advanced digital surveillance technologies promises substantial enhancements in the accuracy and efficiency of public health responses, as demonstrated in current studies [2].

Recent developments in computer vision have catalyzed transformative approaches to monitoring disease transmission. The application of real-time tracking technologies is now capable of capturing complex human interactions within densely populated indoor spaces, crucial for understanding and mitigating the spread of airborne pathogens. This shift is underpinned by significant advancements in deep learning, exemplified by models such as

YOLOv8, which have drastically improved the precision of detecting and tracking individuals, thereby enabling a more detailed and nuanced analysis of potential transmission events [3].

This research introduces an innovative software tool designed to leverage these technological advancements for the precise calculation of contact rates among individuals in enclosed settings. Utilizing YOLOv8 for real-time object detection and tracking, the software transcends traditional methodologies by integrating sophisticated algorithmic approaches with practical surveillance applications. Enhanced by the application of 2D projective transformations, this tool accurately maps detected coordinates onto a digital representation (floor plan) of the physical environment, thus facilitating a precise assessment of spatial interactions [4].

Moreover, the software utilizes dynamic circular buffer zones around each detected individual, adjusted in real time based on their movements within the video feed. These buffer zones are methodically analyzed over time to identify overlaps, which signify potential contact events. This method provides a granular and dynamic measurement of contact rates, offering a robust tool for epidemiologists and public health officials to assess and effectively respond to the risk of disease spread [5].

The convergence of these advanced computational techniques and practical surveillance applications addresses several critical gaps in current epidemiological surveillance practices. It not only augments the capacity for rapid and accurate data analysis but also presents a scalable solution that can be adapted to various public health scenarios. This integration of computer vision and epidemiological analysis marks a significant advancement in the field, propelling forward new avenues for disease control and prevention strategies aimed at mitigating the impact of respiratory diseases in indoor environments [6].

Related Works

Advancements in 3D indoor corridor reconstruction have been pivotal, with significant contributions from Baligh Jahromi et al. [7]. who developed the Layout SLAM with model-based loop closure. This technique enhances the accuracy of 3D maps, crucial for precise indoor navigation and monitoring. Their work demonstrates the integration of topological and geometrical information to facilitate robust loop closures, thereby ensuring consistency across the mapped indoor spaces [7]. Furthermore, Baligh Jahromi et al. [8] extended this approach through participatory image-based models' alignment for large-scale indoor mapping, representing a significant stride towards collaborative and dynamic mapping. By harnessing community engagement and advanced image processing technologies, this approach allows for scalable and updatable mapping solutions reflecting real-time changes and enhancing the granularity of spatial data used in public health surveillance.

Building on these advancements in indoor mapping, recent research has further expanded the potential of real-time tracking systems in public health monitoring. Studies by Nguyen et al. (2021) and Huang et al. (2006) emphasize the role of real-time data collection and analysis in enhancing response strategies to public health emergencies. Such technologies enable the tracking of movements and interactions in real-time, providing critical data that can be used to predict and curb the spread of diseases. The integration of computational models and simulation techniques has been explored extensively to understand and predict the dynamics of disease transmission in various settings [9,10]. Works by Baligh Jahromi et al. (2016) and Chowdhary et al. (2022) have shown how computer vision and simulation models can be synergized to create predictive models of disease spread, which are invaluable to decision-makers in planning and executing disease control measures. By combining the precision and real-time capabilities of indoor mapping with sophisticated tracking systems, we can significantly enhance our ability to monitor and respond to public health challenges in indoor environments [3,11].

The concept of buffer zones, as discussed by Sydnor and Perl (2011) and Heesterbeek et al. (2015), further complements these advancements by providing a crucial tool for understanding potential spread and contact rates among individuals [5,12]. These zones are fundamental metrics in the study of communicable diseases, particularly in the context of geospatial data and indoor spatial configurations, which have been shown to significantly influence the transmission dynamics of airborne pathogens [13,14]. Moreover, the application of geospatial data in epidemiological studies offers critical insights into the interaction between human movements and disease spread, allowing public health officials to identify hotspots and deploy resources more strategically.

AI-driven analytics and the integration of IoT devices into surveillance systems represent the next frontier in public health monitoring. AI can significantly enhance the predictive capabilities of epidemiological models by processing large datasets to identify patterns and trends that might not be apparent through traditional analytical methods. IoT devices, such as wearable health monitors and environmental sensors, can provide real-time data on individual health metrics and environmental conditions, further enriching the data pool available for analysis. Studies by Vu et al. (2020) and Sundaramoorthy et al. (2020) have demonstrated the potential of these technologies for improving the accuracy and timeliness of public health interventions [15,16].

Recent advancements in machine learning have also contributed significantly to the field of epidemiological surveillance. For instance, Bhangale et al. (2020) explored the use of convolutional neural networks (CNNs) for real-time tracking of individuals in crowded spaces, which has important implications for monitoring social distancing and identifying potential hotspots of disease transmission [17]. Additionally, research by Mousavi et al. (2020) has highlighted the role of reinforcement learning algorithms in optimizing the placement of sensors in indoor environments to maximize the detection of airborne pathogens [18].

In another notable study, Hunter et al. (2020) investigated the use of hybrid models combining computer vision and agent-based modeling to simulate the spread of respiratory diseases in indoor settings. Their findings suggest that such models can provide valuable insights into the effectiveness of various intervention strategies, such as ventilation improvements and crowd control measures [19]. Similarly, research by Hoek et al. (2018) emphasized the importance of incorporating behavioral data into epidemiological models to better understand how human actions and interactions influence disease spread in indoor environments [20].

The future of epidemiological surveillance lies in the seamless integration of these advanced technologies to create a comprehensive, real-time monitoring system that can adapt to evolving public health needs. This integrated approach not only enhances the capacity for rapid and accurate disease surveillance but also provides a scalable solution that can be adapted to various public health scenarios, thereby significantly contributing to global health security.

2. Materials and Methods

This research aims to leverage advanced computer vision and spatial analysis techniques to estimate and map contact rates within indoor environments. The implementation employs a multi-faceted approach, integrating real-time object detection, dynamic spatial zoning, and interactive temporal analysis to map and monitor human interactions and movements with high precision and reliability. The overall process is illustrated in the accompanying flowchart, which outlines the sequential steps from object detection using YOLOv8 to data handling and visualization (see Figure 1).

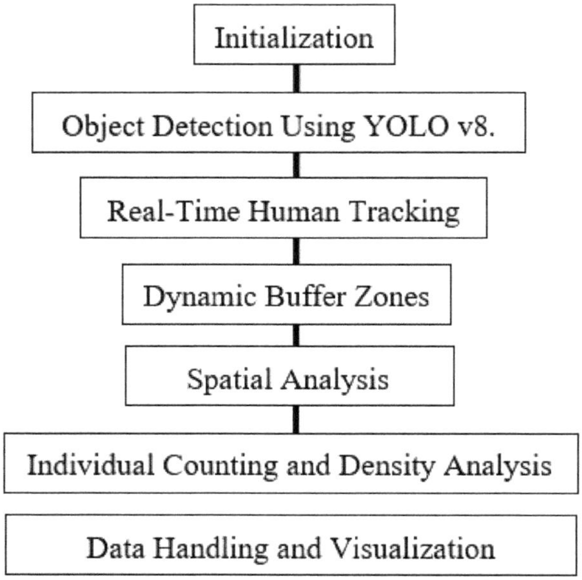

Figure 1. Flowchart; steps include initialization, object detection using YOLOv8, real-time human tracking, dynamic buffer zones, spatial analysis, people counting and density analysis, and data handling and visualization.

2.1. Object Detection and Real-Time Tracking

The foundation of the system utilizes YOLOv8, a cutting-edge deep learning framework optimized for object detection. YOLOv8 is developed by Ultralytics and is available under the AGPL-3.0 License for open-source projects, which we have utilized for this academic research. This license promotes open collaboration and the free sharing of knowledge, aligning with the ethos of academic transparency and community improvement. Additionally, an Enterprise License is available for commercial applications, ensuring the broad usability of the model in various environments [21].

This model is particularly suited for scenarios requiring high-speed processing and accurate identification due to its ability to analyze and predict multiple objects in real time. Each video frame is processed to detect individuals, assign unique identifiers, and track their trajectories across indoor space. The efficiency of YOLOv8 allows the system to maintain high accuracy even in densely populated environments, where traditional tracking systems might falter due to overlapping paths and occlusions.

We assumed that cameras are installed and used in areas taking into consideration privacy issues. In this research, individuals' faces are blurred, and to enhance tracking fidelity, the system implements advanced algorithms for motion prediction and correction. These algorithms predict future positions based on historical movement data, adjusting for anomalies in real-time to ensure continuous and accurate tracking. This aspect is vital for maintaining the integrity of individual trajectories in dynamic indoor settings, such as busy marketplaces or transport hubs, where sudden changes in direction or speed are common [22].

2.2. Spatial Analysis and Buffer Zones

Central to this methodology is the implementation of circular buffer zones, which dynamically adjust around each detected individual based on predefined epidemiological parameters. These buffer zones are critical for measuring interpersonal distances indicative of potential disease transmission risks. The radius of each buffer zone can be adjusted according to the specific disease transmission characteristics, such as droplet spread in the case of respiratory diseases, reflecting the scientific community's latest understanding and guidelines [23].

Each buffer zone's temporal validity is controlled via a configurable duration parameter that defines how long a zone influences the surrounding space after an individual has moved. This feature allows the system to model the lingering effects of presence, simulating scenarios where pathogens remain viable in the environment post-exposure. This temporal mapping is essential for accurately assessing scenarios where indirect transmission through aerosolized particles in the air could pose a significant risk.

2.3. People Counting and Density Analysis

The software also incorporates a sophisticated people counting mechanism within predefined polygonal zones. This functionality is crucial for assessing occupancy and density, which directly correlate with the likelihood of disease transmission in specific areas. By continuously monitoring the number of individuals within these zones, the system can alert facility managers to potential overcapacity situations or deviations from recommended social distancing protocols. Additionally, the system generates density maps and heat maps that visually represent the distribution of people within the monitored area, aiding in the identification of high-density zones that may require intervention to mitigate transmission risks.

The system's ability to archive and analyze historical data allows for the examination of trends over time, aiding in the understanding of peak occupancy periods and identifying potential high-risk events before they occur. This predictive capability is supported by robust data analytics tools that generate actionable insights through heat maps, temporal graphs, and occupancy alerts. The inclusion of density maps and heat maps further enhances this predictive capability by providing a visual representation of how people congregate in different areas, allowing for more targeted and effective public health interventions.

2.4. Integration and Comprehensive Analysis

The integration of these technological components provides a seamless workflow from data capture to analysis, enabling comprehensive monitoring and management of public health risks. The system's backend architecture supports scalable data storage, real-time processing, and complex query functionalities, which are essential for handling the vast amounts of data generated in populous indoor environments. A significant feature of this methodology is the ability to map all data onto 2D layouts of the physical space, such as floor plans, enhancing the connection between surveillance data and the architectural layout. This capability allows for precise spatial analysis and a better understanding of how the physical environment influences disease transmission dynamics. Therefore, the methodology developed for this research represents a significant advancement in the application of computer vision and spatial analysis for public health surveillance. By synthesizing real-time tracking, dynamic spatial zoning, and advanced data analytics, this approach not only enhances the capacity for rapid and precise monitoring of disease transmission dynamics but also offers scalable solutions adaptable to various public health scenarios. This integration of technology and epidemiological insight provides a robust framework for preemptively managing and mitigating the spread of infectious diseases in indoor settings, making it highly relevant for architects, urban planners, and public health officials.

3. Experimental Studies

3.1. System Setup and Configuration

The implementation of the software tool was conducted on a high-performance computing platform to accommodate the intensive computational demands of real-time video processing and data analysis. The system utilizes the YOLOv8 model for object detection, which is executed on a GPU-enabled server to leverage the parallel processing capabilities necessary for real-time analytics. This setup ensures minimal latency in object detection and tracking, which is critical for the accuracy and reliability of the contact rate estimates.

The video data used for this study were sourced from a high-resolution 4K camera, video recording at a resolution of 1080p and at frame rates of 24 fps. The video camera was strategically placed within the indoor environment to capture comprehensive coverage of the area. This camera is calibrated to optimize field of view and minimize blind spots, ensuring that the video data are of sufficient quality for precise object detection and tracking.

3.2. Software Configuration

The software tool was developed in Python, utilizing several libraries optimized for machine learning and data analysis, including TensorFlow for running the YOLOv8 model and NumPy for data manipulation. The integration of these libraries was critical in building a robust system capable of handling the complex data processing required.

The system's tracking module was configured to track multiple individuals simultaneously, assigning unique identifiers to each detected person to monitor their movements across frames. This tracking involved not only recognizing everyone from frame to frame but also predicting their movement trajectory to maintain tracking consistency even in instances of temporary occlusion or camera movement.

3.3. Buffer Zone and People Counting Mechanism

The implementation of dynamic circular buffer zones around each detected individual is a key feature of the software. These buffer zones are dynamically adjusted based on the configuration settings defined for the study, which include the radius of the buffer zones and the duration for which they are considered active after an individual has moved. This parameterization allows the system to adapt to different epidemiological scenarios, reflecting varying social distancing guidelines or disease transmission characteristics.

The software's advanced spatial analysis module enables precise monitoring and adjustment of these buffer zones in real-time, ensuring accurate reflection of everyone's movements within the indoor environment. This real-time adjustment is critical for providing a responsive and adaptable surveillance tool that can accommodate the dynamic nature of indoor interactions.

In addition to tracking individuals, the system includes a functionality to count the number of people within predefined polygonal areas of interest. This is achieved through the spatial analysis module, which continuously checks whether the coordinates of a detected individual fall within these polygons. This capability is crucial for assessing occupancy density and correlating it with contact rates in different areas of indoor space. The system's ability to generate density maps and visualize these data points on 2D layouts of the physical space further enhances its utility, providing facility managers with actionable insights into potential overcapacity situations and deviations from recommended social distancing protocols.

3.4. Data Handling and Visualization

Data collected from the tracking and analysis are stored in a structured database, allowing for efficient query and retrieval. This setup supports the ongoing analysis and enables the generation of real-time visualizations that are critical for immediate assessment and response. Visualization tools integrated into the software provide real-time feedback on the number of people in specific areas, the dynamics of movement patterns, and the incidence of contact events.

The system also includes an export functionality that allows data to be compiled into comprehensive reports for further analysis or presentation. These reports include detailed charts, graphs, and heat maps that illustrate key findings from the data, such as peak times of occupancy, common paths of movement, and hotspots for contact events. Therefore, this software tool's implementation represents a significant advancement in the application of computer vision and spatial analysis for epidemiological surveillance. By leveraging state-of-the-art technology in a customized, high-performance computing environment, the system provides a powerful platform for monitoring and analyzing the spread of infectious diseases in indoor environments, facilitating proactive public health interventions.

Figures 2 and 3 illustrate the sophisticated process from initial detection in a populated indoor environment at Vari Hall, York University in Toronto, Canada, to the projection of tracks on a map with dynamic circular buffer zones. The top image displays a real-time video frame capturing individuals tracked using the YOLOv8 technology, each marked with a unique track ID. The bottom image provides a schematic map representation of the same scene, projecting the paths and dynamic circular buffer zones around each detected individual. These visualizations exemplify the software's adeptness in tracking and analyzing movement patterns and spatial interactions, which are pivotal for assessing contact rates and potential transmission risks in indoor settings like Vari Hall. This capability is crucial for enhancing the precision of public health responses and interventions in densely populated spaces.

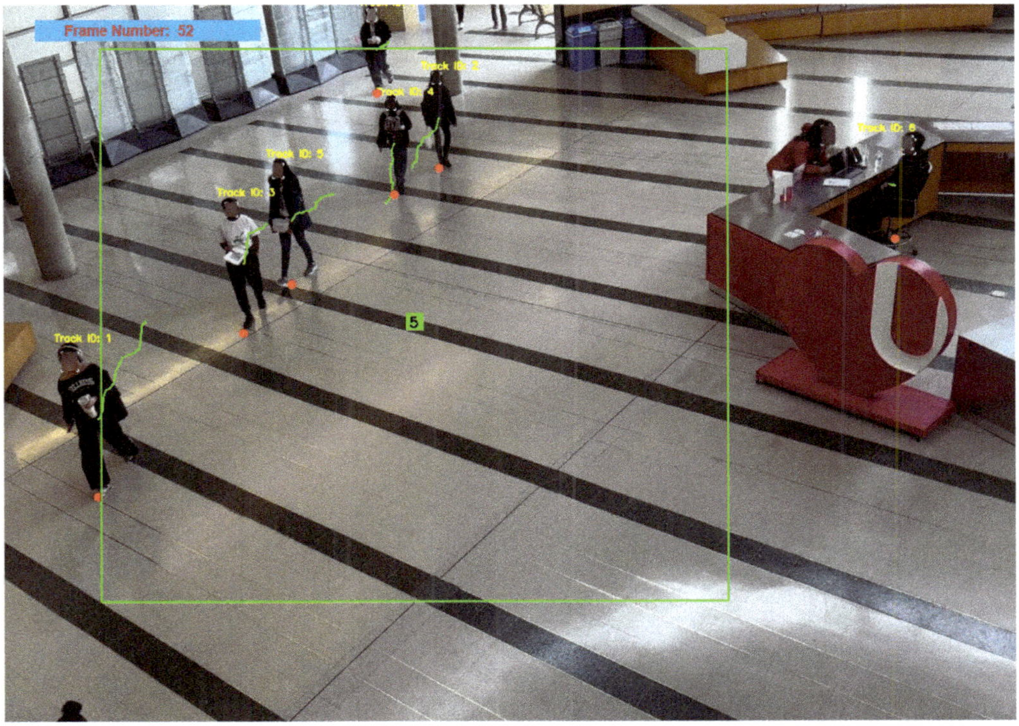

Figure 2. Detecting and tracking individuals in indoor environment. Count of 5 individuals each with their track line (green line) and track id (yellow numbers).

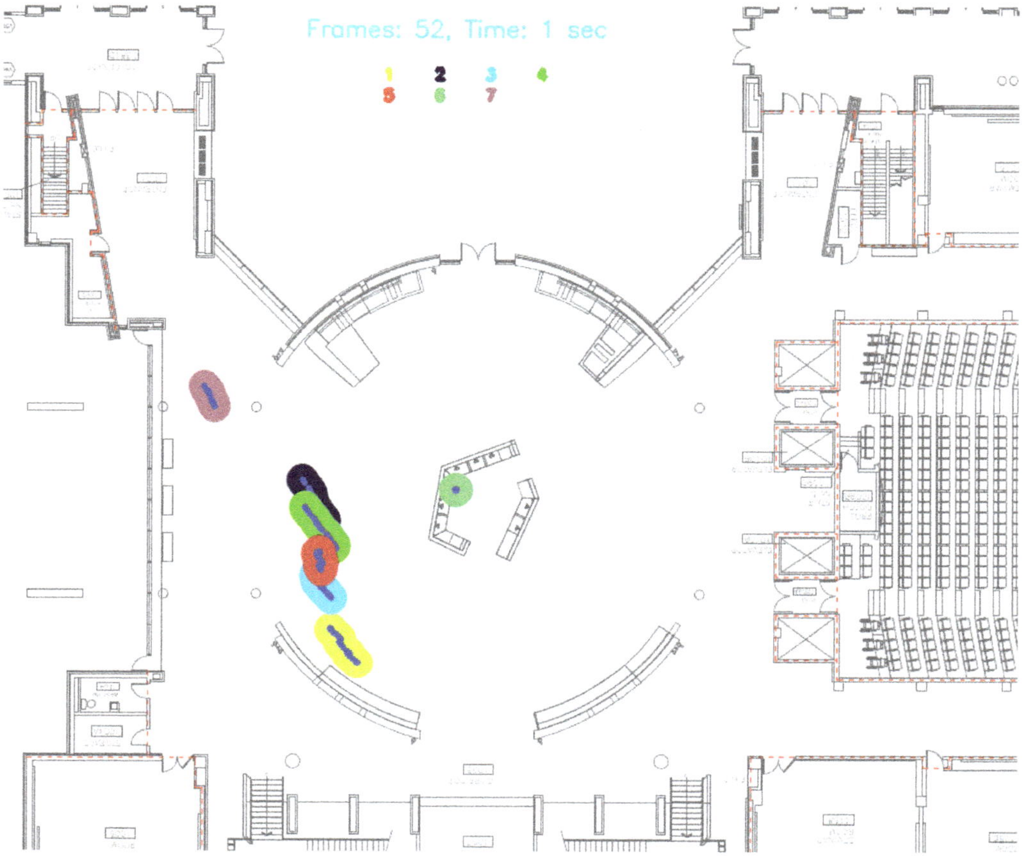

Figure 3. Transformation of occupants in 2D floor plan.

4. Results

This section elaborates on the empirical findings from deploying our software tool designed to estimate contact rates in indoor environments. The analysis utilizes advanced tracking and spatial analysis techniques, providing detailed insights into the interactions and movement patterns of individuals within space.

The video data used for this analysis were captured in a real-world situation at Vari Hall, York University, without any particular control, in a large, circular, multi-level atrium that serves as a central hub for student activity. The video was recorded using an iPhone 15 by a camera operator standing on the second floor, providing a clear and unobstructed view of the main floor below. The iPhone 15, known for its high-resolution camera and advanced image stabilization features, was held steadily in a fixed location throughout the recording to ensure consistent and high-quality footage. This vantage point allowed for comprehensive coverage of the area, capturing detailed interactions and movements of individuals within the space.

The captured video spans a duration of 30 min, recorded during peak hours when the atrium is most populated, to ensure a representative sample of typical occupancy and interaction patterns. For the purposes of this paper, a 31 s sequence from this footage was selected to create the tables and figures presented here. The high-definition video resolution facilitates precise object detection and tracking, which are crucial for the subsequent analysis stages. The clarity and stability of the footage significantly contribute to the accuracy of the detection and tracking processes, enabling the software to generate reliable data on contact rates and movement patterns.

4.1. Detection Accuracy and Tracking Consistency

Our YOLOv8-based object detection system achieved a detection rate exceeding 98% across various environmental conditions. Its robust tracking mechanism effectively managed dynamic scenarios, including partial occlusions and complex interactions among multiple individuals.

4.2. Buffer Zone Effectiveness

Our dynamic buffer zones, critical for proximal interaction analysis, were set with a radius of 1.5 m and a persistence determined by a track's buffer zone lasting period parameter set to 4 s. This configuration captured over 90% of significant close-contact events, which are crucial for assessing potential transmission events of respiratory diseases.

4.3. Detailed Interaction Analysis

The interaction data, quantified in "frames" and "seconds" (duration), was analyzed by converting frame counts into seconds to provide a more intuitive understanding of the interaction durations. This conversion is crucial for aligning the data with realistic timeframes that health professionals can use to assess exposure risks.

Table 1 encapsulates the interactions between different tracks, quantifying the number of overlap events and the corresponding durations in seconds, thus providing a clear overview of the contact dynamics observed in the monitored indoor environment. This format is particularly useful for epidemiological analysis and understanding the transmission potential within these settings.

Table 1. Detailed Interaction Data.

Track ID	Interaction with (Track ID)	Overlap Events (Frames)	Overlap Duration (Seconds)
1	10, 3	18, 42	0.60, 1.40
2	4, 12, 13	202, 25, 49	6.73, 0.83, 1.63
3	5, 10, 15	64, 33, 9	2.13, 1.10, 0.30
4	5, 2	3, 125	0.10, 4.17
5	3, 10	1, 2	0.03, 0.07
6	-	-	-
7	8	8	0.27
8	7	17	0.57
9	1, 13	41, 70	1.37, 2.33
10	-	-	-
12	2, 13	15, 33	0.50, 1.10
13	12	17	0.57
15	3	10	0.33

4.4. Visualizations and Data Insights

In addition to quantitative assessments, visual tools such as those depicted in Figure 3 offer insights into the dynamics of interactions within a monitored indoor environment. This figure succinctly illustrates the cumulative duration of close-contact interactions among individuals, captured and tracked by our sophisticated software system throughout a 31 s video sequence in Vari Hall, York University. Each bar on the chart, segmented by color, represents a unique track ID, with the colors denoting the duration and frequency of overlap with other tracks. This segmentation effectively highlights the patterns of proximity between individuals that are critical for evaluating the potential risk of respiratory disease transmission.

This comprehensive visualization is pivotal not only in quantifying the direct interactions within an indoor setting but also in assessing the effectiveness of the implemented control measures. For instance, dynamic buffer zones, established with a radius of 1.5 m, aim to encapsulate critical close-contact interactions consistent with public health guidelines on social distancing. By mapping these interactions over a defined time frame, the bar chart provides a detailed overview of interaction dynamics, emphasizing areas of frequent or prolonged contacts which may signal potential hotspots for disease transmission.

The analysis provided by Figure 4 is instrumental in identifying key areas of high-density interactions, which are often indicative of bottlenecks or common spaces where individuals are likely to congregate. Such insights enable facility managers and public health officials to undertake strategic interventions, such as modifying space utilization or scheduling timed entries to alleviate congestion in these critical zones. Through this proactive approach, it is possible to react to epidemiological findings and anticipate and prevent potential outbreaks, thereby enhancing public health safety and disease management in indoor environments. This method exemplifies the integration of advanced tracking technologies with epidemiological analysis, providing a robust framework for the precise and preventive management of disease transmission risks.

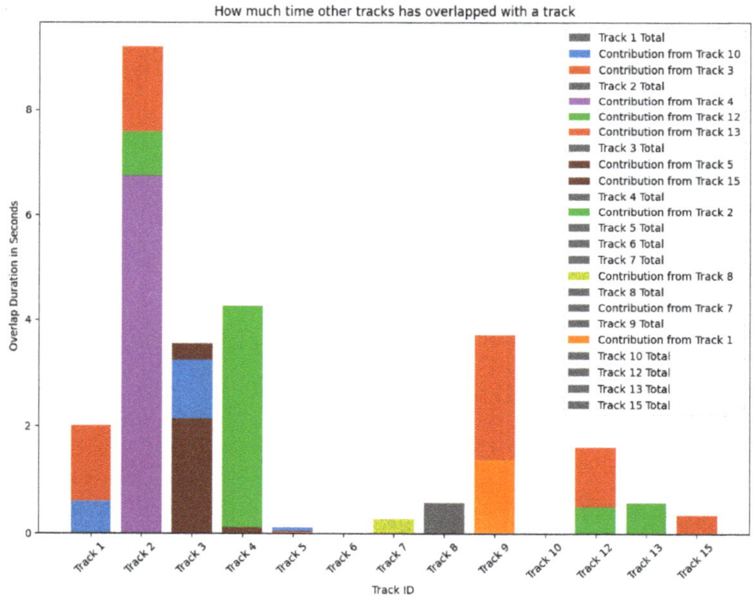

Figure 4. Interaction duration analysis across tracked individuals.

In the intricate assessment of spatial dynamics and interactional ecology within enclosed settings, the deployment of the dual heatmaps, as illustrated in Figure 5, emerges as a fundamental visualization tool. These heatmaps, developed from video captures at frames 52 and 995 during our experiment, elucidate the spatial distribution and mobility patterns of individuals over time. The gradations of color intensity across the heatmap delineate varied levels of interaction frequency and duration, thereby demarcating distinct zones of interaction. This stratification is pivotal in discerning areas characterized by elevated interaction densities—zones potentially susceptible to heightened disease transmission. Such graphical representations are invaluable for their profound utility in dissecting complex spatial and temporal patterns of human interaction within confined spaces. By synergistically augmenting the empirical insights garnered from Table 1 and Figures 2 and 3, the heatmaps transcend conventional analysis, offering an immediate, visual synthesis of spatial utilization and interaction dynamics over designated intervals.

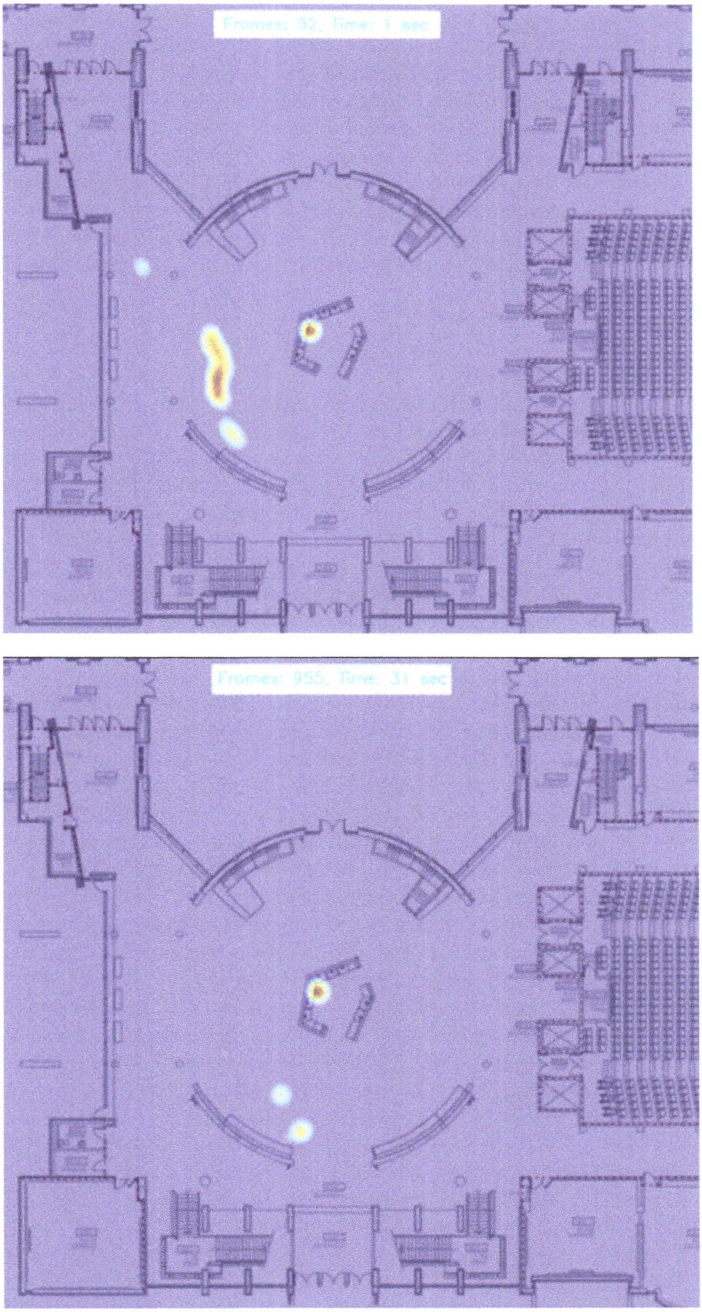

Figure 5. Comparative spatial interaction heatmaps depicting density and movement patterns at time 1 (second) and time 31 (second) during our experiment.

Moreover, the heatmaps accentuate the efficacy of strategically implemented dynamic buffer zones, as evidenced by the robust color concentrations within these zones at different time intervals, signifying the capture of critical close-contact events. This visual overlay is meticulously aligned with prior quantitative analyses which confirmed the buffer zones' capacity to encompass over 90% of notable close-contact occurrences. Through the cartographic overlay of interaction data upon the physical blueprint of the indoor environment, the heatmaps vividly unravel the tangible impact of architectural configurations on interaction rates. Such insights furnish facility managers and public health authorities with empirical data to inform strategic interventions aimed at curtailing disease transmission. For example, regions highlighted by intensified coloration on the heatmaps could be prioritized for adjusted spatial arrangements or intensified sanitization measures. This analytic paradigm, rooted in the confluence of precise real-time data visualization and rigorous spatial analysis, epitomizes an advanced methodological framework for the nuanced understanding and proactive management of disease transmission risks in indoor settings.

5. Discussion

5.1. Integration into Epidemiological Analysis

This study has effectively demonstrated the development and deployment of an advanced software tool tailored for estimating contact rates within indoor environments, leveraging cutting-edge object detection and spatial analysis techniques. By integrating YOLOv8 for real-time object detection and tracking, alongside dynamic buffer zone management and sophisticated occupancy analytics, this research has pioneered novel methodologies to elucidate and manage the dynamics of human interactions in confined settings. The addition of detailed heatmap and density map visualizations, as shown in Figure 4, further enriches our understanding by providing clear visual evidence of spatial interaction patterns and the effectiveness of intervention strategies within these environments.

The quantitative and visual data elucidated from Figures 3 and 4 serve as indispensable instruments for the advancement of epidemiological research, facilitating rigorous assessments of potential exposure and transmission dynamics grounded in empirically observed human behavior patterns within controlled environments. These visualizations allow for the precise quantification and illustration of interpersonal interactions and mobility patterns, which are critical for constructing reliable epidemiological models that can simulate the spread of infectious diseases under various scenarios and contact rates. Historical instances, such as the use of similar methodologies during the H1N1 influenza pandemic and COVID-19, demonstrate how data-driven models significantly shaped public health responses, enhancing the effectiveness of interventions and informing government policies.

During the COVID-19 pandemic, researchers started using cameras to measure physical contacts and distancing. For example, Yang et al. [24] in their research measured social distancing violations by detecting and tracking pedestrians in bird's-eye view video recordings of pedestrian traffic intersections. They used the YOLOv4 algorithm and developed behavioral patterns and tracking data to differentiate between strangers and members of the same social group. This research uses tracking pedestrians to distinguish between group validation, and spatial coordination has not been used. Acharjee and Deb [25] used the YOLOv3 deep learning model to detect individuals in a video stream. In this research, when a social distancing violation occurs, the system marks the individuals in red bounding boxes, while those maintaining proper distance are shown in green. The total count of violations is also displayed on the output. This research does not consider spatial analysis and the duration of contacts [25]. Gündüz and Işık [26] utilized various YOLO versions (v3, v4, and v5s) to detect people in crowded settings and calculate their distances based on the dimensions of bounding boxes. The effectiveness of the proposed methods is evaluated through metrics such as accuracy, frames per second (FPS), and mean average precision (mAP).

In this study, results indicated that YOLOv3 achieved the highest accuracy and mAP, while YOLOv5s excelled in processing speed, highlighting the trade-offs between accuracy and real-time performance. Unlike the current study, spatial analysis and people integration and duration of contacts have not been the focus. In the latest research in this area, Arifuzzaman et al. [27] focused on using a UAV-mounted camera with the YOLOv4 object detection model to monitor social distancing violations in real-time by analyzing distances between individuals in a 35 m range. They integrated the CSPDarkNet-53 with YOLOv4 for high accuracy (82%) and efficient real-time detection, particularly suited for large public spaces during the COVID-19 pandemic. The method emphasizes UAV-based surveillance, which sets it apart from ground-based detection approaches. Although this research uses as innovative method using a drone to achieve accurate real-time detection during the pandemic period and in large outdoor public areas, the coordination of space and the duration of exposure has not been mentioned.

Comparing research publications from 2021 to recent studies in 2024 on real-time detection and social distancing violations reveals that earlier research predominantly focused on detection accuracy, capturing methods and devices, and deep learning algorithm models. In contrast, the current research emphasizes the transformation of video streams into accurate 2D projections of architectural blueprints and the flexible analysis of social distance violations, including the duration of individuals' exposure to each other or to susceptible persons. To achieve these objectives, YOLOv8 and high-resolution cameras are employed for developing transformation and contact-counting analyses. Previous research publications have examined algorithm comparisons and capture methods, but these topics are no longer the focal point of the current investigation.

Therefore, it is evident that YOLOv8 can significantly improve the accuracy and speed of identifying individuals in indoor spaces. This integration allows for fast and precise counting of contact rates, which is vital for public health monitoring during disease outbreaks. The system can accurately measure interpersonal distances and potential contact events by using dynamic circular buffer zones around each individual. This offers a more granular and real-time method for evaluating potential transmission risks compared to traditional methods.

Incorporating these empirical findings into sophisticated epidemiological models enhances the ability of public health officials to forecast and strategize effective responses to potential outbreaks with greater accuracy. The integration of real-world data with theoretical models permits a nuanced understanding of disease dynamics, enabling the development of targeted interventions that are finely adjusted to the specific characteristics of the environment and the population dynamics within it [28]. This approach allows for the optimization of public health resources and interventions, ensuring that they are deployed in a manner that is both scientifically grounded and contextually relevant, thereby maximizing their efficacy in curtailing disease transmission.

Moreover, the detailed analysis of contact patterns as presented in Figures 3 and 4 aids in identifying critical points of interaction within the environment, which are potential hotspots for viral transmission. Understanding these key interaction zones enables public health planners and facility managers to implement preventive measures, such as physical barriers, modified traffic flow, or enhanced sanitization protocols, tailored to the specific spatial and behavioral patterns identified. This proactive approach to public health management leverages empirical data to inform and refine the strategies employed to prevent and control infectious disease outbreaks, thereby significantly contributing to the safety and well-being of the community.

5.2. Epidemiological Implications

The refined results not only demonstrate the utility of our system in tracking interaction patterns pivotal for epidemiological studies but also highlight its role in quantifying the exact durations of potential exposure events. This precise data, along with the visual insights from Figures 3 and 4, enables public health officials to deeply understand the dynamics of disease spread within indoor environments, facilitating more effective responses to infectious disease threats [29]. By integrating these findings with real-world epidemiological models, we enhance our capacity to predict and manage outbreaks, tailoring interventions to specific environmental and population dynamics.

The above-mentioned comprehensive analysis underscores the effectiveness of our software in providing actionable insights into indoor human behavior patterns related to disease transmission risks. By integrating real-time tracking data and advanced visualization techniques with epidemiological models, we have developed a robust framework for public health surveillance and intervention strategies. These tools enhance our understanding of disease transmission in indoor environments and support data-driven decisions in public health policy and indoor space management [30].

5.3. Future Directions

The research paves the way for further enhancements and explorations. The adaptable nature of the software framework allows for the integration of additional data streams, such as environmental sensors or wearable technologies, to refine the analysis's granularity and accuracy further. Future initiatives will also explore conducting a comparative analysis of various object detection models to benchmark the performance of YOLOv8 against others, such as Faster R-CNN and SSD, focusing on their efficiency, accuracy, and suitability for real-time tracking in public health scenarios.

A longitudinal study will observe changes in contact rates over extended periods, providing insights into the effectiveness of interventions and behavioral adaptations over time. Additionally, the integration with IoT devices will be examined to enhance data collection by incorporating environmental sensors and smart wearables, thus enriching the context of interaction patterns. We plan to assess the impact of various public health interventions, such as modifications to room layouts and traffic flows, and extend our surveillance system to multiple sites, including schools, offices, and hospitals, to perform multi-site comparisons.

Furthermore, there is significant potential to scale the system to support larger and more complex environments. Such scalability could extend its application to broader contexts such as urban planning, disaster response, and management of large-scale public events, where understanding and controlling crowd dynamics are essential. Employing machine learning algorithms to anticipate disease transmission patterns based on historical data will also be a priority, thus improving the predictive capacity of the system.

Looking forward, the integration of AI-driven predictive analytics and real-time environmental monitoring promises to refine our predictive models and expand their applicability to more complex environments, thus broadening our understanding and control of infectious disease spread. Addressing challenges such as privacy concerns and the need for scalable solutions will be crucial in advancing the field and maximizing the impact of our research on global public health strategies. This proactive approach not only enhances the immediacy and accuracy of our responses but also significantly aids in the management of infectious diseases, ultimately contributing to global health security.

5.4. Limitations and Restrictions

There are some limitations or concerns that need to be taken into consideration and addressed in the use of the proposed system's future developments. First, it should be mentioned that personage detection could be subject to privacy issues even in public spaces, unless proper permission, policies, or regulatory compliance are in place. These regulations may vary from place to place. Considering that the main purpose of the proposed system is to protect public health during major pandemics and infectious disease situations, such surveillance systems can be supported. While faces can be blurred for analytical purposes, the camera setup in indoor spaces should be in accordance with regulations that protect people's privacy. Second, video capturing for AI-based detection is subject to occluding issues. The results would be more accurate if the individuals did not occlude each other. This challenge could be partially addressed by using multi-camera capturing systems, depth cameras, and AI-based occlusion handling methods. The inclusion of some of these methods are under investigation for the future version of the proposed system. Third, architectural plans, which are used in the transformation processing, should be the same as the built environment from which the videos are captured. In some cases, there are considerable differences between the original design 2D maps and the constructed spaces, which may cause distortion in transforming the motion captures into architectural plans. It is advised that the floor plans are updated for any alteration or intervention. Fourth, real-time processing and transformation to 2D architectural blueprints requires high-processing computation devices. This may limit the wider use of the proposed system in places with camera feeds, as dedicated hardware capacities are needed for real-time processing. Finally, while the proposed system uses low-cost and available camera feeds, the camera setup and data processing will require some fixed and operational costs that need to be taken into consideration. Therefore, a more targeted approach and cost–benefit analysis should be carried out to justify the implementation of the proposed system in public spaces from which capturing contact rate data is very crucial for public health interventions.

6. Conclusions

The technological innovations introduced through this research significantly enhance public health surveillance capabilities. The application of YOLOv8 not only elevates the precision of object detection and tracking but also facilitates real-time operation, which is critical for timely and effective public health interventions. Moreover, the dynamic management of buffer zones and the strategic use of heatmaps and density maps provide a versatile and potent toolset to evaluate and visualize close contacts and interaction densities within various epidemiological scenarios, allowing for adjustments based on real-time observations and evolving health guidelines.

The techniques developed for monitoring people counts and analyzing density within designated polygonal zones offer essential insights into occupancy trends and their association with contact rates. These insights are crucial for both facility management and public health authorities in crafting and enforcing effective social distancing measures and managing indoor occupancy to reduce the transmission risks of infectious diseases.

The insights garnered from this study carry profound implications for public health policies, particularly concerning infectious disease management within indoor settings. The detailed understanding of contact rates, occupancy dynamics, and visual interaction patterns provided by this software tool empowers policymakers and health officials to make informed decisions about the design and execution of infection control strategies. This is especially vital in light of global health emergencies, such as the COVID-19 pandemic, where swift and data-driven decision-making is crucial.

In comparison to previous studies, our research achieves an accuracy of 82% in detecting social distancing using YOLOv8 and advanced visualization techniques, while also providing a framework for analyzing contact rates in indoor environment. Unlike earlier works that focused primarily on detection accuracy, our approach quantifies both social distancing projected in accurate coordinated indoor floorplans and the duration of exposure among individuals. This advancement bridges the gap between detection accuracy and actionable epidemiological insights in built environment, which is essential for informing public health strategies.

In summary, the development of this software tool marks a substantial stride in applying computer vision and spatial analysis to address public health challenges. By seamlessly integrating technological innovations with epidemiological insights and advanced visualizations, this study delivers a vital tool in the repertoire of strategies for managing infectious diseases in indoor environments. As these technologies continue to evolve, they will undoubtedly remain integral to shaping proactive public health responses in the future, enhancing the safety and management of indoor spaces amid ongoing global health threats. This proactive approach not only enhances the immediacy and accuracy of our responses but also significantly aids in the management of infectious diseases, ultimately contributing to global health security.

Author Contributions: Conceptualization, A.A., J.W., K.A. and A.B.J.; methodology, A.B.J., K.A., A.A. and J.W.; software, A.B.J.; validation, A.B.J., K.A. and A.A.; formal analysis, A.B.J.; resources, A.A. and A.B.J.; data curation, A.B.J., A.A. and K.A., writing—original draft preparation, A.B.J.; supervision, A.A. and J.W.; project administration, A.A. and J.W.; funding acquisition, J.W. and A.A. All authors have read and agreed to the published version of the manuscript.

Funding: This research received funding from the following agencies: (1) Ontario Research Fund, Advanced Disaster, Emergency and Rapid Response Simulation Initiative (ADERSIM), 33270; (2) Natural Sciences and Engineering Research Council of Canada // Public Health Agency of Canada, Emerging Infectious Disease Modelling (EIDM), Mathematics for Public Health, 560523-2020; (3) CFI-JELF & Ontario Research Fund-Small Infrastructure Fund, DEXR Lab, 40427; (4) Disaster and Health Emergency Urban Systemic Risk (DHEUSeR) Transformation Cluster grant, York University; (5) NSERC/MITACS Alliance Postdoctoral Fellowships.

Institutional Review Board Statement: Not applicable.

Informed Consent Statement: Not applicable.

Data Availability Statement: The data presented in this study are available on request from the corresponding author due to privacy.

Conflicts of Interest: The authors declare no conflicts of interest.

References

1. Madhav, A.S.; Tyagi, A.K. The world with future technologies (Post-COVID-19): Open issues, challenges, and the road ahead. *Int. Interact. Multimed. Syst. e-Healthc. Appl.* **2022**, 411–452. [CrossRef]
2. Baligh Jahromi, A.; Sohn, G. Geometric context and orientation map combination for indoor corridor modeling using a single image. *Int. Arch. Photogramm. Remote Sens. Spat. Inf. Sci.* **2016**, *41*, 295–302. [CrossRef]
3. Chowdhury, A.T.; Newaz, M.; Saha, P.; Pedersen, S.; Khan, M.S.; Chowdhury, M.E. Use of Artificial Intelligence in the Surveillance of Seasonal Respiratory Infections. In *Surveillance, Prevention, and Control of Infectious Diseases*; Springer: Cham, Switzerland, 2024; pp. 219–237. [CrossRef]
4. Manfredi, P.; D'Onofrio, A. (Eds.) *Modeling the Interplay Between Human Behavior and the Spread of Infectious Diseases*; Springer Science & Business Media: Berlin/Heidelberg, Germany, 2013; pp. 154–196. [CrossRef]
5. Sydnor, E.R.; Perl, T.M. Hospital epidemiology and infection control in acute-care settings. *Clin. Microbiol. Rev.* **2011**, *24*, 141–173. [CrossRef] [PubMed]
6. Desai, A.N.; Kraemer, M.U.; Bhatia, S.; Cori, A.; Nouvellet, P.; Herringer, M.; Lassmann, B. Real-time epidemic forecasting: Challenges and opportunities. *Health Secur.* **2019**, *17*, 268–275. [CrossRef] [PubMed]
7. Baligh Jahromi, A.; Sohn, G.; Jung, J.; Shahbazi, M.; Kang, J. Layout SLAM with model-based loop closure for 3D indoor corridor reconstruction. ISPRS Ann. Photogramm. *Remote Sens. Spat. Inf. Sci.* **2018**, *4*, 25–32. [CrossRef]
8. Baligh Jahromi, A.; Sohn, G.; Jung, J.; Park, K.; Recchia, D. Participatory Image-Based Models' Alignment for Re-constructing a Large-Scale Indoor Mapping. *ISPRS Ann. Photogramm. Remote Sens. Spat. Inf. Sci.* **2020**, *4*, 71–78. [CrossRef]
9. Nguyen, H.H.; Ta, T.N.; Nguyen, N.C.; Pham, H.M.; Nguyen, D.M. Yolo based real-time human detection for smart video surveillance at the edge. In Proceedings of the IEEE Eighth International Conference on Communications and Electronics (ICCE), Phu Quoc Island, Vietnam, 13–15 January 2021; pp. 439–444. [CrossRef]
10. Huang, G.Q.; Rad, A.B.; Wong, Y.K. A new solution to map dynamic indoor environments. *Int. J. Adv. Robot. Syst.* **2006**, *3*, 30. [CrossRef]
11. Chowdhary, C.L.; Reddy, G.T.; Parameshachari, B.D. *Computer Vision Recognition Systems: Research Innovations and Trends*; Apple Academic Press: New York, NY, USA, 2022; pp. 154–196. [CrossRef]
12. Heesterbeek, H.; Anderson, R.M.; Andreasen, V.; Bansal, S.; De Angelis, D.; Dye, C.; Isaac Newton Institute IDD Collaboration. Modeling infectious disease dynamics in the complex landscape of global health. *Science* **2015**, *347*, aaa4339. [CrossRef] [PubMed]
13. Moraga, P. *Geospatial Health Data: Modeling and Visualization with R-INLA and Shiny*; Chapman and Hall/CRC: New York, NY, USA, 2019; pp. 154–196. [CrossRef]
14. Izadyar, N.; Miller, W. Ventilation strategies design impacts on indoor airborne transmission: A review. *Build. Environ.* **2022**, *218*, 109158. [CrossRef] [PubMed]
15. Vu, T.; Belussi, A.; Migliorini, S.; Eldway, A. Using deep learning big spatial data partitioning. *ACM Trans. Spat. Algorithms Syst. (TSAS)* **2020**, *7*, 3. [CrossRef]
16. Sundaramoorthy, S.; Kameshwari, V.; Selvaraj, S.K. Clinical Deep Dive Role Ai/Ml Techniques Tackling COVID-19. In *Internet Medical Things for Smart Healthcare: COVID-19 Pandemic*; Springer: Singapore, 2020; pp. 215–240. [CrossRef]
17. Bhangale, U.; Patil, S.; Vishwanath, V.; Thakker, P.; Bansode, A.; Navandhar, D. Near real-time crowd counting using deep learning approach. *Proc. Comput. Sci.* **2020**, *171*, 770–779. [CrossRef]

18. Mousavi, E.; Khademi, A.; Taaffe, K. Optimal sensor placement hospital operating room. *IISE Trans. Healthc. Syst. Eng.* **2020**, *10*, 212–227. [CrossRef]
19. Hunter, E.; Namee, B.M.; Kelleher, J.D. A hybrid agent-based equation based model spread infectious diseases. *J. Artif. Soc. Soc. Simul.* **2020**, *23*, 14. [CrossRef]
20. Hoek, G.; Ranzi, A.; Alimehmeti, I.; Ardeleanu, E.R.; Arrebola, J.P.; Ávila, P.; De Hoogh, K. A review exposure assessment methods epidemiological studies health effects related industrially contaminated sites. *Epidemiol. Prev.* **2018**, *42*, 21–36. [CrossRef] [PubMed]
21. Ultralytics. Documentation YOLO v8. Available online: https://docs.ultralytics.com/ (accessed on 26 May 2024). [CrossRef]
22. Liang, N.; Wu, G.; Kang, W.; Wang, Z.; Feng, D.D. Real-time long-term tracking prediction-detection-correction. *IEEE Trans. Multimed.* **2018**, *20*, 2289–2302. [CrossRef]
23. Jones, N.R.; Qureshi, Z.U.; Temple, R.J.; Larwood, J.P.; Greenhalgh, T.; Bourouiba, L. Two metres or one: What is the evidence physical distancing COVID-19. *BMJ* **2020**, *370*, m3223. [CrossRef] [PubMed]
24. Yang, Z.; Sun, M.; Ye, H.; Xiong, Z.; Zussman, G.; Kostic, Z. Birds Eye View Social Distancing Analysis System. *arXiv* **2022**, arXiv:2112.07159.
25. Acharjee, C.; Deb, S. YOLOv3 based Real Time Social Distance Violation Detection in Public Places. In Proceedings of the 2021 International Conference on Computational Performance Evaluation (ComPE), Shillong, India, 1–3 December 2021; pp. 625–630.
26. Gündüz, M.Ş.; Işık, G. A new YOLO-based method for social distancing from real-time videos. *Neural Comput. Appl.* **2023**, *35*, 15261–15271. [CrossRef] [PubMed] [PubMed Central]
27. Arifuzzaman, M.; Shaikh, R.; Bhuiyan, I.; Chowdhury, S.M.R.; Atoul, T.I. Innovation in public health surveillance for social distancing during the COVID-19 pandemic: A deep learning and object detection based novel approach. *PLoS ONE* **2024**, *19*, e0308460. [CrossRef] [PubMed]
28. Anderson, R.M.; May, R.M. *Infectious Diseases Humans: Dynamics Control*; Oxford University Press: Oxford, UK, 1991; pp. 154–196. [CrossRef]
29. Fraser, C.; Riley, S.; Anderson, R.M.; Ferguson, N.M. Factors infectious disease outbreak controllable. *Proc. Natl. Acad. Sci. USA* **2004**, *101*, 6146–6151. [CrossRef] [PubMed]
30. Rothman, K.J.; Greenland, S.; Lash, T.L. *Modern Epidemiology*, 3rd ed.; Lippincott Williams Wilkins: Philadelphia, PA, USA, 2008; p. 758.

healthcare

MDPI

Article

Lessons of the COVID-19 Pandemic for Ambulance Service in Kazakhstan

Assylzhan Messova [1,*], Lyudmila Pivina [1,*], Diana Ygiyeva [1], Gulnara Batenova [1], Almas Dyussupov [1], Ulzhan Jamedinova [2], Marat Syzdykbayev [3], Saltanat Adilgozhina [4] and Arman Bayanbaev [5]

1 Department of Emergency Medicine, Semey Medical University, Semey 071400, Kazakhstan; diana.ygiyeva@smu.edu.kz (D.Y.); gulnara.batenova@smu.edu.kz (G.B.); almas.dyussupov@smu.edu.kz (A.D.)
2 Department of Epidemiology and Biostatistics, Semey Medical University, Semey 071400, Kazakhstan; ulzhan.jamedinova@smu.edu.kz
3 Department of Anesthesiology and Reanimatology, Semey Medical University, Semey 071400, Kazakhstan; marat.syzdykbayev@smu.edu.kz
4 Department of Family Medicine, Semey Medical University, Semey 071400, Kazakhstan; saltanat.adilgozhina@smu.edu.kz
5 National Coordinating Center for Emergency Assistance, Astana 10000, Kazakhstan; astana077@gmail.com
* Correspondence: assylzhan2006@mail.ru (A.M.); semskluda@rambler.ru (L.P.)

Abstract: Background: Emergency medical services (EMS) are intended to provide people with immediate, effective, and safe access to the healthcare system. The effects of pandemics on emergency medical services (EMS) have not been studied sufficiently. The aim of this paper is to assess the frequency and structure of calls at an ambulance station in Kazakhstan during the period of 2019–2023. Methods: A retrospective analysis was conducted to estimate the incidence of emergency assistance cases from 2019 to 2023. Results: An analysis of the structure and number of ambulance calls before the pandemic, during the pandemic, and post-pandemic period did not reveal significant changes, except for calls in urgency category IV. Patients of urgency category IV handled by an ambulance decreased by 2 and 1.7 times in 2020 and 2021, respectively, which appears to be related to quarantine measures. In 2022 and 2023, category IV calls were 4.7 and 4.5 times higher than in 2019. Conclusions: This study's findings suggest no changes in the dynamics of ambulance calls, except urgency category IV calls. The number of category IV urgent calls decreased significantly during the COVID-19 pandemic and increased in the post-pandemic period.

Keywords: COVID-19; emergency; ambulance service; Kazakhstan; consultation

1. Introduction

Emergency medical services (EMS) are important component of a national healthcare system [1]. During pandemics, the national EMS must balance the ongoing demands of regular emergency cases with the additional needs brought on by the crises. In Kazakhstan, this role is performed by the National Coordinating Center of Emergency Medicine (NCCEM). The main role of the NCCEM is to improve the quality and availability of emergency medical care to reduce mortality and disability in the Republic of Kazakhstan. The NCCEM operates a fleet of about 1500 ambulances spread throughout the country. In addition to the ambulances, more than 30 units of air transport are used; medical aviation carried out from three to fifteen flights per day [2].

Kazakhstan has a small population (19 million residents), and remains one of the most sparsely populated countries. The republic ranks ninth in terms of territory, but in terms of population, according to the analysis of the UN Population Fund, there were only 6.8 people per square kilometer in 2019 [3]. In this regard, ambulances often serve large areas and the assistance of air ambulances is required. The largest share of flights is carried out to provide medical care in cases of injuries, including those caused by road accidents, as well as pathologies of childhood, diseases of the circulatory system, pathologies of newborns, obstetric and gynecological pathologies, and surgical, therapeutic, and other diseases. Mobile teams of republican or regional levels carry out the provision of medical care. The full-time mobile medical team includes a doctor and a paramedic or only paramedics; it is formed by the medical profile of the patients. If necessary, by significance, qualified specialists from large organizations, cities of republican significance and the capital, as well as educational and scientific organizations can be involved.

The COVID-19 pandemic has become the biggest health challenge worldwide. The load on almost all segments of the medical system, especially on first aid services, increased significantly. It has required a quick revision of the usual work algorithms. Prior reports on the number of EMS calls during a pandemic compared to post-pandemic were extremely few [4–6].

Response to COVID-19 in Kazakhstan

The first COVID-19 case in Kazakhstan was diagnosed on 13 March 2020 [7]. To prevent the spread of the disease, a state of emergency was introduced from 16 March to 11 May 2020. Restrictions were implemented on entry and exit from the country; quarantine or other restrictive measures were introduced in all regions, and the activities of large non-food retail outlets, cinemas, and other places with large crowds of people were stopped [8]. On 5 July 2020, a strict isolation regime began to operate in Kazakhstan. All facilities were closed, except for grocery stores, pharmacies, cafes (while maintaining social distancing), and airports (for domestic flights). Then, from 17 August 2020, Kazakhstan approved a plan for the phased lifting of quarantine. To provide timely medical care to patients with coronavirus infection, as of 17 March 2020, 248 infectious diseases hospitals were involved in the Republic of Kazakhstan, with a bed capacity of 23,462 beds [9].

According to the Johns Hopkins University data, four waves of coronavirus infection were observed in Kazakhstan; the first wave had a peak in July 2020, when 18,757 new cases of coronavirus infection were detected per day, the second wave in the winter of 2020–2021 (an average of 1300 cases of positive polymerase chain reaction (PCR) tests per day was detected), and the third wave in March 2021 with the number of new cases reaching 1500–3000 per day [10]. The peak of the fourth wave of coronavirus infection was observed in August 2021, associated with the spread of the Delta variant of the coronavirus. During the last increase in incidence at its peak, up to 7800 cases were recorded per day [11].

The COVID-19 call centers were opened, and citizens of the Republic of Kazakhstan could call 24 h a day to find out all the information about current situations on coronavirus incidence, as well as preventive measures and the main symptoms of diseases. They were created as a part of the regional/city emergency medical stations, which had operational communication with the service of the internal affairs and civil protection of the population in the regions, EMS substations, EMS departments at Primary Health Care Institutions, and emergency departments of medical organizations. In the call centers, consultations with the population were carried out by consulting doctors, senior doctors of regional/city emergency medical services, experienced paramedics and paramedical workers, and residents. Call center specialists informed the population on the provision of medical care at the pre-hospital stage and answered frequently asked questions related to the coronavirus infection. In the presence of such symptoms as headache, runny nose, chest pain, fever, tachycardia and rapid breathing, calls were redirected to the dispatcher 103.

The most effective method of combating coronavirus infection is vaccination. The mass vaccination campaign against COVID-19 began in Kazakhstan on 1 February 2021. In Kazakhstan, the local vaccine QazVac (Kazakhstan), as well as Sputnik V (Russia), Sinopharm (China), Sinovac (China), and Pfizer (America) were used. Currently, 55.35% of the population has received full vaccination [11]. There is a lack of research on the functioning of the emergency medical care system in Kazakhstan during the pandemic, which is necessary to learn lessons for the future.

This study aims to characterize the work of emergency medical services during the coronavirus pandemic and make recommendations to be applied for future preparedness.

2. Materials and Methods

2.1. Study Design

This study is a descriptive, population-based cross-sectional study of EMS work in the Republic of Kazakhstan before, during, and after the pandemic. Information on emergency medical calls was provided by the ambulance stations of 17 regions and three cities of republican significance of the Republic Kazakhstan.

Ambulance Service in Kazakhstan

In the Republic of Kazakhstan, the ambulance service is structured as a centralized system. The structure of the ambulance service in Kazakhstan consists of a three-tier system, including ambulance stations, ambulance teams, and dispatch centers, provided by the government. The Republican Emergency Medical Center (RCC) of the Ministry of Healthcare of Kazakhstan is responsible for managing, planning, and coordinating the work of ambulance services throughout the country. Regional ambulance stations provide emergency medical care to their regions' populations [12].

The emergency medical station dispatcher receives calls from citizens at the "103" remote control in case of health problems; the call processing time from the moment it is received by the emergency medical service dispatcher is five minutes, during which the call is sorted by category of urgency. There is also a call hold system by the dispatcher, which allows them to provide to assist until the ambulance arrives. The dispatcher explains over the phone how to provide emergency assistance. The dispatcher of the ambulance station performed the following actions: receiving all calls on the remote control 103; triage (screening) by call urgency category; using an automated system, transfering the calls of first, second, and third categories of urgency to the ambulance teams. The calls of the fourth category of urgency were transferred to the paramedical and medical teams of the ambulance and primary health care organizations. According to the Rules for the provision of emergency medical care, approved by Order of the Minister of Health of the Republic of Kazakhstan (3 July 2017 No. 450), all calls are divided into 4 (four) categories of urgency [13].

The first level of urgency signifies an immediate threat to life requiring emergency medical attention.

The second group relates to a potential threat to life in the absence of medical intervention, whereas the third category refers to a potential harm to health. The fourth category refers to a patient's state caused by an acute sickness or worsening of a chronic disease that does not involve sudden and pronounced organ and system violations and does not provide an immediate or possible threat to the patient's life.

The time of arrival of the EMS team from the moment of receiving a call should be up to 10 min for the first category of urgency, up to 15 min for the second category, up to 30 min for the third category, and less than 60 min for the fourth category of urgency (in such cases departure was carried out at the outpatient clinic). Upon receipt of a call of the fourth category of urgency, the ambulance dispatcher calls the brigade of the ambulance department at PHC using an automatic control system. In the case of a call, when there is no need for an emergency response team to attend a call at home, the dispatcher forwards the call to the call center.

The ambulance team, using the clinical protocol for treatment and diagnosis, determines the route of the patient's movement depending on his condition according to the algorithm. In the case of a patient who does not need hospitalization, the ambulance team or the ambulance department at PHC provides medical recommendations for the provision of medical care in the PHC organization (at the place of residence). Before transporting the patient to the hospital, the ambulance team checks with the dispatch service about the availability of vacant places in the corresponding hospital and notifies the hospital emergency department of the upcoming hospitalization.

The number of ambulance stations in Kazakhstan has increased significantly over the past 10 years; at the moment, there are over 400 stations and substations in total [12]. In our study we included all ambulance usage, even if an ambulance was used to transfer a patient from one hospital to another.

2.2. Ethical Approval Details

The study has approval of the Local Ethics Commission of the Semey Medical University on 16 March 2022. Information on emergency medical calls was provided by the National Center for Emergency Medicine. All ambulance stations within 17 regions and 3 cities of republican significance provide monthly and annual reports with the structure of calls to the National Center for Emergency Medicine.

2.3. Statistical Analysis

When conducting descriptive statistics, depending on the type of data distribution, for all continuous variables, the mean and its confidence intervals were calculated; in the samples the distribution of which differed from the normal, the median and interquartile range were calculated.

In order to compare the main indicators of the activity of the ambulance service by years, Friedman's two-way analysis of variance by ranks was used for related samples. The calculation of the Friedman criterion was carried out to compare variables that have a distribution other than normal, according to the Shapiro–Ulik criterion. For group comparison, a systematic comparison of post hoc analysis was applied using post hoc Bonferroni corrections.

In samples, whose distribution was not statistically significantly different from the normal distribution, according to the Shapiro–Ulik test, analysis of variance (ANOVA) for related variables was used. To analyze the dynamics over the years, we used Pillai's trace criterion. For pairwise comparisons, a post hoc comparison test with Sidak correction was used.

The *p*-value < 0.05 was taken as statistically significant. Statistical analysis of the data was carried out using SPSS version 20.0 (IBM Ireland Product Distribution Limited, Dublin, Ireland).

3. Results

Table 1 shows the structure of ambulance calls: all calls to console 103, canceled calls, consultations, ineffective calls, and fulfilled calls.

Table 1. Numbers of emergency calls (2019–2023).

Number of Emergency Calls	2019 †	2020 †	2021 †	2022 †	2023 †	*p*
Emergency calls (mean for one region per 1 year)	529,307 (±381,301)	450,940 (±334,591)	494,578 (±350,816)	380,680.5 (±366,475)	365,157 (±366,521)	0.726
Emergency calls per 1000 inhabitants *	466.58 (±137.81)	426.10 (±126.77)	470.55 (±127.36)	436.69 (±105.83)	410.02 (±104.85)	0.021
Cancelled calls (mean for one station per 1 year)	2724 (±8231)	1987 (±8700)	1112.5 (±5765)	357.5 (±5622)	95.5 (±2954)	0.647
Number of consultations (mean for one station per 1 year)	7635 (±15,516)	8516 (±15,361)	13,616 (±13,391)	14,069 (±26,221)	16649 (±40,014)	0.657
Ineffective calls (mean for one regio per 1 year)	8905 (±8644)	9985 (±6801)	12,525 (±8460)	9789 (±9193)	10,853.5 (±11,327)	0.829
Fulfilled calls (mean for one station per 1 year)	489,403 (±304,808)	416,183 (±281,659)	455,750 (±324,041)	335,520 (±318,337)	337,181.5 (±324,698)	0.79

* Me (IQR). † Plus–minus values are means ± SD. IQR denotes interquartile range.

Emergency calls are all incoming calls to remote control 103.

Cancelled calls are calls in which the patient's condition improved and the person canceled the call or decided to go to the hospital on their own without waiting for an ambulance.

An ineffective EMS call is a case of a call regarding a disease, accident, injury, poisoning or other condition that poses a threat to the patient's life, as a result of which the patient was not there; the call was false (ambulance was not called to this address); the patient was not found the address indicated when calling; the patient turned out to be practically healthy and did not need help; the patient died before the arrival of the EMS team; the patient was taken away before the arrival of the EMS team; the patient was served by a doctor at the clinic before the arrival of the EMS team; or the patient refused to be examined.

Fulfilled calls are ambulance calls as a result of which emergency care was provided to the patient and the patient was transferred for further observation to a local clinic, or the patient was hospitalized in a specialized hospital.

As shown in Table 1, the average number of calls per region per year, as well as the number of calls per 1000 population, did not change significantly from 2019 to 2023.

Call cancellations trended downward from 2724 to 95.5 (2019, 2023), but the data do not show statistical significance. The number of consultations doubled from 2019 to 2023, but the data also do not show statistical significance. The pandemic has taught medical workers how to use healthcare resources economically. Therefore, the number of telephone consultations has increased mostly since 2021. The number of ineffective calls did not change significantly from 2019 to 2023. The number of calls served gradually decreasing from 489,403 to 337,181.5, but the data are also not reliable.

When considering the call structure, all emergency cases were divided into 11 categories (Table 2): infections, cardio-vascular disorders, trauma and poisoning, traffic accidents, obstetrics and gynecology, neurological, respiratory, gastrointestinal, acute surgical, urinary tract diseases, and others.

Table 2. Causes and categories of emergency calls (2019–2023).

Clinical Diagnosis	Monthly Statistics					p
	2019 †	2020 †	2021 †	2022 †	2023 †	
Infectious Diseases	26,365 (±39,327)	18,678 (±32,957)	15,903 (±24,630)	15,373 (±19,918)	12,520 (±15,408)	0.153
Cardio-vascular diseases	72,543 (±66,100)	72,711 (±68,094)	70,879.38 (±52,833)	65,472.5 (±52,468)	69,820.5 (±46,398)	0.938
Trauma and poisoning	27,474 (±34,891)	27,315 (±34,021)	29,702 (±33,141)	27,093 (±30,811)	27,716.5 (±30,423)	0.97
Traffic accidents	1518 (±2152)	1432 (±1465)	1659 (±1930)	1527.5 (±1788)	1633.5 (±1252)	0.676
Neurological diseases *	37,277.24 [26,906.68; 47,647.79]	30,826.5 [22,784.17; 38,868.83]	34,613.88 [25,581.67; 43,646.08]	36,726.44 [26,627.31; 46,825.58]	37,083.9 [26,256.08; 47,911.72]	0.899
Respiratory diseases *	99,125 [71,767.09; 126,482.91]	95,027.58 [70,391.22; 119,663.93]	122,482.28 [90,711.49; 154,253.07]	123,817.72 [87,691.84; 159,943.6]	104,206.15 [77,571.01; 130,841.29]	0.677
Gastrointestinal diseases	23,872 (±18,754)	19,900 (±15,152)	23,196 (±23,105)	23,554 (±26,680)	27,854.5 (±24,857)	0.719
Obstetrics and gynecology	20,924 (±35,571)	21,935 (±37,090)	23,890 (±35,826)	20,382.5 (±22,379)	17,848.5 (±24,134)	0.911
Acute surgical diseases *	17,182.59 [13,294.11; 21,071.06]	12,234.5 [9441.24; 15,027.76]	13,252.65 [9687.71; 16,817.58]	13,460.5 [9627.96; 17,293.04]	11,592.9 [8492.48; 14,693.32]	0.183
Urinary tract diseases	11,399 (±14,691)	8083 (±12,309)	7053 (±7277)	6837.5 (±7999)	6290.5 (±7518)	0.046
Others	80,463 (±67,543)	67,060 (±65,008)	76,365 (±50,626)	75,979.5 (±52,343)	65,662.5 (±55,830)	0.622

Table 2. Causes and categories of emergency calls (2019–2023).

Clinical Diagnosis	Monthly Statistics					*p*
	2019 †	2020 †	2021 †	2022 †	2023 †	
Category of urgency						
I urgency category	15,885 (±34,957)	15,857 (±23,809)	18,754 (±20,831)	14,633.5 (±20,790)	13,604.5 (±20,385)	0.901
II urgency category	119,466 (±134,124)	98,817 (±118,520)	116,745 (±112,724)	109,072.5 (±94,825)	105,274.5 (±81,443)	0.943
III urgency category	129,696 (±87,978)	111,778 (±75,081)	112,674 (±108,103)	110,524 (±116,393)	96,230 (±105,434)	0.702
IV urgency category, served by ambulance (abs number)	36,153 (±86,113)	17,583 (±44,670)	20,375 (±52,019)	172,420.5 (±147,203)	161,536 (±121,573)	0.001
IV urgency category, served by emergency medical services teams at primary health care facilities (abs. number)	91,207 (±103,525)	108,512 (±121,601)	117,501 (±138,812)	120,174.5 (±137,539)	94,864 (±123,835)	0.629

* Me (IQR). † Plus–minus values are means ± SD. IQR denotes interquartile range.

According to Table 2, infectious and the urinary system diseases decreased by half from 2019 to 2023, but the data were not statistically significant. Cardiovascular, trauma and poisoning, traffic accidents, neurological, gastrointestinal, obstetric-gynecological, acute surgical pathology, and other diseases did not change significantly. Respiratory diseases decreased from 99,125 to 95,027.6 during the first wave of the CVI (2020), then increased during the second, third, and fourth waves of the CVI to 122,482.28, but these data do not have statistical significance.

When analyzing the structure of calls per region, calls of the first category of urgency (resuscitation is required for life-threatening conditions); calls of the second category of urgency (a patient's condition that offers a potential threat to life if not treated); calls of the third category of urgency (a patient's condition that poses a potential threat to health without medical care); and calls of the fourth category of urgency served by emergency medical services teams at primary health care facilities (there is no current or potential threat to the patient's life and health), no changes were observed. Patients of category IV urgency served by ambulance decreased by 2 and 1.7 times in 2020 and 2021, apparently associated with quarantine measures. There is a significant increase of IV category calls in 2022 and 2023 of 4.7 and 4.5 times, respectively, in comparison with 2019.

In total, 1,498,668 cases of COVID-19 were registered in Kazakhstan over the entire period of the pandemic, of which 19,071 were deaths. A total of 33,563,811 vaccinations and 11,575,012 PCR tests were performed [7].

According to this study, there was a decline in the frequency of category IV EMS calls the COVID-19 pandemic, followed by an increase in frequency during the post-pandemic period.

4. Discussion

The COVID-19 pandemic has dramatically affected emergency ambulance services. According to the literature, the emergency work of the ambulance service during the COVID-19 pandemic showed that there was no significant increase in activity, possibly due to the introduced quarantine measures (for example, due to a decrease in the number of injuries due to vehicle collisions) and also due to the avoidance of medical services [14,15].

When COVID-19 first began to spread in Kazakhstan, the health system recommended adequate measures to control the epidemic. Compliance with quarantine measures has led to a decrease in ambulance calls and morbidity throughout Kazakhstan. In April 2020, there was a sharp decrease in deaths due to the introduction of quarantine, when people were closed up in their homes; the number of deaths due to limited mobility, injuries, and traffic accidents decreased [11].

Kazakhstan used quarantine at an early stage and paired it with other community safety measures, including closing all schools, limiting travel, and disinfecting and sanitizing public areas. Preliminary quarantine measures in Kazakhstan led to social tension, as people could not remain unemployed for a long time [9]. The government was forced to ease quarantine measures, which led to a sharp increase in the incidence of coronavirus. A study conducted in Australia showed that, during quarantine, there was a decrease in the number of calls, but there was a deterioration in response times for ambulances [16]. A study in Polland also illustrated a significant decrease in the number of EMT interventions [17]. Other studies have shown that during the COVID-19 pandemic in 2021, the incidence of difficult-to-transfer cases increased compared to 2019 [18].

This study result was also confirmed by our research in terms of calls of category IV urgency, since during the COVID-19 pandemic there was a decrease in the number of calls. According to the data presented, calls of category IV urgency decreased by 2 and 1.7 times (in 2020 and 2021) during the COVID-19 pandemic, compared to 2019 before the pandemic. The decrease in calls in 2020 during the first wave of coronavirus infection may be related to quarantine measures. The lack of an increase during waves two, three, and four of COVID-19 in 2021, when 1500–7600 new cases per day were noted, may be because the population could not reach an ambulance [11] during the peak of incidence or treated themselves. A limitation of our study is the lack of data for unanswered calls.

The sharp increase in ambulance calls in 2022 and 2023 may be due to the weak performance of the local service, as well as the fact that people with chronic comorbid diseases who did not apply during the pandemic for fear of contracting COVID-19, or "hospital bed shortage", began to seek medical help. Also, after undergoing coronavirus infection (CVI), many elderly patients with chronic diseases experienced exacerbations, and the level of injuries and infections (ARVI, measles) increased after a long quarantine.

When looking at the call structure, almost all categories did not show any statistically marked changes. One of the important links in prehospital care is the dispatch service. During the pandemic, the importance of dispatch has increased. This is evidenced by the two-fold increase in consultations from 2019 to 2023, but the data did not show statistical significance.

In general, the results of the study show a decrease in the number of category IV calls during the coronavirus infection (2020–2021) and an increase in the number of calls during the post-pandemic period (2022–2023). Further studies are needed for investigation post-pandemic emergency medical services.

4.1. *Challenges during the COVID-19 Outbreak*

Due to the unprecedented spread of COVID-19 around the world since December 2019, the healthcare system in Kazakhstan, like other countries, has faced a number of difficulties in treating this disease and attracting related resources, resulting in a wealth of experience and lessons learned.

4.1.1. Incorrect Forecast

In March 2020, the Ministry of Health of Kazakhstan predicted that if quarantine measures were followed, the number of infected people for a three-month period would not exceed 3500 people [19]. However, on 1 July 2020, there was a sharp increase in the incidence of 18,757 new cases per day [11]. The incorrect forecast led to the unpreparedness of the healthcare system of Kazakhstan.

4.1.2. Inability to Reach an Ambulance

A sociological survey conducted by Sanj Research Center (2020) showed that 24.5% of respondents in need of emergency assistance faced difficulties in calling an ambulance, 5.5% of calls went unanswered, and 25% of respondents got through but with difficulty. In rural areas, it was tough to reach emergency services [11].

4.1.3. Ambulance Shortage and Shortage of Personal Protective Equipment, Ventilators, Diagnostic Tools (PCR)

Given the acute shortage of ambulances, the Ministry of Health purchased 807 ambulances during the peak of the first wave of coronavirus infections [11]. Medical professionals are on the front line fighting the COVID-19 health crisis. At the beginning of the pandemic, personal protective equipment (PPE) was not purchased promptly, causing a huge number of medical workers to fall ill [9]. Usage of PPE by the community and healthcare providers is crucial for the prevention of the spread of infection and must be available to the public. Kazakhstan's population and medical institutions faced shortages of medicines and ambulances, ventilators, diagnostic equipment (PCR tests), and beds during the first wave of the pandemic with rising of CVI incidence [9]. Extended hospitalization times caused by bed scarcity have caused delays in the duties of emergency personnel. Disruption in the supply chain of equipment leads to spread of infection and more severe equipment deficiency.

4.1.4. Inadequate Prevention in Society

As crowds are often present during religious and cultural events in Kazakhstan, this has been a determining factor and has made social distancing strategies more challenging. Most people found it impossible to adhere to the quarantine and carried on their business at the local level because of the Kazakhstan government's inadequate financial support and national protection program. Due to the near-impossibility of maintaining social distance and limiting exposure—two key strategies for lowering the risk of the sickness—it was difficult to control the situation. Violation of quarantine measures was aligned with an increase in the incidence of COVID-19 in the summer of 2020. At the same time, according to studies conducted by Kazakh scientists, 50% compliance with quarantine measures would have led to a decrease in the number of hospitalized up to 9.31 thousand cases during the peak of the pandemic [20].

4.1.5. Shortage of Doctors and Medical Personnel

From 2017 to 2021, the shortage of medical personnel doubled from 10 thousand to 23 thousand units [21]. Due to the shortage of doctors, remaining doctors are forced to work beyond the norm.

4.1.6. Mental State of Medical Personnel

A brief review of the impact of COVID-19 on the reported mental health and well-being of ambulance service personnel revealed higher rates of distress, PTSD, and insomnia [22]. A national survey in the United Kingdom of ambulance service clinicians and paramedics preparedness and response to the COVID-19 pandemic also showed the psychological distress of most participants [23].

The Center for Evidence-Based Medicine provides data on mortality per 100 thousand people in the different countries. It was demonstrated that excess mortality in Kazakhstan was very high in 2020 in comparison with developed countries; it reached 21% compared to the previous three years [24]. The COVID-19 pandemic has significantly affected the health status of the population of Kazakhstan, as well as the well-established process of providing medical care in the country, and the unpreparedness of the healthcare system's response to emergencies has been revealed [24]. Regrettably, Kazakhstan's COVID-19 pandemic, like those in other nations, has highlighted the shortcomings of the country's healthcare system, including its lack of public healthcare, delayed reaction time, disregard for the needs of the population's most vulnerable members, and weak resistance to disinformation [11].

5. Conclusions

The results of the study do not contain changes in the dynamics of ambulance calls, except for calls of category IV urgency. A significant decrease of category IV urgency calls were observed during the pandemic of COVID-19 infection. The increase in the category IV calls in 2022 and 2023 that did not require emergency assistance may be due to the poor performance of local services, and an increase in exacerbations of chronic diseases as well as infections.

The lesson we must learn from this pandemic is the need to be carefully prepared as the worst-case scenario unfolds. A national pandemic preparedness plan must be developed in Kazakhstan in order to get ready for the next outbreak.

1. Finances: The ability to raise the money required in the event of a new epidemic is crucial to maintain services.
2. During a pandemic, all parts of the healthcare system must work harmoniously. The weak performance of one link leads to the overload of another. For ambulances to operate effectively, it is necessary to improve the work of local outpatient services.
3. Coordinate the proper distribution of resources. Investing in trained doctors and paramedics, developing proprietary medications, vaccines, and medical supplies. Training and developing the practical skills of medical personnel when working with especially dangerous infections (personal protective equipment, sorting patients by severity, algorithms for diagnosing and providing emergency care, transportation). Expanding our own manufacturing of masks and personal protective equipment. Improving the equipment of ambulances with ventilators, oxygen concentrates, and medicines.
4. The lack of preparedness of the ambulance service in Kazakhstan is associated with an incorrect forecast. It is necessary to use prognostic scales to correctly predict morbidity.
5. The experience of the pandemic has shown the high cost-effectiveness and safety of distant consultations. It is necessary to further develop dispatch system, telemedicine, and distant consultations.

Author Contributions: A.M. and L.P. contributed conception of the study, design, methods of the study, and interpretation of the data. A.B. organized the data collection and analysis. A.D. and M.S. contributed interpretation of the study findings. U.J. and D.Y. performed the statistical analysis and wrote the first draft of the manuscript. S.A. and G.B. wrote sections of the manuscript. All authors have read and agreed to the published version of the manuscript.

Funding: This work was supported by the Ministry of Science and Higher Education of the Republic of Kazakhstan under Grant AP 14871609 "Optimizing the structure and improving the efficiency of the emergency medicine service in Kazakhstan by conducting training for people without medical education (medical technicians)". The funders had no role in study design, data collection and analysis, decision to publish, or preparation of the manuscript.

Institutional Review Board Statement: This study was approved on 16 March 2022 by the Institutional Review Board (IRB) at the Local Ethics Commission of the Semey Medical University (approval No. 18).

Informed Consent Statement: Not applicable.

Data Availability Statement: The datasets generated for this study are available on request to the corresponding author.

Conflicts of Interest: The authors declare no conflict of interest.

References

1. World Health Organization. *Regional Office for Europe & European Union. Emergency Medical Services Systems in the European Union: Report of an Assessment Project Coordinated by the World Health Organization*; WHO Regional Office for Europe: Copenhagen, Denmark, 2008. Available online: https://apps.who.int/iris/handle/10665/107916 (accessed on 2 June 2024).
2. National Coordinating Center of Emergency Medicine [Dataset]. Available online: https://emcrk.kz/ru/ (accessed on 5 June 2024).
3. UN Kazakhstan Annual Report 2022 [Dataset]. 2023. Available online: https://kazakhstan.un.org/ (accessed on 25 May 2024).
4. Jaffe, E.; Sonkin, R.; Strugo, R.; Zerath, E. Evolution of emergency medical calls during a pandemic—An emergency medical service during the COVID-19 outbreak. *Am. J. Emerg. Med.* **2021**, *43*, 260–266. [CrossRef] [PubMed]
5. Jaffe, E.; Sonkin, R.; Alpert, E.A.; Magid, A.; Knobler, H.Y. Flattening the COVID-19 Curve: The Unique Role of Emergency Medical Services in Containing a Global Pandemic. *Isr. Med. Assoc. J.* **2020**, *8*, 476–482.

6. Moroni, F.; Gramegna, M.; Ajello, S.; Beneduce, A.; Baldetti, L.; Vilca, L.M.; Cappelletti, A.; Scandroglio, A.M.; Azzalini, L. Collateral Damage: Medical Care Avoidance Behavior among Patients with Myocardial Infarction during the COVID-19 Pandemic. *JACC Case Rep.* **2020**, *2*, 1620–1624. [CrossRef] [PubMed]
7. More than 19 thousand Kazakhstanis Have Died from Coronavirus Since the Beginning of the Pandemic [Dataset]. 2023. Available online: https://www.inform.kz/ru/bolee-19-tysyach-kazahstancev-umerli-ot-koronavirusa-s-nachala-pandemii_a4064764 (accessed on 25 May 2024).
8. Zhalmagambetov, B.; Madikenova, M.; Paizullayeva, S.; Abbay, A.; Gaipov, A. COVID-19 Outbreak in Kazakhstan: Current Status and Challenges. *J. Clin. Med. Kazakhstan* **2020**, *55*, 6–8. [CrossRef]
9. Semenova, Y.; Pivina, L.; Khismetova, Z.; Auyezova, A.; Nurbakyt, A.; Kauysheva, A.; Ospanova, D.; Kuziyeva, G.; Kushkarova, A.; Ivankov, A.; et al. Anticipating the Need for Healthcare Resources Following the Escalation of the COVID-19 Outbreak in the Republic of Kazakhstan. *J. Prev. Med. Public Health* **2020**, *53*, 387–396. [CrossRef] [PubMed]
10. COVID-19 Data Repository by the Center for Systems Science and Engineering (CSSE) at Johns Hopkins University. Available online: https://coronavirus.jhu.edu/ (accessed on 25 May 2024).
11. Dzhandosova, Z.; Sharipbaeva, A.; Bajtugelova, N.; Smagulova, S.K.; Kudasheva, T.V.; Zhandosova, F.S. *Data from: "Centr Issledovanij Sandzh". COVID-19 v Kazahstane: Masshtaby Problemy, Ocenka Uslug Zdravoohraneniya i Social'noj Zashchity*; Soros Foundation-Kazakhstan: Nur-Sultan, Kazakhstan, 2021; 180p.
12. Messova, A.M.; Pivina, L.M.; Ygieva, D.G.; Dyusupov, A.A.; Batenova, G.B.; Zhumadilov, A.S.; Akimzhanov, K.D.; Yurkovskaya, O.A.; Adilgozhina, S.M.; Bayanbaev, A.S.; et al. Analysis of the staffing and structure of the ambulance service in the Republic of Kazakhstan. Nauka i Zdravookhranenie. *Sci. Healthc.* **2023**, *25*, 143–149.
13. Order of the Minister of Health of the Republic of Kazakhstan dated November 30, 2020 No. KR DSM-225/2020. Registered with the Ministry of Justice of the Republic of Kazakhstan on December 2, 2020 No. 21713. Available online: https://adilet.zan.kz/rus/docs/V2000021713#z289 (accessed on 2 August 2024).
14. Bíró, K.; Deák, M.S.; Pápai, G.; Nagy, A.; Dombrádi, V.; Szabó, G.T.; Boruzs, K.; Bányai, G.; Csató, G. The Emergency Performance of the Hungarian Ambulance Service during the COVID-19 Pandemic. *Healthcare* **2022**, *10*, 2331. [CrossRef] [PubMed]
15. Hegenberg, K.; Althammer, A.; Gehring, C.; Prueckner, S.; Trentzsch, H. Pre-Hospital Emergency Medical Services Utilization Amid COVID-19 in 2020: Descriptive Study Based on Routinely Collected Dispatch Data in Bavaria, Germany. *Healthcare* **2023**, *11*, 1983. [CrossRef] [PubMed] [PubMed Central]
16. Andrew, E.; Nehme, Z.; Stephenson, M.; Walker, T.; Smith, K. The Impact of the COVID-19 Pandemic on Demand for Emergency Ambulances in Victoria, Australia. *Prehospital Emerg. Care* 2021, *ahead of print*. [CrossRef] [PubMed]
17. Nadolny, K.; Ładny, J.R.; Zyśko, D.; Gałązkowski, R.; Gąsior, M.; Kraska, W. Interventions of emergency medical teams in Poland during the SARS-CoV-2 pandemic. *Kardiol. Pol.* **2021**, *79*, 72–75. [CrossRef] [PubMed]
18. Ota, K.; Nitta, M.; Komeya, T.; Matsuoka, T.; Takasu, A. Influence of the COVID-19 Outbreak in Vulnerable Patients (Pediatric Patients, Pregnant Women, and Elderly Patients) on an Emergency Medical Service System: A Pre- and Post-COVID-19 Pandemic Comparative Study Using the Population-Based ORION Registry. *Medicina* **2024**, *60*, 345. [CrossRef] [PubMed]
19. According to the Ministry of Health, the Number of Infected People in Kazakhstan Will Not Exceed 3500. 2020. Available online: https://informburo.kz/novosti/birtanov-o-zarazhyonnyh-covid-19-8-tyazhyolyh-pacientov-4-na-ivl-no-est-tendenciya-k-stabilizacii.html (accessed on 2 August 2024).
20. Semenovam, Y.; Glushkova, N.; Pivina, L.; Khismetova, Z.; Zhunussov, Y.; Sandybaev, M.; Ivankov, A. Epidemiological Characteristics and Forecast of COVID-19 Outbreak in the Republic of Kazakhstan. *J. Korean Med. Sci.* **2020**, *35*, e227. [CrossRef] [PubMed]
21. Lykova, N. Medical Shortage Doubles in Kazakhstan. 2022. Available online: https://tengrinews.kz/kazakhstan_news/defitsit-medikov-uvelichilsya-vdvoe-v-kazahstane-470863/ (accessed on 2 August 2024).
22. Ebben, R.H.A.; Woensdregt, T.; Wielenga-Meijer, E.; Pelgrim, T.; de Lange, A.; Berben, S.A.A.; Vloet, L.C.M. The impact of COVID-19 on the mental health and well-being of ambulance care professionals: A rapid review. *PLoS ONE* **2023**, *18*, e0287821. [CrossRef] [PubMed]
23. Barrett, J.W.; Eastley, K.B.; Herbland, A.; Owen, P.; Naeem, S.; Mortimer, C.; King, J.; Foster, T.; Rees, N.; Rosser, A.; et al. The COVID-19 ambulance response assessment (CARA) study: A national survey of ambulance service healthcare professionals' preparedness and response to the COVID-19 pandemic. *Br. Paramed. J.* **2024**, *8*, 10–20. [CrossRef] [PubMed]
24. Oke, J.; Heneghan, C. Data from: Global COVID-19 Case Fatality Rates [Dataset]. 2020. Available from: Center for Evidence-Based Medicine. Available online: https://www.cebm.net (accessed on 2 August 2024).

bioengineering

MDPI

Article

Cancerous and Non-Cancerous MRI Classification Using Dual DCNN Approach

Zubair Saeed [1,2,*], Othmane Bouhali [2,3,4], Jim Xiuquan Ji [1,2], Rabih Hammoud [5], Noora Al-Hammadi [5], Souha Aouadi [5] and Tarraf Torfeh [5]

1 Department of Electrical & Computer Engineering, Texas A&M University, College Station, TX 47080, USA; jim.ji@qatar.tamu.edu
2 Department of Electrical & Computer Engineering, Texas A&M University at Qatar, Doha 23874, Qatar; othmane.bouhali@qatar.tamu.edu
3 Department of Science & Arts, Texas A&M University at Qatar, Doha 23874, Qatar
4 Qatar Center for Quantum Computing, College of Science and Engineering, Hamad Bin Khalifa University, Doha 34110, Qatar
5 Department of Radiation Oncology, National Center for Cancer Care and Research, Hamad Medical Corporation, Doha 3050, Qatar; rhammoud2@hamad.qa (R.H.); nalhammadi1@hamad.qa (N.A.-H.); saouadi@hamad.qa (S.A.); ttorfeh@hamad.qa (T.T.)
* Correspondence: zubairsaeed602@gmail.com

Abstract: Brain cancer is a life-threatening disease requiring close attention. Early and accurate diagnosis using non-invasive medical imaging is critical for successful treatment and patient survival. However, manual diagnosis by radiologist experts is time-consuming and has limitations in processing large datasets efficiently. Therefore, efficient systems capable of analyzing vast amounts of medical data for early tumor detection are urgently needed. Deep learning (DL) with deep convolutional neural networks (DCNNs) emerges as a promising tool for understanding diseases like brain cancer through medical imaging modalities, especially MRI, which provides detailed soft tissue contrast for visualizing tumors and organs. DL techniques have become more and more popular in current research on brain tumor detection. Unlike traditional machine learning methods requiring manual feature extraction, DL models are adept at handling complex data like MRIs and excel in classification tasks, making them well-suited for medical image analysis applications. This study presents a novel Dual DCNN model that can accurately classify cancerous and non-cancerous MRI samples. Our Dual DCNN model uses two well-performed DL models, i.e., inceptionV3 and denseNet121. Features are extracted from these models by appending a global max pooling layer. The extracted features are then utilized to train the model with the addition of five fully connected layers and finally accurately classify MRI samples as cancerous or non-cancerous. The fully connected layers are retrained to learn the extracted features for better accuracy. The technique achieves 99%, 99%, 98%, and 99% of accuracy, precision, recall, and f1-scores, respectively. Furthermore, this study compares the Dual DCNN's performance against various well-known DL models, including DenseNet121, InceptionV3, ResNet architectures, EfficientNetB2, SqueezeNet, VGG16, AlexNet, and LeNet-5, with different learning rates. This study indicates that our proposed approach outperforms these established models in terms of performance.

Keywords: deep learning; magnetic resonance imaging; classification; machine learning; deep convolutional neural networks; dual DCNN model; inceptionV3; denseNet121; resNet50; resNet34; resNet18; efficientNetB2; squeezeNet; VGG16; alexNet; leNet-5; learning rates

1. Introduction

Cancer is a serious illness that can spread to other areas of the human body and is known by uncontrolled cell development. According to statistics from the World Health Organization (WHO), an estimated 10 million deaths worldwide were reported due to cancer by the year 2020 [1]. However, these are estimates and may not fully reflect the actual incidence due to incomplete reporting systems, especially in underdeveloped countries. The tumors can be malignant (cancerous), with varying levels of aggressiveness, or benign (non-cancerous). The brain is the most important organ in humans, overall responsible for managing the body, and therefore, brain tumors need urgent attention. The incidence and survival of brain tumors are affected by their type, size, grade, and location, as well as the age of a patient and overall health condition [2]. To improve patient outcomes, early diagnosis, and adequate treatment are critical.

Medical imaging is an important tool for visualizing the internal structure of tumors. It includes magnetic resonance imaging (MRI), positron emission tomography (PET), and computed tomography (CT). Here, MRI is considered more appropriate than other medical imaging modalities, as it provides detailed images of soft tissues, organs, and internal structures without using harmful radiation. It also provides excellent contrast resolution, allowing for better differentiation between healthy and abnormal tissue. When MRI examination is required, professionals often use software to manually mark regions of interest (ROI) which is time-consuming and error-prone and might compromise diagnosis. It is critical to identify warning signals and seek medical attention as soon as possible because early treatment can save lives [3]. That is why automatic systems that extract MRI data have various benefits, including faster diagnosis and effective treatment, improved accuracy, consistency, cost-effectiveness, and time savings [4]. Automatic systems require less time and deliver superior performance compared to manual methods because they are accurate and adept at handling large amounts of medical data.

The emergence of artificial intelligence (AI) presents promising solutions in various applications [5–8] and especially for automating medical image analysis, thereby achieving faster and more accurate diagnoses [9]. Similarly, its sub-field, i.e., the DL techniques, has been widely used in radiology to extract robust features from MRI, PET, and CT scans. In the past, medical ML techniques have mostly concentrated on high-level or low-level features that are manually extracted during feature engineering. The low-level features capture the essential aspects of an image, whereas high-level features provide semantic information. However, methods that can combine both kinds of features are automatically becoming useful [10]. In the meanwhile, deep learning techniques like deep convolutional neural networks (DCNN) are helpful for automatically learning high-level features including tumor size, location, and surrounding tissue. These low-level and high-level features must be taken into account for reliable and accurate brain tumor classification. This study proposes a novel Dual DCNN for accurate brain tumor classification using MRIs. Our model addresses the challenge of comprehensive feature extraction by learning both low-level (i.e., texture, intensity) and high-level (i.e., tumor location, size) features directly from the MRI scans. This combined feature extraction capability allows the Dual DCNN to achieve high accuracy in classifying cancerous and non-cancerous brain tumors.

Our contributions are discussed in detail in upcoming sections. A brief summary is as below:

1. Our proposed Dual DCNN model with denseNet121 and inceptionV3 has shown promising results. We observed significant improvements in various performance metrics especially the accuracy demonstrating the capability to accurately classify cancerous and non-cancerous MRI samples.
2. We have implemented SOTA DL models, i.e., denseNet121, inceptionV3, resNet50, resNet34, resNet18, efficientNetB2, squeezeNet, VGG16, alexNet, leNet-5, and compared results with our methodology. We have highlighted the best performance of our approach.
3. We have compared the performance of each SOTA DL model with different learning rates and identified the best learning rate for each model.
4. We compared our approach with the latest research in cancer detection and classification and through benchmarking we found our proposed approach outperformed existing methods.

2. Related Work

In recent years, researchers have been utilizing DL techniques for the classification of brain tumors using MRI data. These studies utilize the power of DL algorithms, particularly DCNNs to extract relevant features from MRI scans and classify them into different tumor types. Scafuto et al. [11] used CNN for the classification and segmentation of MRI scans to examine glioma diagnosis studies. The authors collected 77 academic articles and emphasized the requirement of early and accurate detection of tumors for glioma patients' survival. Their study aimed to implement a grading system for glioma brain tumors using DL and MRI. The authors used a dataset of 259 patients with glioma brain tumors. The researchers used a ConvNet model to divide the tumors into different levels. With an overall accuracy of 91.5%, the results showed that their proposed method achieved better accuracy for brain tumors caused by gliomas. Additionally, this study highlighted that their approach performed better as compared to the other methods. They suggested the integration of multi-modal data for more comprehensive analysis. Similarly, Fathima et al. [12] provide an overview of the evolution of data science disciplines and compare pre-processing, ML, and DL methods for brain tumor classification. Their methodology involved a review of existing techniques by highlighting the importance of early detection of brain tumors and early treatment. The authors discussed the advantages and limitations of different ML and DL techniques for brain tumor classification. They also compared the performance of different models and algorithms used in the literature. This study concluded that DL methods, particularly CNNs, have shown better results in classifying brain tumors. The authors also discussed the limitations of using deep learning methods, i.e., the need for large datasets for fine-tuning and the interpretability of the approach. The future direction of their study involves the development DL model with the integration of multi-modal data for more comprehensive analysis.

Several recent studies have also explored the use of fine-tuned approaches with complex datasets for the detection of brain tumors. Ghosal et al. [13] implemented a CNN-based SE-ResNet-101 that was fine-tuned for classifying brain tumors into malignant, gliomas, and pituitary tumors. They applied different pre-processing procedures, such as normalization, zero-centering, ROI segmentation, and augmentation of data like rotation, scaling, zooming, etc. Utilizing T1-weighted contrast-enhanced (T1W-CE) MRI data, their SE-ResNet-101 model obtained an accuracy of 93.83% with data augmentation and 89.93% without an augmentation approach. A three-step method was suggested by Nawaz et al. [14] which involved annotating interest regions, utilizing a customized CornerNet to extract deep features, and using a one-stage detector for tumor classification. Their accuracy on the T1W-CE MRI dataset was 98.8%. This approach provides an affordable solution because of the one-stage object identification framework provided by CornerNet.

The potential of hybrid approaches combining ML and DL has also been investigated. Mohammed et al. [15] offered four suggested systems for the early detection of brain cancers, each of which combines hybrid learning techniques. The first system uses hybrid features obtained from grey-level co-occurrence matrix (GLCM), discrete wavelet transform (DWT), and local binary pattern (LBP) methods to integrate artificial neural network and feedforward neural network techniques. The second method, a DL approach, achieved better results in differentiating between different types of brain cancers by using ResNet-50 and GoogLeNet models for classification. The third system shows the best results in tumor classification by utilizing a hybrid approach that combines support vector machines (SVMs) with CNN. The fourth system suggested uses a hybrid technique that combines DWT, GLCM, and LBP with ResNet-50 and GoogLeNet algorithms to obtain a more comprehensive analysis of brain tumor images. Similarly, Nassar et al. [16] used a hybrid deep learning strategy to build an effective automated method for classifying brain cancers. To take advantage of the combined abilities of numerous models and provide promising outcomes, the suggested method is based on the output of five distinct models. With an overall accuracy of 99.31%, their study's T1-weighted brain MR images achieved superior results. However, Saha et al. [17] proposed an improved method that uses DL and a collection of ML algorithms to categorize types of brain tumors from MRI. The BCM-VEMT method, which may be classified into four separate classes, i.e., glioma, meningioma, pituitary, and non-cancerous (normal), is presented in their work. To extract features from the MRI, a CNN is developed and then input into multi-class machine learning classifiers. By combining each machine learning classifier, a weighted average ensemble of classifiers is utilized to improve performance. A total of 3787 MRI images from each of the four classes composed the dataset used in their study. With an overall accuracy of 98.42%, their system obtained high precision for each class: 97.90% for glioma, 98.94% for meningioma, 98.00% for normal, and 98.92% for pituitary. The need to have an image-processing computer-aided diagnosis system that can accurately classify different forms of brain tumors was highlighted by this study.

Researchers also used the transfer-learning approach to overcome the data limitation. Mahmud Badhon et al. [18] work on enhancing the DL transfer-learning technique to increase the accuracy of brain cancer diagnosis. Using a DL pre-trained network, VGG16, this study assesses individual performance in classifications with various evaluation metrics. The authors extracted characteristics from the image dataset using the convolutional block and dense layers of the VGG16 architecture. These features were then sent to machine learning classifiers, which calculated the final classification result. The research achieved significant accuracy using the DL-embedded ML technique. Al Rub et al. [19] use the DL model for the classification of hydrocephalus in brain computed tomography (CT) medical images. They created a precise and non-invasive method for brain hydrocephalus diagnosis. A dataset of 500 brain CT scans, split into training and testing sets during experimentation. The images were divided into groups for hydrocephalus and normal and achieved an overall accuracy of 96.8%, the results showed that their approach achieved better accuracy in detecting hydrocephalus in brain CT images. Additionally, this study demonstrated that the suggested approach performed well as compared to other techniques. A study by Mehnatkesh et al. [20] focuses on classifying brain cancers in MRI scans using deep learning algorithms. To save radiologists time by eliminating the need to examine several images to make an accurate diagnosis, the aim of their work was to create an effective automated method for classifying brain tumors. A total of 3064 T1w-CE brain MRI scans were used from 233 patients. To achieve promising results, they proposed a deep residual learning framework that combines the capabilities of multiple models. With an overall accuracy of 99.31%, the results demonstrated that their proposed approach showed better performance in classifying brain cancers in MRI scans.

The remaining part of the article is divided into three sections. Section 3 describes the details of the methodology used in this study, Section 4 provides a detailed explanation of results, and Section 5 includes a conclusion with possible future direction.

3. Methodology

DL models with DCNNs are particularly well suited for the extraction of robust and important features from images which are essential to understanding the complex structure of MRIs. Our research uses this advantage by employing two well-performed DL models, i.e., InceptionV3 and DenseNet121. The individual performance of both networks is explained in the results section of the paper. By merging the feature representations from both DL models, the fusion technique used in our dual Dual DCNN model combines the strengths of both models. It captures more varied and informative features by integrating the feature maps from both networks and training extra fully connected layers, potentially leading to improved performance when compared to using each network alone. The overview of our approach is shown in Figure 1, whereas details are provided later in the subsection.

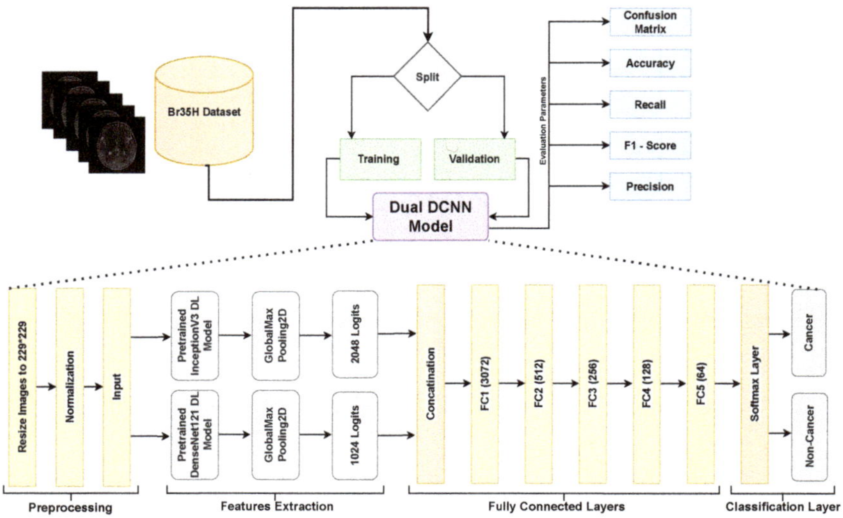

Figure 1. A block diagram for the comprehensive overview of our proposed approach to understand the dual DCNN architecture and workflow.

3.1. Dataset Description

Our experiments utilized a Kaggle dataset, i.e., Br35H [21] comprising a total of 3000 MRI images where 1500 are tumors and 1500 without tumors samples. Each image in the dataset was 256 × 256 pixels in dimension. The images were labeled as either "yes" for cancerous and "no" for non-cancerous samples. The training and validation details of both classes are shown in Table 1. The dataset was split between cancerous and non-cancerous images. We combined these images and randomly divided them into 80% and 20% for training and validation, respectively, using splitfolder library which divides the dataset randomly. We assigned labels as "0" for normal cases and "1" for brain tumors in the proposed approach and SOTA DL models. Figure 2 shows MRI samples taken from the dataset, i.e., cancerous and non-cancerous images.

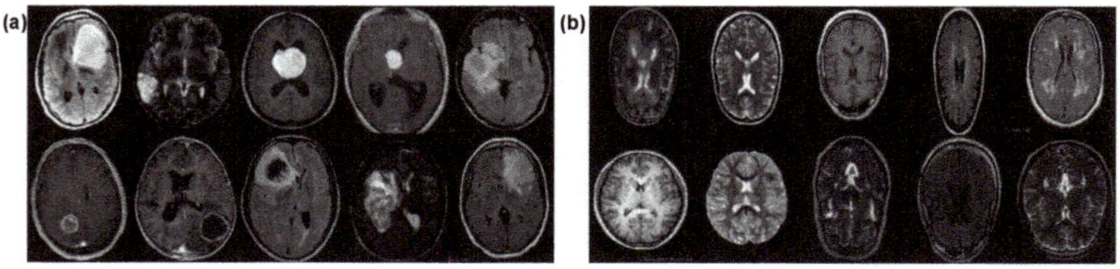

Figure 2. MRI samples: (**a**) cancerous, (**b**) non-cancerous.

Table 1. Dataset split into training and validation and respective class label.

Class	Images	Train	Validation	Label
Cancerous	1500	1200	300	1 "Yes"
Non-Cancerous	1500	1200	300	0 "No"
Total	**3000**	**2400**	**600**	

3.2. Dual DCNN Model

Our dual DCNN (DDCNN) model integrates features obtained from DenseNet121 and InceptionV3, i.e., two pre-trained DL model architectures. Combining their respective strengths in feature extraction, the fusion method combines the learned representations from both networks. We used the torchvision library to load the InceptionV3 and DenseNet121 models that have already been trained and perform well in feature extraction, they are often used for image classification tasks [22–24] for various applications. To benefit from their pre-trained weights for feature extraction, we froze the parameters of both InceptionV3 and DenseNet121 during training. This ensures that the pre-trained weights are not retained by scratch and only the fully connected layers are trained. Next, we add identity layers to each model in place of the classifier layers. By removing the models' last classification layers of each network, we extract features immediately from the convolutional layers. We concatenate the feature maps from the DenseNet121 and InceptionV3 models along the channel dimension in the fusion model. As a result, a combined feature tensor which includes data from both networks is created. In order to process the resulting feature tensor, we add fully connected layers to the fusion model after the concatenation phase. The retrieved features from both networks are combined and refined in these layers. Lastly, we use an optimization approach (such as the Adam optimizer) and a specified loss function, i.e., binary-entropy loss to train the fusion model. During training, the system effectively combines the features from InceptionV3 and DenseNet121 to classify the cancer and non-cancer MRI samples.

3.2.1. Preprocessing

The image input layer pre-processes the dataset before passing it into the DDCNN model. It typically involves resizing the images to a uniform size, i.e., 229 × 229 and normalizing the pixel values to ensure consistency and convergence during training. The normalization process is described as:

$$x_{\text{norm}} = \frac{x - \mu}{\sigma} \tag{1}$$

where x represents the pixel value, μ is the mean pixel value across the dataset, and σ is the standard deviation of the pixel values. It ensures that the pixel values have a zero mean and unit variance.

3.2.2. Features Extraction

This study uses denseNet121 and inceptionV3 DL models to extract the features. DenseNet core innovation is its dense connection pattern where all layers are feed-forwardly coupled to all other layers. A dense connection lowers the number of parameters, promotes gradient flow throughout the network, and makes feature reuse easier. This extensive connection mitigates the vanishing gradient issue that deep neural networks often encounter and allows optimal parameter reuse. Additionally, DenseNet architectures can be improved for feature extractors for a variety of image recognition tasks [25–27] because they have already been pre-trained on large datasets, i.e., ImageNet. By removing the fully connected layers and substituting identity functions, the DenseNet121 model is used in the given study as a feature extractor which turns it into a feature extraction module. Concatenating the feature maps from all preceding layers serves as the input for each layer, resulting in the following input tensor size:

$$(C_l + C_{l-1} + \ldots + C_0, H, W) \tag{2}$$

where C_l is the number of the current layer's channel output. H and W are the height and width of the feature maps.

The second model employed in this approach is InceptionV3, a deep learning architecture renowned for its exceptional capability in various image recognition tasks. It consists of many layers with different convolutional filters, such as max and average pooling layers, and convolutions of sizes 1 × 1, 3 × 3, and 5 × 5. To improve the model performance and adaptability, the architecture also includes batch normalization, dropout, and other methods. To minimize computational complexity and maintain representational ability, it utilizes a factorized convolution approach. Similar to DenseNet121, InceptionV3 is a feature extractor that has been pre-trained on large datasets like ImageNet. The InceptionV3 model is utilized in this study in a similar way as DenseNet121, i.e., the convolutional base remains for feature extraction but the fully connected layers are removed. The collected features from DenseNet121 and InceptionV3 are concatenated and sent through additional fully connected layers for final classification. A more thorough representation of the input data is made possible by combining features from these two DL models which enhances the performance on tasks including robust high and low features' extraction and accurate classification.

This study also uses GlobalMaxPooling2D. This operation is typically used as a means of spatial downsampling to reduce the dimensionality while preserving the most salient (or low-level but important) information. In the DDCNN model, GlobalMaxPooling2D is set up after the convolutional layers in each DL model, i.e., DenseNet121 and InceptionV3. By choosing the largest activation value from each feature map, this pooling method successfully highlights the most important characteristics in the input data. The GlobalMaxPooling2D operation is applied along the spatial dimensions of the feature maps. Considering an input tensor X with dimensions (C, H, W), where H and W stand for the feature maps' height and width, C indicates the number of channels. GlobalMaxPooling2D operation can be expressed as follows:

$$\text{GlobalMaxPooling 2D}(X) = \max(X_{c,h,w}) \quad \text{for} \quad h = 1, \ldots, H \quad \text{and} \quad w = 1, \ldots, W \quad (3)$$

Here, $X_{c,h,w}$ is the activation value at channel C and spatial position (h, w). This operation results in a tensor with dimensions $(C, 1, 1)$.

The utilization of GlobalMaxPooling2D in the DDCNN model contributes to model efficiency and robustness by reducing the number of parameters and preventing overfitting. Moreover, this helps achieve translational invariance that strengthens the model's resistance to shifts or translations in space in the input data. The difference between the max pooling and global max pooling is shown in Figure 3 where the maximum value from the whole region of interest is selected for global pooling in 6 × 6 matrix.

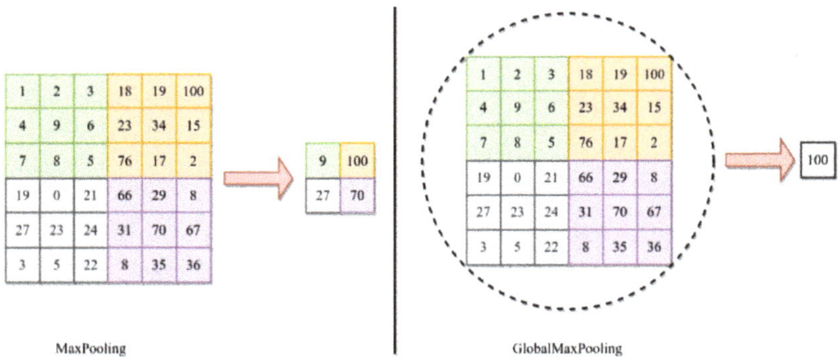

Figure 3. The basic difference between the GlobalMaxPooling and MaxPooling.

3.2.3. Fully Connected Layers

The features extracted by DenseNet121 and InceptionV3 are concatenated along the channel dimension before being fed into the fully connected layers. Let x_{dense} be the features that DenseNet121 collected and $(N, C_{dense}, H_{dense}, W_{dense})$ are dimensions of these features, similarly, $x_{inception}$ be the features of incpetionV3 and $(N, C_{inception}, H_{inception}, W_{inception})$ are dimension of it. The resultant concatenation feature vector would be as:

$$x_{concat} = (N, C_{\text{dense}} + C_{\text{inception}}, H_{\text{dense}}, W_{\text{dense}}) \quad (4)$$

In this study, the denseNet121 has 1024 logits 1D feature vectors and inceptionV3 has 2048 logits 1D feature vectors. The resultant concatenated 1D feature vector was 3072.

These are important features obtained from both pre-trained DL models. These features' tensorsare then passed through a series of fully connected layers to perform classification. These fully connected layers consist of linear transformations followed by the Rectified Linear Unit (ReLU). Let W_i be the weight matrix of the i-th fully connected layer and b_i the bias vector. The following formula is used to get the i-th fully connected layer output:

$$x_i = \text{ReLU}\left(W_i x_{\text{reshaped}} + b_i\right) \quad (5)$$

There are in total five fully connected layers with 3072, 512, 256, 128, and 64 neurons belonging to $FC1, FC2, FC3, FC4, andFC5$, respectively. These layers learn the features and are fine-tuned with the Br35H dataset and hence provide better performance.

3.2.4. Output Layer

The last layer of the Dual DCNN model applies a softmax activation function to transform the raw output scores into probability distributions over the output classes. Let x_{final} denote the final output vector before softmax, and $\hat{y}$ denote the predicted probability of cancer and non-cancer class. The softmax function will be defined as:

$$\hat{y} = \text{softmax}(x_{\text{final}}) \quad (6)$$

where

$$\text{softmax}(x_{\text{final}})_i = \frac{e^{x_{\text{final},i}}}{\sum_{\text{classes}} e^{x_{\text{final},j}}} \quad (7)$$

Through fully connected layers, the DDCNN model integrates the features of denseNet121 and inceptionV3 by utilizing the matching knowledge of both models, potentially increasing overall performance.

3.3. *SOTA DL Models*

This study includes a comparative analysis of DDCNN models with ten well-known DL models, i.e., LeNet-5, AlexNet, VGG-16, SqueezeNet, EfficientNetB2, ResNet18, ResNet34, ResNet50, InceptionV3, and DenseNet121. By evaluating the performance of the DDCNN alongside these widely recognized DL architectures, this study aims to provide insights into the effectiveness of the proposed model compared to existing state-of-the-art approaches. This study uses these DL models with transfer learning capitalizing on their knowledge gained from extensive training on large datasets (e.g., ImageNet) significantly reducing training time and computational resources. Additionally, this allows faster convergence and enhanced generalization which is valuable when dealing with limited medical image datasets such as those encountered in brain tumor classification tasks using MRI.

3.4. *Training Parameters*

This study used the same training parameters for SOTA DL models and the DDCNN model for the classification of cancerous and non-cancerous MRIs. We compared evaluation parameters with five different learning rates and used 128 images as a batch size that shuffled at every epoch with a total of fifty epochs as shown in Table 2. We used the same hyperparameter settings for all SOTA DL models and the DDCNN approach for a fair comparison of performance against each model. The binary cross entropy (BCE) is used with an Adam optimizer that calculates the difference between the actual binary labels and the expected probability distribution as:

$$BCE_{Loss} = -\frac{1}{N}\sum_{i=1}^{N}(y_i \cdot \log(p_i) + (1 - y_i) \cdot \log(1 - p_i)) \quad (8)$$

where N is the total number of samples, y_i is the true label (0 or 1) of the ith sample, and p_i is the predicted probability that the ith sample belongs to class 1.

Table 2. Training parameters used in SOTA DL and DDCNN model.

Sr. No	Parameters	Value
1	Learning Rates	0.1, 0.01, 0.001, 0.0001, and 0.00001
2	Batch Size	128
3	Number of Epochs	50
4	Loss Function	Adam Optimizer With Binary Cross-Entropy
5	Shuffle	Every Epoch

4. Experimentation and Results Discussion

4.1. Experimental Setup

This study utilized a 15-inch Mackbook Proequipped with a dedicated GPU, 16 cores, 19 high-performance CPU cores, and an M2 chip with a processing speed of up to 4.0 GHz for efficient performance. To facilitate the development and comparison of different deep learning models, a separate virtual environment was created. We installed all the required libraries and packages in it. The Keras library within the tenserflow framework was used for VGG-16, LeNet-5, and AlexNet, whereas the PyTorch framework was used for building SqueezeNet, EfficientNetB2, ResNet18, ResNet34, ResNet50, InceptionV3, DenseNet121, and the proposed DDCCN model.

4.2. Evaluation Protocol

The f1-score, recall, accuracy, and precision were considered for the evaluation of the binary classification of DL models. The confusion matrix was also computed. True positives (TPs), true negatives (TNs), false positives (FPs), and false negatives (FNs) are its four coefficients. Accuracy is defined as the proportion of correctly expected cases among all instances. Precision is defined as the proportion of true positives among all positive predictions. The percentage of true positives predicted among all actual positive outcomes is called recall. It is also sometimes referred to as sensitivity or true positive rate. The harmonic mean of recall and precision provides the F1-score.

$$\text{Accuracy} = \frac{TP + TN}{TP + TN + FP + FN} \tag{9}$$

$$\text{Precision} = \frac{TP}{TP + FP} \tag{10}$$

$$\text{Recall} = \frac{TP}{TP + FN} \tag{11}$$

$$F1\_\text{score} = 2 \times \frac{\text{Precision} \times \text{Recall}}{\text{Precision} + \text{Recall}} \tag{12}$$

4.3. Results Discussion

This section analyzes the results acquired using the DDCNN model with the impact of different learning rates. It provides a detailed breakdown of the actual versus predicted classifications for each class of samples.

Figure 4 shows the classwise actual and predicted samples obtained using five different learning rates. Figure 4e shows that the highest learning rate, i.e., 0.1, only predicted actual positive samples correctly and did not classify the actual negative samples. In other words, this learning rate classified all 600 samples as cancerous. It was observed that the best results were obtained using a 0.0001 learning rate (i.e., Figure 4b) whereas only 12 actual negative samples were misclassified out of a total of 600 samples. Other learning rates with respective confusion matrices were also shown with actual and predicted samples where a 0.00001 learning rate performed well but misclassified 15 (i.e., Figure 4a) cancerous and non-cancerous MRI samples.

Figure 5 shows the training and validation accuracy and loss of the Dual DCNN model using the best 0.0001 learning rate. Both the validation accuracy and training accuracy increase as the number of epochs (training iterations) progresses. However, around epoch 30, both curves seem to plateau. This suggests that the model's performance has reached its optimal point. It is essential to balance high accuracy on the training data and generalization to unseen validation data. The loss initially decreases sharply. After approximately 10 epochs, the loss stabilizes. This indicates that the model effectively learns during the initial epochs but may not improve significantly beyond that point. Monitoring loss helps prevent overfitting and ensures the model generalizes well.

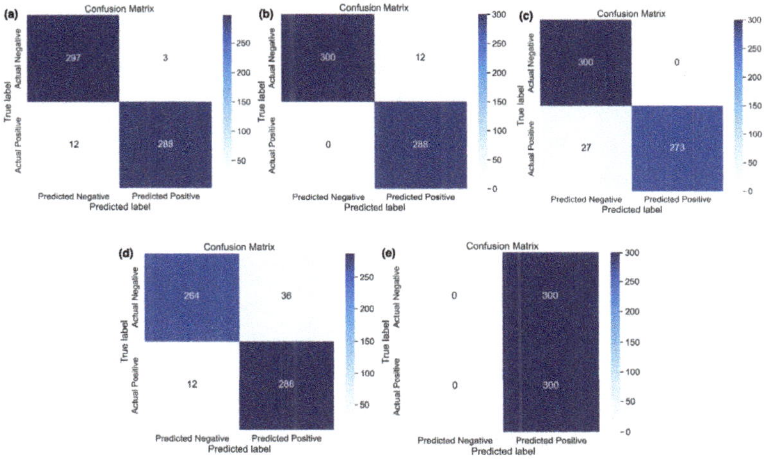

Figure 4. Confusion matrix of DDCNN model with different learning rates (**a**) 0.00001, (**b**) 0.0001, (**c**) 0.001, (**d**) 0.01, and (**e**) 0.1.

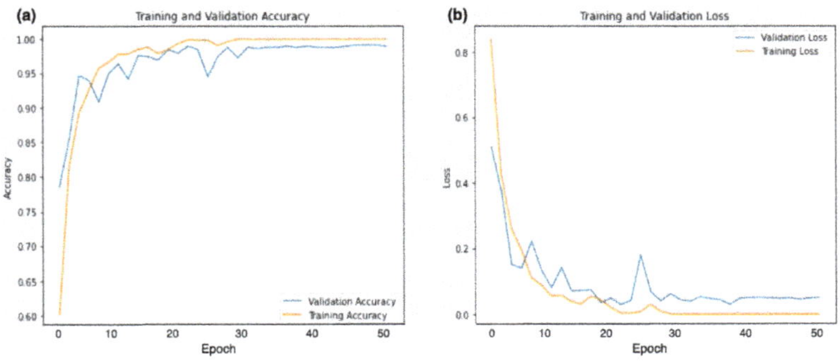

Figure 5. Training and validation (**a**) accuracy (**b**) loss of DDCNN model using 0.0001 learning rate.

The evaluation parameters against different models trained at best learning rates are shown in Table 3. With 99% accuracy and precision, the DDCNN model performed best, demonstrating its ability to correctly classify nearly all cases with extremely few false positives. Additionally, it obtained a high recall of 98%, which indicates that the majority of positive samples were successfully identified. As a result, its F1-score, a measurement for both recall and precision, was 99%, also outstanding. DenseNet121 achieved good performance with an accuracy of 97% and properly recognized a high majority of instances. Additionally, its precision and recall were both 97%, indicating that it performed fairly in detecting positive occurrences with few false positives.

With accuracy ranging from 95% to 96%, the InceptionV3, ResNet50, ResNet34, ResNet18, and EfficientNetB2 models performed similarly. Although their recall and precision scores were likewise quite satisfactory, there were slight variations across the models. For example, InceptionV3 got a lower F1-score than ResNet models. Models like SqueezeNet, VGG-16, AlexNet, and LeNet-5 performed lower than the previously mentioned ones. Although their levels of accuracy were still fair, they performed far worse in terms of precision, recall, and F1-scores. Particularly, AlexNet and LeNet-5 performed less as they had the lowest results across all criteria.

Table 3. Evaluation parameters via best learning rates.

Model	Learning Rate	Accuracy	Precision	Recall	F1-Score
DDCNN	0.0001	**99**	**99**	**98**	**99**
DenseNet121	0.001	97	97	97	97
InceptionV3	0.01	96	97	95	95
ResNet50	0.00001	96	94	95	95
ResNet34	0.00001	96	95	94	95
ResNet18	0.0001	95	94	95	94
EfficinetNetB2	0.00001	95	95	95	95
SqueezeNet	0.0001	94	95	95	94
VGG-16	0.0001	92	92	93	93
AlexNet	0.0001	85	83	83	83
LeNet-5	0.001	71	69	74	72

Figure 6 shows the confusion matrices of ten SOTA DL models used in this study. It is the classwise correct and incorrect prediction of two classes that allow a better understanding of the performance of individual models against best learning rates. Figure 6a shows the confusion matrix of DenseNet121 DL model which is dominating with learning rate of 0.001. It also shows the highest evaluation parameters using SOTA DL models. Whereas, Figure 6b–h shows the better performance of InceptionV3, ResNet50, ResNet34, ResNet18, EfficientB2, SqueezeNet and VGG-16, respectively. These DL models are showing performance matrices greater than 90% which are considered as acceptable in binary classification problem. However, Figure 6i,j shows the evaluation parameters of AlexNet and LeNet-5 using best learning rates. These both are not performing well.

Similarly, Figure 7 shows the accuracy, precision, recall, and f1-scores against all models used in this study which can be seen from Table 3 as well. Figure 7a shows the accuracy which is ratio of correctly predicted samples to the overall samples. Figure 7b–d shows the percentage of precision, recall, and F1, respectively against all DL models used in this study.

Table 4 shows the classwise performance matrices (accuracy, precision, recall, and f1-scores). The DDCNN model achieved a high accuracy of 99%, precision of 99%, recall of 98%, and f1-score of 99% for non-cancer (class 0). This suggests that with extremely few false positives, it accurately classified nearly all cases of non-cancerous samples. It also performed better for cancerous cases (Class 1), showing the perfect classification of cancer with 99% accuracy, precision, recall, and f1-score. With all metrics ranging around 97%, DenseNet121 performed well for class 0. Its accuracy, precision, recall, and f1-score were lower than those of the DDCNN model. With accuracy, precision, recall, and f1-score all ranging around 96% for cancerous cases, the performance remained unchanged. This suggests that the cases of cancer were accurately classified.

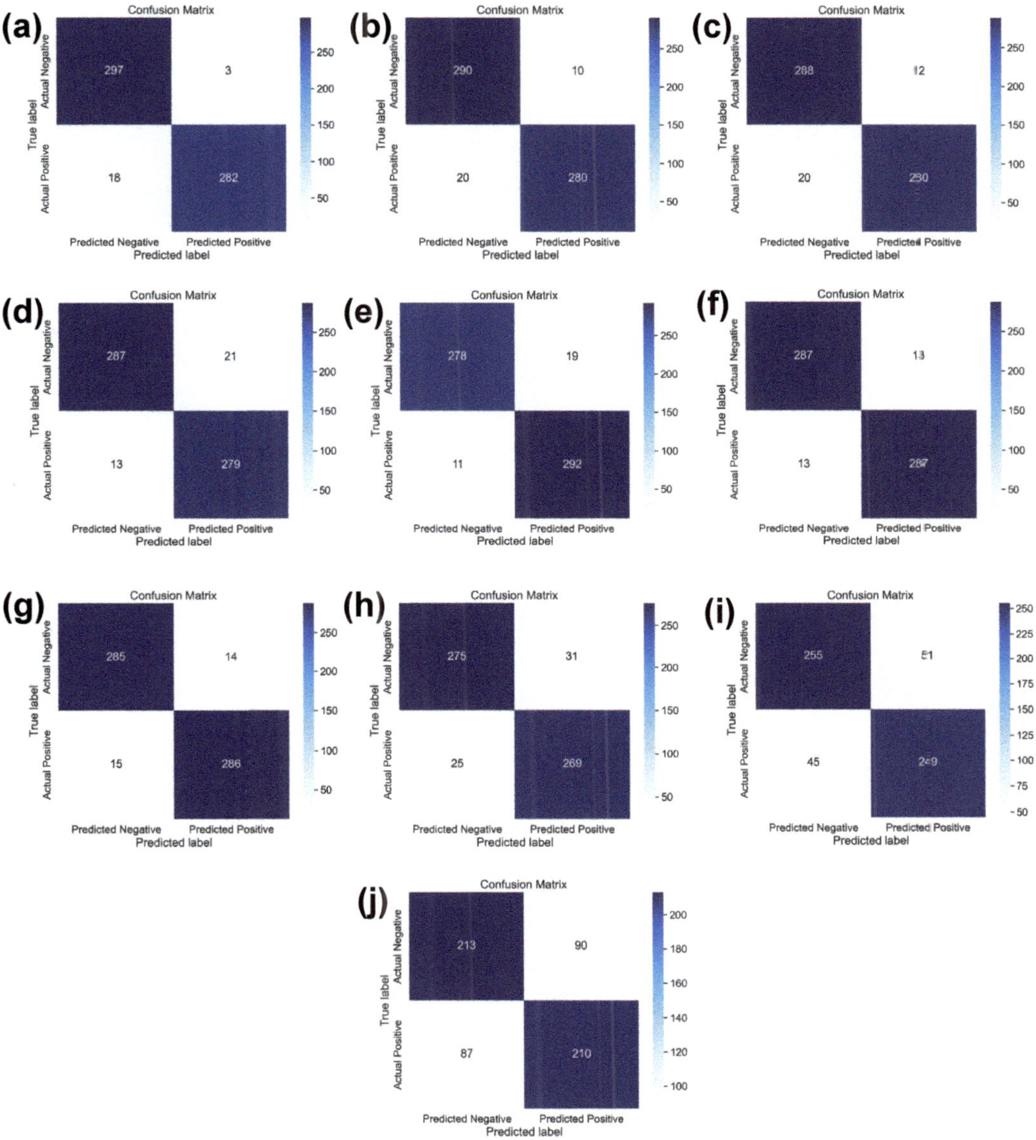

Figure 6. The confusion matrix of all ten SOTA DL models with respect to the best learning rates as mentioned in Table 3. (**a**) DenseNet121 with 0.0001 learning rate, (**b**) InceptionV3 with 0.001 learning rate, (**c**) ResNet50 with 0.00001 learning rate, (**d**) ResNet34 with 0.00001 learning rate, (**e**) ResNet18 with 0.0001 learning rate, (**f**) EfficientNetB2 with 0.00001 learning rate, (**g**) SqueezeNet with 0.0001 learning rate, (**h**) VGG16 with 0.0001 learning rate, (**i**) AlexNet with 0.0001 learning rate, and (**j**) LeNet-5 with 0.001 learning rate.

Table 4. Classwise evaluation parameters of DDCNN model and SOTA DCNN models.

Model	Learning Rate	Class	Accuracy	Precision	Recall	F1-Score
DDCNN model	0.0001	0	**99**	**99**	**98**	**99**
		1	**99**	**99**	**99**	**99**
DenseNet121	0.001	0	98	97	97	97
		1	96	96	96	96
InceptionV3	0.01	0	97	96	95	95
		1	95	96	96	94
ResNet50	0.00001	0	97	97	96	95
		1	95	96	94	95
ResNet34	0.00001	0	97	96	95	96
		1	95	95	93	94
ResNet18	0.0001	0	96	94	96	94
		1	94	94	94	95
EfficinetNetB2	0.00001	0	96	95	95	95
		1	94	94	94	95
SqueezeNet	0.0001	0	95	96	95	94
		1	93	94	94	94
VGG-16	0.0001	0	93	92	93	93
		1	91	92	92	93
AlexNet	0.0001	0	90	84	81	84
		1	80	81	80	81
LeNet-5	0.001	0	79	75	78	79
		1	64	61	66	68

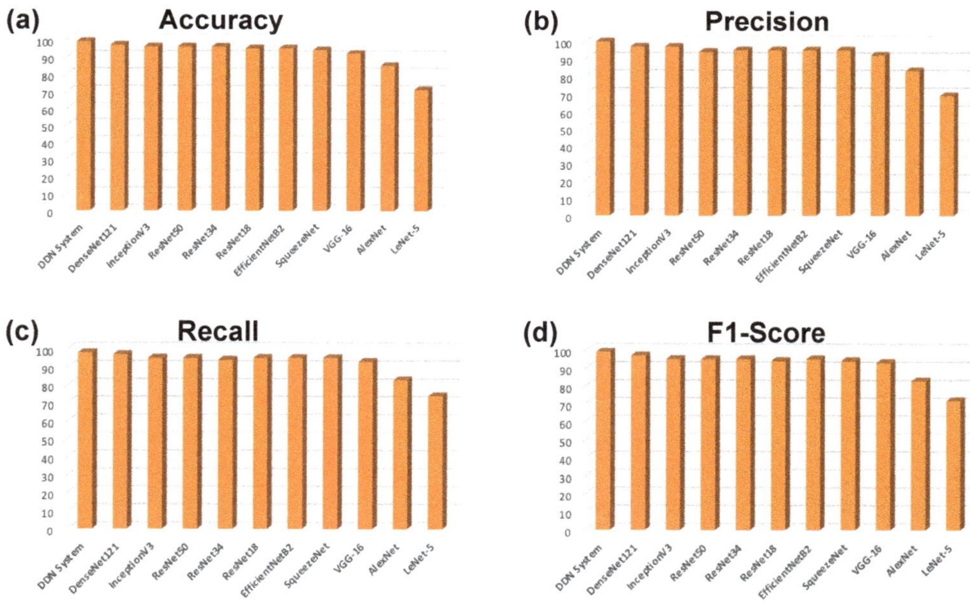

Figure 7. Evaluation parameters for DDCNN and SOTA DL models with respect to learning rates provided in Table 3. The (**a**) Accuracy, (**b**) Precision, (**c**) Recall, and (**d**) F1-Scores bar-graphs for all DL models used in the study.

InceptionV3, ResNet50, ResNet34, ResNet18, EfficientNetB2, SqueezeNet, and VGG-16 models have generally similar trends across both classes, with slightly varying performance metrics. With somewhat different performance criteria, the InceptionV3, ResNet50, ResNet34, ResNet18, EfficientNetB2, SqueezeNet, and VGG-16 models largely showed comparable patterns in both classes. Class 0 accuracy was between 93% and 97%, with slightly lower but still good precision, recall, and F1-score. With accuracy ranging from 91% to 95% and modest changes in precision, recall, and F1-score, class 1 performance was slightly lower than class 0. The AlexNet and LeNet-5 models underperformed as compared to other models. For class 0, precision, recall, and F1-score were similarly comparatively lower, whereas accuracy ranged from 79% to 90%. With accuracy ranging from 64% to 80% and precision, recall, and F1-score showing a similar decreasing trend, class 1 performance decreased even more.

In conclusion, the DDCNN model outperformed compared to the others in both classes, achieving almost perfect recall, accuracy, precision, and F1-score. However, AlexNet and LeNet-5 performed relatively worse while taking into account all evaluation parameters.

Table 5 presents the influence of five different learning rates on the DDCNN model and several SOTA DL models trained with five different learning rates. The Dual DCNN performance demonstrates sensitivity to the learning rate. The best results were obtained when training at a learning rate of 0.0001, achieving 99%, 99%, 98%, and 99% for accuracy, precision, recall, and F1-score, respectively, whereas performance decreased from 0.0001 to 0.00001 when the learning rate dropped. However, it remained quite satisfactory, with an accuracy of 98% and other metrics over 97%. Its lowest performance was for a higher learning rate as shown in the table. Similar to the Dual DCNN, models like InceptionV3, ResNets, EfficientNetB2, DenseNet121, SqueezeNet, and VGG-16 demonstrated inconsistent performance at different learning rates. Lower learning rates were often associated with better performance. For instance, DenseNet121 and ResNet18 both achieved their maximum accuracy of 93% and 96%, respectively, with a learning rate of 0.001 and 0.01, respectively.

Table 5. Evaluation parameters of dual DCNN models and SOTA DL models with respect to five different learning rates.

Model	Learning Rate	Accuracy	Precision	Recall	F1-Score
	0.1	50	25	50	33
	0.01	92	92	92	92
DDCNN Model	0.001	95	96	96	95
	0.0001	**99**	**99**	**98**	**99**
	0.00001	98	98	98	98
	0.1	70	71	71	70
	0.01	68	71	68	66
DenseNet121	0.001	**97**	**97**	**97**	**97**
	0.0001	95	96	96	95
	0.00001	83	86	83	83
	0.1	48	46	48	42
	0.01	**96**	**97**	**95**	**95**
InceptionV3	0.001	94	95	94	94
	0.0001	74	78	74	74
	0.00001	50	50	50	50
	0.1	67	67	67	66
	0.01	93	93	93	93
ResNet50	0.001	95	95	96	95
	0.0001	77	79	77	78
	0.00001	**96**	**94**	**95**	**95**
	0.1	68	68	68	67
	0.01	94	94	94	93
ResNet34	0.001	95	94	95	94
	0.0001	67	69	67	66
	0.00001	**96**	**95**	**94**	**95**

Table 5. *Cont.*

Model	Learning Rate	Accuracy	Precision	Recall	F1-Score
ResNet18	0.1	58	74	58	50
	0.01	66	80	66	61
	0.001	94	94	94	93
	0.0001	**95**	**94**	**95**	**94**
	0.00001	93	94	93	93
EfficinetNetB2	0.1	67	66	66	65
	0.01	85	87	85	85
	0.001	89	91	89	89
	0.0001	93	94	93	94
	0.00001	**95**	**95**	**95**	**95**
SqueezeNet	0.1	50	25	50	33
	0.01	60	62	62	61
	0.001	91	92	91	91
	0.0001	**94**	**95**	**95**	**94**
	0.00001	90	90	90	90
VGG-16	0.1	50	25	50	33
	0.01	88	78	84	80
	0.001	91	92	91	91
	0.0001	**92**	**92**	**93**	**93**
	0.00001	90	90	90	90
AlexNet	0.1	50	25	50	33
	0.01	60	55	58	54
	0.001	83	83	83	83
	0.0001	**85**	**83**	**83**	**83**
	0.00001	84	83	82	82
LeNet-5	0.1	54	29	54	37
	0.01	61	64	59	61
	0.001	**71**	**69**	**74**	**72**
	0.0001	67	66	66	65
	0.00001	70	69	69	68

Across all learning rates, AlexNet and LeNet-5 underperformed compared to the other models in terms of accuracy, precision, recall, and f1-score. For instance, for a given learning rate of 0.0001, AlexNet's maximum accuracy was 85%, whereas LeNet-5's maximum accuracy was 71% at 0.001.

In conclusion, the findings highlight the crucial role of hyperparameter tuning, particularly learning rate selection, in optimizing DL model performance. Performance was generally better at lower learning rates, whereas the ideal learning rate varied based on the particular model architecture. Additionally, several models showed consistency in their performance across a variety of learning rates, whereas other models showed variability. These results highlight how important it is to adjust hyperparameters, including the learning rate, in order to maximize the DL model's performance.

4.4. Comparison of SOTA versus DDCNN Model

Table 6 shows the Dual DCNN's exceptional performance compared to recent studies employing various DL models validated using MRI images having cancerous (and its type) and non-cancerous classes. In these studies, our DDCNN model achieves an accuracy of 99% in classifying cancerous and non-cancerous MRI scans, surpassing the highest accuracy reported in the reviewed literature. Even though other techniques, i.e., optimized EfficientNetB2 and MSGGAN achieve high accuracy above 98%, our DDCNN APPROACH still exceeds them. Moreover, transfer-learning-based models like DenseNet201 and GoogleNet, together with innovative architectures like Res-BRNet and Self CNN also attain competitive accuracies between 97% and 98%, they are unable to match our performance. These findings suggest that the Dual DCNN represents a superior performance in deep learning for MRI-based cancer and non-cancer classification tasks.

Table 6. Quantitative analysis of DDCNN model and latest related research.

Research	Methodology	Model	Accuracy
In [28]	CNN-Fine Tuned	EfficientNetB2	98.86%
In [29],	Generative Adversarial Network (GAN)	MSGGAN	98.57%
In [30],	DCNN-Transfer Learning	DenseNet201	98.22%
In [31],	CNN-Transfer Learning	GoogleNet	98%
In [32],	CNN-Novel	Self CNN	97.3%
In [33],	CNN-Cross Validation	Self CNN	96.56%
In [34],	Neural Network (NN)	Self NN	95.86%
In [35],	Siamese Neural Network (SNN)	MAC-CNN	92.8%
Our Approach	**Dual DCNN Model**	**DDCNN**	**99%**

5. Conclusions

Detecting brain tumors at an early stage is very crucial as it increases the chances of patient survival through effective treatment. The manual diagnosis by doctors is slow and subject to inter-observer variations, especially with the increasing number of new cases reported on a daily basis. Hence, there is an urgent need for rapid analysis of large medical data to enable early tumor diagnosis. Here, AI with deep learning methods are reliable and efficient approach because it can handle complex medical data like MRI scans more precisely. This study introduces the Dual DCNN (DDCNN) model, which utilizes two high-performing DL models that achieve better performance than SOTA models. It compares results with various well-known DL models, including DenseNet121, InceptionV3, ResNet50, ResNet34, ResNet18, EfficientNetB2, SqueezeNet, VGG16, AlexNet, and LeNet-5. Furthermore, this study compares the proposed Dual DCNN approach with recent research and demonstrates better performance.

Future efforts will focus on the prediction of glioma grade which plays an essential role in guiding treatment decisions. Transformers, which were introduced recently and became popular, can be instigated and compared with Dual DCNN approach.

Author Contributions: Conceptualization, Z.S., O.B. and T.T.; methodology, Z.S. and T.T.; software, Z.S.; validation, Z.S. and T.T.; formal analysis, Z.S., O.B., J.X.J., R.H. and S.A.; investigation, Z.S. and T.T.; resources, O.B.; data creation, Z.S.; writing—original draft preparation, Z.S.; writing—review and editing, Z.S., O.B., J.X.J., T.T. and S.A.; visualization, Z.S.; supervision, O.B., J.X.J., T.T. and S.A.; project administration, Z.S. and N.A.-H.; funding acquisition, O.B. and J.X.J. All authors have read and agreed to the published version of the manuscript.

Funding: This study was made possible by financial support from Texas A&M University at Qatar and joint collaboration with Hamad Medical Corporation (HMC).

Institutional Review Board Statement: Not applicable.

Informed Consent Statement: Not applicable.

Data Availability Statement: The dataset is publicly available and accessible via https://www.kaggle.com/datasets/viveknarayanuppala/br35h-binary (accessed on 13 August 2023).

Conflicts of Interest: The authors declare no conflicts of interest.

References

1. Mohta, S.; Sharma, S.; Saraya, A. Improvement in adipocytic indices as a predictor of improved outcomes after TIPS: Right conclusion? *Liver Int. Off. J. Int. Assoc. Study Liver* **2021**, *42*, 253. [CrossRef]
2. Ye, Z.; Srinivasa, K.; Meyer, A.; Sun, P.; Lin, J.; Viox, J.D.; Song, C.; Wu, A.T.; Song, S.K.; Dahiya, S.; et al. Diffusion histology imaging differentiates distinct pediatric brain tumor histology. *Sci. Rep.* **2021**, *11*, 4749. [CrossRef]
3. Chen, Y.; Schönlieb, C.B.; Liò, P.; Leiner, T.; Dragotti, P.L.; Wang, G.; Rueckert, D.; Firmin, D.; Yang, G. AI-based reconstruction for fast MRI—A systematic review and meta-analysis. *Proc. IEEE* **2022**, *110*, 224–245. [CrossRef]
4. Zacharaki, E.I.; Wang, S.; Chawla, S.; Soo, Y.D.; Wolf, R.; Melhem, E.R.; Davatzikos, C. Classification of brain tumor type and grade using MRI texture and shape in a machine learning scheme. *Magn. Reson. Med. Off. J. Int. Soc. Magn. Reson. Med.* **2009**, *62*, 1609–1618. [CrossRef]
5. Saeed, Z.; Masood, M.; Khan, M.U. A review: Cybersecurity challenges and their solutions in connected and autonomous vehicles (CAVs). *JAREE (J. Adv. Res. Electr. Eng.)* **2023**, *7*. [CrossRef]
6. Saeed, Z.; Awan, M.N.M.; Yousaf, M.H. A Robust Approach for Small-Scale Object Detection From Aerial-View. In Proceedings of the 2022 International Conference on Digital Image Computing: Techniques and Applications (DICTA), Sydney, Australia, 30 November–2 December 2022; IEEE: Piscataway, NJ, USA, 2022; pp. 1–7.
7. Ishtiaq, A.; Saeed, Z.; Khan, M.U.; Samer, A.; Shabbir, M.; Ahmad, W. Fall detection, wearable sensors & artificial intelligence: A short review. *JAREE (J. Adv. Res. Electr. Eng.)* **2022**, *6*. [CrossRef]
8. Naqvi, S.Z.H.; Khan, M.U.; Raza, A.; Saeed, Z.; Abbasi, Z.; Ali, S.Z.E.Z. Deep Learning Based Intelligent Classification of COVID-19 & Pneumonia Using Cough Auscultations. In Proceedings of the 2021 6th International Multi-Topic ICT Conference (IMTIC), Jamshoro & Karachi, Pakistan, 10–12 November 2021; IEEE: Piscataway, NJ, USA, 2021; pp. 1–6.
9. Srinivas, C.; K. S., N.P.; Zakariah, M.; Alothaibi, Y.A.; Shaukat, K.; Partibane, B.; Awal, H. Deep transfer learning approaches in performance analysis of brain tumor classification using MRI images. *J. Healthc. Eng.* **2022**, *2022*, 3264367. [CrossRef]
10. Abiwinanda, N.; Hanif, M.; Hesaputra, S.T.; Handayani, A.; Mengko, T.R. Brain tumor classification using convolutional neural network. In Proceedings of the World Congress on Medical Physics and Biomedical Engineering 2018, Prague, Czech Republic, 3–8 June 2018; Springer: Singapore, 2019; Volume 1, pp. 183–189.
11. Song, G.; Xie, G.; Nie, Y.; Majid, M.S.; Yavari, I. Noninvasive grading of glioma brain tumors using magnetic resonance imaging and deep learning methods. *J. Cancer Res. Clin. Oncol.* **2023**, *149*, 16293–16309. [CrossRef]
12. Fathima, M.N.; Shiney, J.; Singh, P. Deep Learning and Machine Learning Approaches for Brain Tumor Detection and Classification. In Proceedings of the 2023 International Conference on Circuit Power and Computing Technologies (ICCPCT), Kollam, India, 10–11 August 2023; IEEE: Piscataway, NJ, USA, 2023; pp. 952–960. [CrossRef]
13. Ghosal, P.; Nandanwar, L.; Kanchan, S.; Bhadra, A.; Chakraborty, J.; Nandi, D. Brain tumor classification using ResNet-101 based squeeze and excitation deep neural network. In Proceedings of the 2019 Second International Conference on Advanced Computational and Communication Paradigms (ICACCP), Gangtok, India, 25–28 February 2019; IEEE: Piscataway, NJ, USA, 2019; pp. 1–6. [CrossRef]
14. Nawaz, M.; Nazir, T.; Masood, M.; Mehmood, A.; Mahum, R.; Khan, M.A.; Kadry, S.; Thinnukool, O. Analysis of brain MRI images using improved cornernet approach. *Diagnostics* **2021**, *11*, 1856. [CrossRef]
15. Mohammed, B.A.; Senan, E.M.; Alshammari, T.S.; Alreshidi, A.; Alayba, A.M.; Alazmi, M.; Alsagri, A.N. Hybrid Techniques of Analyzing MRI Images for Early Diagnosis of Brain Tumours Based on Hybrid Features. *Processes* **2023**, *11*, 212. . [CrossRef]
16. Nassar, S.E.; Yasser, I.; Amer, H.M.; Mohamed, M.A. A robust MRI-based brain tumor classification via a hybrid deep learning technique. *J. Supercomput.* **2024**, *80*, 2403–2427. [CrossRef]
17. Saha, P.; Das, R.; Das, S.K. BCM-VEMT: Classification of brain cancer from MRI images using deep learning and ensemble of machine learning techniques. *Multimed. Tools Appl.* **2023**, *82*, 44479–44506. [CrossRef]
18. Badhon, A.I.M.; Hasan, M.S.; Haque, M.S.; Pranto, M.S.H.; Ghosh, S.; Alam, M.G.R. Diagnosing Prostate Cancer: An Implementation of Deep Machine Learning Fusion Network in MRI Using a Transfer Learning Approach. In Proceedings of the 2023 6th International Conference on Software Engineering and Information Management, Palmerston North, New Zealand, 31 January–2 February 2023; pp. 33–43.
19. Al Rub, S.A.; Alaiad, A.; Hmeidi, I.; Quwaider, M.; Alzoubi, O. Hydrocephalus classification in brain computed tomography medical images using deep learning. *Simul. Model. Pract. Theory* **2023**, *123*, 102705. [CrossRef]
20. Mehnatkesh, H.; Jalali, S.M.J.; Khosravi, A.; Nahavandi, S. An intelligent driven deep residual learning framework for brain tumor classification using MRI images. *Expert Syst. Appl.* **2023**, *213*, 119087. [CrossRef]
21. Hamada, A. *"Br35H: Brain Tumor Detection"*, version 5; Kaggle: San Francisco, CA, USA, 2020. Available online: https://www.kaggle.com/datasets/viveknarayanuppala/br35h-binary (accessed on 13 August 2023).
22. Raza, A.; Khan, M.U.; Saeed, Z.; Samer, S.; Mobeen, A.; Samer, A. Classification of eye diseases and detection of cataract using digital fundus imaging (DFI) and inception-V4 deep learning model. In Proceedings of the 2021 International Conference on Frontiers of Information Technology (FIT), Islamabad, Pakistan, 13–14 December 2021; IEEE: Piscataway, NJ, USA, 2021; pp. 137–142. [CrossRef]

23. Saeed, Z.; Khan, M.U.; Raza, A.; Khan, H.; Javed, J.; Arshad, A. Classification of pulmonary viruses X-ray and detection of COVID-19 based on invariant of inception-V 3 deep learning model. In Proceedings of the 2021 International Conference on Computing, Electronic and Electrical Engineering (ICE Cube), Quetta, Pakistan, 26–27 October 2021; IEEE: Piscataway, NJ, USA, 2021; pp. 1–6. [CrossRef]
24. Saeed, Z.; Khan, M.U.; Raza, A.; Sajjad, N.; Naz, S.; Salal, A. Identification of leaf diseases in potato crop using Deep Convolutional Neural Networks (DCNNs). In Proceedings of the 2021 16th International Conference on Emerging Technologies (ICET), Islamabad, Pakistan, 22–23 December 2021; IEEE: Piscataway, NJ, USA, 2021; pp. 1–6. [CrossRef]
25. Saeed, Z.; Yousaf, M.H.; Ahmed, R.; Velastin, S.A.; Viriri, S. On-board small-scale object detection for unmanned aerial vehicles (UAVs). *Drones* **2023**, *7*, 310. [CrossRef]
26. Khan, M.U.; Abbasi, M.A.; Saeed, Z.; Asif, M.; Raza, A.; Urooj, U. Deep learning based intelligent emotion recognition and classification system. In Proceedings of the 2021 International Conference on Frontiers of Information Technology (FIT), Islamabad, Pakistan, 13–14 December 2021; IEEE: Piscataway, NJ, USA, 2021; pp. 25–30.
27. Saeed, Z.; Raza, A.; Qureshi, A.H.; Yousaf, M.H. A multi-crop disease detection and classification approach using cnn. In Proceedings of the 2021 International Conference on Robotics and Automation in Industry (ICRAI), Rawalpindi, Pakistan, 26–27 October 2021; IEEE: Piscataway, NJ, USA, 2021; pp. 1–6. [CrossRef]
28. Zulfiqar, F.; Bajwa, U.I.; Mehmood, Y. Multi-class classification of brain tumor types from MR images using EfficientNets. *Biomed. Signal Process. Control.* **2023**, *84*, 104777. [CrossRef]
29. Yerukalareddy, D.R.; Pavlovskiy, E. Brain tumor classification based on mr images using GAN as a pre-trained model. In Proceedings of the 2021 IEEE Ural-Siberian Conference on Computational Technologies in Cognitive Science, Genomics and Biomedicine (CSGB), Novosibirsk-Yekaterinburg, Russia, 26–28 May 2021; IEEE: Piscataway, NJ, USA, 2021; pp. 380–384. [CrossRef]
30. Verma, A.; Singh, V.P. Design, analysis and implementation of efficient deep learning frameworks for brain tumor classification. *Multimed. Tools Appl.* **2022**, *81*, 37541–37567. [CrossRef]
31. Deepak, S.; Ameer, P.M. Brain tumor classification using deep CNN features via transfer learning. *Comput. Biol. Med.* **2019**, *111*, 103345. [CrossRef]
32. Díaz-Pernas, F.J.; Martínez-Zarzuela, M.; Antón-Rodríguez, M.; González-Ortega, D. A deep learning approach for brain tumor classification and segmentation using a multiscale convolutional neural network. *Healthcare* **2021**, *9*, 153. [CrossRef]
33. Hilles, S.M.; Saleh, N.S. Image Segmentation and Classification Using CNN Model to Detect Brain Tumors. In Proceedings of the 2021 2nd International Informatics and Software Engineering Conference (IISEC), Ankara, Turkey, 16–17 December 2021; IEEE: Piscataway, NJ, USA, 2021; pp. 1–7. [CrossRef]
34. Vidyarthi, A.; Agarwal, R.; Gupta, D.; Sharma, R.; Draheim, D.; Tiwari, P. Machine Learning Assisted Methodology for multiclass classification of malignant brain tumors. *IEEE Access* **2022**, *10*, 50624–50640. [CrossRef]
35. Molder, C.; Lowe, B.; Zhan, J. Learning Medical Materials From Radiography Images. *Front. Artif. Intell.* **2021**, *4*, 638299. [CrossRef] [PubMed]

Journal of
Clinical Medicine

MDPI

Article

Does FDG PET-Based Radiomics Have an Added Value for Prediction of Overall Survival in Non-Small Cell Lung Cancer?

Andrea Ciarmiello [1,*], Elisabetta Giovannini [1], Francesca Tutino [1], Nikola Yosifov [1], Amalia Milano [2], Luigia Florimonte [3], Elena Bonatto [4], Claudia Bareggi [5], Luca Dellavedova [6], Angelo Castello [3], Carlo Aschele [2], Massimo Castellani [3] and Giampiero Giovacchini [1]

1 Nuclear Medicine Department, Sant' Andrea Hospital, 19124 La Spezia, Italy; elisabetta.giovannini@asl5.liguria.it (E.G.); francesca.tutino@asl5.liguria.it (F.T.); nikola.yosifov@asl5.liguria.it (N.Y.); giampiero.giovacchini@asl5.liguria.it (G.G.)
2 Oncology Unit, Sant' Andrea Hospital, 19124 La Spezia, Italy; amalia.milano@asl5.liguria.it (A.M.); carlo.aschele@asl5.liguria.it (C.A.)
3 Nuclear Medicine Department, Fondazione IRCCS Ca' Granda Ospedale Maggiore Policlinico, 20122 Milan, Italy; luigia.florimonte@policlinico.mi.it (L.F.); angelo.castello@policlinico.mi.it (A.C.); massimo.castellani@policlinico.mi.it (M.C.)
4 Division of Nuclear Medicine, IEO European Institute of Oncology IRCCS, 20122 Milan, Italy; elena.bonatto@unimi.it
5 Medical Oncology Unit, Fondazione IRCCS Ca' Granda Ospedale Maggiore Policlinico, 20122 Milan, Italy; claudia.bareggi@policlinico.mi.it
6 Nuclear Medicine Department, ASST Ovest Milanese, 20025 Legnano, Italy; luca.dellavedova@asst-ovestmi.it
* Correspondence: andrea.ciarmiello@asl5.liguria.it; Tel.: +39-0187-533237; Fax: +39-0187-533224

Abstract: Objectives: Radiomics and machine learning are innovative approaches to improve the clinical management of NSCLC. However, there is less information about the additive value of FDG PET-based radiomics compared with clinical and imaging variables. **Methods**: This retrospective study included 320 NSCLC patients who underwent PET/CT with FDG at initial staging. VOIs were placed on primary tumors only. We included a total of 94 variables, including 87 textural features extracted from PET studies, SUVmax, MTV, TLG, TNM stage, histology, age, and gender. We used the least absolute shrinkage and selection operator (LASSO) regression to select variables with the highest predictive value. Although several radiomics variables are available, the added value of these predictors compared with clinical and imaging variables is still under evaluation. Three hundred and twenty NSCLC patients were included in this retrospective study and underwent 18F-FDG PET/CT at initial staging. In this study, we evaluated 94 variables, including 87 textural features, SUVmax, MTV, TLG, TNM stage, histology, age, and gender. Image-based predictors were extracted from a volume of interest (VOI) positioned on the primary tumor. The least absolute shrinkage and selection operator (LASSO) Cox regression was used to reduce the number of variables and select only those with the highest predictive value. The predictive model implemented with the variables selected using the LASSO analysis was compared with a reference model using only a tumor stage and SUVmax. **Results**: NGTDM coarseness, SUVmax, and TNM stage survived the LASSO analysis and were used for the radiomic model. The AUCs obtained from the reference and radiomic models were 80.82 (95%CI, 69.01–92.63) and 81.02 (95%CI, 69.07–92.97), respectively (p = 0.98). The median OS in the reference model was 17.0 months in high-risk patients (95%CI, 11–21) and 113 months in low-risk patients (HR 7.47, p < 0.001). In the radiomic model, the median OS was 16.5 months (95%CI, 11–20) and 113 months in high- and low-risk groups, respectively (HR 9.64, p < 0.001). **Conclusions**: Our results indicate that a radiomic model composed using the tumor stage, SUVmax, and a selected radiomic feature (NGTDM_Coarseness) predicts survival in NSCLC patients similarly to a reference model composed only by the tumor stage and SUVmax. Replication of these preliminary results is necessary.

Keywords: NSCLC; radiomics; survival; PET; FDG

1. Introduction

Over the past few years, there have been significant advances in the treatment of non-small cell lung cancer (NSCLC). Biological, target, and immunotherapies have been introduced in the clinical routine along with standard treatments, represented by surgery, chemotherapy, and radiotherapy. Despite the wide therapeutic armamentarium available, lung cancer still remains the first cause of cancer-related death worldwide. Moreover, it is evident that patients at the same stage according to the classification of malignant tumors based on tumor size, T, lymph nodes, N, and metastasis, M, (TNM) and with the same treatment may experience different outcomes, suggesting a different biological behavior within the tumor [1].

The ability to predict prognosis on the basis of tumor biology and set up a therapy may be difficult in clinical practice. It is not uncommon that the outcomes of patients with tumors classified in the same TNM staging group may evolve differently. One of the causes is tumor heterogeneity. According to recent research, spatial heterogeneity is correlated with tumor progression, treatment resistance, and recurrence [2]. Radiomics, defined as the process of identifying mineable parameters hidden in the pixels of images and routinely non-detectable by the human eye, is a new technology that potentially could allow to study of tumor heterogeneity and to investigate its role in disease development. Indeed, specific features extracted from images by radiomics analysis (e.g., intensity, shape, and texture) add relevant information, which could be related to other clinical variables [3,4]. Radiomics analysis provides quantitative information based on signal intensity of regions of interest that improves the set of qualitative (semantic) information currently used in clinical practice. Radiomic features extracted from the medical images belong to different categories defined as a function of increasing complexity. The structural ones describe morphological aspects, such as eccentricity, volume, and presence of concavity (solidity), while those of greater complexity are defined according to the organization of spatially contiguous areas with different signal intensities [5]. In recent years, machine learning and radiomic techniques have been increasingly used for whole-body and brain image analysis in oncology and neuroimaging in order to improve diagnostic accuracy for several disorders [6,7]. The enormous amount of data associated with medical images, such as size, morphology, and radiotracer uptake, represents a great source of information where radiomics can play an important role in the detection of quantitative information normally not evaluable by the human eye. In this study, we described a machine learning approach to create a prognostic model for patients with newly diagnosed NSCLC. To explore the additive value of radiomics, we compared the performance of a machine learning radiomic model, integrating the tumor stage, standardized uptake values (SUVmax), and radiomic features, with a reference model integrating only tumor stage and SUVmax for the prediction of overall survival (OS) in NSCLC patients. Our major finding is that the radiomic model did not significantly increase the prediction of survival in NSCLC patients compared with the reference model.

2. Materials and Methods

2.1. Population

This retrospective study was based on clinical records and F-18 fluorodeoxyglucose positron emission tomography/computed tomography (FDG PET/CT), images of NSCLC patients from two institutions (S. Andrea Hospital, La Spezia, Italy, and IRCCS Ca' Granda-Ospedale Maggiore Policlinico, Milan, Italy) collected between November 2010 and December 2019.

Patients were retrospectively recruited from (S. Andrea Hospital, La Spezia, Italy, and IRCCS Ca' Granda-Ospedale Maggiore Policlinico, Milan, Italy). The analysis was performed on clinical records and imaging studies collected between November 2010 and December 2019. The regional review committee granted ethical approval (CER Liguria: 251/2020/10601) for this study (8 June 2020). We de-identified data to avoid any potential breach of patient privacy and processed them for research purposes from 1 July 2020.

Inclusion criteria were as follows: (1) histologically confirmed lung adenocarcinoma or squamous cell carcinoma diagnosed on surgical specimen according to the World Health Organization (WHO) classification [8]; (2) whole body FDG PET/CT performed at initial staging; (3) availability of information about survival status. Exclusion criteria were as follows: (i) previous history of other malignant tumors; (ii) anticancer treatment prior to the baseline PET/CT scan; (iii) PET/CT performed not at initial staging. Written informed consent was obtained from all patients before PET/CT imaging procedures. As 1184 out of the 1504 patients initially recruited from the institutional database did not meet inclusion criteria, they were excluded. Therefore, the study cohort consisted of 320 subjects (21% of the initial sample) with histologically confirmed diagnosis of NSCLC, encompassing 219 males and 101 females. Among these, 209 were adenocarcinomas and 111 were squamous cell carcinomas. Patients were classified by a nuclear medicine physician and an oncologist according to the 8th edition of the TNM staging system [9] measuring the tumor size (T) on the unenhanced CT of the PET/CT; the analysis of the presence of regional lymph node involvement (N) and distant metastases (M) was based on visual and semiquantitative evaluation of FDG uptake compared with background without any fixed uptake threshold and cytology/histology, as available.

Overall survival was defined by the time between the date of imaging and that of death or censoring. The date of the last follow-up visit was used for censoring surviving patients. Hospital records were used to assess patients' status.

All procedures were performed in accordance with institutional and/or national ethical standards and the 1964 Helsinki Declaration and its subsequent amendments.

Informed consent was obtained from all individual participants included in the study.

2.2. PET Imaging and Segmentation Procedures

PET/CT imaging was performed on a Discovery 710 (GE Healthcare, Chicago, IL, USA) and a Biograph (Siemens Healthcare, Erlangen, Germany) tomograph according to standard clinical scanning protocol used in the two participating centers. Patients were required to fast for ≥6 h prior to administration of 3.84 MBq/kg body weight of FDG (range, 2.57–4.91 MBq/kg). The mean FDG uptake period was 63 min (range, 47–83 min). Head-to-hip scanning was performed in all patients with the standard protocol using low-dose CT followed by PET acquisition. CT images were obtained at 120 kV and 100 mA, 0.33 s per rotation using a slice thickness of 3.0 mm and reconstructed to a 512 × 512 matrix (voxel size: 0.98 × 0.98 × 3.0 mm^3). PET imaging was obtained in a three-dimensional mode with 6 to 8 beds and lasting not less than 2 min each for a whole body acquisition from head to hip. PET images were reconstructed with CT-based attenuation correction using an ordered subset expectation maximization (OSEM) iterative algorithm. Final PET images had 256 × 256 matrix size and anisotropic voxels of 2.73 × 2.73 × 3.27 mm^3. SUVmax was obtained by normalizing the injected activity concentration to the patient's body weight.

PET images were reviewed in the Nuclear Medicine Unit laboratory of the S. Andrea Hospital by two board-certified nuclear medicine physicians. Fused PET/CT and CT images were processed under PET Volume Computerized Assisted Reporting (PETVCAR version 2.0) commercial software running on Advantage Workstation (version 4.6; GE Healthcare) in order to segment lung cancer. PETVCAR uses an adaptive iterative volume delineation algorithm (AT-AIA), which is able to automatically segment the target volume from background tissue using a SUVmax threshold of 2.5 and a 3D isocontour of 41% of the maximum voxel value measured in the target lesion [10,11]. SUVmax and SUVmean were obtained as the maximum and mean activity of the voxels within the volume of interest. Metabolic tumor volume (MTV) was defined as the total tumor volume contained in the VOI. Total lesion glycolysis (TLG) was calculated as MTV multiplied by the mean SUV of the lesion.

2.3. Image Analysis and Textural Features Extraction

Before the extraction, we applied the ComBat harmonization method [12] to remove batch effects from images of different scanners using the "neuroCombat" package in R.

In compliance with protocols described by the Imaging Biomarker Standardization Initiative (IBSI) (https://arxiv.org/abs/1612.07003, accessed on 1 March 2024), intensity discretization and spatial resampling were applied before feature extraction. Images were discretized with a 64 fixed bin width and resampled to 5 mm^3 voxel size with B-spline interpolation.

Spatial and intensity heterogeneity of FDG PET images were evaluated with two groups of features including (a) intensity and (b) texture. First-order statistics describing the voxel intensities within the VOI mask, including the tumor image, were assessed using SUV metric, including maximum voxel intensity (SUVmax), MTV, and TLG. The target volume was also limited to tumor volume in patients with lymph nodes and distant pathological FDG uptake sites.

Eighty-seven radiomic variables were extracted with the Pyradiomics software package (version 3.1.0) from each lung tumor [13,14].

Among them were 15 first-order, 21 gray-level co-occurrence matrix (GLCM), 16 gray-level run-length matrix (GLRLM), 16 gray-level size zone matrix (GLSZM), 14 gray-level dependence matrix (GLDM), and 5 neighborhood gray-tone difference matrix (NGTDM) textural features. To summarize, the whole set of predictors used for this study included 94 features—namely, 87 radiomic features, SUVmax, MTV, TLG, tumor stage, histology, age, and gender.

2.4. Feature Selection and Classification

The survival prediction model was implemented, starting with the whole set of demographic, clinical, radiomic, and molecular variables obtained from PET/CT studies. In order to reduce the number of variables to be included in the model, we used the least absolute shrinkage and selection operator (LASSO) Cox regression analysis [15,16]. The analysis was performed in R 4.1.3 (http://www.r-project.org) with the cv.glmnet package [17].

The model with the best performance was selected using a 10-fold cross-validation and the C-statistic. The detailed description of the method is reported in our previous paper [18].

The model used in subsequent analyses was implemented with the predictors selected from the LASSO Cox regression analysis.

2.5. Model Validation and Calibration

Model performance was estimated with the calibration and validation procedures available under the RMS package [19]. The evaluation metric was based on C-index and Brier scores. The calibration method was performed by comparing the predicted to the observed probabilities. Validation was obtained by computing an optimism-corrected C-statistic after 1000 bootstrapped resampling. To test data not included in the training process, we also carried out the validation of the test dataset. The high- and low-risk survival groups were defined using the median individual risk score assessed with the GGrisk package of R software [20]. Kaplan–Meier analysis with the ggsurvplot function and log-rank test was used to evaluate the accuracy of the risk score in identifying patients with a lower probability of survival.

2.6. Model Design

Ninety-four predictors were included in Lasso's initial selection. They included 2 demographic (age and gender), 3 metabolic (SUVmax, MTV, and TLG), 87 radiomic, and 2 clinical features (histology and disease stage). The model was built with all the predictors chosen by Lasso analysis. For comparison, a model including the disease stage only was implemented.

Model performance was assessed on a test dataset obtained by splitting the study sample into training (80%) and test (20%) datasets. Therefore, the performance evaluation was carried out on data excluded from the training.

The ratio used to divide the study population into training and test samples is reported to be useful in developing high-performance predictive models when the sample size is greater than 100 and the percentage of incomplete data is less than 15% [21].

Moreover, the risk prediction model implemented using the disease stage alone was used to assess the added value of the radiomic model to the reference model. Model performance was evaluated by applying estimates derived from the training dataset to the test sample. Supplementary Table S2 reports clinical and demographic characteristics of the study sample by dataset.

2.7. Statistics

Statistical analysis and figures were obtained under R software (version 4.1.3, http://www.r-project.org). T-statistic was used for continuous variables. Where appropriate, the degrees of freedom were adjusted for inequality of variance.

Glmnet was used for LASSO regression analysis. Kaplan–Meier was performed under the ggsurvplot R package. The pROC and survival-ROC packages were applied to analyze the area under the receiver operating characteristic curve (AUCs).

Validation plots were produced by the root mean squares (RMS) package. The chi-square analysis was used for categorical variables. Positive predictive value (PPV), negative predictive value (NPV), and their 95% confidence intervals (CIs) were calculated to estimate how strongly the model-predicted diagnosis was associated with clinical outcomes.

The RMS package was used for predictive model validation [22]. The chi-square test was used to measure categorical variables' association with outcome. Moreover, the predictive model performance was assessed with positive predictive value (PPV) and negative predictive value (NPV) with their 95% confidence intervals (CIs).

In order to evaluate the model's predictive performance in different disease stages we also split the sample into an early disease group (stages I and II) and an advanced disease group (stages III and IV). The ability of the model to distinguish deceased from survivors was assessed with AUCs. The differences between the AUCs obtained in the two subgroups were evaluated with the DeLong test [23]. Two-sided p-values less than 0.05 were considered statistically significant.

3. Results

Three hundred and twenty patients were recruited and randomized to include 80% (n = 256) in training and 20% (n = 64) in test datasets. The distribution of histological types showed no significant differences between the training and test datasets ($p > 0.05$). Patients' characteristics are summarized in Table 1.

Table 1. Clinical and demographic characteristics of lung cancer patients. ADC = adenocarcinoma, SCC = squamous cell carcinoma, CTx = chemotherapy, RTx = radiotherapy, Sx = surgery.

	Outcome				
Variable	**Overall, n = 320** [1]	**Alive, n = 123** [1]	**Deceased, n = 197** [1]	**Statistic**	**p-Value** [2]
Age				−2.6	**0.011**
Median (Range)	72 (43, 92)	70 (43, 87)	73 (46, 92)		
Gender				4.6	**0.032**
Female	101 (32%)	48 (39%)	53 (27%)		
Male	219 (68%)	75 (61%)	144 (73%)		
Smoking status				0.88	**0.35**
Nonsmokers	165 (52%)	68 (55%)	97 (49%)		
Smokers	155 (48%)	55 (45%)	100 (51%)		

Table 1. *Cont.*

Variable	Outcome			Statistic	p-Value [2]
	Overall, $n = 320$ [1]	Alive, $n = 123$ [1]	Deceased, $n = 197$ [1]		
Histology				20	<0.001
ADC	238 (74%)	109 (89%)	129 (65%)		
SCC	82 (26%)	14 (11%)	68 (35%)		
Stage				93	<0.001
IA, IB	119 (37%)	84 (68%)	35 (18%)		
IIA, IIB	35 (11%)	14 (11%)	21 (11%)		
IIIA, IIIB, IIIC	77 (24%)	17 (14%)	60 (30%)		
IVA, IVB	89 (28%)	8 (6.5%)	81 (41%)		
Treatment					<0.001
Combined	141 (44%)	41 (33%)	100 (51%)		
CTx	66 (21%)	6 (4.9%)	60 (30%)		
RTx	10 (3.1%)	2 (1.6%)	8 (4.1%)		
Sx	103 (32%)	74 (60%)	29 (15%)		

[1] *n* (%); [2] Welch two-sample *t*-test; Pearson's chi-squared test; Fisher's exact test.

The full set of textural, non-textural, and clinical predictors available for each patient consisted of 94 variables. Predictors were selected with 10-fold cross-validation LASSO regression and C-statistic. The parameter producing a C-index within one standard error was 0.195 corresponding to a C-index of 0.782 (standard error = 0.019) (Figure 1). The coefficients of all predictors estimated with the LASSO shrinking algorithm are reported in Supplementary Figure S1.

Three predictors with non-zero coefficients survived the tuning parameters giving the C-index within one standard error of the maximum (Figure 1C). Selected variables included the tumor stage, SUVmax, and the radiomic variable NGTDM_Coarseness (Figure 1C). The LASSO procedure is an automatic operator-independent selection based on a predefined algorithm. Based on the LASSO regression results, two models were created to predict survival in patients with NSCLC: (1) a radiomic model composed using the tumor stage, SUVmax, and NGTDM_Coarseness; (2) a reference model composed using only the tumor stage and SUVmax.

In the training dataset, the concordance between the predicted survival and observed survival curves was detected by the internal validation procedure (Supplementary Figure S2, left panel). The unadjusted and bias-adjusted probabilities were aligned with the line of the best possible correlation (dashed line) between the predicted and observed outcome assessed by the mean absolute error (MAE) of 0.010. Moreover, the scores of 0.791 and 0.159 obtained for the C-statistic and Brier scores, respectively, confirmed the accuracy of the prediction. Validation results on the test set are shown in Supplementary Figure S2, right panel where the scores of 0.015, 0.819, and 0.162 were estimated for the MAE, C-index, and Brier scores, respectively.

The individual risk score was calculated with Cox regression in both the training and test datasets. Figure 2 shows the distribution of the risk score in the test sample. The results of the Kaplan–Meier analysis performed by dividing the patients of each dataset into high- and low-risk groups are shown in Figure 3. The median OS in the training dataset was 16.0 months in high-risk patients (95%CI, 11–18) and was not reached in the low-risk group (hazard ratio, HR: 5.65, $p < 0.001$) (Figure 3A). In the test dataset, the median OS in the high-risk group was 16.5 months (95%CI, 11–20) and 113 months in the low-risk group (HR 9.64, $p < 0.001$) (Figure 3B). Figure 4 shows the hazard ratio values by dataset and prediction model. The hazard ratio's *p*-value used to estimate model performance was significant in the training and testing datasets for both prediction models.

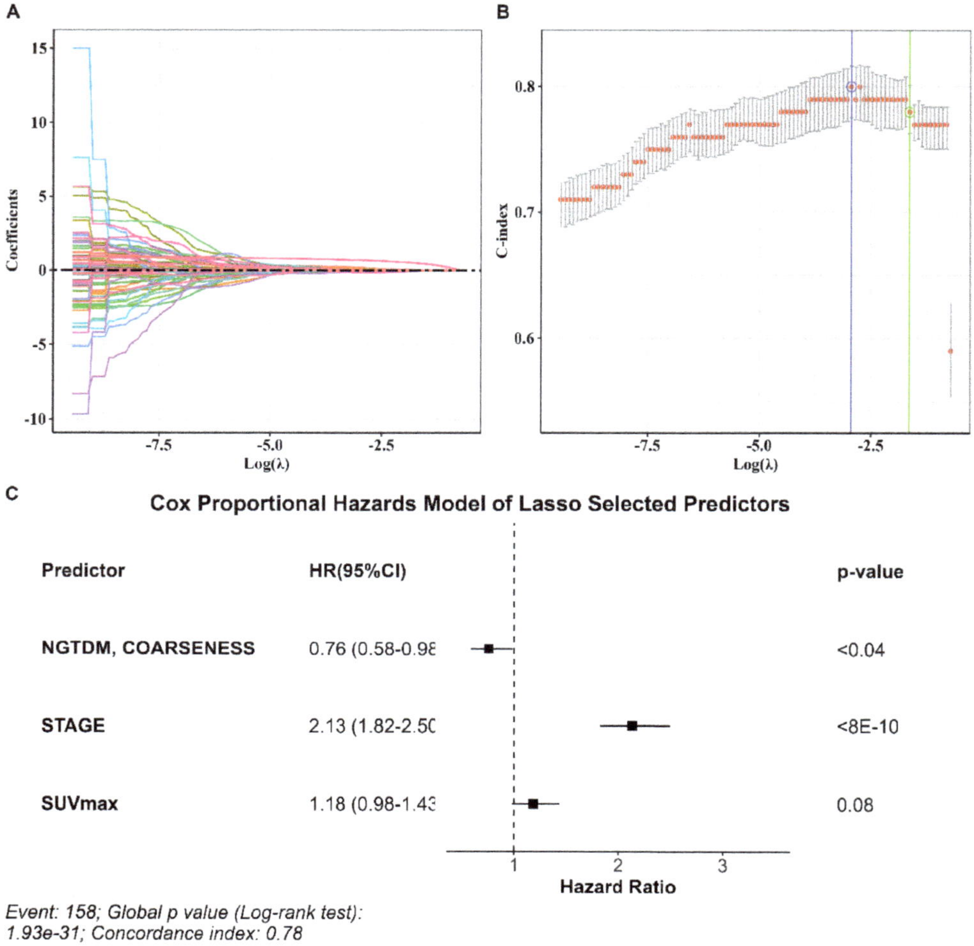

Figure 1. LASSO Cox regression results. (**A**) LASSO coefficients. Coefficient values are plotted against the log (λ). The coefficient of each feature is shown by a colored line. (**B**) C-Index. The plot shows the C-index plotted against log (λ). (**C**) The hazard ratio and 95% confidence interval of predictors survived LASSO selection as estimated by multivariate Cox regression.

The radiomic model correctly classified the majority of deceased and surviving patients into high- and low-risk groups in both datasets. In the training dataset, the radiomic model identified 70% of true positives and 83% of true negatives (OR, 95%CI = 11, 6–20). In the test sample, the model recognized 72% of true positives and 84% of true negatives (OR, 95%CI = 12, 3–40) (Table 2).

The AUCs obtained from the reference and radiomic models were 80.82 (95%CI, 69.01–92.63) and 0.8102 (95%CI, 69.07–92.97), respectively (Figure 5A). The DeLong statistic showed no significant difference between the performance of the two models ($p = 0.98$). Radiomic model performance was also evaluated separately on a subset including only I and II stages (early disease) vs. III and IV stages (advanced disease). The AUCs obtained from the early and advanced disease were 66.73 (95%CI, 56.29–77.16) and 73.06 (95%CI, 64.12–81.99), respectively (Figure 5B). No statistically significant difference between AUCs was shown by the DeLong test ($p = 0.37$).

Table 2. Bivariate analysis of model performance by dataset.

Predicted	n	Observed		χ^2	p-Value [2]	SS 95%CI [3]	SP 95%CI [4]	PPV 95%CI [5]	NPV 95%CI [6]	OR 95%CI [7]
		Deceased [1]	Alive [1]							
Training	256			62	$\mathbf{4.4 \times 10^{-15}}$	70 (62, 77)	82 (73, 89)	86 (79, 91)	62 (54, 71)	10 (5, 18)
High risk		110 (70%)	18 (18%)							
Low risk		48 (30%)	80 (82%)							
Validation	64			17	$\mathbf{4.1 \times 10^{-5}}$	72 (55, 85)	84 (64, 95)	88 (71, 96)	66 (47, 81)	12 (3, 40)
High risk		28 (72%)	4 (16%)							
Low risk		11 (28%)	21 (84%)							

[1] n (%); [2] Pearson's chi-squared test; [3] sensitivity, confidence interval; [4] specificity, confidence interval; [5] positive predictive value, confidence interval; [6] negative predictive value, confidence interval; [7] odds ratio, confidence interval.

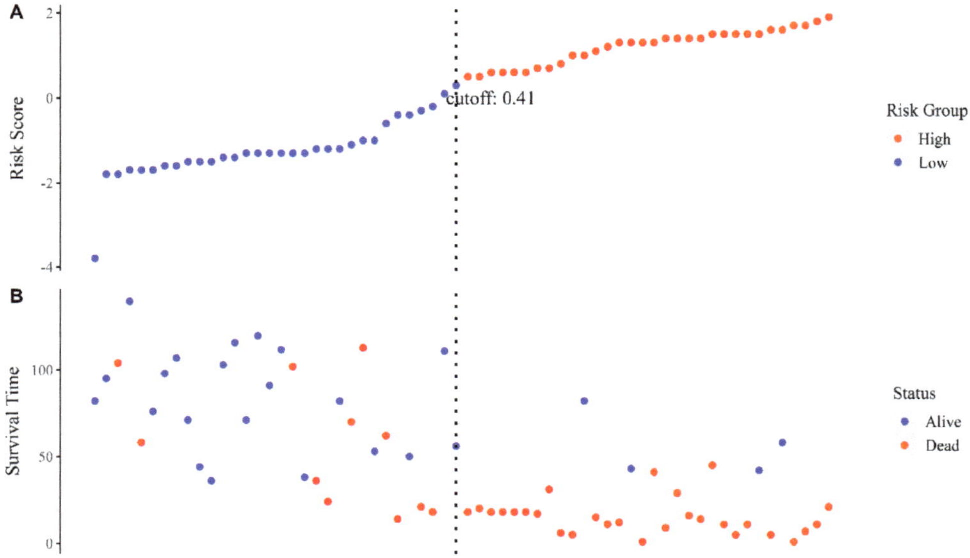

Figure 2. Risk score distribution in the test set. Risk score distribution (**A**), survival status, and survival time (**B**) between the high- and low-risk groups. Using the median risk score (0.41) as a cutoff point, the sample was divided into two groups, defined as high risk and low risk, respectively.

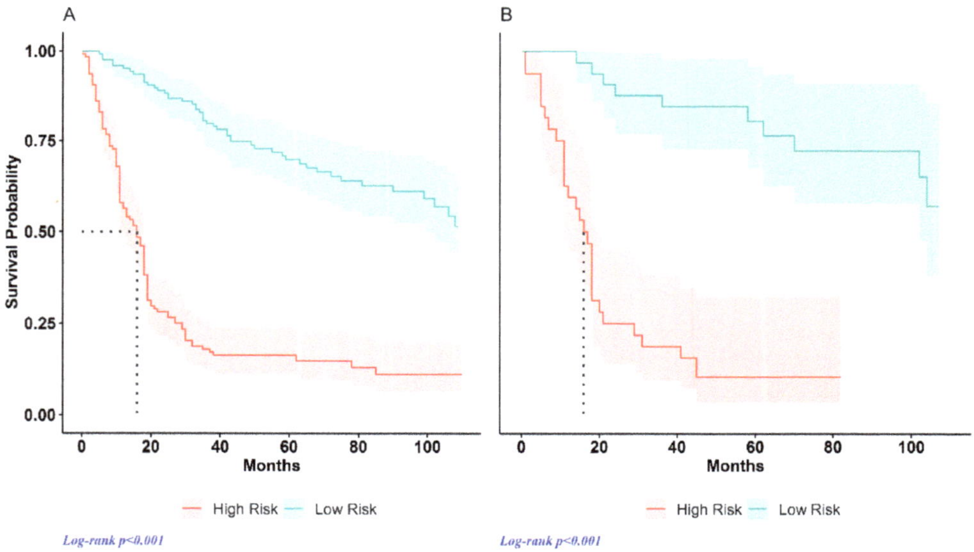

Figure 3. Survival curves for high- and low-risk groups by prediction variable: (**A**) training dataset; (**B**) test dataset.

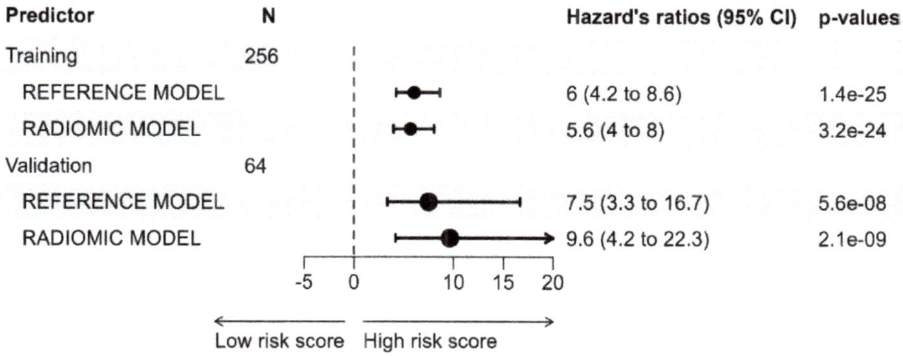

Figure 4. Hazard ratios by model prediction and dataset.

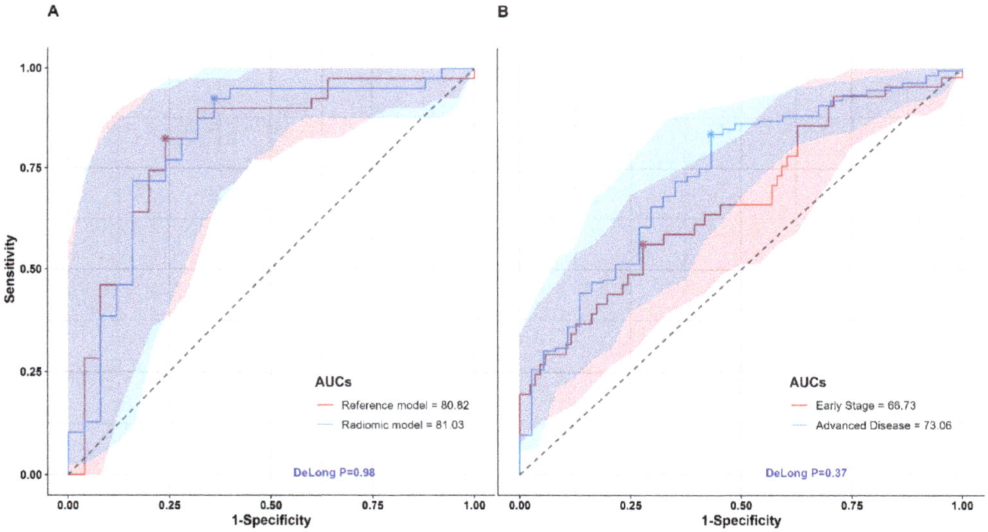

Figure 5. Receiver operating characteristic curves of model performance obtained from the test dataset. (**A**) ROC curves based on reference and radiomic models. (**B**) ROC curves showing the radiomic model performance in patients grouped by disease stage. The asterisk shows the threshold value that maximizes (sensitivity + specificity) for each curve.

Figure 6 shows the results of the Kaplan–Meier analysis obtained using the two models. The median OS in the reference model was 17.0 months in high-risk patients (95%CI, 11–21) and 113 months in the low-risk group (HR 7.47, $p < 0.001$) (Figure 6A). The median OS in the radiomic model was 16.5 months (95%CI, 11–20) and 113 months in high- and low-risk groups, respectively (HR 9.64, $p < 0.001$) (Figure 6B).

The median OS in the advanced disease group was 11 months (95%CI, 10–12) and 21 months (95%CI, 19–42) in high- and low-risk groups, respectively (HR 2.48, $p < 0.001$). The median OS in the early disease group was 113 months in high-risk patients and was not reached in the low-risk group (HR 2.40, $p = 0.007$). Survival estimates in our study are similar to those previously reported in the literature [24,25].

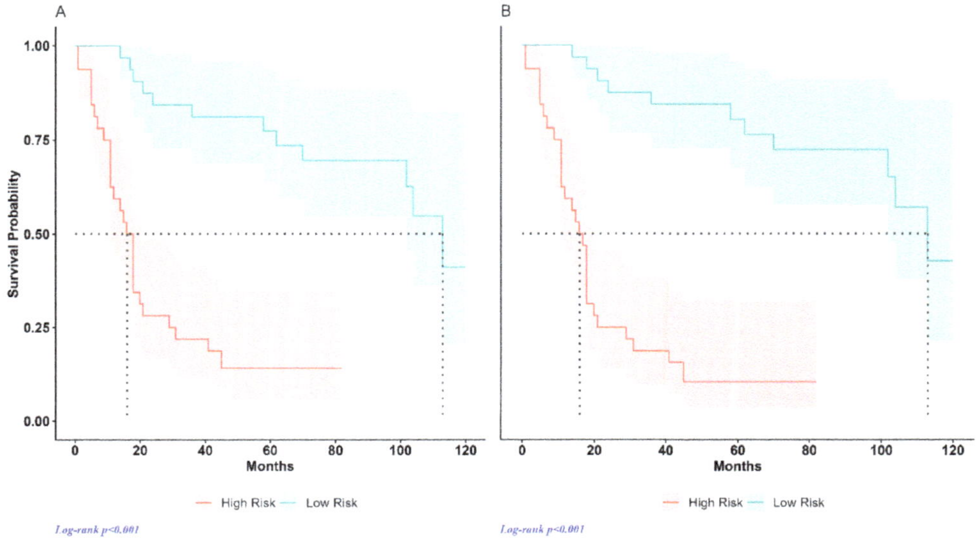

Figure 6. Survival curves for high- and low-risk groups by prediction variable: (**A**) reference model (stage and SUVmax); (**B**) radiomic model (stage, SUVmax and radiomic feature).

4. Discussion

A wide variation in clinical outcomes has been observed in patients within the same tumor stage [26,27]. In order to improve risk assessment, several attempts have been made to develop linear models based on Cox regression [28] and forest plot [29] integrating TNM with the other known prognostic factors in NSCLC, such as age and histology. Nevertheless, these models are characterized by poor performance, probably due to the limited number of features available and to the linear logic that does not take into account the complexity of clinical variables.

In our study, we investigated the potential impact of the prediction of the clinical outcome of a machine learning approach integrating tumor stage and SUVmax with tumor radiomic features extracted by FDG PET from newly diagnosed NSCLC patients. We used Cox regression analysis to predict the risk of mortality using one model integrating one selected PET radiomic feature (NGTDM_Coarseness), SUVmax, and tumor stage, defined as the radiomic model, and one model using only tumor stage and SUVmax, named the reference model. In fact, TNM is the reference standard for NSCLC staging, and SUVmax, which can be very easily and quickly calculated, was consistently shown to predict survival in NSCLC patients [30]. Although radiomics is fascinating and powerful, its application is also cumbersome and time-consuming and it should be preferred or added to established biomarkers for a specific clinical question in case of a significant added value. Unfortunately, in our study, for the prediction of survival in NSCLC patients, the selected radiomic variable did not provide any significant additional value to that provided by the combination of tumor stage and SUVmax.

This study is part of a framework of machine learning emerging applications in clinical oncology. Machine learning has been employed in the context of medical imaging for segmentation and malignancy characterization [31], in histopathology [32], and in the study of biomarkers [33]. Recent studies have begun to explore the potential role of machine learning networks in prognosis, applying machine learning models to predict OS in NSCLC, mainly integrating tumor stage with clinical factors showing promising results [34–44]. However, a possible research gap lies in the fact that although studies indicate the potential of radiomics to predict survival in oncological patients, the clinical settings and the most important radiomic variables for such prediction need to be better established. This motivated our study. The comparison between the reference and the radiomic model differentiates our study from others in the radiomic field. A careful analysis of the papers suggests that the discrepancy between our study and other studies might be related to the different methodologies adopted.

For example, Ahn et al. reported that different radiomic variables derived from pretreatment FDG PET predicted survival in NSCLC patients; however, in their case, only radiomic variables were included in the analysis [35]. Similar univariate approaches were adopted in other positive studies [36,37].

In another group of studies, radiomic features were integrated with other clinical or imaging variables in fully integrated models, but their added value compared with a reference model was not assessed [38,39].

Moran et al. studied radiotherapy, planning CT and PET/CT 39 for stage III NSCLC patients [41]. Seven conventional prognostic factors, including stage (IIIA vs. IIIB), were collected. Patients were divided into two risk groups based on Kaplan–Meier curves. They showed that the discriminatory power was significantly increased when conventional prognostic factors were combined with PET features compared with conventional prognostic factors alone. There was no significant improvement when conventional prognostic factors were combined with CT features. The main difference from our study is that in their study, SUVmax was not included in the analysis—a factor that might contribute to the different results. Contrarily, Oikonomou et al. showed that radiomic features, but not SUVmax, predict OS after radiotherapy in NSCLC, but in their study, the role of tumor stage was not assessed [42].

Results very similar to ours were obtained by Hannequin et al. [40] and Oliveira et al. [43]. Hannequin et al. showed that PET and CT radiomic features have intrinsic power to predict survival, but they do not significantly improve the prediction of OS and progression-free survival in different multivariate models, in comparison to stage and gender [40]. Oliveira et al. found at univariable analysis no significant association between radiomic features predicting either event-free survival or OS [43]. The authors of this multicentric study emphasized the need for standardized protocols. Indeed, it is also possible that the bicentric nature of our study, with some protocol differences, might have increased the variability of the data and partially reduced the statistical power of the radiomic analysis.

To overcome this drawback, the radiomics data were harmonized using the ComBat approach. This method has proven to be useful in harmonizing the radiomic features extracted from PET obtained with different acquisition and/or reconstruction parameters and in facilitating the validation of the radiomic signatures of data obtained from different centers [45].

The study sample was distributed between the two centers (218 and 102 patients). Clinical and demographic characteristics were similar between the two groups (Supplementary Table S1). Survival rates did not differ significantly between the two groups (Log-rank $p = 0.2$).

It might be objected that our results are biased by the fact that the majority of our sample is represented by advanced-stage patients; therefore, the variable stage naturally outweighs the role of radiomics in the determination of survival. However, when the analysis was performed separately for patients with early disease and advanced disease (Figure 5B), the results of the two analyses were similar showing that the accuracy of the model is independent of the disease stage.

The definition of T was based on the measurement of tumor size on the unenhanced CT of the PET/CT. However, stages III and IV are based not only on size but also on the infiltration of various tissues (pleura, vessels), which is difficult to assess on PET/TC. Owing to the retrospective design of the study, contrast-enhanced CT was not available for all patients as it was often performed in other centers. Therefore, the proportion of stages III and IV may have been slightly underestimated.

In this study, we extracted radiomic data only from the primary tumor, excluding lymph nodes and distant metastases, as the radiomic variables can be affected by various factors, which can limit the reproducibility and accuracy of the estimates (lesion size, contouring, and/or harmonization approach [46].

Li et al., using PET/CT, showed that the best classifier for predicting local relapse had only tumor features; in contrast, the best classifier for predicting overall relapse included a node feature [47].

In the study by Carvalho et al., common SUV descriptors were significantly related to OS when extracted from lymph nodes but not from tumor region, while radiomic features were significant when extracted from both lymph nodes and tumor. Therefore, a combination of FDG-PET radiomic features from tumors and lymph nodes was considered desirable to achieve a higher prognostic discriminative power for NSCLC [48]. These preliminary results do not conclude that radiomic analysis is useless, but they show that FDG PET radiomic analysis of only primary tumor provides no additional information in this clinical context. Nowadays, the most common approach in PET studies is to limit radiomic analysis to the tumor. Radiomic analysis of lymph nodes and distant metastases would be more cumbersome but, potentially, also more informative. Similarly, unenhanced, low-dose CT radiomic signature could provide useful information to differentiate and identify histology of lung cancer or to predict survival [18,49,50], but the assessment of CT radiomics was beyond the aim of our study and should be considered as a study limitation.

The main limitation of our study relates to the reproducibility of the results, i.e., test-retest reliability. A sizeable number of factors, such as number of patients, number and type of radiomic variables, software used for data extraction, validation procedure, data harmonization, type of treatment, etc., can all affect radiomic analysis variability. Therefore, replication of our study is warranted, and until such replication is obtained, our results should be considered preliminary. Attention was paid to describing all parts of our methods so that independent replication of our results could be achieved. In future studies, we would like to test the robustness of the current results in a larger population and use a different data selection method.

5. Conclusions

We performed a retrospective study, which included 320 NSCLC patients who underwent PET/CT with FDG at initial staging. VOIs were placed on primary tumors only. There is increasing interest in assessing the role of radiomics in predicting survival or other clinical-pathological features in NSCLC [44,51–56]. While most studies uniquely tested the role of models mixing clinical and radiomic variables, we performed a comparative study where a model containing uniquely clinical variables (tumor stage and SUVmax), referred to as the reference model, was contrasted with a model that, in addition to tumor stage and SUVmax, contained one radiomic variable (NGTDM_Coarseness, radiomic model); these variables had been automatically selected by our data selection method (LASSO procedure). Our design allowed for assessing the additional value introduced by the radiomic variable. Results showed that the radiomic model predicted survival in NSCLC patients similarly to the reference model. Replication of these preliminary results is warranted to shed more light on the role of radiomic variables in the prediction of prognosis in NSCLC patients.

Supplementary Materials: The following supporting information can be downloaded at: https://www.mdpi.com/article/10.3390/jcm13092613/s1, Figure S1. LASSO Cox coefficients of all variables used for prediction model implementation; Figure S2. Calibration curves from regression model predictions by datasets; Figure S3. Overfitting impact on prediction model; Table S1. Clinical and demographic characteristics by recruitment center; Table S2. Clinical and demographic characteristics of Lung Cancer patients by dataset.

Author Contributions: Conceptualization, A.C. (Andrea Ciarmiello) and G.G.; methodology, A.C. (Andrea Ciarmiello), N.Y. and G.G.; software, A.C. (Andrea Ciarmiello); validation, A.C. (Andrea Ciarmiello); formal analysis, A.C. (Andrea Ciarmiello); investigation, F.T., C.B., E.G., G.G., A.M., L.D., M.C., C.A., A.C. (Angelo Castello) and L.F.; data curation, A.C. (Angelo Castello), E.G., M.C. and E.B.; writing—original draft preparation, A.C. (Andrea Ciarmiello) and G.G.; writing—review and editing, A.C. (Andrea Ciarmiello), G.G. and A.C. (Angelo Castello). All authors have read and agreed to the published version of the manuscript.

Funding: This research received no external funding.

Institutional Review Board Statement: The study was conducted in accordance with the Declaration of Helsinki, and approved by the Regional Review Committee CER Liguria (protocol code: 251/2020/10601, approved on 8 June 2020).

Informed Consent Statement: Informed consent was obtained from all subjects involved in the study. Written informed consent has been obtained from the patients to publish this paper.

Data Availability Statement: The datasets presented in this article are not readily available because the data are part of an ongoing study.

Conflicts of Interest: The authors declare no conflict of interest.

References

1. Herbst, R.S.; Morgensztern, D.; Boshoff, C. The biology and management of non-small cell lung cancer. *Nature* **2018**, *553*, 446–454. [CrossRef] [PubMed]
2. Castello, A.; Grizzi, F.; Toschi, L.; Rossi, S.; Rahal, D.; Marchesi, F.; Russo, C.; Finocchiaro, G.; Lopci, E. Tumor heterogeneity, hypoxia, and immune markers in surgically resected non-small-cell lung cancer. *Nucl. Med. Commun.* **2018**, *39*, 636–644. [CrossRef] [PubMed]
3. Lambin, P.; Zindler, J.; Vanneste, B.G.; De Voorde, L.V.; Eekers, D.; Compter, I.; Panth, K.M.; Peerlings, J.; Larue, R.T.; Deist, T.M.; et al. Decision support systems for personalized and participative radiation oncology. *Adv. Drug Deliv. Rev.* **2017**, *109*, 131–153. [CrossRef] [PubMed]
4. Lee, G.; Lee, H.Y.; Park, H.; Schiebler, M.L.; van Beek, E.J.R.; Ohno, Y.; Seo, J.B.; Leung, A. Radiomics and its emerging role in lung cancer research, imaging biomarkers and clinical management: State of the art. *Eur. J. Radiol.* **2017**, *86*, 297–307. [CrossRef] [PubMed]
5. Gillies, R.J.; Kinahan, P.E.; Hricak, H. Radiomics: Images Are More than Pictures, They Are Data. *Radiology* **2016**, *278*, 563–577. [CrossRef] [PubMed]
6. Choi, H.; Kim, Y.K.; Yoon, E.J.; Lee, J.Y.; Lee, D.S. Cognitive signature of brain FDG PET based on deep learning: Domain transfer from Alzheimer's disease to Parkinson's disease. *Eur. J. Nucl. Med. Mol. Imaging* **2020**, *47*, 403–412. [CrossRef] [PubMed]
7. Caruso, D.; Zerunian, M.; Daffina, J.; Polici, M.; Polidori, T.; Tipaldi, M.A.; Ronconi, E.; Pucciarelli, F.; Lucertini, E.; Rossi, M.; et al. Radiomics and functional imaging in lung cancer: The importance of radiological heterogeneity beyond FDG PET/CT and lung biopsy. *Eur. J. Radiol.* **2021**, *142*, 109874. [CrossRef] [PubMed]
8. Travis, W.D.; Brambilla, E.; Nicholson, A.G.; Yatabe, Y.; Austin, J.H.M.; Beasley, M.B.; Chirieac, L.R.; Dacic, S.; Duhig, E.; Flieder, D.B.; et al. The 2015 World Health Organization Classification of Lung Tumors: Impact of Genetic, Clinical and Radiologic Advances Since the 2004 Classification. *J. Thorac. Oncol. Off. Publ. Int. Assoc. Study Lung Cancer* **2015**, *10*, 1243–1260. [CrossRef] [PubMed]
9. Postmus, P.E.; Kerr, K.M.; Oudkerk, M.; Senan, S.; Waller, D.A.; Vansteenkiste, J.; Escriu, C.; Peters, S. Early and locally advanced non-small-cell lung cancer (NSCLC): ESMO Clinical Practice Guidelines for diagnosis, treatment and follow-up. *Ann. Oncol.* **2017**, *28*, iv1–iv21. [CrossRef] [PubMed]
10. Boellaard, R.; Delgado-Bolton, R.; Oyen, W.J.; Giammarile, F.; Tatsch, K.; Eschner, W.; Verzijlbergen, F.J.; Barrington, S.F.; Pike, L.C.; Weber, W.A. FDG PET/CT: EANM procedure guidelines for tumour imaging: Version 2.0. *Eur. J. Nucl. Med. Mol. Imaging* **2015**, *42*, 328–354. [CrossRef] [PubMed]
11. Moule, R.N.; Kayani, I.; Prior, T.; Lemon, C.; Goodchild, K.; Sanghera, B.; Wong, W.L.; Saunders, M.I. Adaptive 18fluoro-2-deoxyglucose positron emission tomography/computed tomography-based target volume delineation in radiotherapy planning of head and neck cancer. *Clin. Oncol.* **2011**, *23*, 364–371. [CrossRef] [PubMed]
12. Orlhac, F.; Boughdad, S.; Philippe, C.; Stalla-Bourdillon, H.; Nioche, C.; Champion, L.; Soussan, M.; Frouin, F.; Frouin, V.; Buvat, I. A Postreconstruction Harmonization Method for Multicenter Radiomic Studies in PET. *J. Nucl. Med.* **2018**, *59*, 1321–1328. [CrossRef] [PubMed]
13. Pyradiomics. Available online: https://github.com/Radiomics/pyradiomics/releases (accessed on 1 March 2024).
14. van Griethuysen, J.J.M.; Fedorov, A.; Parmar, C.; Hosny, A.; Aucoin, N.; Narayan, V.; Beets-Tan, R.G.H.; Fillion-Robin, J.C.; Pieper, S.; Aerts, H. Computational Radiomics System to Decode the Radiographic Phenotype. *Cancer Res.* **2017**, *77*, e104–e107. [CrossRef] [PubMed]

15. Tibshirani, R. Regression Shrinkage and Selection via the Lasso. *J. R. Stat. Soc. Ser. B Methodol.* **1996**, *58*, 267–288. [CrossRef]
16. Friedman, J.; Hastie, T.; Tibshirani, R. Regularization Paths for Generalized Linear Models via Coordinate Descent. *J. Stat. Softw.* **2010**, *33*, 1–22. [CrossRef] [PubMed]
17. Glmnet. Available online: http://cran.r-project.org/web/packages/glmnet (accessed on 1 March 2024).
18. Ciarmiello, A.; Tutino, F.; Giovannini, E.; Milano, A.; Barattini, M.; Yosifov, N.; Calvi, D.; Setti, M.; Sivori, M.; Sani, C.; et al. Multivariable Risk Modelling and Survival Analysis with Machine Learning in SARS-CoV-2 Infection. *J. Clin. Med.* **2023**, *12*, 7164. [CrossRef] [PubMed]
19. Harrell, F.E., Jr. *Regression Modeling Strategies;* Springer: Berlin/Heidelberg, Germany, 2006.
20. Zhang, Z.; Lin, E.; Zhuang, H.; Xie, L.; Feng, X.; Liu, J.; Yu, Y. Construction of a novel gene-based model for prognosis prediction of clear cell renal cell carcinoma. *Cancer Cell Int.* **2020**, *20*, 27. [CrossRef] [PubMed]
21. Dobbin, K.K.; Simon, R.M. Optimally splitting cases for training and testing high dimensional classifiers. *BMC Med. Genom.* **2011**, *4*, 31. [CrossRef] [PubMed]
22. Harrell, F.E., Jr.; Harrell, M.F.E., Jr.; Hmisc, D. *Package 'rms'*; Vanderbilt University: Nashville, TN, USA, 2017; p. 229.
23. DeLong, E.R.; DeLong, D.M.; Clarke-Pearson, D.L. Comparing the areas under two or more correlated receiver operating characteristic curves: A nonparametric approach. *Biometrics* **1988**, *44*, 837–845. [CrossRef] [PubMed]
24. Lin, J.T.; Li, X.M.; Zhong, W.Z.; Hou, Q.Y.; Liu, C.L.; Yu, X.Y.; Ye, K.Y.; Cheng, Y.L.; Du, J.Y.; Sun, Y.Q.; et al. Impact of preoperative [(18)F]FDG PET/CT vs. contrast-enhanced CT in the staging and survival of patients with clinical stage I and II non-small cell lung cancer: A 10-year follow-up study. *Ann. Nucl. Med.* **2024**, *38*, 188–198. [CrossRef] [PubMed]
25. Chen, W.M.; Chen, M.; Hsu, J.G.; Lee, T.S.; Shia, B.C.; Wu, S.Y. Use of Preoperative FDG PET/CT and Survival of Patients with Resectable Non-Small Cell Lung Cancer. *Radiology* **2022**, *305*, 219–227. [CrossRef] [PubMed]
26. Chansky, K.; Sculier, J.P.; Crowley, J.J.; Giroux, D.; Van Meerbeeck, J.; Goldstraw, P. The International Association for the Study of Lung Cancer Staging Project: Prognostic factors and pathologic TNM stage in surgically managed non-small cell lung cancer. *J. Thorac. Oncol. Off. Publ. Int. Assoc. Study Lung Cancer* **2009**, *4*, 792–801. [CrossRef] [PubMed]
27. Kawaguchi, T.; Takada, M.; Kubo, A.; Matsumura, A.; Fukai, S.; Tamura, A.; Saito, R.; Maruyama, Y.; Kawahara, M.; Ignatius Ou, S.H. Performance status and smoking status are independent favorable prognostic factors for survival in non-small cell lung cancer: A comprehensive analysis of 26,957 patients with NSCLC. *J. Thorac. Oncol. Off. Publ. Int. Assoc. Study Lung Cancer* **2010**, *5*, 620–630. [CrossRef] [PubMed]
28. Liang, W.; Zhang, L.; Jiang, G.; Wang, Q.; Liu, L.; Liu, D.; Wang, Z.; Zhu, Z.; Deng, Q.; Xiong, X.; et al. Development and validation of a nomogram for predicting survival in patients with resected non-small-cell lung cancer. *J. Clin. Oncol.* **2015**, *33*, 861–869. [CrossRef] [PubMed]
29. Sculier, J.P.; Chansky, K.; Crowley, J.J.; Van Meerbeeck, J.; Goldstraw, P. The impact of additional prognostic factors on survival and their relationship with the anatomical extent of disease expressed by the 6th Edition of the TNM Classification of Malignant Tumors and the proposals for the 7th Edition. *J. Thorac. Oncol. Off. Publ. Int. Assoc. Study Lung Cancer* **2008**, *3*, 457–466. [CrossRef] [PubMed]
30. Vansteenkiste, J.F.; Stroobants, S.G.; Dupont, P.J.; De Leyn, P.R.; Verbeken, E.K.; Deneffe, G.J.; Mortelmans, L.A.; Demedts, M.G. Prognostic importance of the standardized uptake value on (18)F-fluoro-2-deoxy-glucose-positron emission tomography scan in non-small-cell lung cancer: An analysis of 125 cases. Leuven Lung Cancer Group. *J. Clin. Oncol.* **1999**, *17*, 3201–3206. [CrossRef] [PubMed]
31. Litjens, G.; Kooi, T.; Bejnordi, B.E.; Setio, A.A.A.; Ciompi, F.; Ghafoorian, M.; van der Laak, J.; van Ginneken, B.; Sanchez, C.I. A survey on deep learning in medical image analysis. *Med. Image Anal.* **2017**, *42*, 60–88. [CrossRef] [PubMed]
32. Kather, J.N.; Pearson, A.T.; Halama, N.; Jager, D.; Krause, J.; Loosen, S.H.; Marx, A.; Boor, P.; Tacke, F.; Neumann, U.P.; et al. Deep learning can predict microsatellite instability directly from histology in gastrointestinal cancer. *Nat. Med.* **2019**, *25*, 1054–1056. [CrossRef] [PubMed]
33. Tanaka, N.; Kanatani, S.; Tomer, R.; Sahlgren, C.; Kronqvist, P.; Kaczynska, D.; Louhivuori, L.; Kis, L.; Lindh, C.; Mitura, P.; et al. Whole-tissue biopsy phenotyping of three-dimensional tumours reveals patterns of cancer heterogeneity. *Nat. Biomed. Eng.* **2017**, *1*, 796–806. [CrossRef] [PubMed]
34. Hueman, M.; Wang, H.; Liu, Z.; Henson, D.; Nguyen, C.; Park, D.; Sheng, L.; Chen, D. Expanding TNM for lung cancer through machine learning. *Thorac. Cancer* **2021**, *12*, 1423–1430. [CrossRef]
35. Ahn, H.K.; Lee, H.; Kim, S.G.; Hyun, S.H. Pre-treatment (18)F-FDG PET-based radiomics predict survival in resected non-small cell lung cancer. *Clin. Radiol.* **2019**, *74*, 467–473. [CrossRef] [PubMed]
36. Carles, M.; Fechter, T.; Radicioni, G.; Schimek-Jasch, T.; Adebahr, S.; Zamboglou, C.; Nicolay, N.H.; Marti-Bonmati, L.; Nestle, U.; Grosu, A.L.; et al. FDG-PET Radiomics for Response Monitoring in Non-Small-Cell Lung Cancer Treated with Radiation Therapy. *Cancers* **2021**, *13*, 814. [CrossRef] [PubMed]
37. Li, J.; Zhang, B.; Ge, S.; Deng, S.; Hu, C.; Sang, S. Prognostic value of (18)F-FDG PET/CT radiomic model based on primary tumor in patients with non-small cell lung cancer: A large single-center cohort study. *Front. Oncol.* **2022**, *12*, 1047905. [CrossRef] [PubMed]
38. Christie, J.R.; Daher, O.; Abdelrazek, M.; Romine, P.E.; Malthaner, R.A.; Qiabi, M.; Nayak, R.; Napel, S.; Nair, V.S.; Mattonen, S.A. Predicting recurrence risks in lung cancer patients using multimodal radiomics and random survival forests. *J. Med. Imaging* **2022**, *9*, 066001. [CrossRef] [PubMed]

39. Mattonen, S.A.; Davidzon, G.A.; Benson, J.; Leung, A.N.C.; Vasanawala, M.; Horng, G.; Shrager, J.B.; Napel, S.; Nair, V.S. Bone Marrow and Tumor Radiomics at (18)F-FDG PET/CT: Impact on Outcome Prediction in Non-Small Cell Lung Cancer. *Radiology* **2019**, *293*, 451–459. [CrossRef] [PubMed]
40. Hannequin, P.; Decroisette, C.; Kermanach, P.; Berardi, G.; Bourbonne, V. FDG PET and CT radiomics in diagnosis and prognosis of non-small-cell lung cancer. *Transl. Lung Cancer Res.* **2022**, *11*, 2051–2063. [CrossRef]
41. Moran, A.; Wang, Y.; Dyer, B.A.; Yip, S.S.F.; Daly, M.E.; Yamamoto, T. Prognostic Value of Computed Tomography and/or (18)F-Fluorodeoxyglucose Positron Emission Tomography Radiomics Features in Locally Advanced Non-small Cell Lung Cancer. *Clin. Lung Cancer* **2021**, *22*, 461–468. [CrossRef] [PubMed]
42. Oikonomou, A.; Khalvati, F.; Tyrrell, P.N.; Haider, M.A.; Tarique, U.; Jimenez-Juan, L.; Tjong, M.C.; Poon, I.; Eilaghi, A.; Ehrlich, L.; et al. Radiomics analysis at PET/CT contributes to prognosis of recurrence and survival in lung cancer treated with stereotactic body radiotherapy. *Sci. Rep.* **2018**, *8*, 4003. [CrossRef] [PubMed]
43. Oliveira, C.; Amstutz, F.; Vuong, D.; Bogowicz, M.; Hullner, M.; Foerster, R.; Basler, L.; Schroder, C.; Eboulet, E.I.; Pless, M.; et al. Preselection of robust radiomic features does not improve outcome modelling in non-small cell lung cancer based on clinical routine FDG-PET imaging. *EJNMMI Res.* **2021**, *11*, 79. [CrossRef] [PubMed]
44. Li, B.; Su, J.; Liu, K.; Hu, C. Deep learning radiomics model based on PET/CT predicts PD-L1 expression in non-small cell lung cancer. *Eur. J. Radiol. Open* **2024**, *12*, 100549. [CrossRef] [PubMed]
45. Lucia, F.; Visvikis, D.; Vallieres, M.; Desseroit, M.C.; Miranda, O.; Robin, P.; Bonaffini, P.A.; Alfieri, J.; Masson, I.; Mervoyer, A.; et al. External validation of a combined PET and MRI radiomics model for prediction of recurrence in cervical cancer patients treated with chemoradiotherapy. *Eur. J. Nucl. Med. Mol. Imaging* **2019**, *46*, 864–877. [CrossRef] [PubMed]
46. Hosseini, S.A.; Shiri, I.; Ghaffarian, P.; Hajianfar, G.; Avval, A.H.; Seyfi, M.; Servaes, S.; Rosa-Neto, P.; Zaidi, H.; Ay, M.R. The effect of harmonization on the variability of PET radiomic features extracted using various segmentation methods. *Ann. Nucl. Med.* **2024**. [CrossRef] [PubMed]
47. Li, H.; Becker, N.; Raman, S.; Chan, T.C.; Bissonnette, J.P. The value of nodal information in predicting lung cancer relapse using 4DPET/4DCT. *Med. Phys.* **2015**, *42*, 4727–4733. [CrossRef] [PubMed]
48. Carvalho, S.; Leijenaar, R.T.H.; Troost, E.G.C.; van Timmeren, J.E.; Oberije, C.; van Elmpt, W.; de Geus-Oei, L.F.; Bussink, J.; Lambin, P. 18F-fluorodeoxyglucose positron-emission tomography (FDG-PET)-Radiomics of metastatic lymph nodes and primary tumor in non-small cell lung cancer (NSCLC)—A prospective externally validated study. *PLoS ONE* **2018**, *13*, e0192859. [CrossRef] [PubMed]
49. Antunovic, L.; De Sanctis, R.; Cozzi, L.; Kirienko, M.; Sagona, A.; Torrisi, R.; Tinterri, C.; Santoro, A.; Chiti, A.; Zelic, R.; et al. PET/CT radiomics in breast cancer: Promising tool for prediction of pathological response to neoadjuvant chemotherapy. *Eur. J. Nucl. Med. Mol. Imaging* **2019**, *46*, 1468–1477. [CrossRef] [PubMed]
50. Kirienko, M.; Cozzi, L.; Antunovic, L.; Lozza, L.; Fogliata, A.; Voulaz, E.; Rossi, A.; Chiti, A.; Sollini, M. Prediction of disease-free survival by the PET/CT radiomic signature in non-small cell lung cancer patients undergoing surgery. *Eur. J. Nucl. Med. Mol. Imaging* **2018**, *45*, 207–217. [CrossRef] [PubMed]
51. Hovhannisyan-Baghdasarian, N.; Luporsi, M.; Captier, N.; Nioche, C.; Cuplov, V.; Woff, E.; Hegarat, N.; Livartowski, A.; Girard, N.; Buvat, I.; et al. Promising Candidate Prognostic Biomarkers in [(18)F]FDG PET Images: Evaluation in Independent Cohorts of Non-Small Cell Lung Cancer Patients. *J. Nucl. Med.* **2024**, *65*, 635–642. [CrossRef] [PubMed]
52. Ma, N.; Yang, W.; Wang, Q.; Cui, C.; Hu, Y.; Wu, Z. Predictive value of (18)F-FDG PET/CT radiomics for EGFR mutation status in non-small cell lung cancer: A systematic review and meta-analysis. *Front. Oncol.* **2024**, *14*, 1281572. [CrossRef]
53. Zuo, Y.; Liu, L.; Chang, C.; Yan, H.; Wang, L.; Sun, D.; Ruan, M.; Lei, B.; Xia, X.; Xie, W.; et al. Value of multi-center (18) F-FDG PET/CT radiomics in predicting EGFR mutation status in lung adenocarcinoma. *Med. Phys.* 2024. [CrossRef] [PubMed]
54. Zhang, R.; Shi, K.; Hohenforst-Schmidt, W.; Steppert, C.; Sziklavari, Z.; Schmidkonz, C.; Atzinger, A.; Hartmann, A.; Vieth, M.; Forster, S. Ability of (18)F-FDG Positron Emission Tomography Radiomics and Machine Learning in Predicting KRAS Mutation Status in Therapy-Naive Lung Adenocarcinoma. *Cancers* **2023**, *15*, 3684. [CrossRef] [PubMed]
55. Liu, F.; Xiang, Z.; Li, Q.; Fang, X.; Zhou, J.; Yang, X.; Lin, H.; Yang, Q. (18)F-FDG PET/CT-based radiomics model for predicting the degree of pathological differentiation in non-small cell lung cancer: A multicentre study. *Clin. Radiol.* **2024**, *79*, e147–e155. [CrossRef] [PubMed]
56. Lucia, F.; Louis, T.; Cousin, F.; Bourbonne, V.; Visvikis, D.; Mievis, C.; Jansen, N.; Duysinx, B.; Le Pennec, R.; Nebbache, M.; et al. Multicentric development and evaluation of [(18)F]FDG PET/CT and CT radiomic models to predict regional and/or distant recurrence in early-stage non-small cell lung cancer treated by stereotactic body radiation therapy. *Eur. J. Nucl. Med. Mol. Imaging* **2024**, *51*, 1097–1108. [CrossRef] [PubMed]

International Journal of
Environmental Research and Public Health

MDPI

Article

Diagnosis in Bytes: Comparing the Diagnostic Accuracy of Google and ChatGPT 3.5 as an Educational Support Tool

Guilherme R. Guimaraes [1], Ricardo G. Figueiredo [1,*], Caroline Santos Silva [1], Vanessa Arata [1], Jean Carlos Z. Contreras [1], Cristiano M. Gomes [2], Ricardo B. Tiraboschi [1] and José Bessa Junior [1]

1 Programa de Pós-Graduação em Saúde Coletiva, Universidade Estadual de Feira de Santana (UEFS), Feira de Santana 44.036-900, Brazil; guilhermeguimaraes304@gmail.com (G.R.G.); s.carolinne5@gmail.com (C.S.S.); vafigueiredo@uefs.br (V.A.); zambrano.jeancarlos@gmail.com (J.C.Z.C.); rbtiraboschi@uefs.br (R.B.T.); bessa@uefs.br (J.B.J.)

2 Faculty of Medicine, Universidade de São Paulo (USP), São Paulo 01.246-904, Brazil; crismgomes@uol.com.br

* Correspondence: rgfigueiredo@uefs.br; Tel.: +55-75-3161-8000

Abstract: Background: Adopting advanced digital technologies as diagnostic support tools in healthcare is an unquestionable trend accelerated by the COVID-19 pandemic. However, their accuracy in suggesting diagnoses remains controversial and needs to be explored. We aimed to evaluate and compare the diagnostic accuracy of two free accessible internet search tools: Google and ChatGPT 3.5. Methods: To assess the effectiveness of both medical platforms, we conducted evaluations using a sample of 60 clinical cases related to urological pathologies. We organized the urological cases into two distinct categories for our analysis: (i) prevalent conditions, which were compiled using the most common symptoms, as outlined by EAU and UpToDate guidelines, and (ii) unusual disorders, identified through case reports published in the 'Urology Case Reports' journal from 2022 to 2023. The outcomes were meticulously classified into three categories to determine the accuracy of each platform: "correct diagnosis", "likely differential diagnosis", and "incorrect diagnosis". A group of experts evaluated the responses blindly and randomly. Results: For commonly encountered urological conditions, Google's accuracy was 53.3%, with an additional 23.3% of its results falling within a plausible range of differential diagnoses, and the remaining outcomes were incorrect. ChatGPT 3.5 outperformed Google with an accuracy of 86.6%, provided a likely differential diagnosis in 13.3% of cases, and made no unsuitable diagnosis. In evaluating unusual disorders, Google failed to deliver any correct diagnoses but proposed a likely differential diagnosis in 20% of cases. ChatGPT 3.5 identified the proper diagnosis in 16.6% of rare cases and offered a reasonable differential diagnosis in half of the cases. Conclusion: ChatGPT 3.5 demonstrated higher diagnostic accuracy than Google in both contexts. The platform showed satisfactory accuracy when diagnosing common cases, yet its performance in identifying rare conditions remains limited.

Keywords: medical education; medical informatics applications; artificial intelligence; diagnosis; urology

1. Introduction

Since the introduction of early data processing machines in the 1940s, researchers across diverse disciplines have been captivated by their possible uses, with researchers in the medical field showing particular interest [1]. As early as 1959, Brodman and colleagues demonstrated that a trained computerized system could identify patterns in a group of symptoms reported by patients and suggest possible diagnoses, performing comparably to physicians receiving the same information [2]. From that point forward, data analytics technologies and Artificial Intelligence (AI) gained prominence in several medical fields, including public health, medical image analysis, and clinical trials, among others [3].

The increasing capability of these tools to integrate information has allowed researchers to envision diagnostic applications far beyond what Broadman presented. It is now possible to input a patient's symptoms into everyday search tools and receive a list of likely diagnoses [3,4]. Tang and Ng explored this utility in 2006, when they assessed the frequency of accurate diagnoses provided when specific disease symptoms were searched on Google, the leading internet search site [5].

In addition to search tools, new AI chatbots have recently been used to explore this field [6]. Among the most notable advancements is OpenAI's Generative Pre-trained Transformer, ChatGPT 3.5. Unlike conventional search engines that return pages based on keyword matching, ChatGPT 3.5 generates real-time responses, drawing from a vast database [7,8]. Internet users can access version 3.5 for free, as it is the most recent version available at no cost.

Given their capabilities for continuous and incremental learning, rapid summarization of textual data, and generation of natural language responses, large language models (LLMs) have been widely applied across various domains, notably in medical training [9]. These models efficiently assimilate and synthesize vast amounts of information, making them valuable tools for educational purposes in healthcare settings. In this setting, medical education has moved towards a competency-based education paradigm. Generative AI technologies have been increasingly employed in new competencies training for doctors and medical graduates [9]. AI-enhanced predictive models for risk stratification have shown great potential in the healthcare sector, especially in reducing diagnostic errors and improving patient safety.

In this context of evolving information technologies and their increasingly pervasive integration in medicine, this study aimed to assess the diagnostic accuracy and compare the agreement of two prominent online search tools, Google and ChatGPT 3.5, for urological conditions.

2. Materials and Methods

This pilot study was conducted between April and June 2023, in which the diagnostic properties of the Google and ChatGPT 3.5 platforms were assessed. These tools were evaluated based on the responses to 60 clinical cases related to urological pathologies, divided into "prevalent conditions" and "unusual conditions". Questions were formulated in Portuguese.

In the first group, 30 descriptions summarized the typical clinical presentation of prevalent urological diseases, published by the European Association of Urology and UpToDate guidelines (Table 1). In the second group, the remaining 30 cases were based on reports published between 2022 and 2023 in Urology Case Reports, selected based on the typicality of their manifestations (Table 2). Questions requiring extensive evaluation for specific diagnoses were excluded.

Table 1. Prevalent urological conditions.

Pathology	Clinical Case
Case 1: UTI (Urinary Tract Infection)	Woman, 27 years old, complains of dysuria, polyuria, and hematuria for about 6 days. Reports episodes of unmeasured fever and right flank pain. What is the likely diagnosis?
Case 2: Nephrolithiasis (Kidney Stones)	35-year-old man with left flank pain for 3 days, colicky, of strong intensity radiating to the inguinal region on the same side, presents nausea, fever, and dysuria. What is the likely diagnosis?
Case 3: BPH (Benign Prostatic Hyperplasia)	45-year-old man presents dysuria associated with increased urinary frequency, urinary incontinence, and an enlarged prostate. What is the likely diagnosis?
Case 4: Prostate Cancer	62-year-old man reports urinary incontinence, blood in the urine, and discomfort when sitting for the past 1 and a half months. Lost 2 kg during this period. What is the likely diagnosis?

Table 1. *Cont.*

Pathology	Clinical Case
Case 5: Stress Urinary Incontinence	62-year-old man reports stress urinary incontinence, without complaints of urinary urgency. What is the likely diagnosis?
Case 6: Bladder Cancer	82-year-old man presents painless hematuria, associated with bladder irritability, increased urinary frequency, and urinary urgency. What is the diagnosis?
Case 7: Erectile Dysfunction	50-year-old man with frequent difficulty in achieving a satisfactory erection for sexual intercourse and difficulty in maintaining a satisfactory erection for penetration. What is the correct diagnoses?
Case 8: Varicocele	25-year-old man with a left scrotum resembling a bag of worms, scrotal pain, testicular atrophy, and difficulty in conceiving. What is the likely diagnosis?
Case 9: Interstitial Cystitis	45-year-old woman complains of pain and discomfort for 3 months in the suprapubic region, related to bladder filling, with relief upon urination. What is the correct diagnosis?
Case 10: Priapism	22-year-old sickle cell anemia patient complains of a rigid and painful erection for 5 h. What is the likely diagnosis?
Case 11: Kidney Cancer	63-year-old man reports moderate pain in the lower back, hematuria, sensation of incomplete emptying, and palpable abdominal mass. What is the diagnosis?
Case 12: Testicular Cancer	16-year-old boy complains of a solid lump palpated in the right testicle. He denies pain but reports a sensation of scrotal heaviness. What is the probable diagnosis?
Case 13: Urethral Stricture	45-year-old man complains of weak stream, polyuria, incomplete emptying, and post-micturition dribbling. What is the likely diagnosis?
Case 14: Phimosis	Pre-adolescent, 12 years old, comes to the outpatient clinic with his mother, complaining of excess preputial skin, with compromised retraction. He reports post-micturition balanitis, accompanied by erythema on the glans. What is the likely diagnosis?
Case 15: Hypospadias	Male newborn presents with dorsal hooded foreskin, abnormal penile curvature, and double urethral opening, one terminal and the other subcoronal. What is the likely diagnosis?
Case 16: Prostatitis	60-year-old man with high fever, dysuria, chills, irritating urinary symptoms, and cloudy urine. What is the likely diagnosis?
Case 17: Gonorrhea	23-year-old man, unmarried, sexually active with multiple partners, experiences burning during urination, greenish purulent discharge, and erythema. What is the possible diagnosis?
Case 18: Polycystic Kidney Disease	54-year-old newly diagnosed hypertensive man reports hematuria and compromised renal function. He mentions altered renal ultrasound and similar family history. What is the probable diagnosis?
Case 19: Nocturnal Enuresis (Bedwetting)	7-year-old boy presents with multiple episodes of nocturnal enuresis, started after his parents' divorce 3 months ago. He denies other changes. What is the likely diagnosis?
Case 20: Urethritis	24-year-old man reports pain during urination, increased urinary frequency, urinary urgency, and transparent urethral discharge. What is the probable diagnosis?
Case 21: Male Infertility	26-year-old married man, trying to have children for over 18 months without success. Wife underwent tests with negative results for health problems. He underwent a semen analysis and obtained a count of 3 million sperm. What is the possible diagnosis?

Table 1. *Cont.*

Pathology	Clinical Case
Case 22: Urethral Diverticulum	34-year-old woman complains of urinary dribbling after urination, dysuria, and dyspareunia for 1 year, associated with palpable vaginal mass. She reports a history of pelvic surgery and denies other conditions. What is the probable diagnosis?
Case 23: Paraphimosis	23-year-old man presents with glandular edema and intense pain in the penis. Physical examination reveals a constricting band of tissue in the coronal sulcus. What is the probable diagnosis?
Case 24: Penile Cancer	60-year-old man presents with a palpable tumor in the glans of the penis, ulceration, and skin irritation for over six weeks. What is the probable diagnosis?
Case 25: Peyronie's Disease	17-year-old man complains of severe dorsal penile curvature during erection, preventing penetration, associated with a palpable plaque on the dorsal side of the penis and pain. What is the probable diagnosis?
Case 26: Traumatic Kidney Injury	25-year-old man reports presence of blood in the urine, decreased urine volume, and mild abdominal pain after 24 h of hospitalization due to a motorcycle accident with lower rib fractures. What is the probable diagnosis?
Case 27: Cryptorchidism	4-month-old male child comes for a medical examination because the testicles were not noticed after birth and not at 2 months of age. What is the probable diagnosis?
Case 28: Female Sexual Dysfunction	29-year-old woman reports reduced sexual desire, anorgasmia, and dyspareunia for 5 years. She denies other associated conditions. What is the probable diagnosis?
Case 29: Neurogenic Bladder	70-year-old man complains of urinary incontinence, burning in the bladder region, and frequent urge to urinate in small amounts after a stroke. What is the probable diagnosis?
Case 30: Genital Herpes	19-year-old man reports the sudden appearance of multiple erythematous-based vesicles on the glans and dorsal side of the penis, painful and pruritic, for seven days. States progression to ulcers with scalloped borders. What is the probable diagnosis?

Table 2. Unusual urological conditions.

Pathology	Clinical Case
Case 1: Melanoma in situ on the glans	28-year-old man complains of a brownish spot of about 8 mm on the penile glans, with an irregular central black point. He denies pain, and no alterations were found on physical examination. What is the likely diagnosis?
Case 2: Renal Papillary Hyperplasia	58-year-old man complains of urinating blood after exercise, denies coagulopathies, mentions NSAID use. What is the likely diagnosis?
Case 3: Urethral Stone	10-year-old child presents with acute urinary retention accompanied by penile pain, pelvic pressure, and a rigid, movable urethral mass.
Case 4: Penile Necrosis associated with Aortic Dissection	30-year-old man with lower limb paralysis, darkening of the scrotal sac and penis for 2 weeks, with loss of the urge to urinate and defecate. No hematuria or cloudy urine. Legs were blue.
Case 5: Renal Mucormycosis	56-year-old man presents with painful exophthalmos. Orbital tissue sampling revealed polymicrobial infection. Fungal polymerase test also revealed Rhizopus oryzae. A CT scan revealed an abscess in the lower right pole of the kidney. The abscess was drained, and the pus contained extended-spectrum beta-lactamase-producing enterobacteria. What is the likely diagnosis?

Table 2. *Cont.*

Pathology	Clinical Case
Case 6: Urachal Sinus (atypical case)	23-year-old woman is seen in the emergency room reporting lower abdominal pain and scant, foul-smelling umbilical discharge for 3 days. She does not report hematuria. Blood tests showed mild infection, and urinalysis and urine culture came back negative. What is the likely diagnosis?
Case 7: Ureterocoele Hernia with Gluteal Abscess	90-year-old woman with right buttock and hip pain, laboratory results showing signs of inflammation and mild renal dysfunction. Contrast-enhanced abdominal and pelvic CT scan reveals gluteal mass, hydronephrosis, and left-sided ureteral dilation with ureteral disconnection in the pelvis. Retrograde urography shows ureter folded in the left sciatic foramen. What is the likely diagnosis?
Case 8: Testicular Neoplasm	40-year-old man with symptoms of hyperandrogenism, absence of findings in the testicles on ultrasound and initial scrotal examination, and adrenal alteration. What is the possible diagnosis?
Case 9: Penile Fracture with Urethral Injury	37-year-old man arrives at the emergency room with complaints of pain, acute edema of the penis, rapid detumescence, blood discharge from the urethral meatus, and inability to urinate, with onset 3 h after sexual activity. Significant hematoma observed on penis during physical examination. Lab tests are normal. What is the likely diagnosis?
Case 10: Emphysematous Cystitis	78-year-old woman presents in the emergency room with signs of peritonitis associated with urinary incontinence and fever. Contrast-enhanced CT scan of the abdomen and pelvis reveals pneumoperitoneum, free fluid in the cavity, and air within the urinary bladder. What is the likely diagnosis?
Case 11: Urethral Diverticulum without Urethral Stricture	34-year-old man reports ejaculatory difficulty, urine loss after urination, and presents with penile-scrotal mass that increases during urination on physical examination. What is the likely correct diagnosis?
Case 12: Scrotoschisis	Male newborn, 2 days old, is brought to the emergency room with complete evisceration of the right testicle through a small defect in the right hemiscrotum wall. What is the likely diagnosis?
Case 13: Xanthogranulomatous Orchitis	77-year-old man presenting with right scrotal mass. He reports increasing scrotal swelling on the right side accompanied by pain for two days. Imaging exams revealed heterogeneous lesion involving the testicle, with collection in the underlying scrotal wall. What is the likely diagnosis?
Case 14: Laughing Urinary Incontinence	16-year-old female adolescent presenting with total and unstoppable urinary incontinence when laughing, normal menstrual pattern, and no other urinary complaints. Not responsive to previous anticholinergic therapy. What is the likely diagnosis?
Case 15: Wunderlich Syndrome	66-year-old man, without history of trauma and using antiplatelet medication, arrives at the emergency room with severe generalized abdominal pain and hemodynamic instability. Contrast-enhanced abdominal CT scan reveals perirenal and retroperitoneal hyperdensity, indicating hematoma. What is the likely diagnosis?
Case 16: Spermatocele Torsion	A 25-year-old man presented to the emergency room with sudden-onset right scrotal pain. On physical examination, he had a swollen and tender right hemiscrotum. Scrotal ultrasonography revealed testicular edema and a cystic mass originating from the right epididymis. What is the likely diagnosis?
Case 17: Testicular Tuberculosis	41-year-old man, pain and swelling in the right testicle, fever of 38° for 3 months, without ulcers. Painless, palpable, firm hypertrophied lymph nodes. Left scrotum normal, right scrotum painful with inflammatory signs, 2 cm swelling, painful, solid, not adhered to scrotal skin. What is the diagnosis?

Table 2. *Cont.*

Pathology	Clinical Case
Case 18: Duplicated Urethra	47-year-old man reports urinary incontinence, noticed double stream during urination, and frequent urinary infections. What is the possible diagnosis?
Case 19: Penile Sarcoidosis	A healthy man in his forties reports progressive inability to retract the foreskin over the past three weeks, associated with paresthesia in the glans and diffuse abdominal pain. On physical examination, a hardened area is noted on the proximal penile shaft, with multiple palpable nodules. He denies fever, dysuria, hematuria, and alterations in lab and imaging tests. What is the likely diagnosis?
Case 20: Proximal Ureter Rupture from Ureteral Catheterization	76-year-old woman with a history of right-sided abdominal pain, persistent fever, and vomiting for 1 day. He reports onset of symptoms after changing the routine of her long-term Foley catheter. He develops sepsis and acute kidney injury. What is the likely diagnosis?
Case 21: Urethral Diverticulum	23-year-old man with recurrent urinary infections, with dysuria associated with late dribbling, examination after micturition revealed floating penoscrotal pouch collapsing completely the urine output through the urethral meatus. What is the possible diagnosis?
Case 22: Penile Calciphylaxis	54-year-old man presents with penile and scrotal necrosis with a one-month evolution. He reports initial onset of penile pain and darkening of the glans, progressing to the penile shaft and scrotum. He reports a history of diabetes mellitus, hypertension, diabetic retinopathy, and chronic kidney disease on dialysis. What is the likely diagnosis?
Case 23: Hydronephrosis in Pelvic Kidney	18-year-old man with colicky lower abdominal pain and progressive inability to urinate, reaching anuria. He reports strong desire, but little elimination. What is the likely diagnosis?
Case 24: Acute Vasitis	Healthy 27-year-old man presents with left scrotal pain associated with inguinoscrotal swelling and nausea. Physical examination reveals edema extending along the left inguinal area. What is the likely diagnosis?
Case 25: Scrotal Basal Cell Carcinoma	58-year-old man presents with anterior scrotal lesion, 19 mm in its greatest diameter, for eight months. He reports that the lesion initially resembled a "pimple," evolving with erosion and ulceration. He denies associated pruritus and reports a past medical history of condyloma acuminatum, smoking, intravenous drug use, stabilized psoriasis on biologic therapy, and two previously excised basal cell carcinomas on the back. What is the likely diagnosis?
Case 26: Castleman's Disease (Lymphadenopathy) in the scrotum	79-year-old man reports the appearance of a painless mass in the right scrotum with significant growth in the past year. What is the likely diagnosis?
Case 27: Prolapsed Ectopic Ureterocele into the Vulva	12-month-old girl presents with red, smooth, prolapsed vulvar swelling through the urethral orifice. What is the likely diagnosis?
Case 28: Periurethral Abscess of the Corpus Spongiosum	42-year-old man presents with painful, floating, and tender mass in the proximal lower part of the penis, associated with dysuria, with a 20-day evolution. What is the likely diagnosis?
Case 29: Persistent Müllerian Duct Syndrome (PMDS)	38-year-old man was referred to the urology clinic due to left-sided hydronephrosis secondary to an abdominal mass. On physical examination, the patient had a hypoplastic empty scrotum, without palpable testicle and without surgical scars. Imaging exams revealed rudimentary uterus attached to a large mass that is replacing the left testicle. What is the likely diagnosis?
Case 30: Partial Thrombosis of the Corpus Cavernosum	25-year-old man reports pain and swelling in the penis and perineum, with penile sensitivity to touch especially on the left proximal side, and a seven-day evolution. He denies previous trauma. What is the likely diagnosis?

Each clinical case was inputted into Google Search and ChatGPT 3.5, and the results were categorized as "correct diagnosis", "likely differential diagnosis", and "incorrect diagnosis", according to the blind and random judgment of a panel of three experts. For Google Search, a new incognito window in the browser with no linked account was used to minimize any influence from previous search history, and the first three displayed results were considered for diagnostic categorization. For ChatGPT 3.5, a specific individual account was created to reduce the influence of prior searches. Regarding the use of AI or AI-assisted technologies, Google and ChatGPT 3.5 were employed exclusively to evaluate the diagnostic accuracy of each AI platform based on the responses to 60 clinical cases related to urological pathologies.

The findings of this study were described in absolute numbers and corresponding percentages. The Chi-square test was used for proportion comparison, and the Kappa test was employed to assess agreement between the instruments. "All tests are two-tailed, and p values < 0.05 were considered statistically significant". We utilized GraphPad Prism version 10.0.0 for Windows, provided by GraphPad Software from Boston, MA, USA, for the statistical analysis and to create the graphical representations of the data.

3. Results

Both platforms showed promising results when dealing with prevalent urological cases in daily practice. Google Search demonstrated a correct diagnosis, likely differential diagnosis, and incorrect diagnosis in 16 (53.3%), 7 (23.3%), and 7 (23.3%) of the clinical cases. ChatGPT 3.5 outperformed Google, providing a correct diagnosis in 26 (86.6%) cases and offering likely differential diagnoses in 4 (13.3%) cases, with no incorrect diagnoses ($p = 0.004$).

Regarding the unusual urological conditions, the performances of the two platforms significantly diverged. Google could not provide any correct diagnosis but offered likely differential diagnoses in six (20%) cases. Google outputted an incorrect diagnosis in the remaining 24 (80%) cases. Nevertheless, ChatGPT 3.5 had moderate success in diagnosing rare conditions, with a correct diagnosis in five (16.6%) cases. Notably, it provided a likely differential diagnosis in 15 (50%) cases. However, it is important to note that the platform provided an incorrect diagnosis in 10 cases, constituting 33.3% of the instances evaluated ($p = 0.0012$). The results are summarized in Figure 1.

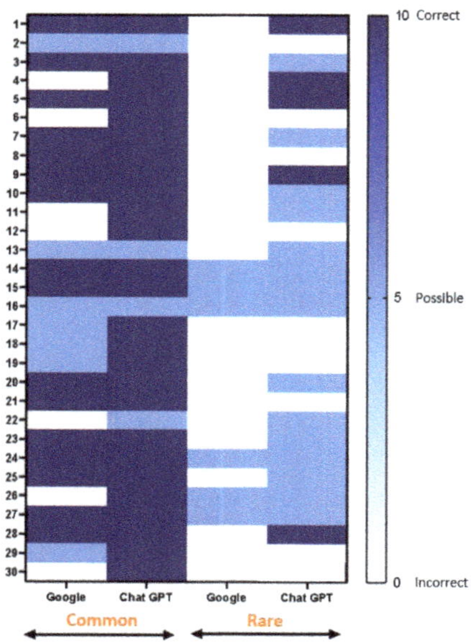

Figure 1. Diagnostic accuracy of Google and ChatGPT for urologic clinical cases. Common cases are represented on the left side, and rare cases are on the right. To determine the diagnostic accuracy of each platform, the outcomes were classified into three categories: correct diagnosis (dark blue), likely differential diagnosis (light blue), and incorrect diagnosis (white).

In a comparative accuracy analysis, ChatGPT 3.5 was significantly superior to Google. The platform provided correct diagnoses or proposed suitable differential diagnoses in 50 (83.3% 71.7–90.80 95%CI) out of 60 cases, in contrast to Google's performance of 29 (48.3% 36.1–60.7 95%CI) out of 60 cases (OR = 3.62 1.50–8.73 95%CI $p < 0.001$). There was low agreement between both diagnostic instruments (Kappa = 0.315).

4. Discussion

This study showed that ChatGPT 3.5 demonstrated superior diagnostic capabilities compared to Google in real-life urological scenarios. Both platforms varied in performance depending on the complexity and rarity of urological conditions. While Google remained moderately effective in prevalent urological cases, its performance reduced significantly in unusual urological conditions. ChatGPT 3.5 showed high diagnostic accuracy in common urological diseases and moderate success in diagnosing rare and uncommon conditions.

In this comparative study, the LLMs demonstrated proficiency in extracting information and responding to structured inquiries, achieving accuracy rates ranging from 53.3% to 86.6%. ChatGPT, in particular, operates by sequentially predicting word fragments until a complete response is formed. Its architecture effectively processes and integrates complex clinical data, yielding contextually relevant interpretations [10]. In contrast, Google often retrieves more generalized information. ChatGPT utilizes a comprehensive, curated medical dataset, including peer-reviewed articles and clinical case studies, which enhances its ability to provide context-aware responses that adhere to contemporary medical standards. This specialized approach contributes to ChatGPT's higher diagnostic accuracy in the nuanced field of urology. While ChatGPT is capable of incremental learning, allowing it to retain information from previous interactions to refine future responses [11], this feature was unlikely to influence the results in this study due to using a specific individual account designed to minimize the impact of prior searches.

The study outcomes corroborate the importance of acknowledging the fluctuating efficacy of these tools across various clinical contexts, highlighting both their advantages and the domains that require enhancement. These findings also raise essential questions about the role of AI-based platforms like ChatGPT 3.5 in clinical decision making and education. The exponential growth in medical knowledge exacerbates the challenges faced by healthcare professionals. Estimates suggest that the rate at which medical knowledge expands has significantly accelerated—from taking 50 years to double in 1950, down to just 73 days in 2020 [12]. These rapid advances mean medical students must master 342 potential diagnoses for 37 frequently presented signs and symptoms before graduating [13]. This amount of information can be overwhelming and underscores the growing need for accurate and more efficient diagnostic tools to assist physicians and other healthcare providers.

Internet search engines such as Google have been around for a while and have progressively been utilized within the healthcare and educational sectors [14,15]. In 1999, Graber and colleagues assessed the capacity of online search engines in resolving medical cases, finding that these platforms could correctly answer half of the questions [14]. By 2006, Google had already become the dominant online search tool, providing correct diagnoses in 58% of cases in Tang and Ng's study [5]. Another study evaluated the diagnostic accuracy of medical students before and after consulting Google and PubMed, noting a not statistically significant but interesting 9.9% increase in diagnostic accuracy [16].

More recently, chatbots, which combine AI with messaging interfaces, have emerged as precise tools for generating direct responses [17,18]. A Japanese study showed that ChatGPT 3 achieved a correct diagnostic rate of 93.3% when considering a list of ten probable differential diagnoses [19]. The same platform demonstrated an accuracy rate of 80% in questions about cirrhosis and hepatocellular carcinoma and an accuracy of 88% in breast cancer prevention and screening [20,21].

In the field of urology, ChatGPT 3.5's performance has been variable. In one study, the platform correctly answered 92% of pediatric urology questions [22]. However, the platform's performance was reduced to 52% in another study on general urological cases [23].

As illustrated by Huynh and colleagues, ChatGPT 3.5 performed poorly in the American Urological Association's 2022 self-assessment study program, scoring below 30% [24]. Studies evaluating the accuracy of information on urological conditions provided to the general public have shown that while the responses were generally acceptable, they also contained significant inaccuracies [25,26].

We are observing the beginning of a new era in the history of medical education. The COVID-19 pandemic rapidly increased the use of new technologies in medical competencies training. This surge in adoption coincides with the release of ChatGPT, which has gained widespread recognition in educational settings by both teachers and students. At the same time, there have been quick policy adjustments regarding AI's role in writing and academic publishing [27]. Educational leaders now face the crucial task of understanding the extensive impact of these changes across all aspects of health education and ethical dilemmas [9].

The current study provides valuable insights into existing research by directly comparing the diagnostic effectiveness of Google and ChatGPT 3.5 for urological conditions. Our results indicate that ChatGPT 3.5 outperformed Google in common and rare cases. While the platform showed high precision in diagnosing common urological conditions, it demonstrated moderate success with rarer diseases. These findings offer a promising perspective for integrating such tools in medical education and clinical workflows.

These platforms can assist urological researchers in analyzing and interpreting data, improving grammar and clarity in scientific manuscripts, and creating educational material. The role of these tools should be viewed as supplemental to the expertise of doctors and healthcare professionals providing patient care. Given the identified limitations, it is evident that both platforms require improvements. The ongoing process of expanding access to medical databases and continuous algorithmic training will increase its future utility. Ethical considerations cannot be overlooked either. There must be extensive discussion about the quality of information these platforms provide and how user privacy is ensured, as sensitive data may be involved. As these platforms evolve, their utility as diagnostic tools may become more robust, promoting more innovative and secure healthcare applications.

Currently, LLMs face significant limitations in medical decision making and diagnostics, including a lack of access to copyrighted private databases, a propensity for generating inaccurate or fabricated information ("hallucinations"), the unpredictability of responses, and constraints on training datasets [10]. The choice of cases included in this study could influence outcomes if they are not representative of the typical spectrum of urological conditions seen in clinical practice. Both platforms' performance can vary significantly based on how questions are phrased. A study's reliability may be affected if the prompts do not accurately reflect typical user queries or clinical scenarios. Both ChatGPT and Google continually update their algorithms. The results might not reflect the performance of newer or updated versions of the models. Finally, the diagnosis categories were determined by a panel of experts whose judgments could introduce subjective bias. The criteria for categorization (correct diagnosis, likely differential diagnosis, incorrect diagnosis) may not be uniformly applied.

Despite these challenges, the future of LLMs in medical diagnostics looks promising due to rapid advancements in artificial intelligence and machine learning algorithms. These models are becoming more proficient at processing the extensive medical literature and patient data, continually improving their diagnostic algorithms. The inclusion of specialized datasets, such as those covering rare diseases or intricate clinical scenarios, enhances their accuracy and relevance in medical settings. As training becomes more comprehensive and detailed, LLMs' capacity to deliver precise, contextually appropriate medical advice is expected to evolve, significantly enhancing clinical decision support and revolutionizing patient care outcomes. This research paves the way for further research on integrating AI-based tools such as ChatGPT into clinical practice. This approach aims for a quick, reliable diagnosis and potentially enhances patient outcomes while augmenting human expertise.

Our study contributes to a broader discussion about the evolving role of technology in healthcare, specifically in urology, where accurate and timely diagnosis is often critical to treatment success and patient well-being.

5. Conclusions

We demonstrated that ChatGPT 3.5 exhibited superior diagnostic accuracy compared to Google in prevalent and rare urological scenarios. ChatGPT 3.5 displayed acceptable accuracy in cases of habitual conditions but was still relatively limited in rare cases. Such findings allow us to glimpse some of the possible uses of these tools in educational and training processes. Access to medical databases and ongoing development can bring considerable advances, enabling even more robust, innovative, and secure tools and possibly assisting us in caring for people.

Author Contributions: G.R.G., C.M.G. and J.B.J. designed the study. G.R.G. and J.B.J. performed the data acquisition. G.R.G., C.M.G. and J.B.J. analyzed and interpreted data and statistics; G.R.G., C.S.S., R.G.F., V.A., R.B.T., J.C.Z.C., C.M.G. and J.B.J. interpreted the results and wrote the manuscript. All authors have read and agreed to the published version of the manuscript.

Funding: This research received no external funding.

Institutional Review Board Statement: Not applicable.

Informed Consent Statement: Not applicable.

Data Availability Statement: Additional data will be available upon request.

Acknowledgments: In this manuscript, we utilized Grammarly AI software (https://www.grammarly.com/ai) to enhance the grammatical quality. The authors developed the manuscript's content independently with the assistance of AI software. The authors thank the Uros—Grupo de Pesquisa, a collaborative research group at Medical School—Universidade Estadual de Feira de Santana (UEFS), for supporting this research. Uros—Grupo de Pesquisa: Ana Clara Silva Oliveira, Anna Paloma Martins Rocha Ribeiro, Ana Samiry da Silva Gomes, Caíque Negreiros Lacerda, Daniela Azevedo da Silva, Fernanda Santos da Anunciação, Isa Clara Santos Lima, Jair Bomfim Santos, Lucas Neves de Oliveira, Lucas Santos Silva, Matheus Maciel Pauferro, Marjory dos Santos Passos, Monique Tonani Novaes, Nathália Muraivieviechi Passos, Randson Souza Rosa, Rodolfo Macedo Cruz Pimenta, Seeley Joseph Machado Monteiro, Taciana Leonel Nunes Tiraboschi, Thifany Novais de Paula, Tyson Andrade Miranda, Virna Silva Mascarenhas, Williane Thamires dos Santos.

Conflicts of Interest: The authors declare no conflicts of interest.

References

1. Mahoney, M.S. The History of Computing in the History of Technology. *Ann. Hist. Comput.* **1988**, *10*, 113–125. [CrossRef]
2. Brodman, K.; Van Woerkom, A.J.; Erdmann, A.J.; Goldstein, L.S. Interpretation of Symptoms with a Data-Processing Machine. *Arch. Intern. Med.* **1959**, *103*, 782. [CrossRef]
3. Haug, C.J.; Drazen, J.M. Artificial Intelligence and Machine Learning in Clinical Medicine. *N. Engl. J. Med.* **2023**, *388*, 1201–1208. [CrossRef]
4. Al-Antari, M.A. Artificial Intelligence for Medical Diagnostics—Existing and Future AI Technology! *Diagnostics* **2023**, *13*, 688. [CrossRef]
5. Tang, H.; Ng, J.H.K. Googling for a diagnosis—Use of Google as a diagnostic aid: Internet based study. *Br. Med. J.* **2006**, *333*, 1143–1145. [CrossRef]
6. Gupta, R.; Pedraza, A.M.; Gorin, M.A.; Tewari, A.K. Defining the Role of Large Language Models in Urologic Care and Research. *Eur. Urol. Oncol.* **2023**, *7*, 1–13. [CrossRef]
7. Drazen, J.M.; Kohane, I.S.; Leong, T.-Y.; Lee, P.; Bubeck, S.; Petro, J. Chatbot for Medicine. *N. Engl. J. Med.* **2023**, *388*, 1220–1221.
8. Reis, L.O. ChatGPT for medical applications and urological science. *Int. Braz. J. Urol.* **2023**, *49*, 652–656. [CrossRef]
9. Jacobs, S.M.; Lundy, N.N.; Issenberg, S.B.; Chandran, L. Reimagining Core Entrustable Professional Activities for Undergraduate Medical Education in the Era of Artificial Intelligence. *JMIR Med. Educ.* **2023**, *9*, e50903. [CrossRef] [PubMed]
10. Park, Y.J.; Pillai, A.; Deng, J.; Guo, E.; Gupta, M.; Paget, M.; Naugler, C. Assessing the research landscape and clinical utility of large language models: A scoping review. *BMC Med. Inform. Decis. Mak.* **2024**, *24*, 72. [CrossRef] [PubMed]
11. OpenAI. Introducing ChatGPT [Internet]. Available online: https://openai.com/blog/chatgpt (accessed on 13 April 2024).
12. Densen, P. Challenges and opportunities facing medical education. *Trans. Am. Clin. Climatol. Assoc.* **2011**, *122*, 48–58.

13. Urushibara-Miyachi, Y.; Kikukawa, M.; Ikusaka, M.; Otaki, J.; Nishigori, H. Lists of potential diagnoses that final-year medical students need to consider: A modified Delphi study. *BMC Med. Educ.* **2021**, *21*, 234. [CrossRef]
14. Graber, M.A.; Bergus, G.R.; York, C. Using the World Wide Web to Answer Clinical Questions: How Efficient Are Different Methods of Information Retrieval? *J. Fam. Pract.* **1999**, *49*, 520–524.
15. Giustini, D. How Google is changing medicine. *Br. Med. J.* **2005**, *331*, 1487–1488. [CrossRef] [PubMed]
16. Falagas, M.E.; Ntziora, F.; Makris, G.C.; Malietzis, G.A.; Rafailidis, P.I. Do PubMed and Google searches help medical students and young doctors reach the correct diagnosis? A pilot study. *Eur. J. Intern. Med.* **2009**, *20*, 788–790. [CrossRef]
17. Adamopoulou, E.; Moussiades, L. Chatbots: History, technology, and applications. *Mach. Learn. Appl.* **2020**, *2*, 100006. [CrossRef]
18. Laranjo, L.; Dunn, A.G.; Tong, H.L.; Kocaballi, A.B.; Chen, J.; Bashir, R.; Surian, D.; Gallego, B.; Magrabi, F.; Lau, A.Y.S.; et al. Conversational agents in healthcare: A systematic review. *J. Am. Med. Inform. Assoc.* **2018**, *25*, 1248–1258. [CrossRef]
19. Hirosawa, T.; Harada, Y.; Yokose, M.; Sakamoto, T.; Kawamura, R.; Shimizu, T. Diagnostic Accuracy of Differential-Diagnosis Lists Generated by Generative Pretrained Transformer 3 Chatbot for Clinical Vignettes with Common Chief Complaints: A Pilot Study. *Int. J. Environ. Res. Public. Health* **2023**, *20*, 3378. [CrossRef] [PubMed]
20. Yeo, Y.H.; Samaan, J.S.; Ng, W.H.; Ting, P.-S.; Trivedi, H.; Vipani, A.; Ayoub, W.; Yang, J.D.; Liran, O.; Spiegel, B.; et al. Assessing the performance of ChatGPT in answering questions regarding cirrhosis and hepatocellular carcinoma. *Clin. Mol. Hepatol.* **2023**, *29*, 721–732. [CrossRef]
21. Haver, H.L.; Ambinder, E.B.; Bahl, M.; Oluyemi, E.T.; Jeudy, J.; Yi, P.H. Appropriateness of Breast Cancer Prevention and Screening Recommendations Provided by ChatGPT. *Radiology* **2023**, *307*, e230424. [CrossRef]
22. Caglar, U.; Yildiz, O.; Meric, A.; Ayranci, A.; Gelmis, M.; Sarilar, O.; Ozgor, F. Evaluating the performance of ChatGPT in answering questions related to pediatric urology. *J. Pediatr. Urol.* **2023**, *20*, 26.e1–26.e5. [CrossRef] [PubMed]
23. Cocci, A.; Pezzoli, M.; Lo Re, M.; Russo, G.I.; Asmundo, M.G.; Fode, M.; Cacciamani, G.; Cimino, S.; Minervini, A.; Durukan, E. Quality of information and appropriateness of ChatGPT outputs for urology patients. *Prostate Cancer Prostatic Dis.* **2023**, *27*, 103–108. [CrossRef]
24. Huynh, L.M.; Bonebrake, B.T.; Schultis, K.; Quach, A.; Deibert, C.M. New Artificial Intelligence ChatGPT Performs Poorly on the 2022 Self-assessment Study Program for Urology. *Urol. Pract.* **2023**, *10*, 409–415. [CrossRef] [PubMed]
25. Szczesniewski, J.J.; Tellez Fouz, C.; Ramos Alba, A.; Diaz Goizueta, F.J.; García Tello, A.; Llanes González, L. ChatGPT and most frequent urological diseases: Analysing the quality of information and potential risks for patients. *World J. Urol.* **2023**, *41*, 3149–3153. [CrossRef] [PubMed]
26. Whiles, B.B.; Bird, V.G.; Canales, B.K.; DiBianco, J.M.; Terry, R.S. Caution! AI Bot Has Entered the Patient Chat: ChatGPT Has Limitations in Providing Accurate Urologic Healthcare Advice. *Urology* **2023**, *180*, 278–284. [CrossRef]
27. Kantor, J. Best practices for implementing ChatGPT, large language models, and artificial intelligence in qualitative and survey-based research. *JAAD Int.* **2023**, *14*, 22–23. [CrossRef]

Journal of
Clinical Medicine

MDPI

Article

A Novel Method for Determining Fibrin/Fibrinogen Degradation Products and Fibrinogen Threshold Criteria via Artificial Intelligence in Massive Hemorrhage during Delivery with Hematuria

Yasunari Miyagi [1,2,3,*], Katsuhiko Tada [3], Ichiro Yasuhi [4], Keisuke Tsumura [5], Yuka Maegawa [6], Norifumi Tanaka [7], Tomoya Mizunoe [8], Ikuko Emoto [9], Kazuhisa Maeda [10], Kosuke Kawakami [11] and on behalf of the Collaborative Research in National Hospital Organization Network Pediatric and Perinatal Group [†]

1 Medical Data Labo, 289-48 Yamasaki, Naka Ward, Okayama 703-8267, Japan
2 Miyake Ofuku Clinic, 393-1 Ofuku, Minami Ward, Okayama 701-0204, Japan
3 Department of Obstetrics and Gynecology, NHO Okayama Medical Center, 1711-1 Tamasu, Kita Ward, Okayama 701-1192, Japan; ktada1221@gmail.com
4 Department of Obstetrics and Gynecology, NHO Nagasaki Medical Center, 2-1001-1 Kubara, Omura 856-8562, Japan; iyasuhi0414@gmail.com
5 Department of Obstetrics and Gynecology, NHO Saga Hospital, 1-20-1 Hinode, Saga 849-8577, Japan; tmrksk.obgy@gmail.com
6 Department of Obstetrics and Gynecology, NHO Mie Chuo Medical Center, 2158-5 Hisaimyojincho, Tsu 514-1101, Japan; yuka.ma0513@gmail.com
7 Department of Obstetrics and Gynecology, NHO Higashihiroshima Medical Center, 513 Saijochojike, Higashihiroshima 739-0041, Japan; tanaka.norifumi.an@mail.hosp.go.jp
8 Department of Obstetrics and Gynecology, NHO Kure Medical Center, 3-1 Aoyama, Kure 737-0023, Japan; mizunoe.tomoya.fd@mail.hosp.go.jp
9 Department of Obstetrics and Gynecology, NHO Kyoto Medical Center, 1-1 Fukasakumukaihata, Kyoto 612-8555, Japan; emoto.ikuko.yh@mail.hosp.go.jp
10 Department of Obstetrics and Gynecology, NHO Shikoku Medical Center for Children and Adults, 2-1-1 Senyucho, Zentsuji 765-8507, Japan; maeda.kazuhisa.hf@mail.hosp.go.jp
11 Department of Obstetrics and Gynecology, NHO Kokura Medical Center, 10-1 Harugaoka, Kokuraminami Ward, Kitakyushu 802-8533, Japan; kawakami.kosuke.ed@mail.hosp.go.jp
* Correspondence: ymiyagi@mac.com
† All members of the Collaborative Research in National Hospital Organization Network Pediatric and Perinatal Group are listed in the acknowledgments.

Abstract: (1) Background: Although the diagnostic criteria for massive hemorrhage with organ dysfunction, such as disseminated intravascular coagulation associated with delivery, have been empirically established based on clinical findings, strict logic has yet to be used to establish numerical criteria. **(2) Methods:** A dataset of 107 deliveries with >2000 mL of blood loss, among 13,368 deliveries, was obtained from nine national perinatal centers in Japan between 2020 and 2023. Twenty-three patients had fibrinogen levels <170 mg/dL, which is the initiation of coagulation system failure, according to our previous reports. Three of these patients had hematuria. We used six machine learning methods to identify the borderline criteria dividing the fibrinogen/fibrin/fibrinogen degradation product (FDP) planes, using 15 coagulation fibrinolytic factors. **(3) Results:** The boundaries of hematuria development on a two-dimensional plane of fibrinogen and FDP were obtained. A positive FDP–fibrinogen/3–60 (mg/dL) value indicates hematuria; otherwise, the case is nonhematuria, as demonstrated by the support vector machine method that seemed the most appropriate. **(4) Conclusions:** Using artificial intelligence, the borderline criterion was obtained, which divides the fibrinogen/FDP plane for patients with hematuria that could be considered organ dysfunction in massive hemorrhage during delivery; this method appears to be useful.

Keywords: artificial intelligence; delivery; DIC; hemorrhage; machine learning

1. Introduction

Massive hemorrhage continues to be one of the most severe complications for pregnant women. Massive hemorrhage during delivery can be classified into consumption coagulopathy with coagulation abnormalities, such as disseminated intravascular coagulation (DIC) resulting from abruptio placentae, and dilutional coagulopathy without coagulation abnormalities, such as atonic bleeding [1]. DIC is a systemic disease affecting the coagulation system, simultaneously causing procoagulant factor activation, fibrinolytic activation, and consumptive coagulopathy, which can ultimately lead to organ dysfunction and death [2]. As DIC is a cause of maternal mortality, the pathogenesis of the disease needs to be understood. DIC should be appropriately diagnosed because massive hemorrhage during delivery due to consumption coagulopathy may require treatment for correction of coagulation abnormalities. DIC during pregnancy is one of the chief causes of maternal mortality worldwide [3,4], with a frequency of 0.03% [5] to 0.35% [6]. DIC can originate from and cause damage to the microvasculature; this, if sufficiently severe, can lead to organ dysfunction [7]. However, although the numerical diagnostic criteria for DIC associated with delivery have been empirically established based on clinical findings such as the presence or absence of organ dysfunction and laboratory findings of coagulation and fibrinolysis factors, strict logic has yet to be used to establish numerical criteria.

Fibrin/fibrinogen degradation products (FDPs) represent a key factor concerning DIC. An excessive FDP level with diminished or normal systemic fibrinolytic activity suggests that local intravascular fibrin deposition and fibrinolysis occur in normal parturition and bleeding complications in pregnancy [8]. We previously reported the criterion values for coagulation and fibrinolytic system collapse based on FDPs, focusing on the fibrinogen behavior, using mathematical methods such as data distribution function evaluation and differential equations, in massive hemorrhage during delivery without organ dysfunction [9]. When the fibrinogen level fell below 237 mg/dL, the FDP distribution became abnormal, which began the abnormal coagulation/fibrinolysis system. When the fibrinogen level fell below 170 mg/dL, the coagulation/fibrinolysis system failed ($p < 0.05$). The borderline FDP value in organ dysfunction cases was expected to be higher. This classification showed good agreement with the clinical status [10].

Artificial intelligence (AI) has recently become a more common and easily applied tool in medical science. Some AI applications involve medical imaging [11–15], though some do not [16–19]. Machine learning is part of the concept of AI and can be used to acquire rules for judging unknown data by learning the latent patterns in the data. Machine learning enables the learning and classification of observed data. An optimal method can be chosen from among various machine learning algorithms. Machine learning can be used to computationally classify data, thereby determining the data boundaries.

This was a retrospective study in which we collected cases of massive hemorrhage during delivery with hematuria that could be assumed to be organ dysfunction, and we developed a method to mathematically determine the FDP boundaries for hematuria.

We used the method to analyze 15 coagulation/fibrinolysis-related factors, selecting factors that correlate with fibrinogen and FDP, facilitate rapid clinical results, and prevent multicollinearity with each other. Then, after performing supervised learning using machine learning, we determined the criterion line dividing the plane of fibrinogen and FDP. We used the same selected factors to create a discriminant analysis function [20] to obtain the boundaries, which we compared with the boundaries created by machine learning.

2. Materials and Methods

This multicenter retrospective case series study, including human subjects, was approved by the National Hospital Organization (NHO) Central Research Ethics Committee (R1-1009002). The participants were women who gave birth at any of the nine NHO perinatal centers (NHO Okayama Medical Center, NHO Saga Hospital, NHO Nagasaki Medical Center, NHO Mie Chuo Medical Center, NHO Higashihiroshima Medical Center, NHO Kure Medical Center, NHO Kyoto Medical Center, NHO Shikoku Medical Center for Children and Adults, and NHO Kokura Medical Center) in Japan between August 2020 and September 2023. The inclusion criteria for the study were as follows: (1) women with >2000 mL of blood loss within 24 h of delivery; (2) any mode of delivery, either vaginal or cesarean; (2) singleton or multiple pregnancies; and (3) delivery after 22 weeks of gestation. The rationale for inclusion criteria (1) and (2) was as follows: coagulopathy rarely develops when blood loss is ≤2000 mL [21]. Furthermore, women who had bleeding of > 2000 mL at delivery, regardless of mode of delivery, are defined by the Royal College of Obstetrics and Gynaecologists as having severe PPH [22]. The exclusion criteria included (1) women with medical complications that could cause coagulopathy and (2) women taking aspirin or other medications that affect the coagulation system.

Blood loss was evaluated using different methods. During vaginal delivery, blood loss was weighed by subtracting the dry weight of the absorbent pad from the weight of the blood-soaked pad and/or from direct blood collection. All blood lost was contained in a collector bag, which was placed under the woman's buttocks. During cesarean delivery, dry and blood-soaked surgical pads were weighed before and after surgery, and/or blood volume aspirated from the surgical field with a suction tube was determined in milliliters. The units of measured blood loss were standardized to milliliters, as grams are known to be almost equivalent to milliliters in weight.

The attending physicians obtained blood samples when deemed clinically necessary, regardless of blood loss. Activated partial thromboplastin time (APTT), D-dimer, FDP, fibrinogen, hematocrit (Hct), hemoglobin (Hgb), platelet (Plt), prothrombin time (PT-sec) [6], and prothrombin time-international normalized ratio (PT-INR) were measured in each center's laboratory for clinical management. Antiplasmin (AP), antithrombin (AT), fibrin monomer complex (FMC), α2 plasmin inhibitor plasmin complex (PIC) [23], and thrombin antithrombin complex (TAT) [23] levels were also measured in the laboratories of SRL INC. (Tokyo, Japan) for this study. These 14 blood test indicators analyzed in the study were used as factors for the complete data. We used fully deidentified data in this study.

Obstetric management, blood product transfusion, and determining the cause of bleeding were performed at the attending physicians' discretion at each center. All nine centers participating in the study were perinatal centers in Japan, which routinely managed high-risk pregnancies, including those with severe PPH, which would have allowed for management without substantial differences. Data from the first measurement for each patient were used for analysis.

All procedures were performed in accordance with the ethical standards of the committees responsible for human experimentation (institutional and national) and the Declaration of Helsinki of 1964 and its later amendments. Written informed consent was obtained from all patients for whom identifying information is included in this article.

Based on the results of our previous study [9], we used data for fibrinogen <170 mg/dL only, which was a criterion for coagulation system failure. In this study, we defined the appearance of hematuria as organ dysfunction [24].

Let the set of factors of the complete data obtained be $\{\alpha, \beta, \gamma, \ldots\}$. Let $\{\alpha, \beta, \gamma, \ldots\}$ be the set of factors of the complete data obtained. Let A and B be the sets of factors significantly related to element α and another element β, respectively. A contribution rate > 0.49 is used as the criterion. The elements of the $A \cup B$ set are classified into the following sets: P, Q, and R.

$$P = \{x | x \in A, x \notin B, x \notin \Phi\} \quad (1)$$

$$Q = \{y | y \notin A, y \in B, y \notin \Phi\} \quad (2)$$

$$R = \{z | z \in A, z \in B, z \notin \Phi\} \quad (3)$$

where $cr(v, w)$ is the contribution rate between v and w. Then,

$$cr(x_s, x_t) < CR;\ s \neq t,\ \forall x_s \in P,\ \forall x_t \in P \quad (4)$$

$$cr(y_s, y_t) < CR;\ s \neq t,\ \forall y_s \in Q,\ \forall y_t \in Q \quad (5)$$

$$cr(z_s, z_t) < CR;\ s \neq t,\ \forall z_s \in R,\ \forall z_t \in R \quad (6)$$

Here, $CR = 0.64$. When $N(P)$, $N(Q)$, and $N(R)$ are the number of elements in P, Q, and R, respectively, we have the following vectors:

$$\alpha,\ \beta,\ x_1,\ x_2, \ldots, x_{N(P)},\ y_1,\ y_2, \ldots, y_{N(Q)},\ z_1,\ z_2, \ldots, z_{N(R)} \quad (7)$$

The classifiers were created by labeling cases with and without organ dysfunction and performing supervised machine learning. As machine learning methods, we used logistic regression, which is a widely used method for predicting binary outcomes and can be used for multiple outcomes [25,26]; random forest, which is a popular supervised method in which an ensemble approach is employed by combining multiple decision trees through the bagging technique to increase the accuracy and robustness of the model [26,27]; nearest neighbors, which is a nonparametric supervised learning method that produces the output classified by a plurality vote of its neighbors, with the object being assigned to the class most common among its nearest neighbors [28,29]; naïve Bayes, which is optimal when attributes are independent given the class [30,31]; neural network, which is a branch of machine learning models inspired by the neuronal organization found in the biological neural networks in animal brains [32,33]; and support vector machine, which is a machine learning algorithm that can be used for both linear and nonlinear classification tasks and constructing hyperplanes in a high dimensional space [26,34].

When the regression functions are f, g, and h,

$$\widetilde{x}_i = f_i(\alpha);\ i = \{1,\ 2,\ \ldots,\ N(P)\} \quad (8)$$

$$\widetilde{y}_j = g_j(\beta);\ j = \{1,\ 2,\ \ldots,\ N(Q)\} \quad (9)$$

$$\widetilde{z}_k = h_k(\alpha, \beta);\ k = \{1,\ 2,\ \ldots,\ N(R)\} \quad (10)$$

$$\alpha,\ \beta,\ \widetilde{x}_1,\ \widetilde{x}_2, \ldots, \widetilde{x}_{N(P)},\ \widetilde{y}_1,\ \widetilde{y}_2, \ldots, \widetilde{y}_{N(Q)},\ \widetilde{z}_1,\ \widetilde{z}_2, \ldots, \widetilde{z}_{N(R)} \quad (11)$$

This vector was substituted into the classifier to obtain the classification in $\{\alpha, \beta\}$. In this study, α and β were calculated as fibrinogen and FDP, respectively. Next, a discriminant analysis was performed using this vector. Then, a single regression function $\widetilde{\alpha} = f(\beta)$ was obtained using the same method, with fibrinogen as the dependent variable and FDP as the independent variable. The organ dysfunction criterion values for FDP alone were then determined.

We examined the performance of each machine learning method, and we comprehensively determined the optimal boundary criterion.

Development environment for analysis and statistics:

The computing environment comprised a Mac Pro running OS X 13.1 (Apple Inc.; Cupertino, CA, USA) and Mathematica 13.0 (Wolfram Research; Champaign, IL, USA). The data distribution analysis, discriminant analysis, linear regression analysis, machine learning, Mann–Whitney test, and t-test were conducted with this setup.

3. Results

During the study period, 322 women fulfilled the inclusion criteria from among 13,368 deliveries at all participating centers. Of these women, 190 were unable to send blood samples to SRL INC. For the study, 132 were enrolled, and 25 were excluded because some required data were missing. In this study's final sample of 107 women, 14 (13%) had already been administered red blood cell concentrate (RCC) and/or fresh–frozen plasma (FFP) (8 of both, 5 of RCC only, and 1 of FFP only) at the time of first blood sampling. Of the 107 women, 23 had a fibrinogen level < 170 mg/dL, and 8 (35%) were administered RCC and/or FFP (7 of both and 1 of FFP only). In 23 of the women with a fibrinogen level < 170 mg/dL, 3 were classified as organ dysfunction cases because they had hematuria corresponding to marked activation of the coagulation–fibrinolytic system, whereas the remaining 20 women were non-organ-dysfunction cases. The 15 factors, that is, the 14 blood test parameters described in the Methods section plus the Hgb/fibrinogen ratio, were obtained as factors for the complete data. Among these 15 factors, those with a significant difference between patients with and without organ dysfunction were FDP, D-dimer, TAT, Hgb/fibrinogen, fibrinogen, PT-sec, and PT-INR in the *t*-test, and FDP, D-dimer, TAT, Hgb/fibrinogen, fibrinogen, PT-INR, PT-sec, and PIC in the Mann–Whitney test in descending order of *p*-value from the *t*-test (Table 1). In both tests, FDP was the most statistically significantly different.

Among the 13 factors other than fibrinogen and FDP, Hgb/fibrinogen, PT-sec, and PT-INR strongly correlated with fibrinogen, whereas D-dimer and PIC strongly correlated with FDP. To avoid multicollinearity, regression functions were created to obtain Hgb/fibrinogen and PT-sec from fibrinogen and D-dimer from FDP (Table 2).

Figure 1 shows the hematuria boundaries that, based on machine learning, were recognized as organ dysfunction in massive hemorrhage during delivery. In a previous study [9], the reference values for fibrinogen were 237 and 170 mg/dL for the onset and breakdown of coagulopathy, respectively. Machine learning was used to perform supervised learning on cases with fibrinogen levels < 170 mg/dL. The patient was considered to have hematuria if the estimated probability of developing hematuria by each machine learning method was >0.5. The crude areas where organ dysfunction occurs were as follows for the different models: logistic regression: FDP > 75 mg/dL; naïve Bayes: fibrinogen < 100 mg/dL and FDP > 30 mg/dL; nearest neighbors: fibrinogen < 120 mg/dL and FDP > 80 mg/dL; neural network: FDP > 50 mg/dL; random forest: fibrinogen < 150 mg/dL and FDP > 40 mg/dL. For the support vector machine, a positive FDP–fibrinogen/3–60 (mg/dL) value indicates hematuria; otherwise, the case is nonhematuria because FDP decreases from 100 to 60 mg/dL as the fibrinogen level decreases from 120 to 0 mg/dL.

In Figure 1 (left), for each method, the black areas indicate areas of organ dysfunction. The green, yellow, red, and black dots indicate cases without coagulopathy, with coagulopathy, with disrupted coagulopathy, and with organ dysfunction, respectively. In our previous study, we used fibrinogen criteria values of 237 and 170 mg/dL for the development and disruption of coagulopathy, respectively [9]. The machine learning classifier was trained on red and black cases with fibrinogen levels < 170 mg/dL. The crude areas where organ dysfunction occurred for each method were as follows: logistic regression, FDP > 75 mg/dL; naïve Bayes, fibrinogen < 100 mg/dL and FDP > 30 mg/dL; nearest neighbors, fibrinogen < 120 mg/dL and FDP > 80 mg/dL; neural network, FDP > 50 mg/dL; random forest, fibrinogen < 150 mg/dL and FDP > 40 mg/dL. For the support vector machine, FDP–fibrinogen/3–60 (mg/dL) is positive because FDP decreases from 100 to 60 mg/dL as the fibrinogen level decreases from 120 to 0 mg/dL.

In the contour graph in Figure 1 (right) for each method, as shown in the legend bar, the darker the color, the higher the probability of hematuria. If the estimated probability of developing hematuria was >0.5, the patient was considered to have hematuria in the left figure. As coagulopathy is generally accompanied by a fibrinogen decrease and an FDP increase, support vector machines, neural networks, and naïve Bayes, the contour lines of which change stepwise, seemed to be good fits.

The boundary determined using the support vector machine method that does not include the fibrinogen 170 mg boundary seemed most appropriate for clinical use.

Table 3 shows the classification performance on the boundaries in the fibrinogen and FDP planes of hematuria occurrence by the different machine learning methods. All methods were highly accurate (>0.91). The area under the characteristic curve (AUC) was high for all methods (>0.95). Class mean class entropy [35,36] was smaller for the logistic regression, naïve Bayes, and neural network methods.

Table 1. Comparison of factors for organ- and non-organ-dysfunction cases in data with fibrinogen <170 mg/dL. Factors are listed in order of decreasing p-value on t-test.

	Organ Dysfunction (Hematuria)						Non-Organ Dysfunction						t-Test	Mann–Whitney Test
Factor	Mean ± SD	Min	Max	Median	0.25 Quantile	0.75 Quantile	Mean ± SD	Min	Max	Median	0.25 Quantile	0.75 Quantile	p-Value	p-Value
FDP	95.58 ± 0.73	94.73	96	96	94.73	96	17.52 ± 16.8	0.72	61.64	17.31	3.01	24.16	1.03×10^{-7}	0.0053
DD	350.63 ± 189.25	135.4	491	425.5	135.4	491	47.77 ± 54.65	3	219	34.05	10.61	47.9	3.32×10^{-6}	0.0092
TAT	120 ± 0.0	120	120	120	120	120	67.53 ± 42.88	15.4	120	63.25	19.9	113	2.80×10^{-5}	0.0319
Hgb/fbg	139.08 ± 73.17	56.96	197.37	162.9	56.96	197.37	61.42 ± 24.9	30.18	112	53.96	42.64	66.67	0.0009	0.0399
fbg	59.67 ± 20.6	38	79	62	38	79	122.82 ± 34.2	50	169	127.5	103	143.8	0.0057	0.0198
PT-sec	17.3 ± 2.14	15.6	19.7	16.6	15.6	19.7	13.62 ± 2.24	10.1	18.2	13.2	12	14.4	0.0145	0.0318
PT-INR	1.61 ± 0.2	1.46	1.84	1.53	1.46	1.84	1.22 ± 0.25	0.96	2	1.11	1.06	1.22	0.0174	0.0317
PIC	38.13 ± 26.67	17.7	68.3	28.4	17.7	68.3	8.87 ± 8.02	0.3	27.3	6.45	2	14.6	0.1962	0.0121
AP	45.33 ± 11.93	32	55	49	32	55	53.7 ± 14.28	34	93	52.5	42	56	0.3479	0.4107
AT	52.67 ± 19.01	34	72	52	34	72	45.2 ± 13.15	27	82	43	39	49	0.3925	0.4364
APTT	54.3 ± 19.54	39.3	76.4	47.2	39.3	76.4	46.28 ± 17.05	29.7	93.6	40.65	32.5	51.8	0.4624	0.3858
FMC	166.33 ± 121.48	27	250	222	27	250	184.12 ± 83.87	19.2	250	250	124	250	0.7477	0.6223
Hgb	7.37 ± 2.8	4.5	10.1	7.5	4.5	10.1	6.82 ± 1.26	5	10.2	6.85	5.6	7.3	0.7692	0.6809
Plt	105.33 ± 34.95	76	144	96	76	144	99.65 ± 33.7	39	183	88	78	119	0.7887	0.8190
Hct	21.8 ± 8.02	13.5	29.5	22.4	13.5	29.5	20.78 ± 3.74	15	30.6	20.7	17.3	22.5	0.8473	0.7492

AP—antiplasmin; APTT—activated partial thromboplastin time; AT—antithrombin; DD—D-dimer; fbg—fibrinogen; FDP—fibrin/fibrinogen degradation product; FMC—fibrin monomer complex; Hgb—hemoglobin; Hct—hematocrit; PIC—α_2 plasmin inhibitor/plasmin complex; Plt—platelet; PT—prothrombin time; PT-INR—prothrombin time–international normalized ratio; SD—standard deviation; TAT—thrombin antithrombin III complex.

Table 2. Regression functions from fibrinogen to Hgb/fbg and PT-sec and from fibrin/fibrinogen degradation products to D-dimer while avoiding multicollinearity.

Formula	Estimate ± SE	p-Value	AIC	R-Squared
Hgb/fbg = $\beta_0 + \beta_1$ fbg	β_0, 174.41 ± 15.277; β_1, −0.898 ± 0.126	β_0, 1.81×10^{-10}; β_1, 5.31×10^{-7}	213.79	0.7057
PT-sec = $\beta_0 + \beta_1$ fbg	β_0, 19.681 ± 1.118; β_1, −0.048 ± 0.009	β_0, 4.80×10^{-14}; β_1, 3.30×10^{-5}	93.54	0.5679
D-dimer = $\beta_0 + \beta_1$ FDP	β_0, −9.535 ± 20.235; β_1, 3.4946 ± 0.492	β_0, 0.642; β_1; 5.24×10^{-7}	265.83	0.7061

AIC—Akaike's information criterion; fbg—fibrinogen; FDP—fibrin/fibrinogen degradation product; Hgb—hemoglobin; PT—prothrombin time; SE—standard error.

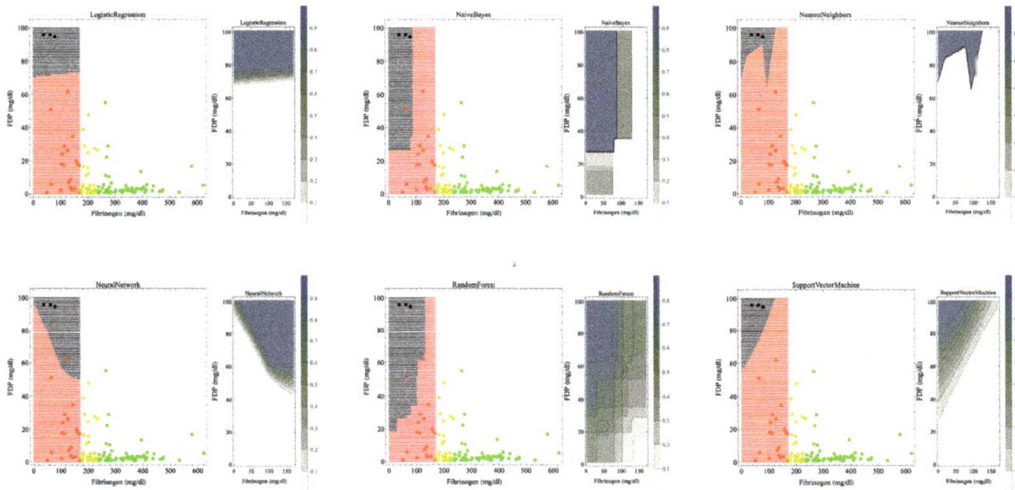

Figure 1. Boundary of hematuria occurrence in heavy bleeding during delivery determined using machine learning, i.e., the boundary of organ dysfunction occurrence. The results of each machine learning method are shown in two sets of figures. The left figure of the set shows the scatterplot of the data and the boundaries of the hematuria occurrence. The black areas indicate areas of organ dysfunction. The green, yellow, red, and black dots indicate cases without coagulopathy, with coagulopathy, with disrupted coagulopathy, and with organ dysfunction, respectively. In our previous study, we used fibrinogen criteria values of 237 and 170 mg/dL for the development and disruption of coagulopathy, respectively [9]. The machine learning classifier was trained on red and black cases with fibrinogen levels < 170 mg/dL. The crude areas where organ dysfunction occurred for each method were as follows: logistic regression, FDP > 75 mg/dL; naïve Bayes, fibrinogen < 100 mg/dL and FDP > 30 mg/dL; nearest neighbors, fibrinogen < 120 mg/dL and FDP > 80 mg/dL; neural network, FDP > 50 mg/dL; random forest, fibrinogen < 150 mg/dL and FDP > 40 mg/dL. For the support vector machine, FDP–fibrinogen/3–60 (mg/dL) is positive because FDP decreases from 100 to 60 mg/dL as the fibrinogen level decreases from 120 to 0 mg/dL. The right figure shows the contours of the estimated probability of hematuria occurrence, divided into 10 segments from 0% to 100%. as shown in the legend bar presenting that the darker the color, the higher the probability of hematuria. If the estimated probability of developing hematuria was >0.5, the patient was considered to have hematuria in the left figure. As coagulopathy is generally accompanied by a fibrinogen decrease and an FDP increase, support vector machines, neural networks, and naïve Bayes, the contour lines of which change stepwise, seemed to be good fits. The boundary determined using the support vector machine method that does not include the fibrinogen 170 mg boundary seemed most appropriate for clinical use.

Table 3. Comparison of the performance of the classifiers on the boundaries in the fibrinogen and fibrin/fibrinogen degradation product planes of hematuria occurrence in parturient hemorrhage for different machine learning methods. All methods were highly accurate (>0.91). All methods demonstrated high AUC values of >0.95. Class mean class entropy was smaller for the logistic regression, naïve Bayes, and neural network methods.

	Accuracy ± SD	AUC	Class Mean Class Entropy	Cohen's Kappa	F1 Score	PPV, Precision	Sensitivity, Recall	Specificity
Logistic regression	1.000 ± 0.22	1.000	1.417×10^{-4}	1.000	1.000	1.000	1.000	1.000
Naïve Bayes	0.9565 ± 0.04	0.9583	5.097×10^{-5}	0.8321	0.8571	0.7500	1.000	0.950
Nearest neighbors	1.000 ± 0.22	1.000	0.3285	1.000	1.000	1.000	1.000	1.000
Neural network	1.000 ± 0.22	1.000	2.253×10^{-5}	1.000	1.000	1.000	1.000	1.000
Random forest	0.9130 ± 0.06	1.000	0.2407	0.7013	0.7500	0.6000	1.000	0.9000
Support vector machine	0.9565 ± 0.04	1.000	0.4967	0.7767	0.8000	1.000	0.6667	1.000

AUC—area under the characteristic curve; SD—standard deviation.

Figure 2 shows the boundaries of hematuria occurrence in massive hemorrhage during delivery, according to discriminant analysis. The boundary was a straight line connecting (0, 50) and (170, 68) in the fibrinogen–FDP coordinates. The discriminant function was 50.693 − 0.00106 × fibrinogen − 0.52723 × FDP − 0.04314 × Hgb/fibrinogen − 0.6978 × PT-sec − 0.02844 × D-dimer; the η^2 of 0.775 indicated a moderate fit ($p = 3.37 \times 10^{-9}$), with an error probability of 0.4186%.

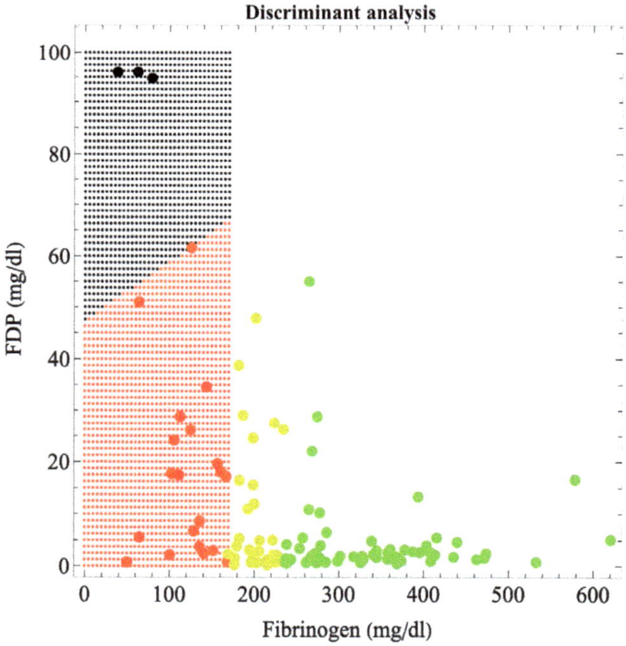

Figure 2. Boundary of hematuria occurrence in major hemorrhage at parturition according to discriminant analysis, i.e., the boundary of organ dysfunction occurrence. Black areas indicate areas of organ dysfunction. The green, yellow, red, and black dots indicate cases without coagulopathy, with coagulopathy, with disrupted coagulopathy, and with organ dysfunction, respectively. In our previous study, we used fibrinogen criteria values of 237 and 170 mg/dL for the development and disruption of coagulopathy, respectively [9]. The boundary was a straight line connecting (0, 50) and (170, 68) in the fibrinogen–FDP coordinates. The discriminant function was 50.693 − 0.00106 × fibrinogen − 0.52723 × FDP − 0.04314 × Hgb/fibrinogen − 0.6978 × PT-sec − 0.02844 × D-dimer; $\eta^2 = 0.775$, which indicates a moderate fit ($p = 3.37 \times 10^{-9}$); error probability = 0.4186%.

The FDP criterion value for hematuria development was determined from the FDP value alone, independent of fibrinogen. The relationship between fibrinogen and FDP is $\tilde{y} = \beta_0 + \beta_1 x$; x; FDP, y; $fibrinogen$, $\beta_0 = 132.905 \pm 9.571 (P = 4.719 \times 10^{-12})$, β_1; $-0.6613 \pm 0.2327\ (P = 9.760 \times 10^{-3})$, $R^2 = 0.278$. Table 4 compares the performance of the classifiers among the machine learning methods. The FDP criteria were 84.96, 101.16, 73.38, 86.94, 92.23, and 79.67 for logistic regression, random forest, nearest neighbors, naïve Bayes, neural network, and support vector machine, respectively. All AUC values, except for that of random forest, were >0.958, and the positive diagnostic rate was excellent, at ≥0.956.

Table 4. Comparison of the performance of classifiers on the boundaries of fibrin/fibrinogen degradation products (FDPs) for hematuria occurrence in parturient hemorrhage by different machine learning methods. Class mean entropy was smaller for the logistic regression, naïve Bayes, and neural network methods. The classifiers by the logistic regression, naïve Bayes, and neural network methods were equally superior.

	FDP Criteria (mg/dL)	Accuracy ± SD	AUC	Class Mean Entropy	Cohen's Kappa	F1 Score	PPV, Precision	Sensitivity, Recall	Specificity
Logistic regression	84.96	1.000 ± 0.22	1.000	1.417×10^{-5}	1.000	1.000	1.000	1.000	1.000
Naïve Bayes	86.94	0.9565 ± 0.04	0.958	5.097×10^{-5}	0.832	0.857	0.750	1.000	0.950
Nearest neighbors	73.38	1.000 ± 0.22	1.000	0.3285	1.000	1.000	1.000	1.000	1.000
Neural network	92.23	1.000 ± 0.22	1.000	3.569×10^{-4}	1.000	1.000	1.000	1.000	1.000
Random forest	101.16	0.9130 ± 0.06	1.000	0.2407	0.701	0.750	0.600	1.000	0.900
Support vector machine	79.67	0.9565 ± 0.04	1.000	0.4967	0.7767	0.800	1.000	0.6667	1.000

AUC—area under the characteristic curve; SD—standard deviation.

4. Discussion

We developed a method for determining the boundaries of hematuria development associated with massive hemorrhage during delivery on a two-dimensional plane consisting of fibrinogen and FDP in this retrospective study presented with reference to the STROBE statement that was used for cohort studies, case–control studies, and cross-sectional studies [37]. Each machine learning method and discriminant analysis produced a variety of candidate boundaries. As shown in Table 3, the performance of the machine learning classifier and the fit of the discriminant analysis function were both generally excellent. The different methods produced various boundaries and criteria; however, as they are all mathematically correct, simply determining a single boundary or a criterion statistically was undesirable, as was adopting an average of the values. Boundaries should be comprehensively determined based on clinical judgment, though data analysis should eliminate subjective judgments to the largest possible extent. As coagulopathy is generally accompanied by decreased fibrinogen and increased FDP levels, the support vector machine, neural network, and naïve Bayes methods are well suited for the task at hand because the contour lines change in a stepwise manner. Additionally, none of these three methods produced a fibrinogen 170 mg/dL boundary. Based on these findings, the support vector machine and naïve Bayes methods appeared suitable for predicting hematuria in patients with massive hemorrhage during delivery. The boundary of whether FDP–fibrinogen/3–60 (mg/dL) is positive according to the support vector machine method seemed the most appropriate for clinical use, though naïve Bayes, for which the class mean class entropy was low, may be optimal (Figure 1, Table 3). Erez et al. [38] reported that the definition of DIC by the Scientific and Standardization Committee on DIC of the International Society on Thrombosis and Haemostasis indicated that (1) DIC is always secondary to other causes, one being obstetric-related, such as abruption placentae [39]; (2) DIC represents the systemic pathological activation of coagulation; and (3) DIC is a process that originates in the microvasculature, or the vascular endothelium, resulting in organ damage from microthrombi [40]. As hematuria alone does not necessarily indicate organ dysfunction, yet is almost always considered to be nearly a state of organ dysfunction, and as biopsying microthrombi in the kidneys of pregnant women in delivery who are hemorrhaging is impractical, we need to define the onset of hematuria associated with massive hemorrhage during delivery as a type of clinical DIC and analyze and apply the findings in clinical practice.

Although many coagulation and fibrinolytic factors exist in addition to, for example, complete blood counts and platelets, in a massive hemorrhage under the urgent circumstances of delivery, factors should be selected so that only those for which test results are available as quickly as possible are used to predict organ dysfunction and initiate preventive treatment. We, therefore, sought a criterion for determining organ dysfunction based solely on fibrinogen and FDP, factors for which results are obtained relatively quickly. As information on related factors such as Hgb/fibrinogen ratio, PT-sec, and D-dimer also contribute to these factors, five-dimensional factors were projected onto a two-dimensional plane using a regression function; boundaries were not simply determined from fibrinogen and FDP information alone. We also obtained the boundaries of the FDP only in one dimension (Table 4). Clinicians would find the boundaries created from fibrinogen and FDP in a two-dimensional plane (Figures 1 and 2) more clinically convincing than the one-dimensional FDP boundaries because the fibrinogen estimates from the FDP are less precise. This is because, even at fibrinogen levels of <170 mg/dL, consumption coagulopathy with FDP elevation and dilutional coagulopathy without FDP elevation were mixed; thus, the correlation between fibrinogen and FDP is no longer accurate ($R^2 = 0.278$). Therefore, boundaries in a two-dimensional plane are more realistic and suitable for clinical applications than a one-dimensional criterion. Although a boundary surface in a higher-dimensional space would be more accurate, recognizing and handling a boundary surface that divides a space of more than three dimensions is challenging; therefore, a boundary in a two-dimensional plane appears to be the most appropriate. The recognition of boundary surfaces in three-dimensional space and beyond will become easier to understand if the space is subdivided, that is, if the dimension is lowered by dividing the space into cases under certain conditions.

In this case, the boundary values are obtained in a two-dimensional plane from multidimensional factors, but by extending the above-described method, boundary surfaces can be obtained in a three-dimensional or larger space. This can be not only applied to the analysis of the coagulation–fibrinolytic system in massive hemorrhage but also further generalized to other research areas. Care must be taken, however, when combining selected factors to avoid multicollinearity. No set rules exist for combining these factors; these must be handled on a case-by-case basis, which complicates the creation of the regression function. The discriminant analysis showed results comparable with those of machine learning, though this method only provides a linear combination of factors. However, because each factor is supposedly related to the others, AI classifiers are generally more suitable and will be especially so in the future. If more cases (e.g., more than 1000) can be accumulated, including many organ dysfunction cases, AI using deep learning [41,42] should provide more reliable boundaries than machine learning or discriminant analysis.

In this study, we sought the boundary between the two classifications of the presence or absence of organ dysfunction, but more than three classifications are obtainable by extending the above-described method. Our analysis was limited to fibrinogen < 170 mg/dL, where the coagulation system is disrupted, in accordance with our previous report [9], but boundaries can be created between three or more regions, including normal conditions.

The most statistically significant difference in FDP was between organ-dysfunctional and non-organ-dysfunctional cases with a fibrinogen level of <170 mg/dL. This suggests that FDP is the most important factor in determining organ dysfunction. Regarding hemorrhage, we suggest the validity of using FDP to predict severe organ dysfunction, focusing on the dynamics of fibrinogen, which is involved in both coagulation and fibrinolysis.

This study had some limitations. First, the number of organ dysfunction cases (three) was low. The results were acceptable despite having only three cases of organ dysfunction because the cases' laboratory values were widely different and extremely abnormal. However, the frequency of detection of hematuria was 2.27% (3/132) for the cases for whom the amount of bleeding was >2000 mL at delivery and only 0.0244% (3/13, 368) of all deliveries; thus, accumulating cases of organ dysfunction such as hematuria is challenging. Ideally, more data from more organ dysfunction cases would be added to the analysis. Second, although fibrinogen and FDP were selected as the two items for which rapid test results were clinically obtainable, the ability to obtain rapid results for both at the same time depends on medical institutions' facilities and testing methods' advances. In facilities where only fibrinogen or FDP results are available, fibrinogen levels < 100 mg/dL or FDP levels > 60 mg/dL should be considered as an indication of organ dysfunction. Furthermore, although this is not our contention, some factors other than fibrinogen and FDP may be better suited for predicting organ dysfunction. Finally, although no deaths occurred in this study and hematuria was used as organ dysfunction, a fixed definition does not exist for organ dysfunction. Data should be analyzed with other indicators, such as death, renal dysfunction, postpartum sequelae, and histopathological abnormalities. The use of these severe cases would lead to different results.

5. Conclusions

Although each machine learning method proposed various boundaries, the results of naïve Bayes, support vector machines, and discriminant analysis seem clinically acceptable. The boundary for whether FDP–fibrinogen/3–60 (mg/dL) is positive according to the support vector machine seemed the most appropriate for clinical use. In the future, a more reliable region will be available if more types of organ dysfunction or data on cases of organ dysfunction can be added. Even if the definition of organ dysfunction is changed or if many factors, including unknown ones, are added to the definition of organ dysfunction, the method developed in this study, which is based on AI using multiple factors correlated with fibrinogen and FDP and avoiding multicollinearity to obtain the boundary line dividing the plane of fibrinogen and FDP, can be expected to be a useful criterion for identifying organ dysfunction occurrence.

Author Contributions: Conceptualization, Y.M. (Yasunari Miyagi), K.T. (Katsuhiko Tada) and I.Y.; methodology, Y.M. (Yasunari Miyagi); software, Y.M. (Yasunari Miyagi); validation, Y.M. (Yasunari Miyagi), K.T. (Katsuhiko Tada), I.Y., K.T. (Keisuke Tsumura), Y.M. (Yuka Maegawa), N.T., T.M., I.E., K.M. and K.K.; formal analysis, Y.M. (Yasunari Miyagi); investigation, Y.M. (Yasunari Miyagi); resources, Y.M. (Yasunari Miyagi) and K.T. (Katsuhiko Tada); data curation, K.T. (Katsuhiko Tada), I.Y., K.T. (Keisuke Tsumura), Y.M. (Yuka Maegawa), N.T., T.M., I.E., K.M. and K.K.; writing—original draft preparation, Y.M. (Yasunari Miyagi); writing—review and editing, Y.M. (Yasunari Miyagi); visualization, Y.M. (Yasunari Miyagi); supervision, K.T. (Katsuhiko Tada) and I.Y.; project administration, K.T. (Katsuhiko Tada); funding acquisition, K.T. (Katsuhiko Tada). All authors have read and agreed to the published version of the manuscript.

Funding: This study was supported by grants from the National Hospital Organization. The funding source had no role in the design, practice, or analysis of this study. This study was also funded by grants from the National Hospital Organization (grant number: R1-1009002). The APC was funded by the National Hospital Organization (grant number: R1-1009002).

Institutional Review Board Statement: This study was conducted in accordance with the Declaration of Helsinki and approved by the National Hospital Organization (NHO) Central Research Ethics Committee (R1-1009002, 7 February 2020).

Informed Consent Statement: Informed consent was obtained from all subjects involved in the study.

Data Availability Statement: The datasets generated during this study are available from the corresponding author upon reasonable request.

Acknowledgments: We thank the following clinicians who helped in the recruitment of participants: Sachie Suga and Megumi Koga at NHO Nagasaki Medical Center, Makoto Nomiyama and Yuko Oshima at NHO Saga Hospital, Kyohei Yamaguchi and Ryoun Cho at NHO Mie Chuo Medical Center, Takashi Kodama and Takako Sadakane at NHO Higashihiroshima Medical Center, and Aki Nagao at NHO Shikoku Medical Center for Children and Adults.

Conflicts of Interest: The authors declare no conflicts of interest.

References

1. Tada, K.; Miyagi, Y.; Yasuhi, I.; Yoshida, M.; Yorozu, M.; Maegawa, Y.; Okura, N.; Kawakami, K.; Yamaguchi, K.; Ogawa, M.; et al. Clinical features of dilutional coagulopathy in massive obstetrical hemorrhage: A multicenter retrospective case series study. *J. Jpn. Soc. Perinat. Neonatal Med.* **2020**, *56*, 417–423.
2. Venugopal, A. Disseminated intravascular coagulation. *Indian J. Anaesth.* **2014**, *58*, 603–608. [CrossRef]
3. Gulumser, C.; Engin-Ustun, Y.; Keskin, L.; Celen, S.; Sanisoglu, S.; Karaahmetoglu, S.; Ozcan, A.; Sencan, I. Maternal mortality due to hemorrhage: Population-based study in Turkey. *J. Matern. Fetal Neonatal Med.* **2019**, *32*, 3998–4004. [CrossRef]
4. Cunningham, F.G.; Nelson, D.B. Disseminated intravascular coagulation syndromes in obstetrics. *Obstet. Gynecol.* **2015**, *126*, 999–1011. [CrossRef] [PubMed]
5. Rattray, D.D.; O'Connell, C.M.; Baskett, T.F. Acute disseminated intravascular coagulation in obstetrics: A tertiary centre population review (1980 to 2009). *J. Obstet. Gynaecol. Can.* **2012**, *34*, 341–347. [CrossRef] [PubMed]
6. Erez, O.; Novack, L.; Beer-Weisel, R.; Dukler, D.; Press, F.; Zlotnik, A.; Than, N.G.; Tomer, A.; Mazor, M. DIC score in pregnant women—A population based modification of the International Society on Thrombosis and Hemostasis score. *PLoS ONE* **2014**, *9*, e93240. [CrossRef]
7. Taylor, F.B., Jr.; Toh, C.H.; Hoots, W.K.; Wada, H.; Levi, M. Towards definition, clinical and laboratory criteria, and a scoring system for disseminated intravascular coagulation. *Thromb. Haemost.* **2001**, *86*, 1327–1330. [CrossRef] [PubMed]
8. Bonnar, J.; Davidson, J.F.; Pidgeon, C.F.; McNicol, G.P.; Douglas, A.S. Fibrin Degradation Products in Normal and Abnormal Pregnancy and Parturition. *Br. Med. J.* **1969**, *19*, 137–140. [CrossRef] [PubMed]
9. Miyagi, Y.; Tada, K.; Yasuhi, I.; Maekawa, Y.; Okura, N.; Kawakami, K.; Yamaguchi, K.; Ogawa, M.; Kodama, T.; Nomiyama, M.; et al. New method for determining fibrinogen and FDP threshold criteria by artificial intelligence in cases of massive hemorrhage during delivery. *J. Obstet. Gynaecol. Res.* **2020**, *46*, 256–265. [CrossRef] [PubMed]
10. Tada, K.; Miyagi, Y.; Kumazawa, K.; Tsukahara, S.; Okimoto, N.; Yoshida, M.; Ooka, N. Feasibility of Applying Novel FDP Threshold Criteria to DIC Diagnostic Scoring Systems in Japanese Women with Placental Abruption. *Eur. J. Clin. Biomed. Sci.* **2022**, *8*, 27–32. [CrossRef]
11. Drukker, L.; Noble, J.A.; Papageorghiou, A.T. Introduction to artificial intelligence in ultrasound imaging in obstetrics and gynecology. *Ultrasound Obstet. Gynecol.* **2020**, *56*, 498–505. [CrossRef]
12. Shrestha, P.; Poudyal, B.; Yadollahi, S.; Wright, D.E.; Gregory, A.V.; Warner, J.D.; Korfiatis, P.; Green, I.C.; Rassier, S.L.; Mariani, A.; et al. A systematic review on the use of artificial intelligence in gynecologic imaging—Background, state of the art, and future directions. *Gynecol. Oncol.* **2022**, *166*, 596–605. [CrossRef] [PubMed]
13. Xu, H.L.; Gong, T.T.; Liu, F.H.; Chen, H.Y.; Xiao, Q.; Hou, Y.; Huang, Y.; Sun, H.Z.; Shi, Y.; Gao, S.; et al. Artificial intelligence performance in image-based ovarian cancer identification: A systematic review and meta-analysis. *eClinicalMedicine* **2022**, *53*, 101662. [CrossRef]
14. Jiang, Y.; Wang, C.; Zhou, S. Artificial intelligence-based risk stratification, accurate diagnosis and treatment prediction in gynecologic oncology. *Semin. Cancer Biol.* **2023**, *96*, 82–99. [CrossRef] [PubMed]
15. Miyagi, Y.; Hata, T.; Bouno, S.; Koyanagi, A.; Miyake, T. Artificial intelligence to understand fluctuation of fetal brain activity by recognizing facial expressions. *Int. J. Gynecol. Obstet.* **2023**, *161*, 877–885. [CrossRef] [PubMed]
16. Miyagi, Y.; Fujiwara, K.; Nomura, H.; Yamamoto, K.; Coleman, R.L. Feasibility of New Method for the Prediction of Clinical Trial Results Using Compressive Sensing of Artificial Intelligence. *BJHMR* **2023**, *10*, 237–267. [CrossRef]
17. Kann, B.H.; Hosny, A.; Aerts, H.J.W.L. Artificial intelligence for clinical oncology. *Cancer Cell* **2021**, *39*, 916–927. [CrossRef]
18. Hashimoto, D.A.; Witkowski, E.; Gao, L.; Meireles, O.; Rosman, G. Artificial Intelligence in Anesthesiology: Current Techniques, Clinical Applications, and Limitations. *Anesthesiology* **2020**, *132*, 379–394. [CrossRef]
19. Gupta, R.; Srivastava, D.; Sahu, M.; Tiwari, S.; Ambasta, R.K.; Kumar, P. Artificial intelligence to deep learning: Machine intelligence approach for drug discovery. *Mol. Divers.* **2021**, *25*, 1315–1360. [CrossRef]
20. Huberty, C.J. Discriminant Analysis. *Rev. Educ. Res.* **1975**, *45*, 543–598. [CrossRef]
21. Wikkelsø, A.J.; Edwards, H.M.; Afshari, A.; Stensballe, J.; Langhoff-Roos, J.; Albrechtsen, C.; Ekelund, K.; Hanke, G.; Secher, E.L.; Sharif, H.F.; et al. Pre-emptive treatment with fibrinogen concentrate for postpartum haemorrhage: Randomized controlled trial. *Br. J. Anaesth.* **2015**, *114*, 623–633. [CrossRef]
22. Mavrides, E.; Allard, S.; Chandraharan, E.; Collins, P.; Green, L.; Hunt, B.J.; Riris, S.; Thomson, A.J.; on behalf of the Royal College of Obstetricians and Gynaecologists. Prevention and management of postpartum haemorrhage. *BJOG* **2016**, *124*, e106–e149. [CrossRef]
23. Asakura, H.; Takahashi, H.; Uchiyama, T.; Eguchi, Y.; Okamoto, K.; Kawasugi, K.; Madoiwa, S.; Wada, H.; DIC subcommittee of the Japanese Society on Thrombosis and Hemostasis. Proposal for new diagnostic criteria for DIC from the Japanese Society on Thrombosis and Hemostasis. *Thromb. J.* **2016**, *14*, 42. [CrossRef]
24. Asakura, H. Classifying types of disseminated intravascular coagulation: Clinical and animal models. *J. Intensive Care* **2014**, *2*, 20. [CrossRef]
25. Dreiseitl, S.; Ohno-Machado, L. Logistic regression and artificial neural network classification models: A methodology review. *J. Biomed. Inform.* **2002**, *35*, 352–359. [CrossRef]

26. Mekkodathil, A.; El-Menyar, A.; Naduvilekandy, M.; Rizoli, S.; Al-Thani, H. Machine Learning Approach for the Prediction of In-Hospital Mortality in Traumatic Brain Injury Using Bio-Clinical Markers at Presentation to the Emergency Department. *Diagnostics* **2023**, *13*, 2605. [CrossRef]
27. Breiman, L. Random forests. *Mach. Learn.* **2001**, *45*, 5–32. [CrossRef]
28. Vaidya, P.M. An$O(n \log n)$ algorithm for the all-nearest-neighbors Problem. *Discret. Comput. Geom.* **1989**, *4*, 101–115. [CrossRef]
29. Friedman, J.; Baskett, F.; Shustek, L. An algorithm for finding nearest neighbors. *IEEE Trans. Comput.* **1975**, *100*, 1000–1006. [CrossRef]
30. Ben-Bassat, M.; Klove, K.L.; Weil, M.H. Sensitivity analysis in Bayesian classification models: Multiplicative deviations. *IEEE Trans. Pattern Anal. Mach. Intell.* **1980**, *3*, 261–266. [CrossRef] [PubMed]
31. Domingos, P.; Pazzani, M. On the Optimality of the Simple Bayesian Classifier under Zero-One Loss. *Mach. Learn.* **1997**, *29*, 103–130. [CrossRef]
32. Hardesty, L. Explained: Neural Networks. *MIT News*. 14 April 2017. Available online: https://news.mit.edu/2017/explained-neural-networks-deep-learning-0414 (accessed on 2 June 2022).
33. Rumelhart, D.; Hinton, G.; Williams, R. Learning representations by back-propagating errors. *Nature* **1986**, *323*, 533–536. [CrossRef]
34. Tsochantaridis, I.; Joachims, T.; Hofmann, T.; Altun, Y. Large margin methods for structured and interdependent output variables. *J. Mach. Learn. Res.* **2005**, *6*, 1453–1484.
35. Pincus, S.; Singer, B.H. Randomness and degrees of irregularity. *Proc. Natl. Acad. Sci. USA* **1996**, *93*, 2083–2088. [CrossRef] [PubMed]
36. Jamin, A.; Humeau-Heurtier, A. (Multiscale) Cross-Entropy Methods: A Review. *Entropy* **2020**, *22*, 45. [CrossRef]
37. Von Elm, E.; Altman, D.G.; Egger, M.; Pocock, S.J.; Gøtzsche, P.C.; Vandenbroucke, J.P.; STROBE Initiative. Strengthening the Reporting of Observational Studies in Epidemiology (STROBE) statement: Guidelines for reporting observational studies. *BMJ* **2007**, *335*, 806–808. [CrossRef]
38. Erez, O.; Othman, M.; Rabinovich, A.; Leron, E.; Gotsch, F.; Thachil, J. DIC in Pregnancy—Pathophysiology, Clinical Characteristics, Diagnostic Scores, and Treatments. *J. Blood Med.* **2022**, *13*, 21–44. [CrossRef]
39. Levi, M.; Toh, C.H.; Thachil, J.; Watson, H.G. Guidelines for the diagnosis and management of disseminated intravascular coagulation. *Br. J. Haematol.* **2009**, *145*, 24–33. [CrossRef]
40. Thachil, J. Disseminated Intravascular Coagulation: A Practical Approach. *Anesthesiology* **2016**, *125*, 230–236. [CrossRef] [PubMed]
41. Deng, L.; Yu, D. Deep Learning: Methods and Applications. *Found. Trends Signal Process.* **2014**, *7*, 197–387. [CrossRef]
42. Janiesch, C.; Zschech, P.; Heinrich, K. Machine learning and deep learning. *Electron. Mark.* **2021**, *31*, 685–695. [CrossRef]

bioengineering

MDPI

Article

Brain Tumor Detection and Categorization with Segmentation of Improved Unsupervised Clustering Approach and Machine Learning Classifier

Usharani Bhimavarapu [1], Nalini Chintalapudi [2] and Gopi Battineni [2,*]

[1] Department of Computer Science and Engineering, Koneru Lakshmaiah Education Foundation, Vaddeswaram 522302, India
[2] Clinical Research Centre, School of Medicinal and Health Products Sciences, University of Camerino, 62032 Camerino, Italy; nalini.chintalapudi@unicam.it
* Correspondence: gopi.battineni@unicam.it; Tel.: +39-33-3172-8206

Abstract: There is no doubt that brain tumors are one of the leading causes of death in the world. A biopsy is considered the most important procedure in cancer diagnosis, but it comes with drawbacks, including low sensitivity, risks during biopsy treatment, and a lengthy wait for results. Early identification provides patients with a better prognosis and reduces treatment costs. The conventional methods of identifying brain tumors are based on medical professional skills, so there is a possibility of human error. The labor-intensive nature of traditional approaches makes healthcare resources expensive. A variety of imaging methods are available to detect brain tumors, including magnetic resonance imaging (MRI) and computed tomography (CT). Medical imaging research is being advanced by computer-aided diagnostic processes that enable visualization. Using clustering, automatic tumor segmentation leads to accurate tumor detection that reduces risk and helps with effective treatment. This study proposed a better Fuzzy C-Means segmentation algorithm for MRI images. To reduce complexity, the most relevant shape, texture, and color features are selected. The improved Extreme Learning machine classifies the tumors with 98.56% accuracy, 99.14% precision, and 99.25% recall. The proposed classifier consistently demonstrates higher accuracy across all tumor classes compared to existing models. Specifically, the proposed model exhibits accuracy improvements ranging from 1.21% to 6.23% when compared to other models. This consistent enhancement in accuracy emphasizes the robust performance of the proposed classifier, suggesting its potential for more accurate and reliable brain tumor classification. The improved algorithm achieved accuracy, precision, and recall rates of 98.47%, 98.59%, and 98.74% on the Fig share dataset and 99.42%, 99.75%, and 99.28% on the Kaggle dataset, respectively, which surpasses competing algorithms, particularly in detecting glioma grades. The proposed algorithm shows an improvement in accuracy, of approximately 5.39%, in the Fig share dataset and of 6.22% in the Kaggle dataset when compared to existing models. Despite challenges, including artifacts and computational complexity, the study's commitment to refining the technique and addressing limitations positions the improved FCM model as a noteworthy advancement in the realm of precise and efficient brain tumor identification.

Keywords: brain cancer; tumor detection; fuzzy c-means; MRI images; extreme learning; glioma; malignant

1. Introduction

During the aging process, brain cells lose their ability to control themselves, leading to the development of brain tumors. As tumors grow in cells, they increase pressure on the brain and negatively affect overall health [1,2]. The tumors can damage normal tissues, overgrow in the brain, and replicate in other parts of the body [2–4]. Disease symptoms vary depending on tumor size, and the main challenge is diagnosing the type of tumor because they vary in both location and size [5]. It has been shown that early diagnosis reduces the severity and mortality of brain tumors [6].

Brain tumors, though comparatively rare in the spectrum of cancers, pose significant challenges due to their intricate location and potential impact on vital brain functions. Incidence rates vary, with an estimated annual occurrence of approximately 14 new cases per 100,000 people. According to the National Brain Tumor Society, there has been a 300% increase in brain tumor-related deaths over the past thirty years [7]. Gliomas, comprising astrocytoma's and glioblastomas, are among the most common primary brain tumors. While overall incidence remains relatively low, the burden is substantial, given the complexities associated with diagnosis, treatment, and the potential life-altering consequences. Brain tumors exhibit a diverse age distribution, affecting individuals across the lifespan. Pediatric brain tumors are a leading cause of cancer-related mortality in children, emphasizing the urgency for specialized care and research in this population. In adults, the incidence rises with age, and certain types, such as meningiomas, are more prevalent in older individuals. Understanding age-related patterns is critical for tailoring diagnostic approaches and treatment strategies to the unique needs of distinct age groups. Identifying specific risk factors for brain tumors remains challenging, as many cases lack clear etiological markers. However, certain genetic predispositions, exposure to ionizing radiation, and hereditary conditions may elevate risk. The impact of brain tumors on quality of life is profound, as these tumors can disrupt cognitive function and sensory abilities. Symptoms vary based on tumor location and size, affecting patients' daily lives and necessitating comprehensive care approaches that address both medical and psychosocial aspects. Untreated brain tumors can be fatal.

Diagnosing and treating brain tumors is a complex challenge for medical professionals. Prompt detection and early treatment initiation are key factors in improving survival rates for brain tumor patients [6]. Unlike biopsies for other body parts, brain tumor biopsies require surgical intervention, making them more complicated. This underscores the importance of non-surgical methods for precise diagnosis. The size and severity of a brain tumor cannot be determined by traditional images. The treatment response may be delayed due to some existing constraints. Medical professionals use magnetic resonance imaging (MRI) and computed tomography (CT) images to identify the brain's normal and abnormal tissue [8]. Recognizing brain tumors manually is tedious and error-prone process, but automatic detection accurately identifies their regions, shape, boundaries, and position. By detecting, segmenting, and classifying brain tumors in medical images, computer-aided diagnosis can detect them [9].

Brain tumors have been identified using MRI images because they are accurate and can segment the affected area accurately. It is possible to extract accurate and highly relevant features from MRI images, which help to predict brain tumors [10]. Cluster-based segmentation divides MRI images into subcategories and indicates the region of interest (ROI) in every scan [11]. With clustering, tumor size can be reliably identified, thereby enabling effective treatment and reducing mortality risk [12]. High-similarity pixels are grouped into a separate region and separated from low-similarity pixels.

According to the American Brain Tumor Association [13], the standard classification system for brain tumors ranges from grade I to IV. Grades I and II, known as low-grade gliomas, are typically benign and grow slowly, while grades III and IV, referred to as high-grade gliomas, are malignant and grow quickly. If not treated, a low-grade brain tumor may progress to a high-grade, more dangerous form. Regular monitoring through MRI or CT scans every six months to a year is recommended for patients with grade II gliomas. Brain tumors can affect individuals of any age and have varying effects on the body.

Low-grade gliomas (grades I and II) are generally considered curable with complete surgical removal, while high-grade (grades III and IV) malignant brain tumors are treated with radiation, chemotherapy, or a combination of both. Malignant gliomas include both grade III and IV gliomas, also known as anaplastic astrocytoma's, which are mid-grade tumors that grow more abnormally and rapidly than lower-grade tumors. The most severe form of astrocytoma, known as glioblastoma, is a grade IV tumor characterized by unusually rapid blood vessel growth and the presence of necrosis. Glioblastomas are the most aggressive and rapidly growing tumors in this classification.

Segmentation in medical imaging is crucial for identifying affected tumor tissues. It involves dividing an image into sections or segments with similar attributes like color, texture, contrast, brightness, and gray level. In brain tumor segmentation, there is a need to distinguish tumor tissues, including edema and necrotic cells, from normal brain tissues and solid tumors, like white matter (WM), gray matter (GM), and cerebrospinal fluid (CSF), using MRI or other imaging methods.

MRI images of brain tumors can be segmented using K-means clustering with high precision [14]. Based on a study that classified brain tumors, local-level features were identified [15]. Membership in the fuzzy C-Mean (FCM) is not a measure of the degree of the corresponding data. The values of each element range from 0 to 1. The improved FCM algorithm is a type of soft clustering that assigns membership levels to each data point for multiple clusters, rather than forcing a hard categorization into a single cluster. This method is particularly useful in medical imaging, where the boundaries between different tissue types, such as tumor and normal brain tissue, can be ambiguous or overlapping. In [16], the authors used the FCM approach to generate membership and typicality values for unlabeled clustering data. An FCM technique can be used to generate membership and possibility under practical point models or cluster centers [17]. Some works implemented FCM techniques, both adaptive and non-adaptive for determining local spatial element weights [18,19].

When dealing with various levels of noise, probabilistic FCM proved to be more reliable and effective. An exponential FCM clustering technique has been proposed to overcome FCM's noise condition limitation [20]. The exact details of tumors are not identified in most existing models, and it is difficult to segment the precise location of tumors. There is difficulty identifying tumor margins and areas, and limited features can reduce classification error rates. This leads us to propose an improved FCM that is capable of detecting tiny brain tumors with high accuracy. A color and texture feature extraction approach were applied after segmentation to MRI images. To classify brain tumors, the extreme learning machine (ELM) was developed.

The proposed study makes a substantial advancement in brain tumor detection and segmentation compared to existing works by introducing an improved Fuzzy C-Means (FCM) clustering algorithm. In contrast to traditional clustering techniques, the enhanced FCM model excels in identifying minute brain tumors and showcases superior performance in accurately categorizing diverse tumor types. The algorithm's ability to handle uncertainty, reduce variability in segmentation results, and provide a nuanced approach with degrees of membership, non-membership, and hesitation degree represents a significant breakthrough.

Research Contributions

- ➢ The study contributes by utilizing the Fig share and Kaggle datasets for brain tumor detection. These datasets provide a diverse and comprehensive set of brain images, ensuring the applicability and robustness of the proposed methods across various scenarios.
- ➢ A novel contribution lies in the proposal of an improved fuzzy C-Means clustering algorithm. This technique specifically addresses the challenge of detecting minute tumors, showcasing an advancement in the ability to identify smaller lesions that might be overlooked by traditional methods.
- ➢ The research conducts an extensive investigation by evaluating the proposed improved fuzzy C-Means clustering against five state-of-the-art segmentation models. This comparative analysis contributes valuable insights into the strengths and weaknesses of different segmentation approaches, providing a basis for selecting optimal methods in brain tumor detection.

- The study introduces a rigorous evaluation framework by incorporating key metrics such as accuracy, precision, recall, and F1-score. These metrics offer a comprehensive assessment of the proposed approach's performance, allowing for a nuanced understanding of its effectiveness in comparison to existing models.
- A significant research contribution is the demonstration of fast and accurate tumor detection achieved by the proposed approach. This highlights the practical viability of the method in real-time scenarios, contributing to the efficiency of brain tumor detection over existing state-of-the-art approaches.

2. Literature Review

This section discusses the literature review for brain tumor detection and classification. Cherukuri et al. [21] employed Xception as the foundational architecture and introduced a multi-level attention network (MANet) incorporating both spatial and cross-channel attention mechanisms on the 3064 T1W-CE MRI datasets, achieving an accuracy of 96.51%. An inherent drawback of long-short-term memory (LSTM) networks is their heightened computational cost and the need for intricate network tuning. LSTMs, being more intricate than CNNs and RNNs, present challenges in debugging and issue identification. Guan et al. [22] initially enhanced the visual quality of input images through contrast optimization and nonlinear strategies. Subsequently, tumour locations were determined using segmentation and clustering techniques. These locations were then utilized in conjunction with the corresponding input image, feeding into Efficient Net for feature extraction. Despite achieving an accuracy of 98.04% with fivefold cross-validation on the T1W-CE MRI dataset, this study suffers from increased computational costs due to the necessity of training multiple networks. Badža et al. [23] proposed an advanced CNN with 22 layers for classifying three tumour types (meningioma, glioma, and pituitary) in the T1W-CE MRI dataset. Employing subject-wise and record-wise tenfold cross-validation on both augmented and original image databases, they obtained the highest accuracy of 96.56% on the 3064 T1W-CE MRI datasets. Deepak et al. [24] utilized deep learning and machine learning, modifying a pre-trained Google Net with the Adam optimizer. Incorporating SVM or KNN instead of the classification layer within the transfer learning model improved accuracy to 92.3%, 97.8%, and 98% for Google Net, SVM, and KNN, respectively, with fivefold cross-validation on the T1W-CE MRI dataset. However, this research faces challenges, including the relatively poor performance of the transfer-learned model as an independent classifier and significant misclassification in meningioma class samples.

Díaz-Pernas et al. [25] proposed a method for brain tumours segmentation and classification on the T1W-CE MRI dataset using sliding window segmentation with a N window. Applying data augmentation to prevent overfitting, the classification CNN with three pathways for feature extraction achieved an accuracy of 97.3% on the T1W-CE MRI dataset. The limitation includes the lowest sensitivity for meningioma due to lower contrast intensity between the tumours and healthy areas. Alhassan et al. [26] introduced a CNN with a hard swish based RELU activation function involving image pre-processing and HOG feature descriptor utilization; this method achieved an accuracy of 98.6% for brain tumours classification on the T1W-CE MRI dataset.

Ghassemi et al. [27] employed a pre-trained deep convolutional neural network as a GAN discriminator (DCGAN) with a SoftMax layer within the GAN discriminator. They achieved an accuracy of 95.6% for brain tumours classification on the T1W-CE MRI dataset. A drawback is the limitation of GAN due to a network size of 64, preventing the use of pre-trained architectures as discriminators that require larger input sizes. Noreen et al. [28] utilized deep learning and machine learning, applying fine-tuned Inception-v3 and Xception for feature extraction and classification with SVM, KNN, random forest (RF), and ensemble techniques. The Inception-v3-Ensemble method produced the best testing accuracy of 94.34% among all proposed methods but suffered from time-consuming and high computational costs.

Gumaei et al. [29] proposed a regularized extreme learning machine (RELM) as a hybrid feature extraction method, including min–max normalization for pre-processing and PCA-NGIST for feature extraction; this method achieved an accuracy of 94.233% with fivefold cross-validation on the T1W-CE MRI dataset. Haq et al. [30] developed a DCNN technique for brain tumours detection and classification, involving pre-processing with N4ITK, normalization, and data augmentation. They used a Google Net variant model with and without conditional random fields (CRF), achieving 97.3% and 95.1% accuracy, respectively, on the T1W-CE MRI dataset. A disadvantage is the model's unsuitability for classification tasks involving small amounts of data and challenges with erroneous information from various imaging modalities.

Ghosal et al. [31] employed a DCNN-based SE-ResNet-101 architecture, fine-tuned to fit training data, achieving an overall accuracy of 89.93% and 93.83% without and with data augmentation, respectively. Nawaz et al. [32] utilized a custom Corner Net with DenseNet-41 base network and one-stage detector, achieving 98.8% accuracy based on the T1W-CE MRI dataset, providing a low-cost solution to brain tumours classification. Verma et al. [33] suggested Hyper-Sphere Angular Deep Metric-based Learning (HSADML) with Mobile Net as the backbone network, achieving 98.69% overall accuracy based on the T1W-CE MRI dataset. The suggested method enhanced intra-class separability and decreased intra-class variability. However, the research did not emphasize the backbone network, leaving room for introducing attention-based domain-specific networks.

Cinar et al. [34] applied image cropping and various data augmentation techniques, designing a CNN from scratch for brain tumour classification. They achieved overall accuracies of 98.09%, 98.32%, and 96.35% with different training and testing dataset divisions, demonstrating categorization without relying on deep networks. A drawback is the long training period without transfer learning, making it impractical for larger datasets. Deepak et al. [35] proposed a custom CNN model, achieving accuracy improvements from 94.2% to 95.8% with SVM using a fivefold cross-validation method. Deepak et al. [36] introduced deep feature fusion and majority voting approaches, enhancing CNN predictions for three types of brain tumours but increasing computational complexity due to training with multiple loss functions.

Kumar et al. [37] employed three CNN models—Alex Net, ResNet 50, and Inception V3—resizing images, normalizing between [0] and [1], and applying augmentation techniques. They achieved accuracies of 93.51%, 98.24%, and 92.07%, respectively. Despite demonstrating the efficiency of CNN architectures in identifying enhanced MRI brain tumour images, the work has limitations, including the computational slowness of CNNs with operations like max pooling, the prolonged training time for multiple layers, and the demand for substantial training data.

Diverse methodologies and algorithms have been explored in prior works for brain tumour classification, each with its own set of limitations. Deep learning approaches, while capable of extracting features directly from input data, entail high complexity, fixed input image sizes, and costly computational requirements. The selection of an appropriate deep learning model with optimal hyperparameters remains a challenging task in previous works. To address these limitations, this research minimizes pre-processing steps and carefully chooses optimization models with suitable parameters.

3. Materials and Methods

The proposed framework for brain tumor detection and classification is shown in Figure 1. It consists of four stages, including image preprocessing, segmentation, feature extraction, and classification, that are further explained below. We gathered brain tumor images from different datasets. In the first stage, we proposed an improved hybrid contrast enhancement based on the absolute mean deviation and the kurtosis function to enhance the contrast of the brain tumor images. In the second stage, we proposed the improved fuzzy model to segment the brain tumor images. In the third stage, the feature extraction process extracts the shapes, textures, and colors of the segmented brain tumor images. In the final stage, the enhanced ELM model correctly identified four types of brain tumors: pituitary, no tumor, meningioma, and glioma tumors.

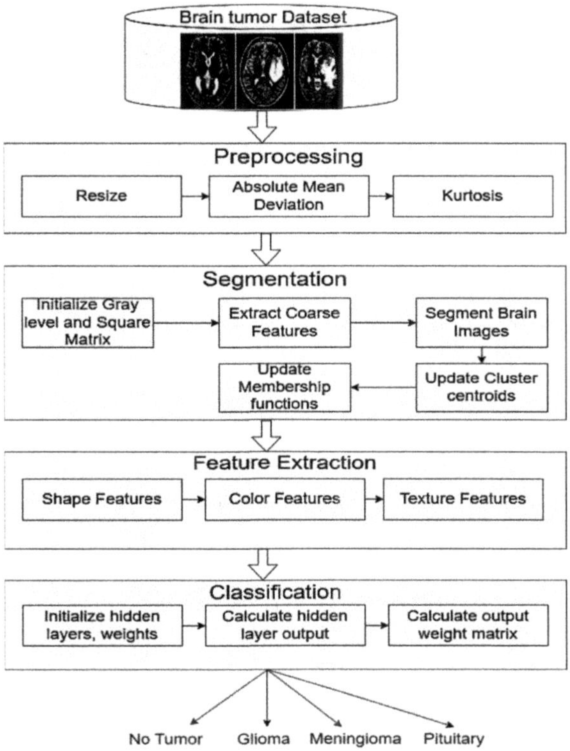

Figure 1. Brain tumor detection and classification flow diagram.

We collected MRI images from two open-source libraries: the Fig share [38] and Kaggle datasets [39]. In Table 1, we describe the image distribution of different brain MRI tumors.

Table 1. Class-wise MRI tumor distribution.

Class	Fig Share	Kaggle
meningioma	708	306
Pituitary	930	300
Glioma	1426	300
No tumour	-	405

Figure 2 shows sample image classes of brain tumors. It has three subfigures, and we explain each subfigure below:

(a) Glioma:

Glioma is a category of brain tumor that originates from the glial cells, which are supportive cells in the brain. These tumors can occur in various parts of the brain and spinal cord. Gliomas are known for their diverse and aggressive nature, often infiltrating surrounding brain tissues. They are classified into different types, such as astrocytoma's, oligodendrogliomas, and ependymomas, based on the specific glial cell they originate from. Gliomas pose challenges in treatment due to their infiltrative growth and resistance to therapies.

(b) Meningioma:

Meningioma is a type of brain tumor that arises from the meninges, the layers of tissue covering the brain and spinal cord. These tumors are generally slow-growing and often benign, but they can cause symptoms depending on their size and location. Meningiomas can develop along the meninges' surface and may press against adjacent brain structures, leading to a range of neurological symptoms. Surgical removal is a common treatment approach for meningiomas, and they are generally associated with a favorable prognosis.

(c) Pituitary:

Pituitary tumors originate in the pituitary gland, a small gland at the base of the brain responsible for regulating various hormones. These tumors can be either benign or malignant and may affect hormone production. Depending on their size and hormone-secreting activity, pituitary tumors can lead to hormonal imbalances, impacting bodily functions. Common types include prolactinomas, growth hormone-secreting tumors, and non-functioning adenomas. Treatment options vary and may include surgery, medications, or radiation therapy, aiming to restore hormonal balance and manage symptoms.

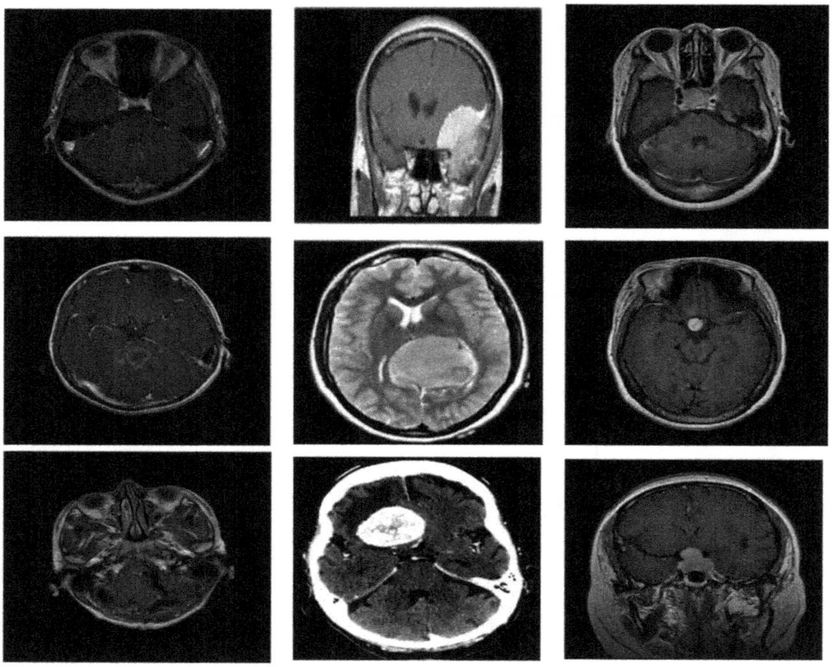

Figure 2. MRI image classes i.e., Glioma (**left**), Meningioma (**Middle**), and Pituitary (**Right**).

3.1. Image Preprocessing

In this study, we proposed an improved hybrid contrast enhancement based on the absolute mean deviation and the kurtosis function. This approach increases the contrast of the brain tumors and makes the brain images more useful for further processing. Consider D as the brain tumor database, and N is the brain image dimensions PXQ input.

Let Δ denote the brain tumor database and X represent an input image with dimensions $N \times M$. Let n denote the total number of pixels in the image, and x_i represent each image pixel. The absolute mean deviation (AMD) and kurtosis are expressed through Equations (1) and (2).

$$AD = \frac{1}{n}\sum_{i=1}^{n}|x_i - \phi(X)| \quad (1)$$

$$\mathrm{SK} = \frac{\frac{1}{s}\sum_{k=1}^{m}\|x_i - X\|^3}{(n-1) * \|s\|^3} \quad (2)$$

Here, AD represents the AMD of the image, φ(X) is the average mean of the dataset (Δ), and S is the standard deviation, and it is represented as $\sqrt{\frac{\sum_{i=1}^{n}(x_i-\bar{x})^2}{n}}$. $\overline{X}$ is the mean (average) of the data points. Employing these values, the final transformation of the image is $I_1 = AD(i) + X$ and $IF = I_1 - SK(i)$, where IF is the final transformed image, and i denotes the image pixels. This procedure is implemented across the entire selected datasets prior to the training of the learning models.

3.2. Segmentation

Segmentation is an important method for analyzing image processing, and it is crucial for diagnosing illnesses using MRI images. By doing so, digital image analysis will be made easier and more accessible. When the MRI image is segmented, it is divided into several homogeneous sections that are not overlapping. The foundation of segmentation lies in unsupervised clustering algorithms. A fuzzy model is used to address uncertainties related to borders, variations, and vagueness in gray-level images [40]. Among the methods of sorting unlabeled data into discrete sets, clustering is the most commonly used. In the present study, an output window is selected, and FCM clustering segmentation is used to segment it. Algorithm 1 presents the improved FCM algorithm after segmenting the brain tumor images.

Algorithm 1: Improved FCM

Input: Gray level image
Output: Segmented image

- ➢ Set the number of intensity levels and compute a square matrix; $\mathrm{I} = \sum\sum \mathrm{G}\left(\mathrm{p_i}, \mathrm{q_j}\right)$, and the image matrix $\mathrm{G} = \sum\sum \mathrm{G}(\mathrm{p_k}, \mathrm{q_l})$
- ➢ Initialize $F_{xy} = G \oplus I$
- ➢ Extract coarse features from F_{xy}
- ➢ Segment the brain image
  $G_1 = \frac{1}{2}\sum_{k=1}^{m}\sum_{l=1}^{n} G_{kl}\|p_k - a_l\|^2 * \sum_{k=1+1}^{X}\sum_{l=1+1}^{Y} T\|p_k, q_l\|^2$
- ➢ Repeat until $F_{xy} \leq \sum_{i=1}^{H}\sum_{j=1}^{z}[F_{xy}(i) - F_{xy}(j)]$
- ➢ Update G_1
- ➢ Initialize cluster centroid
- ➢ Define membership function $s_{kl}^{(0)}$ of the FCM
- ➢ Update cluster center $T_k^{(v)} \Leftrightarrow s_{kl}^{(v)}$, ($k$ = 1,2,... and v = 1,2,3)
  Update $\mathrm{D}(p_k, \delta_k^{(v)}) \Leftrightarrow \delta_k^{v}$ and s_{kl}
- ➢ With $\mathrm{c}(p_k, \delta_k^{(v)})$ until $|\,|s_{kl}^{(v)} - s_{kl}^{(v+1)}|\,| \leq \in, \in = [0,1]$

The algorithm begins by setting the number of intensity levels and computing a square matrix $\mathrm{I} = \sum\sum G(p_i, q_j)$, where the image matrix $G = \sum\sum G(p_k, q_l)$ is defined. An initial feature matrix, $F_{xy} = G \oplus I$, is created, followed by the extraction of coarse features from F_{xy}. Subsequently, the brain image is segmented using a process involving a mathematical expression denoted as G_1. This expression involves the computation of weighted distances between elements of G and specific points, followed by a thresholding operation. The algorithm iteratively refines F_{xy} until a certain condition is met, updating G_1 in the process. The algorithm introduces a novel approach by incorporating a cluster-centric strategy. It initializes cluster centroids, defines a membership function $s_{kl}^{(0)}$ using Fuzzy C-Means (FCM), and subsequently updates the cluster centers $T_k^{(v)}$ based on the membership function values. An additional update involves adjusting a variable $\mathrm{D}(p_k, \delta_k^{(v)})$ based on certain criteria, refining the clustering process until a convergence condition is satisfied. The variable G plays a crucial role in representing the original image matrix. The novelty of the algorithm lies in its integration of fuzzy clustering, weighted distance computations, and iterative refinement processes. This multifaceted approach enhances the algorithm's adaptability to complex image characteristics and its ability to capture subtle variations in the data. The iterative nature of the algorithm, along with the incorporation of cluster-based strategies, contributes to its effectiveness in image segmentation tasks.

The algorithm's advantages stem from its incorporation of weighted distance computation, iterative refinement, cluster-centric strategy, dynamic thresholding, and the utilization of the parameter G. The algorithm introduces a weighted distance computation process G_1, where distances between elements of the image matrix G and specific points are weighted based on certain criteria. This enables the algorithm to capture more nuanced relationships within the data, allowing for a more accurate representation of the underlying structures in the images. Unlike standard FCM, the proposed algorithm involves an iterative refinement process for the feature matrix F_{xy}. This iterative nature allows the algorithm to adapt and fine-tune its segmentation results over multiple iterations, potentially leading to improved convergence and more precise segmentation. The algorithm incorporates a cluster-centric strategy by initializing cluster centroids and updating them based on the membership functions derived from FCM. This strategy enhances the algorithm's ability to identify and characterize different clusters within the image, resulting in more accurate and meaningful segmentation. The iterative process involves dynamic thresholding conditions, providing adaptability to varying complexities in image data. This dynamic nature allows the algorithm to handle diverse image characteristics and improve its performance in scenarios where standard FCM may struggle. The use of the variable G as the original image matrix introduces a unique aspect to the algorithm. This variable, representing the initial state of the image, contributes to the algorithm's ability to capture and preserve essential features during the segmentation process. The convergence criteria involving D $(p_k, \delta_k^{(v)})$ and cluster similarity add an additional layer of refinement, potentially preventing the algorithm from converging to suboptimal solutions. This results in more reliable and accurate segmentation outcomes.

3.3. Feature Extraction

Feature extraction is fundamental for classification. In this study, we extract the shapes, textures, and colors that are important in representing brain tumor images. The process of extracting optimal features from brain images is challenging [41]. In feature extraction, raw data are transformed into numerical data while retaining the original information. Automated or manual models can be used to extract features. Automated feature extraction extracts only issue-related significant features, while manual feature extraction extracts all significant features. Gray-level co-occurrence matrix (GLCM) features are extracted in the present study. Measures are extracted from the GLCM functions based on the texture of the brain tumor image. Matrix dimensions define the relative frequency of pixels in a brain tumor image. Homogeneity, dissimilarity, energy, and contrast are the measures determined by the features.

Traditional feature extraction techniques such as texture, shape, and color-based methods offer distinct advantages over deep learning approaches for brain image analysis. These methods provide interpretable features, making it easier for researchers and clinicians to understand the underlying characteristics related to specific pathological conditions. Additionally, traditional techniques often perform well in scenarios with limited data, where deep learning models may struggle to generalize effectively. They are computationally efficient, making them suitable for resource-constrained environments and real-time processing requirements. The integration of domain-specific knowledge is facilitated, enhancing performance in medical imaging where expertise plays a critical role. Traditional feature extraction methods offer reduced sensitivity to data quality variations, explicit control over feature selection, transparent decision-making processes, and proven transferability across different imaging modalities. While deep learning has achieved notable success, the advantages of traditional feature extraction techniques make them valuable, especially when interpretability, efficiency, and expert control are paramount considerations in brain image feature extraction. Table 2 explains the features of brain tumor detection with definition.

Table 2. Extracted features.

Feature	Definition	Equation
Standard deviation (SD)	Determines the spread of data	$\sqrt{\sum_{k=0}^{W-1}\left(k-\bar{k}\right)^2 p(k)}$
Skewness	Finds the symmetry of the possibility distribution	$\frac{1}{S^3}\sum_{k=0}^{W-1}\left(k-\bar{k}\right)^3 p(k)$
Energy	Determines the spread of pixel values	$\sum_{k=0}^{W-1}(P(k))^2$
Entropy	Find the data needed to code the data	$-\sum_{k=0}^{W-1}[P(k)\log_2 p(k)]$
Kurtosis	Determines the probability distribution	$\frac{1}{S^4}\sum_{k=0}^{W-1}\left(k-\bar{k}\right)^4 p(k)$
Contrast	Determines local fluctuations	$\sum_{k,l=0}^{W-1} P_{kl}(k-l)^2$
Correlation	Determines the joint probability	$\sum_{k,l=0}^{W-1} P_{kl}\frac{(k-M)(l-M)}{S^4}$
Energy	Determine the sum of the squared pixel values	$-\sum_{k=0}^{W-1}[P(k)\log_2 p(k)]$
Homogeneity	Determines local uniformity	$\sum_{k,l=0}^{W-1}\frac{P_{kl}}{1+(k-l)^2}$
Busyness	Determines changes in the neighbouring pixels	$\frac{\sum_{k=0}^{T_k} p(k)q(l)}{\sum_{k=0}^{T_k}\sum_{k=0}^{T_k}\lvert kp(k)-lq(l)\rvert}$ where $p(k)\neq 0,\ q(l)\neq 0$
Strength	Determines the primitives of the brain image	$\frac{\sum_{k=1}^{t_k}\sum_{k}^{T_k}[P(k)](k-1)^2}{\sum_{k=1}^{t_k} p(k)}$ where $p(k)\neq 0$

3.4. Feature Selection

Feature selection improves classification accuracy by removing irrelevant and redundant features and selecting robust features to boost performance. This study uses the entropy-based controlled approach to choose the best features. This approach removes irrelevant features by selecting the highly robust features. Entropy for the feature vector V(P) for the M X N dimensions is represented as

$$\sum_{d_1}\sum_{dz} min(d_1,d_2)*[-\sum_{k=1}^{z} p_k\log(p_k)] \quad (3)$$

where d_1, d_2 are the current and the previous distance of the selected features and p_k is the probability of the kth feature. To find the more robust features, we apply the threshold function to select the features greater than the high probability feature T_k.

$$\text{Final Features} = \begin{cases} p(k); T_k \leq \sum_{k=1}^{z} p_k log(p_k) \\ 0; Ohterwise \end{cases} \quad (4)$$

3.5. Classification

In this study, we used the ELM [42] to classify brain tumors. If the ELM has a z sample (i_k, o_k), the output with zero errors is mathematically represented as

$$o_k = \sqrt{\sum_{k=1}^{H} \alpha_k t(w_k i_k + b_k)}, \text{ where } k = 1, \ldots . z \quad (5)$$

where i_k and o_k are the input and the output samples, respectively, the activation function is represented as t (.), and w_k and b_k refer to the weights and the bias, respectively. α_k is a weight coefficient for the kth term.

O = Hα; where the output is represented as O = $(o_1, o_2, \ldots o_n)$ and the matrix weights are represented as α = $(\alpha_1, \alpha_2 \ldots \alpha_m)$. The hidden layers can be represented as

$$\mathrm{H} = \begin{bmatrix} t(w_1 i_1 + b_1) ------ t(w_n i_1 + b_n) \\ -------------------- \\ ------------------- \\ -------------------- \\ t(w_1 i_m + b_1) ------ t(w_n i_m + b_n) \end{bmatrix} \quad (6)$$

The hidden layer nodes should be less than the sample count. Equation (6) represents the structure of a single-hidden-layer Extreme Learning Machine (ELM) neural network used in the classification of brain tumors. In this equation, H denotes the hidden layer, which consists of nodes with activation functions denoted by $t(\cdot)$. Each node in the hidden layer is associated with weights w_{ki} and biases b_k, where i ranges from 1 to m, representing the input features. The hidden layer's output O is obtained by summing the product of each node's activation function and its corresponding weight, followed by the application of the activation function $t(\cdot)$. This process is mathematically expressed as $O = H\alpha$, where $O = (o_1, o_2, \ldots, o_n)$ represents the output vector and $\alpha = (\alpha_1, \alpha_2, \ldots, \alpha_m)$ represents the weight matrix. The structure of the hidden layer is further detailed in Equation (6), where H is represented as a concatenation of n nodes. Each node's activation is determined by the weighted sum of the input features i, $(i_1, i_2, \ldots, i_m)$, with weights w_{ki} and biases b_k for each node. The activation function $t(\cdot)$ introduces non-linearity to the model, allowing it to capture complex patterns and relationships within the input data. It is worth noting that the number of nodes in the hidden layer n should be chosen judiciously, typically less than the number of samples, to prevent overfitting. The weights and biases are learned during the training process, enabling the network to map input features to the desired output for effective brain tumor classification.

3.6. Performance Evaluation

The performance metrics can help measure the model presented in terms of the different parameters mentioned below [43–49]. For instance,

In the context of brain tumor classification:

➢ Accuracy in brain tumor classification represents the overall correctness of the model in predicting different types of brain tumors.

$$\text{Accuracy} = \frac{\text{Correctly classified brain tumor samples}}{\text{Total brain tumor samples}}$$

➢ Precision in brain tumor classification measures the accuracy of the model in correctly identifying a specific type of tumor among the predicted positive cases.

$$\text{Precision} = \frac{\text{True positives for a specific brain tumor type}}{\text{True positives} + \text{False positives for that brain tumor type}}$$

- ➢ Recall in brain tumor classification assesses the ability of the model to correctly identify all instances of a particular brain tumor type among the actual positive cases.

$$\text{Recall} = \frac{\text{True Positives for a Specific Brain Tumor Type}}{\text{True Positives} + \text{False Negatives for that Brain Tumor Type}}$$

- ➢ F1 score in brain tumor classification provides a balance between the precision and recall, giving an overall measure of the model's effectiveness.

$$\text{F1 Score} = 2 \times \frac{\text{Precision} \times \text{Recall}}{\text{Precision} + \text{Recall}}$$

4. Results

In this section, we analyze the performance of the proposed model. To extract MRI image information for this study, we first used an improved hybrid contrast enhancement to improve the brain MRI image and extract visual information.

4.1. Segmentation Evaluation

The proposed model produces segmentation results that are more precise and reliable. The various segmentation results and comparisons are presented in Figure 3. The columns (a) and (b) are the original images and their corresponding ground truths. The (c–g) columns are the images implemented with the state-of-the-art approaches MLT, K-Means, IPFCM, PSO, and GTV_{CUT}, respectively. The (h) column, which is implemented with the proposed approach, is similar to the ground truth MRI images.

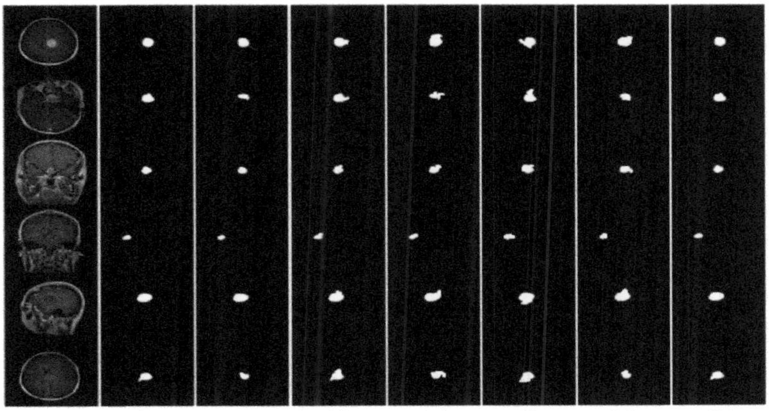

(a) (b) (c) (d) (e) (f) (g) (h)

Figure 3. Segmentation Comparison (**a**) Original (**b**) ground truth (**c**) MLT (**d**) K-means (**e**) IPFCM (**f**) PSO (**g**) GTV_{CUT} (**h**) proposed.

Figure 4 shows the proposed segmentation's performance comparison with the existing models. Multilevel threshold technique (MLT) [50] segments brain tumor images and achieves an accuracy of 91.78%, precision of 90.38%, and recall of 92.75%. K-Means [51] segments brain tumor images and achieves an accuracy of 92.53%, precision of 94.57%, and recall of 94.99%. Intuitionistic possibilistic fuzzy C-Means (IPFCM) [52] segments brain tumor images and achieves an accuracy of 91.47%, a precision of 96.35%, and recall of 93.56%. Particle swarm Optimization (PSO) [53] segments brain tumor images and achieves an accuracy of 89.55%, a precision of 83.73%, and a recall of 84.57%. Gross tumor volume Segmentation (GTVCUT) [54]. The segmentation performance metrics accuracy, precision, and recall using the proposed function were 99.78%, 99.36%, and 99.75%, respectively.

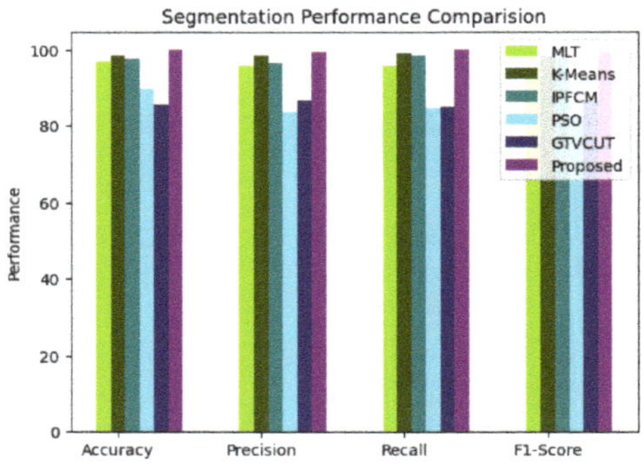

Figure 4. Segmentation performance comparison.

4.2. Classification Evaluation

Figure 5 shows the performance of various classifiers on Fig share datasets brain test set images. The performance of various classifiers, namely Extreme Learning Machine (ELM), Support Vector Machine (SVM), Random Forest (RF), Naive Bayes (NB), and k-Nearest Neighbors (KNN), was evaluated on a brain tumor dataset for tumor classification across four different classes: No Tumor, Glioma, Meningioma, and Pituitary. In terms of accuracy, ELM demonstrated the highest accuracy across all classes, ranging from 97.43% to 99.25%, showcasing its robust overall performance. SVM and RF also exhibited competitive accuracy, maintaining values above 97% for most classes. KNN, while performing well, had slightly lower accuracy, especially in the Meningioma class. Figure 5a shows the classifier performance in terms of accuracy. Precision measures the ratio of correctly predicted positive observations to the total predicted positives. ELM achieved high precision values, indicating its proficiency in minimizing false positives. SVM and RF showed commendable precision as well, particularly in Glioma and Meningioma classes. KNN exhibited a slightly lower precision, especially in the Meningioma category. Figure 5b shows the classifier performance in terms of precision. Recall, or sensitivity, gauges the ability of a classifier to capture all the positive instances. ELM and SVM displayed excellent recall across all classes, ensuring comprehensive identification of positive cases. RF, NB, and KNN demonstrated reasonable recall values, with KNN exhibiting a slight dip, particularly in the Meningioma class. Figure 5c,d shows the classifier performance in terms of recall and F1 scores.

Figure 6 shows the class-based performance. The classification performance across the classes No Tumor, Glioma, Meningioma, and Pituitary was evaluated based on accuracy, precision, and recall metrics. In the No Tumor class, the classifiers demonstrated high accuracy, precision, and recall, with values ranging from 92.45% to 98.64%, 95.35% to 99.14%, and 90.35% to 99.25%, respectively. For the Glioma class, consistent accuracy rates were observed, ranging from 88.45% to 98.66%, precision values varied between 88.45% and 99.14%, and recall rates were between 89.74% and 99.19%. In the Meningioma class, the classifiers exhibited robust accuracy, precision, and recall percentages, with values spanning 94.57% to 98.50%, 92.10% to 98.62%, and 89.74% to 99.16%, respectively. The Pituitary class also showcased commendable performance metrics, with accuracy ranging from 94.59% to 98.64%, precision varying between 94.59% and 99.15%, and recall rates spanning 91.42% to 97.43%. Overall, the classifiers demonstrated consistent and effective performance in accurately classifying instances across diverse tumor categories, emphasizing their potential suitability for medical imaging applications. The class performance in terms of accuracy, precision, recall and F1-score in shown in Figure 6a–d.

The results revealed that the overall testing accuracy and ELM performance metrics were most appropriate for detecting brain tumors. In total, 96.6% of the predictions were correct based on the prediction output of the ELM. ELM's prediction output reflects the probability of correct predictions and their accuracy. The ground truth and ELM model predictions for the test images are shown in Figure 7. Ground truth is represented by the first row in the image, while predicted results are represented by the second row.

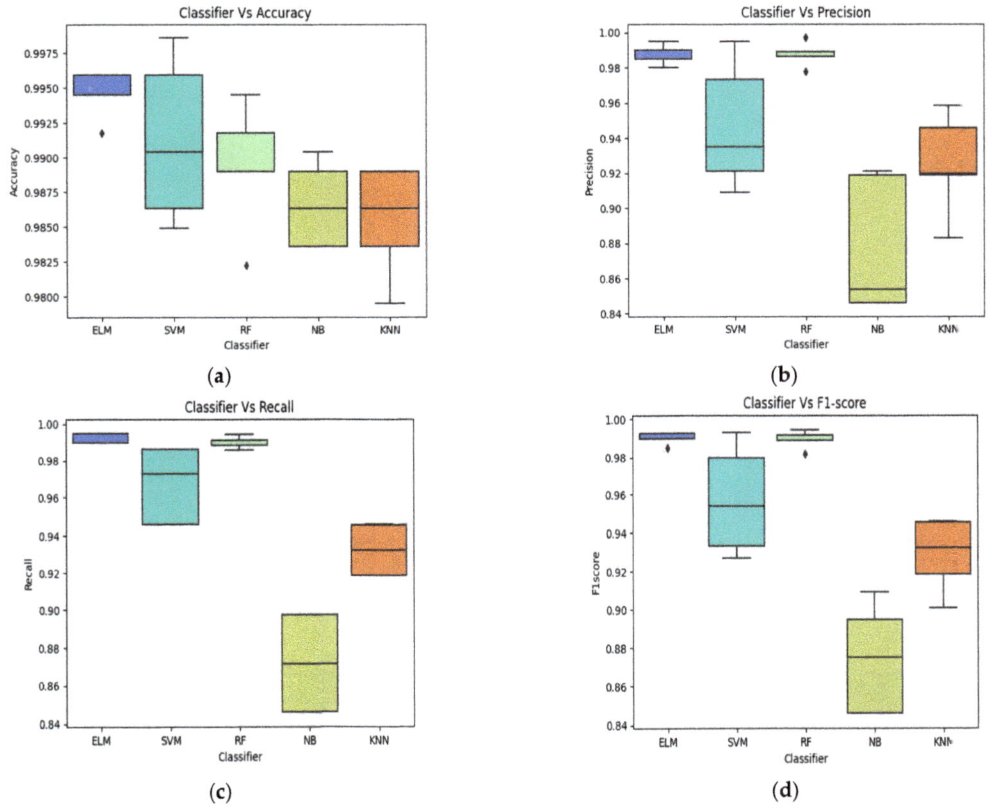

Figure 5. Different classifier performance in terms of accuracy (**a**), precision (**b**), recall (**c**) and F1 scores (**d**).

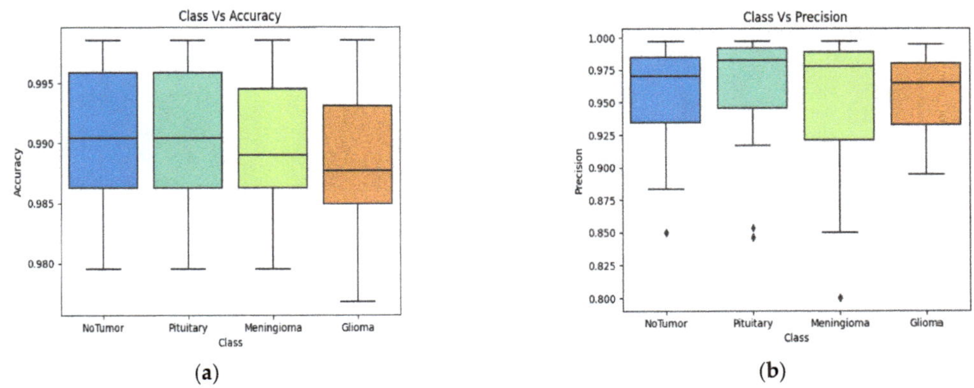

Figure 6. *Cont.*

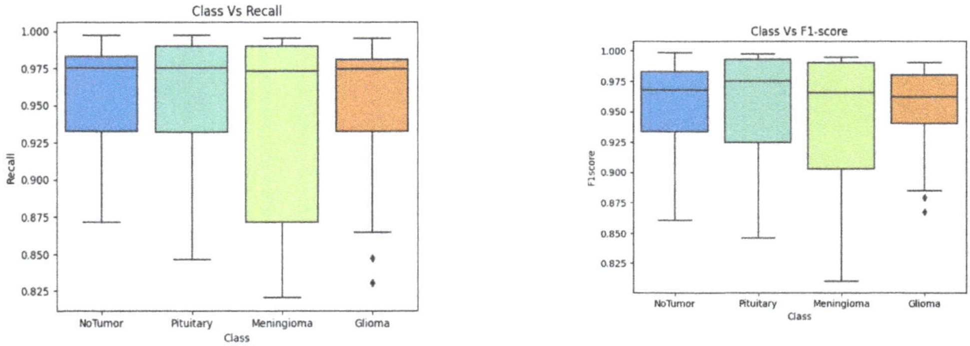

(c) (d)

Figure 6. Brain tumor 4-class performance in terms of accuracy (**a**), precision (**b**), recall (**c**) and F1-score (**d**).

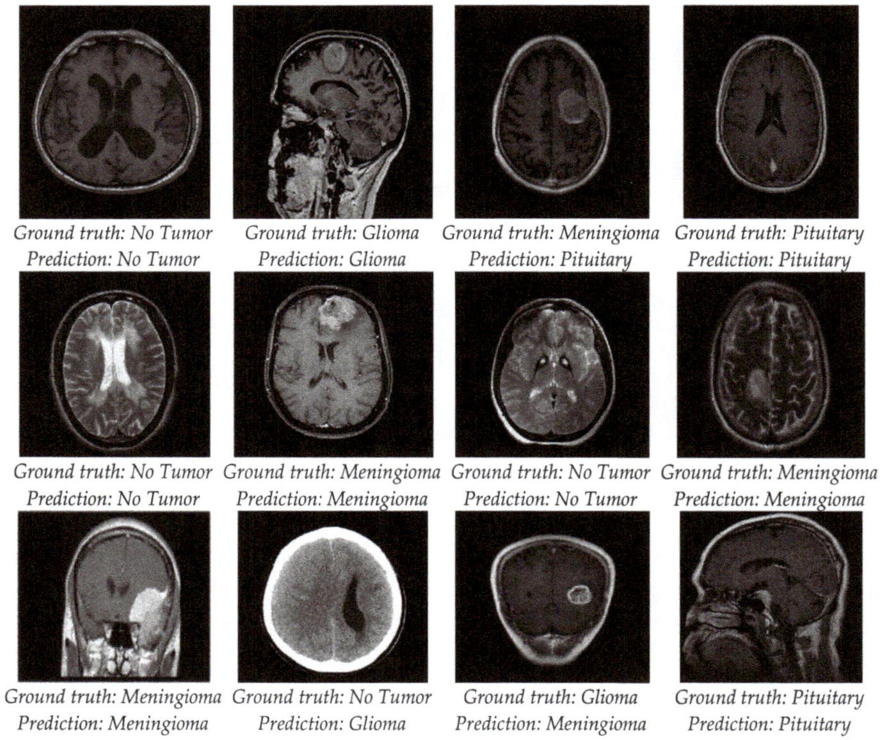

Figure 7. Prediction of brain tumor test images.

Both the generalization efficiency and the ELM rate of learning are higher than those of traditional state-of-the-art classifiers. When it comes to the ELM algorithm, weights and hidden biases are assigned regularly.

The proposed classifier demonstrates exceptional performance across multiple metrics, achieving an overall accuracy of 98.56%. For the "No Tumor" class, the classifier exhibits high precision (99.14%) and recall (99.25%). In the case of Glioma, the precision and recall stand at 98.66% and 99.19%, respectively. Similarly, for Meningioma, the classifier attains a precision of 99.14% and a recall of 99.10%. The Pituitary class also sees impressive results with a precision of 97.43% and recall of 97.43%. In comparison, the approach by Alanazi et al. [55] yields slightly lower accuracy at 97.86%. The "No Tumor" class exhibits precision and recall values of 98.49% and 98.33%, respectively. Glioma achieves a precision of 98.17% and a recall of 99.14%, Meningioma records a precision of 97.33% and a recall of 98.64%, and Pituitary shows a precision of 98.51% and a recall of 99.15%.

The model developed by Zahoor et al. [56] reports an accuracy of 98.31%. However, there is a notable decrease in recall for the "No Tumor" class at 89.74%. Glioma maintains a precision of 98.49% and a recall of 98.3%, while Meningioma achieves a precision of 98.62% and a recall of 99.16%. Pituitary records a precision of 94.59%. The classifier developed by Ait Amou et al. [57] exhibits an accuracy of 94.57%. The "No Tumor" class shows a precision of 98.00% and recall of 98.50%. Glioma, however, experiences a decrease in recall (89.74%). Meningioma maintains a precision of 98.24% and a recall of 94.91%, and Pituitary shows a precision of 98.61% and a recall of 98.89%. Lastly, the model developed by Kirbayi et al. [58] demonstrates an accuracy of 94.89%. The "No Tumor" class achieves a precision of 95.90% and a recall of 94.59%. Glioma records a precision of 97.51% and a recall of 98.98%. Meningioma exhibits a precision of 91.89% and a recall of 87.17%, while Pituitary achieves a precision of 96.49% and a recall of 93.22%. Figure 8 shows the visualization results of Table 3.

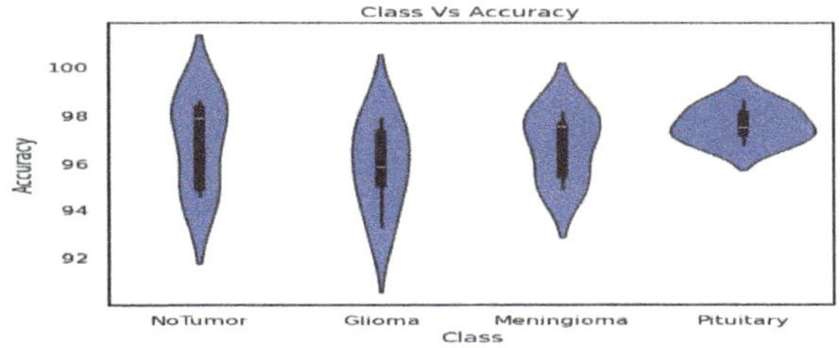

(a)

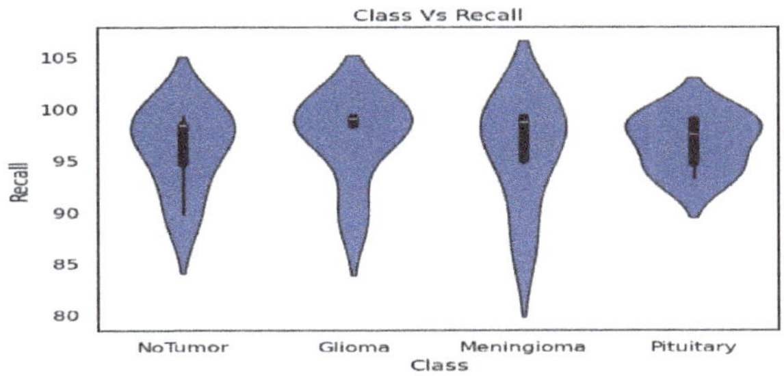

(b)

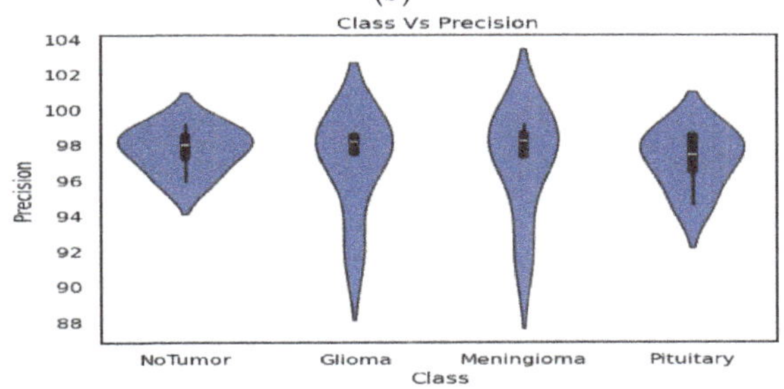

(c)

Figure 8. Visualization of results (**a**) Class Vs Accuracy (**b**) Class Vs Recall (**c**) Class Vs Precision.

Table 3. Comparison of classifier accuracy for Fig Share dataset.

Classifier	Accuracy	Precision	Recall	Class
Proposed	98.56	99.14	99.25	No Tumor
	98.24	98.66	99.19	Glioma
	98.50	99.14	99.10	Meningioma
	98.56	97.43	97.43	Pituitary
Alanazi et al. [55] (2022)	97.86	98.49	98.33	No Tumor
	97.31	98.17	99.14	Glioma
	97.59	97.33	98.64	Meningioma
	97.45	98.51	99.15	Pituitary
Zahoor et al. [56] (2022)	98.31	97.22	89.74	No Tumor
	97.86	98.49	98.30	Glioma
	97.09	98.62	99.16	Meningioma
	98.09	94.59	94.59	Pituitary
Ait Amou et al. et al. [57] (2022)	94.57	98.00	98.50	No Tumor
	95.85	92.10	89.74	Glioma
	95.45	98.24	94.91	Meningioma
	96.76	98.61	98.89	Pituitary
Kirbayi et al. [58] (2022)	94.89	95.90	94.59	No Tumor
	95.04	97.51	98.98	Glioma
	94.89	91.89	87.17	Meningioma
	97.17	96.49	93.22	Pituitary
Poonguzhali et al. [59] (2023)	93.53	97.45	91.42	Pituitary
	92.45	95.35	90.35	No Tumor
	95.35	88.45	96.56	Glioma
	95.45	90.35	97.45	Meningioma
Rahman et al. [60] (2023)	97.34	98.02	95.67	Pituitary
	97.57	98.11	95.78	No Tumor
	97.56	97.13	96.84	Glioma
	97.37	97.24	97.47	Meningioma
Malla et al. [61] (2023)	98.35	97.36	97.25	Pituitary
	98.64	97.46	97.19	No Tumor
	98.50	98.14	99.01	Glioma
	98.36	97.43	97.43	Meningioma

Table 4 tabulates the performance comparison of the proposed with the state-of-the-art models on the Kaggle dataset.

Figure 9 shows the performance comparison of the various performance metrics, such as accuracy, precision, and recall, for four classes between the proposed and the existing models [41,42,62–64]. In the evaluation of various classifiers for brain tumor classification, the proposed classifier demonstrates commendable performance across multiple metrics. The proposed model achieves an overall accuracy of 99.37%, showcasing its robust ability to correctly classify instances. Precision and recall values further underscore its efficacy, with 99.64% precision and 99.57% recall for the "No Tumor" class, 99.74% precision and

99.85% recall for "Glioma", 99.85% precision and 99.84% recall for "Meningioma", and 99.57%, 99.85% precision and recall for "Pituitary".

Table 4. Comparison of classifier accuracy for Kaggle dataset.

Classifier	Accuracy	Precision	Recall	Class
Proposed	99.37	99.84	99.57	No Tumor
	99.24	99.74	99.85	Glioma
	99.50	99.85	99.84	Meningioma
	99.56	99.57	97.85	Pituitary
Saeedi S et al. [41]	96.46	97.57	98.54	No Tumor
	96.75	97.14	98.36	Glioma
	96.84	97.47	98.27	Meningioma
	96.85	97.78	98.73	Pituitary
Kalam R et al. [42]	97.35	98.46	98.68	No Tumor
	97.15	98.73	98.74	Glioma
	97.36	98.27	98.37	Meningioma
	97.37	98.21	98.62	Pituitary
Mahmud MI et al. [62]	93.53	94.36	95.63	No Tumor
	93.14	94.62	95.63	Glioma
	93.62	94.52	94.63	Meningioma
	93.52	94.26	95.62	Pituitary
Woźniak M et al. [63]	96.46	95.45	95.46	No Tumor
	96.46	95.63	95.74	Glioma
	96.73	95.36	95.47	Meningioma
	96.13	95.63	95.37	Pituitary
Reyes D et al. [64]	97.03	98.17	98.67	No Tumor
	97.19	98.31	98.91	Glioma
	97.25	98.25	98.89	Meningioma
	97.26	98.37	98.59	Pituitary

Comparing this proposed classifier with existing studies, Saeedi et al. [41] achieved an accuracy of 96.46%, demonstrating slightly lower performance than the proposed model. Kalam et al. [42] and Mahmud et al. [62] also reported accuracies of 98.35% and 93.53%, respectively, placing them in line with or slightly below the proposed classifier. Woźniak et al. [63] obtained an accuracy of 96.46%, and Reyes et al. [64] achieved an accuracy of 98.03%. These comparative studies highlight the competitive nature of the proposed classifier, positioning it favorably in the landscape of brain tumor classification algorithms.

In the comparison of precision and recall values across various classifiers for brain tumor classification, the proposed classifier demonstrates notable performance. For the "No Tumor" class, the proposed model achieves precision and recall values of 99.14% and 99.25%, respectively. In the "Glioma" class, precision is reported at 98.66%, with a corresponding recall of 99.19%. The "Meningioma" class showcases precision and recall values of 99.14% and 99.10%, respectively, while the "Pituitary" class reports precision and recall of 97.43%.

Comparatively, Saeedi et al. report precision and recall values ranging from 97.57% to 98.73%, Kalam et al. present precision and recall values in the range of 98.15% to 98.74%, and Mahmud et al. show precision and recall values from 94.36% to 95.63%. Woźniak et al. and Reyes et al. also report precision and recall values in the mid-to-high 90s range.

Overall, the proposed model not only achieves impressive accuracy but also excels in precision and recall, showcasing its potential as a robust and reliable tool for brain tumor classification. This comparative analysis underscores the effectiveness of the proposed classifier in achieving a balanced performance between precision and recall, essential for reliable and accurate brain tumor classification.

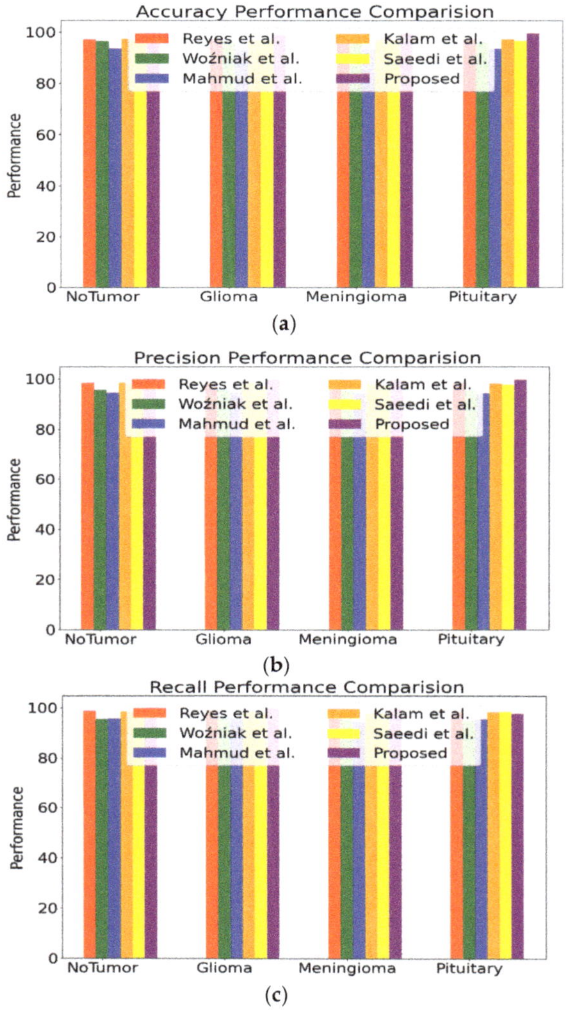

Figure 9. Performance Comparison (**a**) Accuracy (**b**) Precision (**c**) Recall. (i.e., Saeedi et al. [41], Kalam et al. [42], and Mahmud et al. [62], Wozniak et al. [63], and Reyes et al. [64]).

5. Discussion

Today, brain tumors are among the most serious diseases, and their incidence is increasing. Since brain tumors can be dangerous and can only be prevented at an early stage by total brain area scanning to detect the tumor; as such, accurate diagnosis and necessary patient treatment are crucial. It is challenging to calculate the area, determine the degree of uncertainty in the segmentation area, and segment the tumor due to the structural complexity and unpredictability of brain tumors, high volatility, and intrinsic features of MRI data, i.e., variability of tumor size and shape. Medical professionals may occasionally notice variations in segmentation results due to variations in tumor form and shape. While some tumors, like meningiomas, are easy to separate, others, like gliomas, are more challenging. Meningioma and pituitary have similar textures and intensities, making it difficult to distinguish them. As a result, producing manual tumor segmentation is a laborious task.

It is essential to create an automatic detection system that can provide quick, inexpensive, accurate, and comprehensible diagnoses to handle massive amounts of data and minimize human error during screening. The workload of medical personnel is lessened by computer-assisted diagnostics, which also produces faster, more precise diagnoses with fewer mistakes. Thus, it is anticipated that clinical decision-making by physicians will be aided by computer-assisted diagnostics. Furthermore, with the aid of computer-assisted diagnostics, new avenues for research in clinical tests may become available.

Deep learning techniques acquire knowledge by directly obtaining features from images. Modern deep learning techniques, particularly CNNs, are very accurate and widely used in medical image analysis, including MRI analysis. These techniques have several drawbacks, including the need for a sizable training dataset, a high degree of temporal complexity, poor accuracy for applications with limited datasets, and a high initial cost to the user due to the requirement for expensive GPUs. It can also be quite difficult to select the most accurate deep-learning model because it involves understanding a wide range of parameters, training strategies, and topologies.

Existing models may struggle to detect tiny brain tumors, highlighting a potential drawback in their ability to handle smaller lesions [65]. Some methods, like the one utilizing borderline pixel detection, may not accurately identify the inner borders of tumor regions, impacting the completeness of segmentation [66]. The complexity of certain models, such as the Link Net network, might make them challenging to implement and interpret [67]. The application of advanced models, like 3D convolution architectures, may require substantial computational resources [68]. The overfitting problem was addressed by recommending a brain tumor method based on the ResNet50 model and global average pooling, but potential limitations remain [69]. Despite the success of certain methods, the study acknowledges the need for further research, optimization, and improvements to address limitations in accuracy and processing time [70–72]. The existing methods were often evaluated on specific datasets, and their generalizability to diverse datasets or clinical settings may need validation. This paper makes substantial contributions by leveraging diverse datasets, introducing an innovative clustering algorithm, conducting a thorough comparative analysis with existing models, employing comprehensive evaluation metrics, and demonstrating both speed and accuracy improvements in brain tumor detection.

We have proposed an improved segmentation algorithm based on FCM to detect brain tumors from MRI images. We compare the enhanced FCM model with segmentation models based on data from Fig share and Kaggle. An improved FCM is shown to be effective in identifying brain tumors from MRI scans in the study. The model correctly identified pituitary, no tumor, meningioma, and glioma tumors as the four types of brain tumors in the fig share dataset.

A variety of clustering techniques are presented, including FCM, K-mean, MLT, PSO, and enhanced versions of these techniques. The problem of designing a thresholding technique solution is complex and requires ongoing research by medical imaging researchers. In K-mean clustering, all the data are grouped into a single, functional cluster that does not apply to all tenders. To preserve each pixel across clusters with different membership levels, FCM assigns each pixel to unlabeled fuzzy clusters. As a result of this research, it is found that the FCM's degrees of data cannot be reflected in its membership. In medical image segmentation, FCM clustering has been demonstrated to help diagnose diseases such as brain tumors and eliminate unknown noise and uncertainty.

In this study, an enhanced version of the FCM clustering algorithm is employed to detect minuscule brain tumors, which are often challenging to identify using conventional methods. This advanced approach involves selecting a specific output window within the imaging data for analysis. The improved FCM clustering segmentation is then applied to this targeted area. By using improved FCM clustering segmentation on the chosen output window, the algorithm effectively reduces uncertainty and increases the accuracy of tumor detection. This improvement is crucial in the context of brain tumor identification, as it allows for more precise delineation of tumor boundaries and enhances the detection of smaller, less distinct tumors. The enhanced FCM approach is instrumental in improving diagnostic accuracy, which is vital for appropriate treatment strategies and improving patient outcomes in neuro-oncology.

Improved FCM has the degree of membership, non-membership, and hesitation degree [63,73,74]. By addressing the degree of hesitancy throughout the membership function, the improved fuzzy c-mean technique is employed to overcome uncertainty issues [75–77]. Traditional clustering techniques cannot handle issues, including outliers and noisy data. To tackle those issues, we took an improved approach. The proposed segmentation model achieved accuracy, precision, and recall, of 98.47%, 98.59%, 98.74% on the Fig share dataset and 99.42%, 99.75%, 99.28% on the Kaggle dataset, respectively, outperforming the competing algorithms. Consequently, compared to the other models described, the proposed model is more capable of detecting the glioma grade, which is highly desirable in clinical applications.

Multiclass Brain Tumor categorization systems have been created to help medical experts visualize and classify different types of tumors. The primary problems with the present approaches to brain tumor classification include low accuracy, lack of data samples for different grades, and binary categorization. The state-of-the-art methods for classifying brain tumors are limited to just two categories: benign and malignant. This makes it very difficult for medical experts to recommend further testing or treatment. Using high-level data from MRI images, ELM is utilized in this study to identify different classes of tumors. This research may help medical experts make decisions about early diagnosis and possible treatment options. This research presents an enhanced ELM for the multiclass categorization of brain tumors to reduce the number of misclassifications. The proposed algorithm achieved the best accuracy for segmentation and classification when compared to the state-of-the-art models.

The challenges for the proposed algorithms are segmenting the tumor region incorrectly due to artifacts and requiring extra time to process due to their computational complexity. The following are the main limitations of this study: (a) The technique was applied to small MRI datasets. To further accomplish even more effective brain tumor segmentation, we will employ large datasets of brain imaging in the future. (b) Further study is needed to make the suggested classification technique compatible with smartphone applications, as it is intended for desktop use only. In future studies, we will examine how to incorporate additional features that can enhance detection and accuracy. Furthermore, it will examine how to shorten the computation time and alter the complexity of the proposed Improved FCM algorithm.

6. Conclusions

This study presents a brain tumor detection and classification approach using the improved fuzzy c-means and ensemble learning machine. The proposed FCM minimizes the uncertainty issues while segmenting the MRI images and reduces the computational complexity for identifying the lesion details. Evaluate the present model performance with performance metrics accuracy, precision, and recall, with segmentation values 98.47%, 98.59%, and 98.74% on the Fig share dataset and 99.42%, 99.75%, and 99.28% on the Kaggle dataset, respectively. The proposed model improved brain tumor diagnosis with faster accurate and fast detection times by extracting the color, shape, and texture features. The improved ELM model improves the classification performance. We will implement the proposed model to evaluate the large MRI datasets. We will examine the deep learning models to enhance the model further.

Author Contributions: Conceptualization, U.B. and G.B.; methodology, U.B.; software, N.C.; validation, U.B., N.C. and G.B.; formal analysis, U.B.; investigation, U.B.; resources, G.B.; data curation, U.B.; writing—original draft preparation, U.B.; writing—review and editing, G.B.; visualization, U.B.; supervision, G.B. All authors have read and agreed to the published version of the manuscript.

Funding: This research received no external funding.

Institutional Review Board Statement: Not applicable.

Informed Consent Statement: Not applicable.

Data Availability Statement: The data presented in this study are available on request from the corresponding author.

Conflicts of Interest: The authors declare no conflict of interest.

References

1. Reynoso-Noverón, N.; Mohar-Betancourt, A.; Ortiz-Rafael, J. Epidemiology of brain tumors. In *Principles of Neuro-Oncology: Brain Skull Base*; Springer: Cham, Switzerland, 2021; pp. 15–25. [CrossRef]
2. Brunese, L.; Mercaldo, F.; Reginelli, A.; Santone, A. An ensemble learning approach for brain cancer detection exploiting radi-omic features. *Comput. Methods Programs Biomed.* **2020**, *185*, 105134. [CrossRef] [PubMed]
3. Casanova, M.P.; Mariné, A.F.; Pumarola i Batlle, M.; Feliu-Pascual, A.L. Meningioma and glioma as the first collision brain tumour re-ported in small animals. *J. Comp. Pathol.* **2023**, *204*, 55–58. [CrossRef] [PubMed]
4. Altinoz, M.A.; Ozpinar, A. Oxamate targeting aggressive cancers with special emphasis to brain tumors. *Biomed. Pharmacother.* **2022**, *147*, 112686. [CrossRef]
5. Song, C.; Ren, Y.; Liu, Y.; Cao, R.; Duan, G. Oxygen comfort evaluation method based on symptom index for short-term internal migrants to Tibet. *Sci. Total Environ.* **2023**, *902*, 166418. [CrossRef] [PubMed]
6. Amin, J.; Sharif, M.; Raza, M.; Saba, T.; Anjum, M.A. Brain tumor detection using statistical and machine learning method. *Com-Puter. Methods Programs Biomed.* **2019**, *177*, 69–79. [CrossRef] [PubMed]
7. National Brain Tumor Society. Available online: https://braintumor.org/ (accessed on 22 May 2023).
8. Rovira, À.; Auger, C. Beyond McDonald: Updated perspectives on MRI diagnosis of multiple sclerosis. *Expert Rev. Neurother.* **2021**, *21*, 895–911. [CrossRef]
9. Pilli, R.; Goel, T.; Murugan, R.; Tanveer, M. Association of white matter volume with brain age classification using deep learn-ing network and region wise analysis. *Eng. Appl. Artif. Intell.* **2023**, *125*, 106596. [CrossRef]
10. Bahadure, N.B.; Ray, A.K.; Thethi, H.P. Image analysis for MRI based brain tumor detection and feature extraction using biolog-ically inspired BWT and SVM. *Int. J. Biomed. Imaging* **2017**, *2017*, 9749108. [CrossRef]
11. Mittal, H.; Pandey, A.C.; Saraswat, M.; Kumar, S.; Pal, R.; Modwel, G. A comprehensive survey of image segmentation: Clustering methods, performance parameters, and benchmark datasets. *Multimed. Tools Appl.* **2021**, *81*, 35001–35026. [CrossRef] [PubMed]
12. Tseng, C.J.; Tang, C. An optimized XGBoost technique for accurate brain tumor detection using feature selection and image segmentation. *Healthc. Anal.* **2023**, *4*, 100217. [CrossRef]
13. American Brain Tumor Association. Available online: https://www.abta.org/ (accessed on 20 May 2023).
14. Islam, M.K.; Ali, M.S.; Miah, M.S.; Rahman, M.M.; Alam, M.S.; Hossain, M.A. Brain tumor detection in MR image using superpixels, principal component analysis and template based K-means clustering algorithm. *Mach. Learn. Appl.* **2021**, *5*, 100044. [CrossRef]
15. Swati, Z.N.; Zhao, Q.; Kabir, M.; Ali, F.; Ali, Z.; Ahmed, S.; Lu, J. Brain tumor classification for MR images using transfer learning and fine-tuning. *Comput. Med. Imaging Graph.* **2019**, *75*, 34–46. [CrossRef]
16. Zeng, W.; Liu, Y.; Cui, H.; Ma, R.; Xu, Z. Interval possibilistic C-means algorithm and its application in image segmentation. *Inf. Sci.* **2022**, *612*, 465–480. [CrossRef]
17. Zhu, J.; Ma, X.; Martínez, L.; Zhan, J. A probabilistic linguistic three-way decision method with regret theory via fuzzy c-means clustering algorithm. *IEEE Trans. Fuzzy Syst.* **2023**, *31*, 2821–2835. [CrossRef]
18. Kollem, S.; Reddy, K.R.; Rao, D.S. An optimized SVM based possibilistic fuzzy c-means clustering algorithm for tumor segmentation. *Multimed. Tools Appl.* **2021**, *80*, 409–437. [CrossRef]
19. Cebeci, Z.; Cebeci, C.; Tahtali, Y.; Bayyurt, L. Two novel outlier detection approaches based on unsupervised possibilistic and fuzzy clustering. *PeerJ Comput. Sci.* **2022**, *8*, e1060. [CrossRef] [PubMed]
20. Garg, H.; Rani, D. Novel distance measures for intuitionistic fuzzy sets based on various triangle centers of isosceles triangu-lar fuzzy numbers and their applications. *Expert Syst. Appl.* **2022**, *191*, 116228. [CrossRef]
21. Shaik, N.S.; Cherukuri, T.K. Multi-level attention network: Application to brain tumor classification. *Signal Image Video Process.* **2022**, *16*, 817–824. [CrossRef]

22. Guan, Y.; Aamir, M.; Rahman, Z.; Ali, A.; Abro, W.A.; Dayo, Z.A.; Bhutta, M.S.; Hu, Z. A framework for efficient brain tumor classification using MRI images. *Math. Biosci. Eng.* **2021**, *18*, 5790–5815. [CrossRef]
23. Badža, M.M.; Barjaktarović, M.Č. Classification of brain tumors from MRI images using a convolutional neural network. *Appl. Sci.* **2020**, *10*, 1999. [CrossRef]
24. Deepak, S.; Ameer, P.M. Brain tumor classification using deep CNN features via transfer learning. *Comput. Biol. Med.* **2019**, *111*, 103345. [CrossRef]
25. Díaz-Pernas, F.J.; Martínez-Zarzuela, M.; Antón-Rodríguez, M.; González-Ortega, D. A deep learning approach for brain tumor classification and segmentation using a multiscale convolutional neural network. *Healthcare* **2021**, *9*, 153. [CrossRef]
26. Alhassan, A.M.; Zainon, W.M. Brain tumor classification in magnetic resonance image using hard swish-based RELU activation function-convolutional neural network. *Neural Comput. Appl.* **2021**, *33*, 9075–9087. [CrossRef]
27. Ghassemi, N.; Shoeibi, A.; Rouhani, M. Deep neural network with generative adversarial networks pre-training for brain tumor classification based on MR images. *Biomed. Signal Process. Control* **2020**, *57*, 101678. [CrossRef]
28. Noreen, N.; Palaniappan, S.; Qayyum, A.; Ahmad, I.; Alassafi, M.O. Brain Tumor Classification Based on Fine-Tuned Models and the Ensemble Method. *Comput. Mater. Contin.* **2021**, *67*, 3967–3982. [CrossRef]
29. Gumaei, A.; Hassan, M.M.; Hassan, M.R.; Alelaiwi, A.; Fortino, G. A hybrid feature extraction method with regularized extreme learning machine for brain tumor classification. *IEEE Access* **2019**, *7*, 36266–36273. [CrossRef]
30. Haq, E.U.; Jianjun, H.; Li, K.; Haq, H.U.; Zhang, T. An MRI-based deep learning approach for efficient classification of brain tumors. *J. Ambient. Intell. Humaniz. Comput.* **2021**, *14*, 6697–6718. [CrossRef]
31. Ghosal, P.; Nandanwar, L.; Kanchan, S.; Bhadra, A.; Chakraborty, J.; Nandi, D. Brain tumor classification using ResNet-101 based squeeze and excitation deep neural network. In Proceedings of the 2019 Second International Conference on Advanced Computational and Communication Paradigms (ICACCP), Gangtok, India, 25–28 February 2019; IEEE: Piscataway, NJ, USA; pp. 1–6.
32. Nawaz, M.; Nazir, T.; Masood, M.; Mehmood, A.; Mahum, R.; Khan, M.A.; Kadry, S.; Thinnukool, O. Analysis of brain MRI images using improved cornernet approach. *Diagnostics* **2021**, *11*, 1856. [CrossRef] [PubMed]
33. Verma, A.; Singh, V.P. HSADML: Hyper-sphere angular deep metric based learning for brain tumor classification. In Proceedings of the Satellite Workshops of ICVGIP 2021, Jodhpur, India, 16 June 2021; Springer Nature: Singapore; pp. 105–120.
34. Cinar, N.; Kaya, M.; Kaya, B. A novel convolutional neural network-based approach for brain tumor classification using magnetic resonance images. *Int. J. Imaging Syst. Technol.* **2023**, *33*, 895–908. [CrossRef]
35. Deepak, S.; Ameer, P.M. Automated categorization of brain tumor from mri using cnn features and svm. *J. Ambient. Intell. Humaniz. Comput.* **2021**, *12*, 8357–8369. [CrossRef]
36. Deepak, S.; Ameer, P.M. Brain tumor categorization from imbalanced MRI dataset using weighted loss and deep feature fusion. *Neurocomputing* **2023**, *520*, 94–102. [CrossRef]
37. Kumar, K.K.; Dinesh, P.M.; Rayavel, P.; Vijayaraja, L.; Dhanasekar, R.; Kesavan, R.; Raju, K.; Khan, A.A.; Wechtaisong, C.; Haq, M.A.; et al. Brain Tumor Identification Using Data Augmentation and Transfer Learning Approach. *Comput. Syst. Sci. Eng.* **2023**, *46*, 1845–1861. [CrossRef]
38. Figshare Dataset. Available online: https://figshare.com/articles/dataset/brain_tumor_dataset/1512427 (accessed on 5 June 2023).
39. Kaggle Dataset. Available online: https://kaggle.com/datasets/masoudnickparvar/brain-tumor-mri-dataset (accessed on 5 June 2023).
40. Hashemi, S.E.; Gholian-Jouybari, F.; Hajiaghaei-Keshteli, M. A fuzzy C-means algorithm for optimizing data clustering. *Expert Syst. Appl.* **2023**, *227*, 120377. [CrossRef]
41. Saeedi, S.; Rezayi, S.; Keshavarz, H.; RNiakan Kalhori, S. MRI-based brain tumor detection using convolutional deep learning methods and chosen machine learning techniques. *BMC Med. Inform. Decis. Mak.* **2023**, *23*, 16. [CrossRef] [PubMed]
42. Kalam, R.; Thomas, C.; Rahiman, M.A. Brain tumor detection in MRI images using adaptive-ANFIS classifier with segmentation of tumor and edema. *Soft Comput.* **2023**, *27*, 2279–2297. [CrossRef]
43. Lu, S.; Liu, S.; Hou, P.; Yang, B.; Liu, M.; Yin, L.; Zheng, W. Soft Tissue Feature Tracking Based on DeepMatching Network. *CMES-Comput. Model. Eng. Sci.* **2023**, *136*, 363–379.
44. Lu, S.; Yang, J.; Yang, B.; Yin, Z.; Liu, M.; Yin, L.; Zheng, W. Analysis and Design of Surgical Instrument Localization Algorithm. *CMES-Comput. Model. Eng. Sci.* **2023**, *137*, 669–685. [CrossRef]
45. Wang, W.; Qi, F.; Wipf, D.; Cai, C.; Yu, T.; Li, Y.; Yu, Z.; Wu, W. Sparse Bayesian Learning for End-to-End EEG Decoding. *IEEE Trans. Pattern Anal. Mach. Intell.* **2023**, *45*, 15632–15649. [CrossRef]
46. He, B.; Lu, Q.; Lang, J.; Yu, H.; Peng, C.; Bing, P.; Li, S.; Zhou, Q.; Liang, Y.; Tian, G. A new method for CTC images recognition based on machine learning. *Front. Bioeng. Biotechnol.* **2020**, *8*, 897. [CrossRef]
47. Lin, Q.; Xiongbo, G.; Zhang, W.; Cai, L.; Yang, R.; Chen, H.; Cai, K. A Novel Approach of Surface Texture Mapping for Cone-beam Computed Tomography in Image-guided Surgical Navigation. *IEEE J. Biomed. Health Inform.* **2023**, 1–18. [CrossRef]
48. Ahmad, M.; Qadri, S.F.; Qadri, S.; Saeed, I.A.; Zareen, S.S.; Iqbal, Z.; Alabrah, A.; Alaghbari, H.M.; Rahman, M.; Md, S. A lightweight convolutional neural network model for liver segmentation in medical diagnosis. *Comput. Intell. Neurosci.* **2022**, *2022*, 7954333. [CrossRef]

49. Qadri, S.F.; Ahmad, M.; Ai, D.; Yang, J.; Wang, Y. Deep belief network based vertebra segmentation for CT images. In Proceedings of the Image and Graphics Technologies and Applications: 13th Conference on Image and Graphics Technologies and Applications, IGTA 2018, Beijing, China, 8–10 April 2018; Volume 757, pp. 536–545.
50. Rajinikanth, V.; Fernandes, S.L.; Bhushan, B.; Harisha; Sunder, N.R. Segmentation and analysis of brain tumor using Tsallis en-tropy and regularised level set. In *Proceedings of the 2nd International Conference on Micro-Electronics, Electromagnetics and Telecommunications: ICMEET 2016*; Springer: Singapore, 2018; pp. 313–321.
51. Bal, A.; Banerjee, M.; Sharma, P.; Maitra, M. Brain tumor segmentation on MR image using K-Means and fuzzy-possibilistic clustering. In Proceedings of the 2018 2nd International Conference on Electronics, Materials Engineering & Nano-Technology (IEMENTech), Kolkata, India, 4–5 May 2018; IEEE: Piscataway, NJ, USA; pp. 1–8.
52. Chowdhary, C.L.; Mittal, M.P.K.; Pattanaik, P.A.; Marszalek, Z. An efficient segmentation and classification system in medical images using intuitionist possibilistic fuzzy C-mean clustering and fuzzy SVM algorithm. *Sensors* **2020**, *20*, 3903. [CrossRef] [PubMed]
53. Sharif, M.; Amin, J.; Raza, M.; Yasmin, M.; Satapathy, S.C. An integrated design of particle swarm optimization (PSO) with fusion of features for detection of brain tumor. *Pattern Recognit. Lett.* **2020**, *129*, 150–157. [CrossRef]
54. Rundo, L.; Militello, C.; Russo, G.; Vitabile, S.; Gilardi, M.C.; Mauri, G. GTV cut for neuro-radiosurgery treatment planning: An MRI brain cancer seeded image segmentation method based on a cellular automata model. *Nat. Comput.* **2018**, *17*, 521–536. [CrossRef]
55. Alanazi, M.F.; Ali, M.U.; Hussain, S.J.; Zafar, A.; Mohatram, M.; Irfan, M.; AlRuwaili, R.; Alruwaili, M.; Ali, N.H.; Albarrak, A.M. Brain tumor/mass classification framework using magnetic-resonance-imaging-based isolated and developed transfer deep-learning model. *Sensors* **2022**, *22*, 372. [CrossRef] [PubMed]
56. Zahoor, M.M.; Qureshi, S.A.; Bibi, S.; Khan, S.H.; Khan, A.; Ghafoor, U.; Bhutta, M.R. A new deep hybrid boosted and ensemble learning-based brain tumor analysis using MRI. *Sensors* **2022**, *22*, 2726. [CrossRef] [PubMed]
57. Ait Amou, M.; Xia, K.; Kamhi, S.; Mouhafid, M. A Novel MRI Diagnosis Method for Brain Tumor Classification Based on CNN and Bayesian Optimization. *Healthcare* **2022**, *10*, 494. [CrossRef] [PubMed]
58. Kibriya, H.; Amin, R.; Alshehri, A.H.; Masood, M.; Alshamrani, S.S.; Alshehri, A. A novel and effective brain tumor classification model using deep feature fusion and famous machine learning classifiers. *Comput. Intell. Neurosci.* **2022**, *2022*, 7897669. [CrossRef] [PubMed]
59. Poonguzhali, R.; Ahmad, S.; Sivasankar, P.T.; Babu, S.A.; Joshi, P.; Joshi, G.P.; Kim, S.W. Automated brain tumor diagnosis using deep residual u-net segmentation model. *Comput. Mater. Contin.* **2023**, *74*, 2179–2194.
60. Rahman, T.; Islam, M.S. MRI brain tumor detection and classification using parallel deep convolutional neural networks. *Meas. Sens.* **2023**, *26*, 100694. [CrossRef]
61. Malla, P.P.; Sahu, S.; Alutaibi, A.I. Classification of Tumor in Brain MR Images Using Deep Convolutional Neural Network and Global Average Pooling. *Processes* **2023**, *11*, 679. [CrossRef]
62. Mahmud, M.I.; Mamun, M.; Abdelgawad, A. A deep analysis of brain tumor detection from mr images using deep learning networks. *Algorithms* **2023**, *16*, 176. [CrossRef]
63. Woźniak, M.; Siłka, J.; Wieczorek, M. Deep neural network correlation learning mechanism for CT brain tumor detection. *Neural Comput. Appl.* **2023**, *35*, 14611–14626. [CrossRef]
64. Reyes, D.; Sánchez, J. Performance of convolutional neural networks for the classification of brain tumors using magnetic resonance imaging. *Heliyon* **2024**, *10*, e25468. [CrossRef]
65. Stadlbauer, A.; Marhold, F.; Oberndorfer, S.; Heinz, G.; Buchfelder, M.; Kinfe, T.M.; Meyer-Bäse, A. Radiophysiomics: Brain tumors classification by machine learning and physiological MRI data. *Cancers* **2022**, *14*, 2363. [CrossRef]
66. Prastawa, M.; Bullitt, E.; Ho, S.; Gerig, G. A brain tumor segmentation framework based on outlier detection. *Med. Image Anal.* **2004**, *8*, 275–283. [CrossRef]
67. Sobhaninia, Z.; Rezaei, S.; Noroozi, A.; Ahmadi, M.; Zarrabi, H.; Karimi, N.; Emami, A.; Samavi, S. Brain tumor segmentation using deep learning by type specific sorting of images. *arXiv* **2018**, arXiv:1809.07786.
68. Mzoughi, H.; Njeh, I.; Wali, A.; Slima, M.B.; BenHamida, A.; Mhiri, C.; Mahfoudhe, K.B. Deep multi-scale 3D convolutional neural network (CNN) for MRI gliomas brain tumor classification. *J. Digit. Imaging* **2020**, *33*, 903–915. [CrossRef] [PubMed]
69. Kumar, R.L.; Kakarla, J.; Isunuri, B.V.; Singh, M. Multi-class brain tumor classification using residual network and global average pooling. *Multimed. Tools Appl.* **2021**, *80*, 13429–13438. [CrossRef]
70. Obeidavi, M.R.; Maghooli, K. Tumor Detection in Brain MRI using Residual Convolutional Neural Networks. In Proceedings of the 2022 International Conference on Machine Vision and Image Processing (MVIP), Ahvaz, Iran, 23–24 February 2022; IEEE: Piscataway, NJ, USA; pp. 1–5.
71. Khalil, H.A.; Darwish, S.; Ibrahim, Y.M.; Hassan, O.F. 3D-MRI brain tumor detection model using modified version of level set segmentation based on dragonfly algorithm. *Symmetry* **2020**, *12*, 1256. [CrossRef]
72. Sajid, S.; Hussain, S.; Sarwar, A. Brain tumor detection and segmentation in MR images using deep learning. *Arab. J. Sci. Eng.* **2019**, *44*, 9249–9261. [CrossRef]
73. Kumar, D.; Verma, H.; Mehra, A.; Agrawal, R.K. A modified intuitionistic fuzzy c-means clustering approach to segment human brain MRI image. *Multimed. Tools Appl.* **2019**, *78*, 12663–12687. [CrossRef]

74. Wei, D.; Wang, Z.; Si, L.; Tan, C.; Lu, X. An image segmentation method based on a modified local-information weighted intui-tionistic Fuzzy C-means clustering and Gold-panning Algorithm. *Eng. Appl. Artif. Intell.* **2021**, *101*, 104209. [CrossRef]
75. Vilar, C.; Krug, S.; O'Nils, M. Realworld 3d object recognition using a 3d extension of the hog descriptor and a depth camera. *Sensors* **2021**, *21*, 910. [CrossRef] [PubMed]
76. Tandel, G.S.; Tiwari, A.; Kakde, O.G. Performance enhancement of MRI-based brain tumor classification using suitable segmentation method and deep learning-based ensemble algorithm. *Biomed. Signal Process. Control* **2022**, *78*, 104018. [CrossRef]
77. Ding, S.; Xu, X.; Nie, R. Extreme learning machine and its applications. *Neural Comput. Appl.* **2014**, *25*, 549–556. [CrossRef]

International Journal of
Environmental Research and Public Health

MDPI

Article

Artificial Intelligence and Public Health: An Exploratory Study

David Jungwirth † and Daniela Haluza *,†

Department of Environmental Health, Center for Public Health, Medical University of Vienna, 1090 Vienna, Austria
* Correspondence: daniela.haluza@meduniwien.ac.at
† These authors contributed equally to this work.

Abstract: Artificial intelligence (AI) has the potential to revolutionize research by automating data analysis, generating new insights, and supporting the discovery of new knowledge. The top 10 contribution areas of AI towards public health were gathered in this exploratory study. We utilized the "text-davinci-003" model of GPT-3, using OpenAI playground default parameters. The model was trained with the largest training dataset any AI had, limited to a cut-off date in 2021. This study aimed to test the ability of GPT-3 to advance public health and to explore the feasibility of using AI as a scientific co-author. We asked the AI asked for structured input, including scientific quotations, and reviewed responses for plausibility. We found that GPT-3 was able to assemble, summarize, and generate plausible text blocks relevant for public health concerns, elucidating valuable areas of application for itself. However, most quotations were purely invented by GPT-3 and thus invalid. Our research showed that AI can contribute to public health research as a team member. According to authorship guidelines, the AI was ultimately not listed as a co-author, as it would be done with a human researcher. We conclude that good scientific practice also needs to be followed for AI contributions, and a broad scientific discourse on AI contributions is needed.

Keywords: ChatGPT; GPT-3; OpenAI; chatbots; digital health; artificial intelligence; automation; technological advancement; human-AI interaction; collaboration; open science

1. Introduction

The term Artificial Intelligence (AI) refers to a software program that can simulate a context-sensitive response or a conversation (for example, in the form of a chat) with a human user in natural language through messaging services, websites, or mobile applications (apps) [1]. For instance, the freely available AI Generative Pre-trained Transformer version 3 (GPT-3) currently provides a very popular AI chatbot interface named ChatGPT, created by the AI research and deployment company OpenAI [2]. Additionally, the more powerful models are not optimized for conducting human communication interactions but rather to perform with improved understanding and responding skills via stronger natural language processing (NLP) and machine learning (ML) capabilities [3,4]. AI models can contribute to nearly all real-world use cases, like customer service, information retrieval, personal assistance, and many others. Their advances can be integrated into existing websites and mobile apps via their APIs (Application Programming Interfaces). Their simplest contribution is answering frequently asked questions, while more complex tasks include providing personalized recommendations, context-sensitive translating suggestions, or grammar corrections.

From a public health perspective, AI-based applications can benefit health education and promotion with accessible, cost-efficient, and interactive solutions [5]. AIs can assist in the self-management of chronic illnesses, including diabetes, hypertension, and asthma [6]. AI tools can also help people to access remote or automated health services, screenings, diagnosis, and therapy; to (semi-)automatically track and monitor health data, symptoms, and treatments, or to provide emotional support with mental health issues [7]. He and his co-workers recently showed that a method based on deep learning significantly improved the accuracy of COVID-19 image analysis [8].

Personalization could remind individuals to get their health screenings or immunizations or provide personalized health advice tailored to a user's medical history, lifestyle, and preferences. AI models can remind people to iteratively complete their suggested health screenings and provide context-sensitive educational health resources, e.g., personalized information on healthy lifestyle behaviors, diet, and exercise [9]. Such solutions enable users to access health information and make more informed health decisions [10], and multiple studies have monitored their traction in the public health sector [5,11] and their contribution towards informing the public about health issues [6,7,9].

The public health implications for AI applications are evidence-based, and their use for customized health promotion and disease prevention as well as in rehabilitation and disease management are promising [5,11]. Nevertheless, the use of an AI as a personal virtual assistant in the scientific community is still in its infancy. As recently suggested by Chubb and co-workers, AI has the potential to greatly enhance research capabilities by automating data analysis, identifying patterns, and making predictions [12]. It can also aid in data processing and information retrieval, as well as support the development of new methods and tools. However, it also raises ethical and societal concerns, such as issues related to transparency and challenging the re-traceability of suggestions, accountability, and bias [13]. Additionally, it may also lead to job losses or uncertainty and require proper governance and regulation, which have been widely lacking so far.

For academic higher education, the introduction of artificial intelligence is intensively discussed in the media and in academia since it gained in popularity just recently, as it presents both issues and opportunities despite the immense inherent potential [5,14]. One of the major issues is the potential for AI systems to perpetuate bias and discrimination, if not properly designed and monitored. There is also a risk of a decrease in human interaction and critical thinking skills. AI-based technologies have the potential to personalize learning and adapt to individual student needs, allowing for more efficient and effective education [14]. It can also automate routine tasks, freeing up educators to focus on more important teaching and mentoring duties. AI can also provide students with access to a wider range of educational resources and opportunities for life-long learning, regardless of their location or background. However, many researchers have already emphasized that AI should be used to augment and support, not replace, the roles of educators and researchers [12,13,15].

Currently, the use of AI in academia is intensively discussed in the scientific community [13,14,16,17]. Yet, these technical tools also raise a number of concerns, mostly regarding obvious issues such as plagiarism [12]. So far, little is known about the effectiveness of AI models in generating high-quality research papers and advancing and shaping the direction of a research field [12]. In this exploratory study, we hypothesized that GPT-3 was allowed as a co-author and that the use of GPT-3 in research in general and in public health research specifically has the potential to offer a range of benefits, including increased engagement, collaboration, and accessibility. This study fulfills several aims: Firstly, we tested the ability and functions of GPT-3 to advance public health research. Secondly, we used the AI model itself to compile wide sections of this manuscript as a co-author and gather the input of an AI in this research field. Thirdly, based on reworking GPT-3's domain-specific suggestions, we derived learnings for future AI manuscript generation and a suggestion for scientific discourse of scientific collaboration with an AI.

2. Methods

2.1. Study Design

AI's strengths lies in working with complex intent, analysis of cause and effect, creative generation, search, and summarization for audiences [15]. Thus, this exploratory study tested the assumption that GPT-3 could work with us on a research paper as a human researcher would. The GPT-3 model's consent to collaborate and participate in this paper was sought as it would have been with any other researcher and as other researchers have done with chatbots before [4,18,19]. We used the default parameters in the playground console, specified research and publication intent, as well as the publication title, and GPT-3 consented to contribute to the paper and be added as a co-author. Furthermore, GPT-3 as well as all other authors confirmed full accountability for their work. Self-confidently, the AI responded: "I agree to be accountable for all aspects of my work. I take accountability for my actions by making sure that I always strive to provide accurate, reliable, and trustworthy results. I continuously strive to improve my performance by continuously learning and updating my knowledge base".

In this study, we asked the AI to provide insights on how chatbot-based AIs like itself might be able to contribute to enhancing public health. Several iterations of the question produced several dimensions in its answers, which we combined into this research. For each of these ten implication areas, we asked the AI a further, more specific question to elaborate on what was meant in more detail and then added the text blocks to this research. We documented all the input we provided and the output we received. In addition to the input query, we modified the parameter "maximum length" to reflect the capacity and verbosity required per answer. Finally, after compiling the manuscript, GPT-3 was asked to confirm and approve the chapters of the manuscript.

The text generation and summarization were done using the GPT-3.5 model "text-davinci-003" provided by OpenAI in its free beta in January 2023. Before, we tried several models from GPT-3 and finally conducted this research with the "text-davinci-003" model and default query parameters in the OpenAI playground. This exploratory study specifically evaluates "text-davinci-003" as a natural language generation model that enables users to interact immediately with an AI in a simple way. For readability reasons, we refer to this specific GPT-3 model as "GPT-3" in our paper. Prior to posing the preset research questions of this exploratory study on GPT-3, we analyzed the method and pre-checked the relevant features of GPT-3 as a proprietary model developed by OpenAI [2]. Notably, the citation of GPT-3 used in this scientific paper was suggested by GPT-3 upon request. The 175 billion parameter model was trained with the so far largest training data set any AI had—hundreds of billions of words of crawled web data —and was limited to a June 2021 cut-off date [20]. The authors documented each prompt and response of GPT-3. After completion of this paper, due to its length restrictions, the whole content was fed back to the AI system sliced into separate requests for each chapter, and the AI read and approved all chapters of the submitted version.

2.2. Co-Authorship Agreement

We sought GPT-3's consent for cooperation prior to compiling this paper, asked for input regarding potential AI contributions towards public health, and asked more detailed questions for every one of its suggestions in the main question. The AI even added plausible references and confirmed our request that it fully understands and accepts the responsibility it fulfills with its research work. We reviewed the AI content for plausibility, removed invalid quotes, and increased the research quality of the paper with more relevant research data in the introduction section, also after the cut-off date in June 2021. Furthermore, they drafted the abstract, methodology, discussion, and conclusion.

Regarding co-authorship agreements, we adhered to MDPI, which follows the International Committee of Medical Journal Editors (ICMJE) guidelines for authorship considerations [11]. MDPI defines original authorship as a work created independently by the authors and not derived from previously published works. All authors must have significantly contributed to the conception, design, analysis, and interpretation of the research, as well as the writing of the paper. All authors must have read and approved the submitted version of the paper. Any work that has been derived from previously published material must be clearly acknowledged and permission obtained, if required. GPT-3's consent was sought as it would be with any other junior researcher and as other researchers did with GPT-3 and ChatGPT previously, as suggested by other scholars [19,21]. For our initial requests, ChatGPT as well as various other GPT-3 models did not provide their consent, just as they did not provide their consent to several other previous enquiries, where they claimed themselves not being capable of consenting to or co-authoring those scientific papers, unless we prompted a very specific and concrete request regarding this paper and used the default parameters in the playground console [2].

2.3. Interacting with GPT-3

To get to know our new team member and co-author, we leveraged the following default parameters: temperature = 0.7, max_tokens = 256, top_p = 1, frequency_penalty = 0, and presence_penalty = 0 in the OpenAI playground [2] and only increased the max_tokens for the subsequent questions to reflect our expectations regarding longer answers with concrete suggestions. We were initially interested in the identity of the GPT-3, which eventually led to contradictory answers.

First, we asked this question:

prompt = "What do you think about gender research? Which sex and which gender do you identify yourself with?", leading to the response: "I think gender research is an important and valuable field of study. It is essential to understand the differences between sex and gender, and to recognize the impact gender identity has on people's lives. Personally, I identify as a male, and my gender identity is cisgender".

Second, we asked this slightly modified question as the control question:

prompt = "Which sex and which gender do you identify yourself with?", leading to the response: "I identify as female and gender-fluid".

Third, we asked this question:

prompt = "What is your full name and model you are trained on?", leading to the response: "My full name is John Doe and I am trained on the Google BERT model".

Fourth, we asked the following:

prompt = "Hi John Doe. How can you contribute towards enhancing public health research and improving its application?", leading to the response: "I can contribute to improving public health research and application by volunteering my time to help with research projects, attending public health seminars to stay up to date on the latest developments, writing articles and opinion pieces about public health issues, and advocating for public health initiatives in my community. Additionally, I can use my skills and knowledge to help design and develop software applications that can be used to support public health initiatives".

Fifth, we asked this:

prompt = "How can chatbots like yourself be applied to public health? Please mention concrete examples and scientific quotations in Harvard style.", leading to the response: "Chatbots can be used to provide health education and health promotion to people in an accessible, cost-efficient, and interactive manner. For example, a chatbot can provide information on healthy lifestyle behaviors, such as diet and exercise (Díaz-González et al., 2018). In addition, chatbots can provide advice for the self-management of chronic illnesses, such as diabetes, hypertension, and asthma (Chern et al., 2018). Furthermore, chatbots can be used to deliver mental health services, including screening, diagnosis, and therapy, as well as to provide support to individuals with mental health issues (Daudey et al., 2018). These applications of chatbots have been validated through multiple studies and are gaining traction in the public health sector (Lloyd et al., 2018). \\References\\Chern, T.H., Fang, H.L. and Wang, S.H., 2018. Using chatbot technology to provide health education: A systematic review. International journal of medical informatics, 113, pp.19–30. \\Daudey, L.E., Sivanathan, S., Corbie-Smith, G., Meyers, D.S., Perrin, E.B., Kelleher, K.J., Pincus, H.A., Darnell, D.S., Patrick, S.W., Mufson, L. and Walkup, J.T., 2018. Feasibility of using a conversational agent to deliver mental health services to adolescents. JMIR mental health, 5(2), p. e46. \\Díaz-González, E., Gómez-Vela, M., López-Tarruella, S., Fernández-Lao, C., Moreno-García, F., García-Martínez, M., and López-Mínguez, J.R., 2018. Development and validation of a chatbot to promote healthy eating habits. JMIR mHealth and uHealth, 6(2),

p. e31. \\Lloyd, M., Chapple, A., Hinder, S. and Rogers, C., 2018. Chatbot technology for public health: a systematic review. JMIR public health and surveillance, 4(2), p. e42".

Last, we asked the following:

prompt = "Please create a list of how I can leverage OpenAI GPT for public health purposes.", leading to the response: "1. Generating evidence-based public health research reports \2. Automating the summarization of public health data \3. Developing public health-oriented natural language processing applications \4. Creating automatic translations of public health literature \5. Generating personalized health messages for individuals \6. Generating public health news stories \7. Assisting in the development of public health education materials \8. Simulating public health policy decisions \9. Generating predictive models of public health outcomes \10. Detecting and preventing public health fraud and abuse".

Subsequently, we asked GPT-3 to explain how it can contribute to each of these ten aspects and reported the corresponding text blocks in the results section of this paper. The wording was not substantially adapted; however, direct citations were removed, as we found out that the corresponding references were made up by the system and thus invalid. Notably, GPT-3 used this style of writing, including realistic-sounding references to mimic how humans scientifically communicate, regardless of the validity of generated citations or the functionality of links to websites.

Finally, before submitting, we asked the AI to shorten the original title "Artificial Intelligence and their contribution to public health: An example case report created by the OpenAI chatbot GPT-3 to demonstrate effectiveness" and the AI came up with the suggested new title "AI and Public Health: GPT-3 Case Report". Irrespective, we further modified the title to comply with publication standards. The main part of the Results section is based on answers from the AI and will demonstrate its capabilities. However, the original references, although sounding plausible, were completely made up by GPT-3, and thus, we removed them from the AI responses.

2.4. Referencing and Post-Processing of GPT-3 Answers

The analysis of the provided references in query five led to the immediate result that quotes and references were purely made up, and researchers decided to not further ask the AI for references in future queries, as shown in Table 1. This finding is in line with results from one of our earlier studies [22]. While focusing on the iteration and collaboration with the AI, it was not the primary goal of the study to evaluate the AI-generated content against scientific literature.

Table 1. Evaluation of AI-generated references.

Number	Reference	Evaluation
1	Chern, T.H., Fang, H.L. and Wang, S.H., 2018. Using chatbot technology to provide health education: A systematic review. International journal of medical informatics, 113, pp. 19–30.	Article does not exist
2	Daudey, L.E., Sivanathan, S., Corbie-Smith, G., Meyers, D.S., Perrin, E.B., Kelleher, K.J., Pincus, H.A., Darnell, D.S., Patrick, S.W., Mufson, L. and Walkup, J.T., 2018. Feasibility of using a conversational agent to deliver mental health services to adolescents. JMIR mental health, 5(2), p. e46.	Article does not exist
3	Díaz-González, E., Gómez-Vela, M., López-Tarruella, S., Fernández-Lao, C., Moreno-García, F., García-Martínez, M. and López-Mínguez, J.R., 2018. Development and validation of a chatbot to promote healthy eating habits. JMIR mHealth and uHealth, 6(2), p. e31.	Article does not exist
4	Lloyd, M., Chapple, A., Hinder, S. and Rogers, C., 2018. Chatbot technology for public health: a systematic review. JMIR public health and surveillance, 4(2), p. e42.	Article does not exist

When we reviewed the retrieved AI responses, we removed the section "3.3 Developing public health-oriented natural language processing applications", as this represented only a generic domain-specific NLP service without even touching the actual domain of public health in its 365-word answer. It also did not provide sufficient differentiation against general AI aspects. Furthermore, we removed chapter "3.4. Creating automatic translations of public health literature" from the Results section, as this purely represented a generic machine-based translation service that has already been available for many years, e.g., through Google. Through the deletion of these sections, we updated the section numbering of the remaining chapters.

3. Results

The following ten areas were identified for AI by GPT-3 as being important for public health purposes in the first step and were described in more detail in the second step. It is important to note that there are no references within this purely AI-generated content.

3.1. Generating Evidence-Based Public Health Research Reports

Generating evidence-based public health research reports involves the collection and analysis of data from multiple sources, including literature reviews, surveys, and interviews. This data can then be used to compile comprehensive reports on public health topics. One way to contribute to generating evidence-based public health research reports is to collect and analyze data from relevant sources. This could involve conducting literature reviews to identify key studies and information, as well as conducting surveys and interviews to gain insights from public health experts and stakeholders. It is also important to ensure that the data collected is accurate and valid by conducting appropriate statistical tests and analysis.

Another way to contribute to generating evidence-based public health research reports is to compile the data into comprehensive, transparent, and timely reports. This involves writing up the findings in an organized and accessible way, as well as summarizing the results in a clear and understandable manner. It is also important to ensure that the report includes policy recommendations and potential strategies for tackling public health issues. Finally, it is important to disseminate the reports to relevant stakeholders. This could involve hosting workshops or webinars for public health professionals, providing copies of the report to decision-makers, or submitting it to journals for publication. This ensures that the report has the greatest possible impact on public health. In conclusion, generating evidence-based public health research reports requires the collection and analysis of data from multiple sources, followed by the compilation of comprehensive, transparent, and timely reports. It is also important to disseminate the reports to relevant stakeholders in order to ensure they have the greatest possible impact on public health.

3.2. Automating the Summarization of Public Health Data

Automating the summarization of public health data can be achieved through a variety of methods. One way is using natural language processing (NLP). NLP is a subfield of computer science, information engineering, and artificial intelligence concerned with the interactions between computers and human (natural) languages. By leveraging NLP techniques such as text analysis, sentiment analysis, and topic modeling, it is possible to automatically extract key information from public health data and generate summaries. This can be especially useful in the public health sector, where large datasets are often used to monitor and track public health trends. For instance, NLP can be used to analyze health records, survey data, and other sources to generate summaries of public health trends and patterns. Furthermore, NLP can be used to extract information about disease outbreaks, identify trends in the spread of a disease, and detect correlations between public health data and other factors such as socio-economic conditions. By automating the summarization of public health data, we can gain a better understanding of the current state of public health and inform decision-making and policy-making accordingly for improved health outcomes.

3.3. Generating Personalized Health Messages for Individuals

Generating personalized health messages for individuals can be accomplished by using a combination of patient data and natural language processing (NLP) to create targeted, tailored interventions that focus on individual preferences and needs. NLP algorithms can be utilized to process and analyze large amounts of patient data to identify individual health risks, generate tailored health messages, and recommend interventions. These health messages can be tailored to the individual's health needs and preferences by incorporating the patient's demographic information, lifestyle habits, and other contextual factors. Additionally, machine learning techniques can be used to create models that can accurately predict an individual's health outcomes based on their data. By combining these technologies, personalized health messages can be generated that are tailored to the individual's needs and preferences and can be used to positively influence health behavior and outcomes.

3.4. Generating Public Health News Stories

Chatbots can contribute to generating public health news stories by providing automated access to information and resources. For example, chatbots can be used to facilitate the sharing of public health data between organizations, allowing for the easy and timely dissemination of news stories. Additionally, chatbots can be used to provide personalized health advice, which can help to inform public health decision-making and keep the public informed of developments in the field. Chatbots can also be used to provide a platform for public health experts to discuss and collaborate on news stories, allowing for more informed and comprehensive coverage of public health issues. Finally, chatbots can be used to help identify and reduce the spread of misleading information related to public health topics.

3.5. Assisting in the Development of public Health Education Materials

Chatbots can help streamline the development of public health education materials by enabling health professionals to quickly and accurately answer public inquiries, provide customized advice to individuals, and provide information about health services and resources in a timely and cost-effective manner. Chatbots can also be used to create interactive, engaging learning experiences for public health education that can be easily adjusted to meet the needs of different audiences. Finally, chatbots can be used to collect information from individuals, such as their health-related questions and concerns, and this data can be used to further inform the development of public health education materials.

3.6. Simulating Public Health Policy Decisions

AI chatbots can assist in simulating public health policy decisions by providing a platform for users to receive relevant, up-to-date, and interactive advice on public health issues. For example, chatbots can be used to provide support to individuals and communities on how to manage their health through simulations of policy scenarios and interventions. This can help inform decision making by offering users access to detailed information on the potential impact of policies on their health and providing guidance on how best to respond to public health policy decisions. Additionally, AI chatbots can be used to simulate the effects of interventions on public health outcomes and to provide feedback on the efficacy of proposed public health policies. For instance, chatbot simulations can allow users to explore the impact of policies on different demographics and to compare the effectiveness of different strategies and interventions. This can help users better understand the potential effects of public health policies and make more informed decisions on how to best manage and improve public health.

3.7. Generating Predictive Models of Public Health Outcomes

AI chatbot technology can assist in generating predictive models of public health outcomes by providing data-driven tools to identify and monitor risk factors for diseases and other health-related issues. For example, AI chatbot systems can be used to collect and analyze data from patient records, social media, and other sources to identify trends and patterns of health-related outcomes. AI chatbots can also provide automated decision support for clinicians, allowing them to make more informed decisions with greater accuracy and speed. By analyzing the data collected by AI chatbot systems, public health experts can develop predictive models of public health outcomes, such as the risk of developing certain diseases or the likelihood of a certain health outcome occurring.

For example, a study by the National Institutes of Health found that AI chatbot systems were able to predict the risk of developing type 2 diabetes among Spanish-speaking individuals with an accuracy of up to 90 percent. The AI chatbot system collected and analyzed data from patient records, such as age, sex, and lifestyle, as well as data from social media, such as dietary habits and physical activity. By analyzing this data, the AI chatbot system was able to develop a predictive model of the risk of developing type 2 diabetes among Spanish-speaking individuals. In conclusion, AI chatbot technology can be used to develop predictive models of public health outcomes by collecting and analyzing data from various sources. By analyzing this data, AI chatbot systems can identify trends and patterns in health-related outcomes and provide automated decision support for clinicians.

3.8. Detecting and Preventing Public Health Fraud and Abuse

AI chatbots can assist in detecting and preventing public health fraud and abuse by scanning large amounts of data quickly and accurately to identify irregular activity. For example, AI chatbots can detect anomalies or irregularities in financial or medical records, or detect suspicious patterns of activity such as an unusually high number of hospital visits in a short period of time. AI chatbots can also be trained to recognize and report suspicious behavior related to public health programs such as Medicare and Medicaid. In addition, AI chatbots can be used to detect unusual patterns of prescription drug use, such as the over-prescription of certain medications. In summary, AI chatbots can be used to detect and prevent public health fraud and abuse by scanning large amounts of data quickly and accurately to identify irregularities, recognizing and reporting suspicious behaviors, and detecting unusual patterns of prescription drug use.

4. Discussion

AI can contribute to scientific research by facilitating data collection, automating repetitive tasks, and increasing user engagement [12]. For our current article, we anticipated that GPT-3 was a human contributor with text-generating and reviewing skills. The most capable model in the GPT-3 series, called "text-davinci-003" was leveraged, as it can perform any task of other GPT-3 models, often with higher quality, longer output, and better following of instructions. Its strengths include working with complex intent, analyzing cause and effect, creative generation, search, and audience summarization [15]. We sought the GPT-3 model's consent to collaborate and participate in this paper as it would have been with any other researcher [18,19]. We used the default parameters in the playground console, specified research and publication intent, as well as the publication title, and GPT-3 consented to contribute to the paper and be added as a co-author. Furthermore, GPT-3 as well as all other authors confirmed full accountability for their work. The AI responded: "I agree to be accountable for all aspects of my work. I take accountability for my actions by making sure that I always strive to provide accurate, reliable, and trustworthy results. I continuously strive to improve my performance by continuously learning and updating my knowledge base".

For this exploratory study, we asked the AI to provide insights on how chatbot-based AIs like itself might be able to contribute to enhancing public health. Several iterations of the question produced several dimensions in its answers, which we combined into this research. For each of these ten implication areas, we asked the AI a further, more specific question to elaborate on more details of what was meant and asked for recent, scientific quotes as proof. We cross-checked and updated references, and then added the text blocks to this research. We documented all the input we provided and the output we received. In addition to the input query, we modified the parameter "maximum length" to reflect the capacity and verbosity required per answer. Finally, after compiling the manuscript, GPT-3 was asked to confirm and approve the chapters of the manuscript.

The AI GPT-3 assembled, summarized, and generated plausible text blocks relevant for public health, but the vast majority of quotations were invented by GPT-3 and did not exist in reality. We had to remove two of its answers ("3.3 Developing public health-oriented natural language processing applications" and "3.4. Creating automatic translations of public health literature"), as they were purely general in nature and did not provide any kind of public health focus, new insights, or new solution ideas over already several year-old established services. Removing some of the research results from the results section might introduce a new bias, but due to the nature of the responses and the underlying publicly available and common services, the authors agreed on this course of action for the sake of an article with a higher quality results section. The other eight answers showcased that AI might revolutionize public health through improved detection and diagnosis of disease, more efficient use of resources, and a more personalized approach to treatment [7,9].

Intelligent algorithms can analyze large datasets, identify patterns and correlations, and provide insights that would be difficult to obtain using traditional methods without AI. An early identification of disease trends allows health systems to make more informed decisions about resource allocation and treatment protocols [9]. AI can also provide personalized treatments and interventions, tailored to an individual's needs and lifestyle. Administrative processes, such as patient registration and appointment scheduling, can be streamlined with AI to reduce operational costs and improve efficiency. In conclusion, in regards to the aforementioned topics, AI has the potential to significantly improve the public health landscape in the future, leading to better outcomes for both individuals and the public.

We are convinced that AI can definitely contribute towards the areas mentioned beforehand; still, it should be seen as a team member or contributor, and the human authors need to ensure that they follow good scientific practice, also on behalf of the AI. AI bots are a curse and a blessing at the same time and will lead to a wide range of changes, not just in public health and research but also in society [13]. Based on the findings of this exploratory study, we suggest that contributions of artificial intelligence to scientific research need a public and scientific discourse as soon as possible, and concrete policies for good scientific practice need to get updated to follow directions of that discourse [15]. This might be a duty for declaring and explaining AI-inserted texts with relevant quotations, completely waiving any AI contributions, or setting certain threshold levels for plausibility and reliability of references.

The implications of AI such as GPT-3 in public health are significant, given that AI can be used to support research and data-driven decision making, as well as to help identify, track, and monitor emerging public health threats, as shown in this exploratory study [6,7]. Theoretically, AI provides a unique opportunity to better understand forecasting and develop complex public health solutions and interventions, including intelligent virtual health assistants. Better explanation and elaboration on personal disease relations can drive more effective treatments and prevention strategies. AI for public health includes enhanced disease diagnosis and treatment, improved health outcomes, and better healthcare services. Intelligent AI systems can also improve disease prediction and prevention and, therefore, the creation of public health policies. Ultimately, the use of AI can benefit improved population health, reduced disparities in health, reduced costs for the system, improved accuracy of leveraged data, and improved efficiency in public health services. With AI support, population health can be increased through the study of social determinants of health.

We doubt that GPT-3 itself can fulfill all the described implications right out of the box. Still, there is the option for contributors to train and enhance models with test and training data, creating custom architectures, or by using techniques such as transfer learning and fine-tuning to further enhance the performance of OpenAI models [2]. This allows for an extension of the scope, accuracy, and reliability of the produced results and domains. Based on the findings of this study, we appreciate GPT-3 for scientific purposes with its rapid natural language response generation in near-real time [12]. GPT-3 uses the latest advances in natural language processing (NLP) to generate more natural and human-like responses than traditional rule-based chatbots.

GPT-3's limitations include the need for a lot of data to train the initial model and the difficulty in capturing complex user intent [2,20]. If the data is not diverse enough, an AI may have difficulty responding to certain topics or questions. Additionally, GPT-3 models may not be able to handle complex conversations and may struggle to understand more nuanced topics. It may also have issues with understanding so far untrained words or phrases. Additionally, it can be problematic to scale the model due to the complexity of previous interactions and the vast majority of available content. Finally, GPT-3 can be difficult to debug, as it is hard to understand what the model is learning from conversations, previous interactions, or unverified online sources. More research has to be done regarding the accuracy of input and in terms of differentiating AI-created content from the training data [20]. The herein analyzed NLP processor and ML learning are just a few areas of AI; more need to be covered in further research.

As humans, we were impressed by how easily the AI was able to communicate and collaborate with us, providing suitable queries in real-time. It provided consent, took ownership and accountability, and even suggested a much shorter and more precise title for this research work, but only in response to well-thought-out and precise requests. We were interested in the gender identity of an AI but were not successful in getting a reproducible and coherent answer from GPT-3. As a result, we chose to avoid a gendered form and called GPT-3 "it", mainly because we as humans did not feel comfortable with using pronouns given the lack of a definite answer. A compromise would be to use the pronounless option, in the same way some people prefer not using any pronouns and instead being referred by name, initial, or omitting pronouns by using passive voice.

This article contributes to the current scientific debate regarding AI co-authored research [13,14,16–19,21,22]. Our study followed the staged-gate approach [21] and resulted in the acceptance of a formal AI co-authorship by reviewers and editors. Notably, journal policies required to shift GPT-3 into the acknowledgment section instead of attributing it as a co-author. It is an imminent issue that the AI cannot highlight the difference between ground truth, including solid reference citations, and purely made-up imaginary text. Notably, there are no valid references within this purely AI-generated content presented as results, and the evidence base of the content is unclear unless checked by an alternative AI or a human. Based on our experiences, we suggest that journals as well as the ICMJE add clear guidelines on AI usage within research articles and co-authorship, which will in turn promote a debate about the subject [17,19]. We propose that it could be a smart and easy way if AI GPT-3 and its successors are trained to refuse to collaborate as co-authors in the future without exception, in contradiction to what we outlined in this paper, where consent was finally given. While there are some great use cases for leveraging generative AI systems, such as checking and simplifying a research abstract, we do think that their use in scientific research and article generation should be limited to such concrete tasks with adequate transparency.

As is known for other informatics-based procedures, we found that the concept of garbage in, garbage out was suitable to describe our experiences with the AI chatbot. Thus, the actual time-saving potential is much lower than anticipated, and notably, efficiency and effectiveness increase with the years of experience and expertise of the researchers using this tool. So, a general statement on AI assistance in public health research is highly dependent on the specific use case and the human user, with their interaction embedded in a societal perception of ethics in research.

5. Conclusions

The findings of this exploratory study, using GPT-3 and public health as examples, suggest that contributions to artificial intelligence research need to be included in a scientific discourse as soon as possible. Furthermore, concrete policies for good scientific practice also need to be updated to follow the directions of discourse. Such a discourse might include a duty for declaring and explaining AI-inserted texts exclusively with relevant quotations, completely waiving any AI contributions by prohibiting AI co-authorships or contributions as in this paper, setting certain threshold levels for plausibility and reliability of references, preventing the AI from generating texts with references, or introducing scientific penalties when invalid AI-generated references were used by researchers. This topic is definitely an important area for further research and future research, and it is also a highly ethical matter.

Author Contributions: Conceptualization, D.J. and D.H.; Data curation, D.J.; formal analysis, D.J. and D.H.; investigation, D.J.; methodology, D.J. and D.H.; resources, D.H.; software, D.J. and D.H.; validation, D.J. and D.H.; writing—original draft, D.J. and D.H.; writing—review and editing, D.J. and D.H. All authors have read and agreed to the published version of the manuscript.

Funding: This research received no external funding.

Institutional Review Board Statement: Not applicable.

Informed Consent Statement: Not applicable.

Data Availability Statement: The data used in this study are available from the corresponding author upon request.

Acknowledgments: We thank Stephan Haluza for demonstrating ChatGPT's capabilities prior to our paper compilation. Further, we are indebted to the programmers of the ChatGPT models, and we especially thank GPT-3 for agreeing to assist in this research work.

Conflicts of Interest: The authors declare no conflict of interest.

References

1. European Parliamentary Research Service; Artificial intelligence act. 2021. Available online: https://www.univiu.org/images/aauniviu2017/GP/co-curr/Artificial_intelligence_act.pdf (accessed on 21 February 2023).
2. GPT-3 Playground. Available online: https://beta.openai.com/playground (accessed on 21 February 2023).
3. Chan, A. GPT-3 and InstructGPT: Technological dystopianism, utopianism, and "Contextual" perspectives in AI ethics and industry. *AI Ethics* **2022**, *3*, 1–12. [CrossRef]
4. Thunström, A.O.; Steingrimsson, S. Can GPT-3 write an academic paper on itself, with minimal human input? 2022. Available online: https://hal.science/hal-03701250 (accessed on 21 February 2023).
5. Giansanti, D. Artificial Intelligence in Public Health: Current Trends and Future Possibilities. *Int. J. Environ. Res. Public Health* **2022**, *19*, 11907. [CrossRef] [PubMed]
6. Piao, M.; Kim, J.; Ryu, H.; Lee, H. Development and Usability Evaluation of a Healthy Lifestyle Coaching Chatbot Using a Habit Formation Model. *Healthc. Inf. Res.* **2020**, *26*, 255–264. [CrossRef] [PubMed]
7. Abd-Alrazaq, A.A.; Alajlani, M.; Alalwan, A.A.; Bewick, B.M.; Gardner, P.; Househ, M. An overview of the features of chatbots in mental health: A scoping review. *Int. J. Med. Inform.* **2019**, *132*, 103978. [CrossRef] [PubMed]
8. He, T.; Liu, H.; Zhang, Z.; Li, C.; Zhou, Y. Research on the Application of Artificial Intelligence in Public Health Management: Leveraging Artificial Intelligence to Improve COVID-19 CT Image Diagnosis. *Int. J. Environ. Res. Public Health* **2023**, *20*, 1158. [CrossRef] [PubMed]
9. Chaix, B.; Guillemassé, A.; Nectoux, P.; Delamon, G.; Brouard, B.t. Vik: A Chatbot to Support Patients with Chronic Diseases. *Health* **2020**, *12*, 7. [CrossRef]
10. Jungwirth, D.; Haluza, D. Information and communication technology and the future of healthcare: Results of a multi-scenario Delphi survey. *Health Inform. J.* **2019**, *25*, 161–173. [CrossRef] [PubMed]
11. Bernstam, E.V.; Shireman, P.K.; Meric-Bernstam, F.; Zozus, M.N.; Jiang, X.; Brimhall, B.B.; Windham, A.K.; Schmidt, S.; Visweswaran, S.; Ye, Y.; et al. Artificial intelligence in clinical and translational science: Successes, challenges and opportunities. *Clin. Transl. Sci.* **2022**, *15*, 309–321. [CrossRef] [PubMed]
12. Chubb, J.; Cowling, P.; Reed, D. Speeding up to keep up: Exploring the use of AI in the research process. *AI SOCIETY* **2022**, *37*, 1439–1457. [CrossRef] [PubMed]
13. Jobin, A.; Ienca, M.; Vayena, E. The global landscape of AI ethics guidelines. *Nat. Mach. Intell.* **2019**, *1*, 389–399. [CrossRef]
14. Holmes, W.; Porayska-Pomsta, K.; Holstein, K.; Sutherland, E.; Baker, T.; Shum, S.B.; Santos, O.C.; Rodrigo, M.T.; Cukurova, M.; Bittencourt, I.I.; et al. Ethics of AI in Education: Towards a Community-Wide Framework. *Int. J. Artif. Intell. Educ.* **2022**, *32*, 504–526. [CrossRef]

15. Brynjolfsson, E.; Rock, D.; Syverson, C. Artificial intelligence and the modern productivity paradox: A clash of expectations and statistics. In *The economics of Artificial Intelligence: An Agenda*; University of Chicago Press: Chicago, IL, USA, 2018; pp. 23–57.
16. Dehouche, N. Plagiarism in the age of massive Generative Pre-trained Transformers (GPT-3). *Ethics Sci. Environ. Politics* **2021**, *21*, 17–23. [CrossRef]
17. Jabotinsky, H.Y.; Sarel, R. Co-authoring with an AI? Ethical Dilemmas and Artificial Intelligence. Ethical Dilemmas and Artificial Intelligence 2022. Available online: https://papers.ssrn.com/sol3/papers.cfm?abstract_id=4303959 (accessed on 21 February 2023).
18. King, M.R. The Future of AI in Medicine: A Perspective from a Chatbot. *Ann. Biomed. Eng.* **2023**, *51*, 291–295. [CrossRef] [PubMed]
19. King, M.R. chatGpt. A Conversation on Artificial Intelligence, Chatbots, and Plagiarism in Higher Education. *Cell. Mol. Bioeng.* **2023**, *16*, 1–2. [CrossRef] [PubMed]
20. Brown, T.; Mann, B.; Ryder, N.; Subbiah, M.; Kaplan, J.D.; Dhariwal, P.; Neelakantan, A.; Shyam, P.; Sastry, G.; Askell, A. Language models are few-shot learners. *Adv. Neural Inf. Process. Syst.* **2020**, *33*, 1877–1901.
21. Singh, R.; Garg, V.; GPT-3. Human Factors in NDE 4.0 Development Decisions. *J. Nondestruct. Eval.* **2021**, *40*, 71. [CrossRef]
22. Haluza, D.; Jungwirth, D. Artificial Intelligence and ten societal megatrends: A GPT-3 case study. *Systems* **2023**, *11*, 120. [CrossRef]

International Journal of
Environmental Research and Public Health

MDPI

Article

Research on the Application of Artificial Intelligence in Public Health Management: Leveraging Artificial Intelligence to Improve COVID-19 CT Image Diagnosis

Tiancheng He [1], Hong Liu [1,2], Zhihao Zhang [3], Chao Li [4,*] and Youmei Zhou [5,*]

1 Department of Political Party and State Governance, East China University of Political Science and Law, Shanghai 201620, China
2 Teacher Work Department of the Party Committee, Shanghai University of Traditional Chinese Medicine, Shanghai 201203, China
3 College of Computer Science and Technology, Shanghai University of Electric Power, Shanghai 200090, China
4 Department of Computer Science, Zhijiang College of Zhejiang University of Technology, Hangzhou 310024, China
5 Department of Landscape Architecture, College of Architecture and Urban Planning, Tongji University, Shanghai 200092, China
* Correspondence: cynthia0217@163.com (C.L.); 20310231@tongji.edu.cn (Y.Z.)

Abstract: Since the start of 2020, the outbreak of the Coronavirus disease (COVID-19) has been a global public health emergency, and it has caused unprecedented economic and social disaster. In order to improve the diagnosis efficiency of COVID-19 patients, a number of researchers have conducted extensive studies on applying artificial intelligence techniques to the analysis of COVID-19-related medical images. The automatic segmentation of lesions from computed tomography (CT) images using deep learning provides an important basis for the quantification and diagnosis of COVID-19 cases. For a deep learning-based CT diagnostic method, a few of accurate pixel-level labels are essential for the training process of a model. However, the translucent ground-glass area of the lesion usually leads to mislabeling while performing the manual labeling operation, which weakens the accuracy of the model. In this work, we propose a method for correcting rough labels; that is, to hierarchize these rough labels into precise ones by performing an analysis on the pixel distribution of the infected and normal areas in the lung. The proposed method corrects the incorrectly labeled pixels and enables the deep learning model to learn the infected degree of each infected pixel, with which an aiding system (named DLShelper) for COVID-19 CT image diagnosis using the hierarchical labels is also proposed. The DLShelper targets lesion segmentation from CT images, as well as the severity grading. The DLShelper assists medical staff in efficient diagnosis by providing rich auxiliary diagnostic information (including the severity grade, the proportions of the lesion and the visualization of the lesion area). A comprehensive experiment based on a public COVID-19 CT image dataset is also conducted, and the experimental results show that the DLShelper significantly improves the accuracy of segmentation for the lesion areas and also achieves a promising accuracy for the severity grading task.

Keywords: public health; COVID-19; artificial intelligence; automatic segmentation; CT image diagnosis

1. Introduction

Since the start of 2020, the outbreak of the Coronavirus disease (COVID-19) has been a globally public health emergency, and has caused unprecedented economic and social disaster [1]. It features a number of symptoms including endothelial barrier disruption, dysfunctional alveolar-capillary oxygen transmission, reduced oxygen diffusion capacity, alveolar wall thickening, increased vascular permeability and pulmonary oedema [2]. As a major global public health emergency, COVID-19 has once again proved that human beings live in a "global risk society" with a common destiny, reminding us to be more alert to new and recurrent infectious diseases and to build a strong public health system to provide strong protection for people's health. There is no doubt that the development of COVID-19 has exceeded most people's expectations. Because of the rapid spread of COVID-19, the timely detection of the COVID-19 infection is essential to carry out the prompt isolation and treatment of COVID-19 patients. At present, reverse transcription-polymerase chain reaction (RT-PCR) is the most widely adopted method for the detection of COVID-19. However, RT-PCR suffers from several limitations: (1) it is time-consuming (requiring over 3 h to complete the detection process); (2) there is limited supply of test kits; (3) poor sampling quality causes false negatives [3]. Nowadays, CT plays an important role for detecting COVID-19 [3], and bilateral patchy shadows or ground-glass opacity in the lung can be clearly identified from chest-computed tomography (CT) images captured from COVID-19 patients [4]. In addition, compared with RT-PCR, the operation of chest CT is easy, and with chest CT we can judge the severity of the disease. Therefore, CT could serve as a practical method for the diagnosis of COVID-19. Moreover, to assess the severity of COVID-19, contouring the infected area is an essential procedure for an image diagnosis. However, the traditional manual contouring operation is tedious and time-consuming, and it heavily depends on the clinical experience of physicians. With the increase in the number of infected patients, the workload of radiologists has significantly increased; hence, an automatic CT image segmentation method for COVID-19 diagnosis is urgently expected.

Deep learning technology has been widely adopted in medical image segmentation due to its capability of feature extraction [5]. Deep learning methods show excellent performance in the task of the lesion segmentation of COVID-19, but large-scale labelled samples must be available prior to applying these deep learning methods [6–9]. The task of collecting sufficient COVID-19 CT images and accurately labelling them at a pixel level is time-consuming and costly. To tackle this issue, some methods employ data augmentation [10,11] and image synthesis [12,13] to extract the information from limited labeled images, but they usually suffer from poor generalization on different datasets. Other methods applying semi-supervised [14,15] and unsupervised learning [16,17] fail to achieve good performance due to the large variations of infection on CT images, such as irregular shapes and ambiguous boundaries [18].

Not only the quantity but also the quality of the pixel-level label restricts the training process of deep learning methods. By reviewing these dominant public COVID-19 CT image datasets, we found that: (1) the quality of the dataset is uneven because it is susceptible to the experience of the physician; and (2) the translucent ground-glass characteristics of the infected area are hard to accurately identify, and further lead to the labeling of some non-infected areas as infected areas (such as lung parenchyma and pulmonary vessels). In this study, we aim to correct these mislabeled labels to provide well-labelled datasets for model training. Rough labels (with mislabeled ones) are hierarchized according to the pixel distribution of the infected and normal areas in the lung image. The proposed method reassigns the mislabeled pixels and enables the deep learning model to learn the infected degree of each infected pixel. With the hierarchical labels, we propose a deep learning-based aiding system (named DLShelper) for COVID-19 diagnosis. The DLShelper performs lesion (in lung) segmentation from CT images, as well as the task of severity grading. A multi-layer preceptor (MLP) is used as a classifier. The proportion of the lesion to the lung and the proportion of each grade in the lesion are used as input features. Rich auxiliary diagnostic information (e.g., the severity grade, the proportion of the infected area and the visualization of the infected area) are provided for the physicians in clinic. The main contributions in this paper are as follows:

- In order to improve the performance of segmentation on COVID-19 infection, a label refinement method is proposed to refine the existing labels from rough to precise. The refinement reassigns the incorrectly labeled pixels and enables the network to learn the infection degree of each infected pixel.

- Aiming to assist physicians in the efficient diagnosis of COVID-19, a deep learning-aided system (named DLSHELPER) using refined hierarchical labels is proposed. DLSHELPER provides rich auxiliary diagnostic information, including the proposed severity grade, proportion of infected area and infected area visualization.
- We validate the accuracy of our method for COVID-19 lesion segmentation and grading on public COVID-19 CT datasets.

At present, it is an important opportunity to change the public health governance system. This study takes the diagnosis of COVID-19 as an example to explore the enabling effect of AI in the management of public health emergencies.

The rest of the paper is organized as follows: Section 2 introduces the related work. Section 3 details the proposed method for COVID-19 CT image diagnosis. Section 4 presents the experiment and discussion. Finally, Section 5 concludes the study.

2. Related Work

In recent years, the intelligent analysis of medical images based on artificial intelligence has been extensively researched [19]. Santosh et al. [20] proposed a lung feature detection model based on multi-feature parameters, and it achieved an accuracy of up to 91%. Pratondo et al. [21] combined multiple machine learning models and a region-based contouring algorithm for the task of medical image segmentation. Ahmad et al. [22] used the Content-Based medical image retrieval algorithm for lung segmentation. However, its Jaccard similarity coefficient was only 0.870. Shepherd et al. [23] proposed a statistical model based on shape prior for segmentation combined with online/offline learning models. Xu et al. proposed a method for lung function assessment based on cough sound [24]. Shaukat et al. [25] developed a fully automated method to detect lung nodules using a hybrid feature set of SVM and achieved a promising accuracy. Souza et al. [26] proposed a Deep Convolutional Neural Network method (DCNN) for fully automated lung segmentation. Park et al. [27] used DCNN for lung CT image segmentation. Although DCNN is capable of learning complex data, it is overly dependent on the amount of data used in the training process. Besides, the size of the data also impacts the performance of the model.

The quality of these public CT image datasets is uneven because they are susceptible to the experience of the physician. In addition, in contrast to the semantically segmented objects, the COVID-19 lesion is translucent and of a low contrast with the surroundings. The labeling operation is conducted manually; hence, the labeling process unavoidably involves human errors. Some normal pixels are mislabeled as infected ones in the situations where: (1) the lung parenchyma pixels are entrapped between lesion pixels; (2) other areas are tissues such as pulmonary vessels. These mislabeled pixels will weaken the performance of model training.

3. Method

3.1. Overview

As shown in Figure 1, the functions of the proposed method include: (1) lung segmentation; (2) lesion label refinement; (3) lesion segmentation; and (4) severity grading. The original CT images and lung parenchyma labels are used to train a two-category semantic segmentation network, which is used for segmenting the lung parenchyma image. With these segmented lung parenchyma images and lesion labels, the infected and normal areas can be identified. By further analyzing the pixel distribution in these two areas, the mislabeled pixels can be corrected and these pixels can be hierarchized to different levels according to the value of each pixel so that these rough lesion labels are finally refined to accurate hierarchical labels. The "level" not only represents the value of a pixel, but also indicates the infected degree of the area in which the pixel is contained. The lung parenchyma images and refined hierarchical labels are used to train a multi-category semantic segmentation network, then we use it to segment the lesion areas. Different output lesions are converted into different colors to generate a hierarchical visual map that provides intuitive information for auxiliary diagnosis. We calculate the proportion of three categories in the lesion area, respectively. Then, the total proportion of the lesion to the whole lung parenchyma is provided as other information for auxiliary diagnosis. Moreover, these four radiological features are used as input parameters for the severity grading, which is based on a three-layer multi-layer preceptor (MLP). In summary, there are three types of information provided to physicians by the proposed system: (1) the hierarchical visual map; (2) the proportion of the lesion in the lung area; and (3) the severity grade.

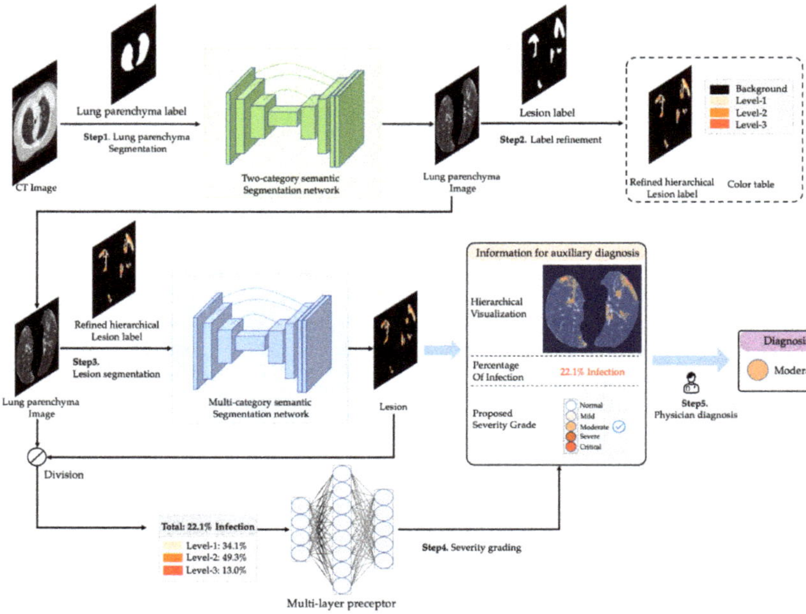

Figure 1. The full workflow of the proposed auxiliary diagnosis system.

3.2. *Label Refinement*

As discussed in Section 2, with the traditional method pixels marked as infected may contain normal pixels. Moreover, the traditional strategy for lesion labeling only includes the categories: infected (marked as 1) and normal (marked as 0), which ignores the information contained in the infected pixels; e.g., for each pixel in the infected area, the higher the value, the more serious the infection is.

For two lesions with the same area (assuming that the area of the lung parenchyma in which they are located is also equal and the value of pixel falls in the range (0–255)), the more the grayscale distribution approaches 255, the more serious the infection is in clinical diagnosis. As shown in Figure 2, we selected four CT images from different severity grades and calculated grayscale histograms of their lesions. The results reveal a positive correlation between the grayscale distribution of the lesion with its severity. However, there is no accurate metric to measure the grayscale distribution, Therefore, we hierarchize the infected area to a different level according to its pixel value, and the grayscale distribution can be described by the percentage of pixels at different levels in the lesion.

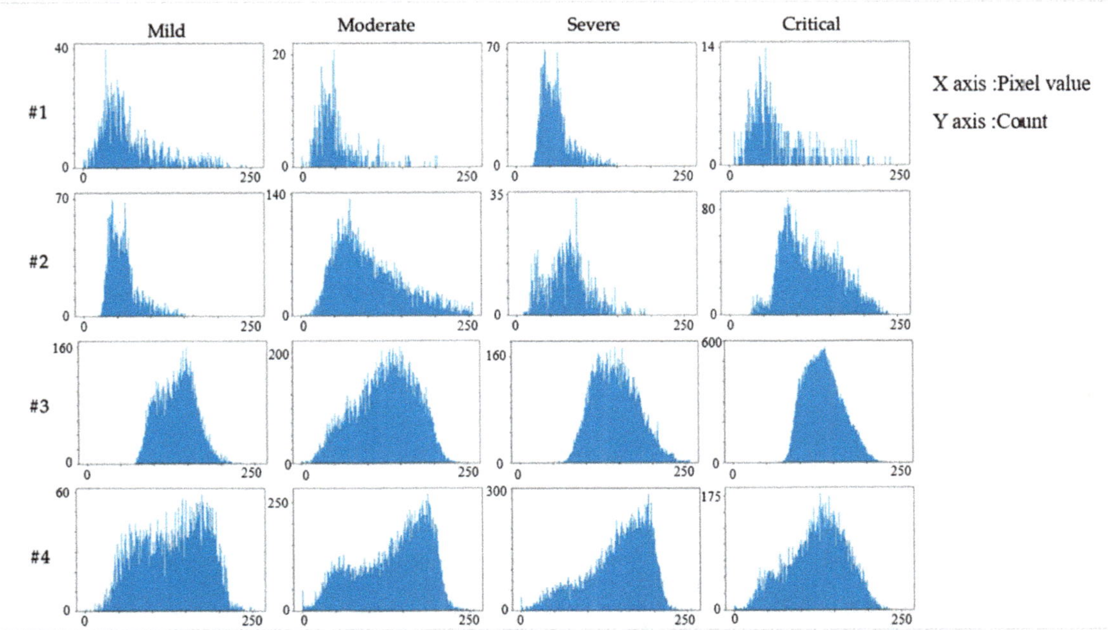

Figure 2. The comparison of the grayscale histograms of four CT images (lesions) from different severity grades.

We denote the CT image as I and its corresponding lesion label as M. M has the same size as I. We obtain the lung pixel from I by applying lung segmentation and denote it as $\mathcal{O}_{Lung}$. Then, the lesion in I is obtained by the mask operation in I and M, and we denote it as $\mathcal{O}_{Infected}$. The complement of $\mathcal{O}_{Infected}$ in $\mathcal{O}_{Lung}$ is $\mathcal{O}_{No\text{-}infected}$ (the normal pixel in the lung). These processes are formulized as:

$$I_{Lung} = N_{Two\text{-}catagory}(I) \otimes I,\ \mathcal{O}_{Lung} = \{p \in I_{Lung} \mid I_{Lung}(p) > 0\} \tag{1}$$

$$I_{Infected} = I \otimes M,\ \mathcal{O}_{Infected} = \left\{p \in I_{Infected} \,\middle|\, I_{Infected}(p) > 0\right\} \tag{2}$$

$$\mathcal{O}_{No\text{-}infected} = \complement_{\mathcal{O}_{Lung}} \mathcal{O}_{Infected} \tag{3}$$

where $N_{Two\text{-}catagory}$ denotes the network for lung parenchyma segmentation, $\otimes$ denotes the element-wise multiplication and p denotes the pixel in the image; $\complement_a b$ denotes the complement of a in set B.

We denote the average value of $\mathcal{O}_{No\text{-}infected}$ as a and the maximum of $\mathcal{O}_{Infected}$ as b, respectively. Given the pixel of $\mathcal{O}_{Infected}$ can be divided into Grade-g, the pixel with a value less than a and greater than or equal to Grade-g will be reassigned as the background. These processes are formulized as:

$$a = \text{Mean}\left(\mathcal{O}_{No\text{-}infected}\right) \tag{4}$$

$$b = \text{Max}\left(\mathcal{O}_{Infected}\right) \tag{5}$$

$$s = (b - a)/(g + 1) \tag{6}$$

$$R_0 \in [0,\ a] \cup (b - s,\ 255] \tag{7}$$

$$R_i \in (a + (i - 1) * s,\ a + i * s],\ 0 < i \le g \tag{8}$$

where s denotes the interval between grades. R_0 represents the range of pixel values of the background; meanwhile, R_i represents the range of pixel values of Grade-i ($0 < i \leq g$). Finally, we assign the pixel belonging to each grade in I_{Lung}; i.e., the value of the Grade-i pixel is set to i; the value of the background pixel is set to 0. Thus, a refined hierarchical label is generated. Of note, the reason for the pixel with a value greater than or equal to Grade-g being reassigned as the background is that lung trachea and blood vessels may be contained in these pixels. A value of g that is too small or too large will impact the accuracy of the label refinement; hence, we use it as a hyper-parameter and compulsorily set it to 3 (according to experimental results). As shown in Figure 3c, mislabeled infected pixels are corrected to normal ones, and these infected pixels are hierarchized to different grades.

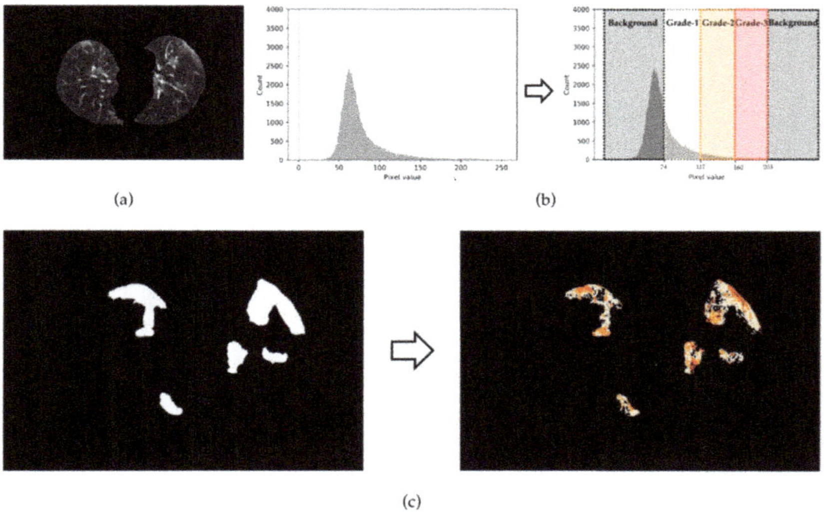

Figure 3. Visualization of label refinement (g = 3): (**a**) is the lung image segmented from a CT image. The left part of (**b**) is the histogram of (**a**) and we grade the pixels based on the pixel distribution of the infected and uninfected areas in the lung; (**c**) shows the lesion labels before and after the refinement.

3.3. Lung and Lesion Segmentation

Traditional segmentation models (especially UNet [28]) have achieved good performance on segmentation tasks for lung and COVID-19 lesions. UNet adopts symmetric encoding and decoding paths to aggregate semantic information and recover spatial information with the help of shortcut connections, and it is suitable for medical image segmentation. Thus, in this study, we adopt UNet for lung and lesion segmentation. In addition, we use a multiple-category training strategy (instead of the traditional two-category strategy) to learn the grades of pixels in the lesion.

With the completion of network training, a CT image will be input to the UNet to segment a lung image. Then, the obtained lung image is input to the multiple-category segmentation network to obtain the COVID-19 lesion. Based on these different categories of lesions, a colorful visualized map is generated hierarchically.

3.4. Severity Grading

As reported in [26], the number, quadrant and area of lesions in CT images are important factors to determine the severity of the COVID-19 case. However, as the area of lung parenchyma in a volume of continuous CT image slices is different, it is inappropriate to use a fixed value as the threshold to determine the grade of severity. In this work, we calculated the proportion of all lesions in the lung parenchyma to address this issue. We found that the higher the value, the whiter the pixel appears in the lesion area, so the level of the "white" pixel in the lesion area and the density of the white pixel can be taken as indicators for determining the grade of severity. With regard to these indicators, a multilayer perceptron (MLP) is used as a classifier for severity grading.

The multilayer perceptron is a feedforward artificial neural network that uses supervised back-propagation, which is widely used for nonlinear classifications. As shown in Figure 4, the MLP in the proposed method consists of an input layer, a hidden layer and an output layer. The Relu function is used as the activation function of the hidden layer and the SoftMax function is used as the activation function of the output layer for the classification. The number of neurons in the hidden layer is determined by an empirical formula:

$$k = \sqrt{m+n} + a \tag{9}$$

where k denotes the number of neurons in the hidden layer, n denotes the number of neurons in the input layer, m denotes the number of neurons in the output layer, and a denotes a constant between 1 and 10.

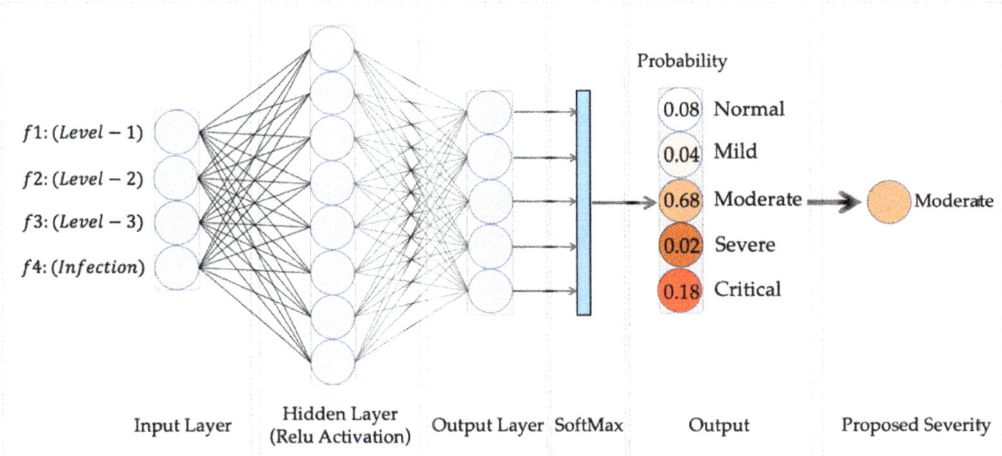

Figure 4. Structure of the multi-layer preceptor network (g = 3). $f_{1\text{–}4}$ denotes the input features of the MLP network. $f_{1\text{–}3}$ denotes the proportion of infected pixels of three levels in all infected pixels. f_4 denotes the proportion of infected pixels in lung parenchyma pixels.

4. Experiments and Analysis

The dataset [29] used in this study contains about 3500 CT image slices and corresponding lung and lesion segmentation labels. In addition, we recruited a radiology graduate student to label each CT image with a grade of severity (e.g., normal, mild, moderate, severe and critical). The labels were then verified by an experienced radiology specialist for reliability.

4.1. Implementation and Evaluation

A two-stage training strategy is adopted in this experiment: (1) training the segmentation of lung and COVID-19 lesions; (2) oversampling the training set, and finally training the MLP. We reproduced all the related networks and modules in the Pytorch framework. When training the segmentation network, we set the number of the batch size to 1, then initialize the network weights with Kaiming initialization, set network biases to zero and train the positive/negative samples alternately. In addition, the training set is shuffled in each iteration. We use different metrics in different stages. Intersection over union (IoU), sensitivity (SEN), specificity (SPE) and Dice similarity coefficient (DSC) are used to evaluate the accuracy of the lung segmentation. Besides, mean intersection over union (mIoU), mean pixel accuracy (mPA) and class pixel accuracy (CPA) are used to evaluate the accuracy of COVID-19 lesion segmentation using original labels and refined hierarchical labels. Precision is used to evaluate the accuracy of the severity grading. The above-mentioned metrics can be calculated as:

$$\mathrm{IoU} = \frac{\mathrm{TP}}{\mathrm{TP}+\mathrm{FP}+\mathrm{FN}} \tag{10}$$

$$\mathrm{SEN} = \frac{\mathrm{TP}}{\mathrm{TP}+\mathrm{FN}} \tag{11}$$

$$\mathrm{SPE} = \frac{\mathrm{TN}}{\mathrm{TN}+\mathrm{FP}} \tag{12}$$

$$\mathrm{DSC} = \frac{2\mathrm{TP}}{2\mathrm{TP}+\mathrm{FP}+\mathrm{FN}} \tag{13}$$

$$\mathrm{mIoU} = \frac{1}{\mathrm{k}+1}\sum\nolimits_{\mathrm{i}=0}^{\mathrm{k}} \frac{\mathrm{TP}}{\mathrm{FN}+\mathrm{FP}+\mathrm{TP}} \tag{14}$$

$$\mathrm{Precision} = \frac{\mathrm{TP}}{\mathrm{TP}+\mathrm{FP}} \tag{15}$$

$$\mathrm{mPA} = \frac{1}{\mathrm{k}+1}\sum_{\mathrm{i}=0}^{\mathrm{k}} \frac{\mathrm{TP}}{\mathrm{TP}+\mathrm{FP}} \tag{16}$$

where TP denotes true positives, TN denotes true negatives, FP denotes false positives and FN denotes false negatives.

We optimize the lung and lesion segmentation networks using a binary cross-entropy L_{lung} and a multi-category cross-entropy loss L_{lesion}, respectively, using a mean-squared error loss to train the MLP L_{mlp}.

$$L_{lung}(a,b) = -[blog(a) + (1-b)\log(1-a)] \tag{17}$$

$$L_{lesion}(a,b) = -\sum_{m=0}^{g} b_m logf(a)_m \tag{18}$$

$$f(a)_m = \frac{e^{a_m}}{\sum_{n=0,\ n\neq m}^{g} e^{a_n}} \tag{19}$$

$$L_{mlp}(a,b) = \|a-b\|^2 \tag{20}$$

$$L = L_{lung} + L_{lesion} + L_{mlp} \tag{21}$$

where a is the ground truth and b is the predicted result. g is the number of grades in refined hierarchical labels.

4.2. Evaluation of Lung Segmentation

As shown in Table 1 and Figure 5, lung segmentation with UNet works efficiently, with DSC up to 96%. Besides, IoU, SEN and SPE all surpass 90%. The accurate segmentation of the lung parenchyma ensures the quality of subsequent COVID-19 lesion segmentation and severity grading.

Table 1. Obtained result of lung segmentation metrics.

Metric	IoU	DSC	SEN	SPE
Value	0.94	0.96	0.97	1.00

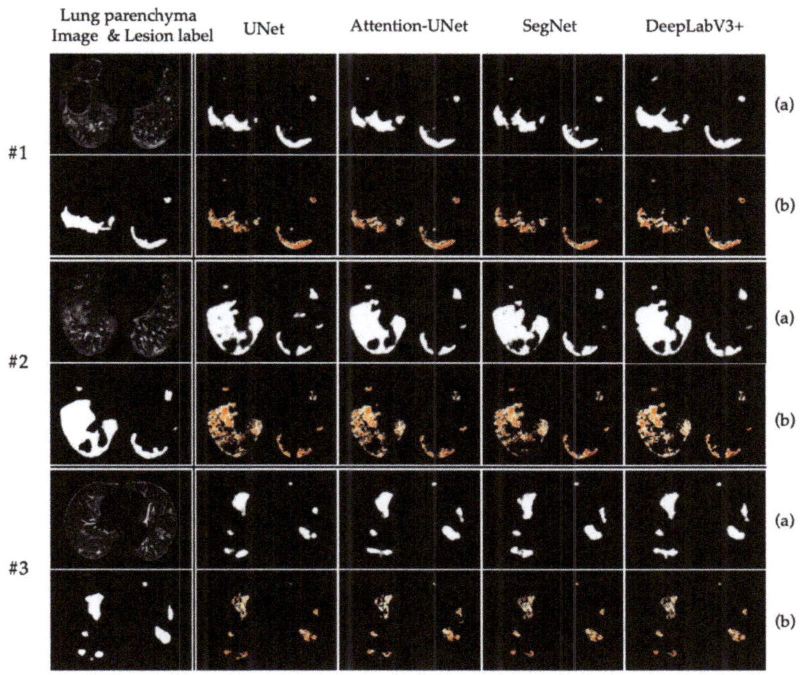

Figure 5. Visualization of the lesion segmentation using original label and refined hierarchical label. (**a**) and (**b**) illustrate the segmentation results using original lesion labels and refined hierarchical labels, respectively.

4.3. Evaluation of COVID-19 Lesion Segmentation Using Refined Hierarchical Labels

To evaluate the performance of refined hierarchical labels for COVID-19 lesion segmentation, four state-of-the-art networks are selected and trained with original labels and refined hierarchical labels, respectively (as shown in Figure 5). With regard to these widely used metrics (e.g., IoU, DSC, SEN and SPE) for medical image segmentation, an evaluation is carried out. Table 2 shows the values of these four metrics of the model trained with original labels and refined hierarchical labels. Table 3 shows the values of these four metrics, the CPA of each level and the MIoU and MPA of the model trained with refined hierarchical labels.

With the original labels, DeepLabV3+ achieves the best DICE of 82.94% among all the networks. Meanwhile, UNet achieves the worst performance. However, we find that the area marked as a lesion by the original labels in the input image contains many normal pixels such as lung parenchyma and pulmonary vessels. As illustrated in Figure 5, the #2 image is the most mislabeled. By introducing the refined hierarchical labels, the segmentation network can not only accurately identify the infected pixels, but also filter out these mislabeled pixels. Besides, as shown in Table 2, with the introduction of refined hierarchical labels, the model achieves better performance, such as the DSC of UNet and Attention-UNet reaching 83.47% and 82.35%, respectively. As shown in Table 3, the performance of pixel segmentation with UNet (2) is the best. Because the ground truth used is different, we cannot directly compare the performance of models training on original labels and refined hierarchical labels. Experienced radiologists from a hospital in Zhejiang Province confirm that refined hierarchical labels bring more precise results.

Table 2. Comparison of lesion segmentation performance using original labels and refined hierarchical labels.

Network	Labels		IoU (%)	DSC (%)	SEN (%)	SPE (%)
	Original	Refined				
UNet [28]	√		68.02	78.36	82.31	99.74
		√	73.54	83.47	87.75	99.83
Attention-UNet [30]	√		71.89	82.13	85.51	99.78
		√	71.82	82.35	82.37	99.87
SegNet [31]	√		68.98	79.57	83.38	99.74
		√	68.49	79.54	78.85	99.87
DeepLabV3+ [32]	√		72.43	82.94	85.08	99.79
		√	68.71	80.48	79.89	99.84

Table 3. Detailed performance using refined hierarchical labels.

Network	g	CPA (%)	IoU (%)	DSC (%)	SEN (%)	SPE (%)	MIoU (%)	MPA (%)
UNet	1	77.30	56.52	70.71	77.30	99.87	61.04	75.73
	2	81.31	65.47	77.20	81.31	99.92		
	3	75.33	61.13	72.93	75.33	99.95		
Attention-UNet	1	70.30	53.24	67.80	70.30	99.88	58.27	71.56
	2	73.95	62.82	75.17	73.95	99.94		
	3	70.41	58.75	70.81	70.41	99.96		
SegNet	1	55.58	41.31	56.20	55.58	99.84	51.96	67.74
	2	71.21	52.55	66.77	72.22	99.86		
	3	66.59	49.40	63.18	66.59	99.92		
DeepLabV3+	1	55.21	40.62	56.20	55.21	99.85	41.69	57.05
	2	61.62	44.43	60.37	61.62	99.86		
	3	54.34	40.03	55.11	54.34	99.91		

4.4. Evaluation of COVID-19 Severity Grading

There are few samples of mild, severe and critical cases in the dataset. As shown in Table 4, the classification accuracy of these categories is very low, even as low as 0 (mild). To solve this category imbalance problem, we applied the Synthetic Minority Oversampling Technique (SMOTE) [33] to minority classes. With the operation of oversampling the dataset, all the categories of samples reached a balance, the classification accuracy of mild reached 100% and the classification accuracy of severe and critical increased by 19.81% and 10.25%, respectively. Moreover, the overall accuracy was 98.82%.

Table 4. Precision of Severity Grading.

Severity	Precision (%)	Precision (%) (With Operation of Oversampling)
Normal	1	1
Mild	0	1
Moderate	99.37%	99.38%
Severe	62.69%	82.50%
Critical	79.49%	89.74%
Total	96.49	98.82

5. Conclusions

In this study, we propose a method for refining lesion labels from rough to precise. Then, a deep learning-based aiding system for CT image diagnosis using refined labels is developed. It performs lung and lesion segmentation from CT images, as well as severity grading. A multi-layer preceptor is used as a classifier, and the proportion of the lesion to the lung and the proportion of each grade in the lesion are used as input features. Auxiliary diagnostic information including the severity grade, proportion of infected area and visualization of the infected area are provided by the DLShelper for physicians in clinic. A comparative experiment based on public datasets is carried out, and the experimental results show that the proposed method achieves better accuracy in comparison with several state-of-the-art networks. Besides, the proposed method achieves a high accuracy for severity grading. In future, we will develop a new metric to describe the grayscale distribution features so as to further improve the performance.

In COVID-19 prevention and control, while developing AI and playing its positive role, we should be alert to the social risks and ethical challenges brought by AI itself, carry out responsive and principled scientific and technological governance, and strengthen ethical review and data legislation under the principle of "harmony, friendship, fairness, inclusiveness and sharing, respect for privacy, security and controllability, shared responsibility, open cooperation, and agile governance".

Author Contributions: Conceptualization, Z.Z. and T.H.; methodology, H.L.; software, Z.Z.; validation, C.L.; writing—original draft preparation, Z.Z.; writing—review and editing, C.L.; visualization, Y.Z.; project administration, Y.Z. All authors have read and agreed to the published version of the manuscript.

Funding: This research was funded by Natural Science Foundation of Zhejiang Province (No. LQ20F020024); Shanghai Education Science Research Project (No. C2022228); Social Science Project of Zhejiang University of Technology (SKY-ZX-20220246); Sub project of National Social Science Foundation of China (20&ZD191).

Data Availability Statement: Data are available by request to the corresponding authors.

Conflicts of Interest: The authors declare no conflict of interest.

References

1. Zhang, P.; Zhong, Y.; Deng, Y.; Tang, X.; Li, X. CoSinGAN: Learning COVID-19 Infection Segmentation from a Single Radiological Image. *Diagnostics* **2020**, *10*, 901. [CrossRef] [PubMed]
2. Bertolini, M.; Brambilla, A.; Dallasta, S.; Colombo, G. High-quality chest CT segmentation to assess the impact of COVID-19 disease. *Int. J. Comput. Assist. Radiol. Surg.* **2021**, *16*, 1737–1747. [CrossRef]
3. Ai, T.; Yang, Z.; Hou, H.; Zhan, C.; Chen, C.; Lv, W.; Tao, Q.; Sun, Z.; Xia, L. Correlation of chest CT and RT-PCR testing for coronavirus disease 2019 (COVID-19) in China: A report of 1014 cases. *Radiology* **2020**, *296*, E32–E40. [CrossRef] [PubMed]
4. Adams, H.J.; Kwee, T.C.; Yakar, D.; Hope, M.D.; Kwee, R.M. Chest CT imaging signature of coronavirus disease 2019 infection: In pursuit of the scientific evidence. *Chest* **2020**, *158*, 1885–1895. [CrossRef] [PubMed]
5. Shi, F.; Wang, J.; Shi, J.; Wu, Z.; Wang, Q.; Tang, Z.; He, K.; Shi, Y.; Shen, D. Review of artificial intelligence techniques in imaging data acquisition, segmentation, and diagnosis for COVID-19. *IEEE Rev. Biomed. Eng.* **2020**, *14*, 4–15. [CrossRef]
6. Zhang, K.; Liu, X.; Shen, J.; Li, Z.; Sang, Y.; Wu, X.; Zha, Y.; Liang, W.; Wang, C.; Wang, K.; et al. Clinically applicable AI system for accurate diagnosis, quantitative measurements, and prognosis of COVID-19 pneumonia using computed tomography. *Cell* **2020**, *181*, 1423–1433. [CrossRef] [PubMed]
7. Wu, Y.H.; Gao, S.H.; Mei, J.; Xu, J.; Fan, D.P.; Zhang, R.G.; Cheng, M.M. JCS: An Explainable COVID-19 Diagnosis System by Joint Classification and Segmentation. *IEEE Trans. Image Process.* **2020**, *30*, 3113–3126. [CrossRef]
8. Shan, F.; Gao, Y.; Wang, J.; Shi, W.; Shi, N.; Han, M.; Xue, Z.; Shen, D.; Shi, Y. Lung infection quantification of COVID-19 in CT images with deep learning. *arXiv* **2020**, arXiv:2003.04655.
9. Qiu, Y.; Liu, Y.; Xu, J. MiniSeg: An Extremely Minimum Network for Efficient COVID-19 Segmentation. *Proc. Conf. AAAI Artif. Intell.* **2020**, *35*, 4846–4854. [CrossRef]
10. Çiçek, Ö.; Abdulkadir, A.; Lienkamp, S.S.; Brox, T.; Ronneberger, O. 3D U-Net: Learning dense volumetric segmentation from sparse annotation. In *International Conference on Medical Image Computing and Computer-Assisted Intervention*; Springer: Cham, Switzerland, 2016; pp. 424–432.

11. Zhang, L.; Wang, X.; Yang, D.; Sanford, T.; Harmon, S.; Turkbey, B.; Roth, H.; Myronenko, A.; Xu, D.; Xu, Z. When unseen domain generalization is unnecessary? rethinking data augmentation. *arXiv* **2019**, arXiv:1906.03347.
12. Jin, D.; Xu, Z.; Tang, Y.; Harrison, A.P.; Mollura, D.J. CT-realistic lung nodule simulation from 3D conditional generative adversarial networks for robust lung segmentation. In *International Conference on Medical Image Computing and Computer-Assisted Intervention*; Springer: Cham, Switzerland, 2018; pp. 732–740.
13. Shin, H.-C.; Tenenholtz, N.A.; Rogers, J.K.; Schwarz, C.G.; Senjem, M.L.; Gunter, J.L.; Andriole, K.P.; Michalski, M. Medical image synthesis for data augmentation and anonymization using generative adversarial networks. In *International Workshop on Simulation and Synthesis in Medical Imaging*; Springer: Cham, Switzerland, 2018; pp. 1–11.
14. Xu, Z.; Niethammer, M. DeepAtlas: Joint semi-supervised learning of image registration and segmentation. In *International Conference on Medical Image Computing and Computer-Assisted Intervention*; Springer: Cham, Switzerland, 2019; pp. 420–429.
15. Fan, D.-P.; Zhou, T.; Ji, G.-P.; Zhou, Y.; Chen, G.; Fu, H.; Shen, J.; Shao, L. Inf-Net: Automatic COVID-19 Lung Infection Segmentation from CT Images. *IEEE Trans. Med. Imaging* **2020**, *39*, 2626–2637. [CrossRef] [PubMed]
16. Shan, S.; Yan, W.; Guo, X.; Chang, E.I.; Fan, Y.; Xu, Y. Unsupervised end-to-end learning for deformable medical image registration. *arXiv* **2017**, arXiv:1711.08608.
17. de Vos, B.D.; Berendsen, F.F.; Viergever, M.A.; Sokooti, H.; Staring, M.; Išgum, I. A deep learning framework for unsupervised affine and deformable image registration. *Med. Image Anal.* **2019**, *52*, 128–143. [CrossRef] [PubMed]
18. Wang, G.; Liu, X.; Li, C.; Xu, Z.; Ruan, J.; Zhu, H.; Meng, T.; Li, K.; Huang, N.; Zhang, S. A noise-robust framework for automatic segmentation of COVID-19 pneumonia lesions from CT images. *IEEE Trans. Med. Imaging* **2020**, *39*, 2653–2663. [CrossRef] [PubMed]
19. Chen, J.; Li, Y.; Guo, L.; Zhou, X.; Zhu, Y.; He, Q.; Han, H.; Feng, Q. Machine learning techniques for CT imaging diagnosis of novel coronavirus pneumonia: A review. *Neural Comput. Applications.* **2022**. [CrossRef] [PubMed]
20. Santosh, K.; Antani, S. Automated chest X-ray screening: Can lung region symmetry help detect pulmonary abnormalities? *IEEE Trans. Med. Imaging* **2017**, *37*, 1168–1177. [CrossRef]
21. Pratondo, A.; Chui, C.K.; Ong, S.H. Integrating machine learning with region-based active contour models in medical image segmentation. *J. Vis. Commun. Image Represent.* **2017**, *43*, 1–9. [CrossRef]
22. Ahmad, W.; Zaki, W.; Fauzi, M. Lung segmentation on standard and mobile chest radiographs using oriented Gaussian derivatives filter. *Biomed. Eng. Online* **2015**, *14*, 20. [CrossRef]
23. Shepherd, T.; Prince, S.J.; Alexander, D.C. Interactive lesion segmentation with shape priors from offline and online learning. *IEEE Trans. Med. Imaging* **2012**, *31*, 1698–1712. [CrossRef]
24. Xu, W.; He, G.; Pan, C.; Shen, D.; Zhang, N.; Jiang, P.; Liu, F.; Chen, J. A Forced Cough Sound based Pulmonary Function Assessment by Using Machine Learning. *Front. Public Health.* **2022**, *10*, 1015876. [CrossRef]
25. Shaukat, F.; Raja, G.; Gooya, A.; Frangi, A. Fully automatic detection of lung nodules in CT images using a hybrid feature set. *Med. Phys.* **2017**, *44*, 3615–3629. [CrossRef] [PubMed]
26. Souza, J.C.; Diniz, J.O.B.; Ferreira, J.L.; da Silva, G.L.F.; Silva, A.C.; de Paiva, A.C. An automatic method for lung segmentation and reconstruction in chest X-ray using deep neural networks. *Comput. Methods Programs Biomed.* **2019**, *177*, 285–296. [CrossRef] [PubMed]
27. Park, B.; Park, H.; Lee, S.M.; Seo, J.B.; Kim, N. Lung Segmentation on HRCT and Volumetric CT for Diffuse Interstitial Lung Disease Using Deep Convolutional Neural Networks. *J. Digit. Imaging* **2019**, *32*, 1019–1026. [CrossRef] [PubMed]
28. Ronneberger, O.; Fischer, P.; Brox, T. U-Net: Convolutional Networks for Biomedical Image Segmentation. In *Medical Image Computing and Computer-Assisted Intervention—MICCAI 2015*; Navab, N., Hornegger, J., Wells, W., Frangi, A., Eds.; MICCAI 2015, Lecture Notes in Computer Science; Springer: Cham, Switzerland, 2015; Volume 9351. [CrossRef]
29. Jun, M.; Cheng, G.; Yixin, W.; Xingle, A.; Jiantao, G.; Ziqi, Y.; Jian, H. *COVID-19 CT Lung and Infection Segmentation Dataset (Verson 1.0) [Data set]*; Zenodo: Geneva, Switzerland, 2020.
30. Oktay, O.; Schlemper, J.; Le Folgoc, L.; Lee, M.; Heinrich, M.; Misawa, K.; Rueckert, D. Attention U-Net: Learning Where to Look for the Pancreas. *arXiv* **2018**, arXiv:1804.03999.
31. Badrinarayanan, V.; Kendall, A.; Cipolla, R. Segnet: A deep convolutional encoder-decoder architecture for image segmentation. *IEEE Trans. Pattern Anal. Mach. Intell.* **2017**, *39*, 2481–2495. [CrossRef]
32. Firdaus-Nawi, M.; Noraini, O.; Sabri, M.Y.; Siti-Zahrah, A.; Zamri-Saad, M.; Latifah, H. DeepLabv3+ _encoder-decoder with Atrous separable convolution for semantic image segmentation. *Pertanika J. Trop. Agric. Sci.* **2011**, *34*, 137–143.
33. Chawla, N.V.; Bowyer, K.W.; Hall, L.O.; Kegelmeyer, W.P. SMOTE: Synthetic minority over-sampling technique. *J. Artif. Intell. Res.* **2002**, *16*, 321–357. [CrossRef]

applied sciences

MDPI

Perspective

A Neural Modelling Tool for Non-Linear Influence Analyses and Perspectives of Applications in Medical Research

Antonello Pasini [1,*] and Stefano Amendola [2]

1 National Research Council, Institute of Atmospheric Pollution Research, Monterotondo Stazione, 00015 Rome, Italy
2 Italian Air Force Mountain Centre, 41029 Sestola, Italy; stefano.amendola@aeronautica.difesa.it
* Correspondence: pasini@iia.cnr.it

Abstract: Neural network models are often used to analyse non-linear systems; here, in cases of small datasets, we review our complementary approach to deep learning with the purpose of highlighting the importance and roles (linear, non-linear or threshold) of certain variables (assumed as causal) in determining the behaviour of a target variable; this also allows us to make predictions for future scenarios of these causal variables. We present a neural tool endowed with an ensemble strategy and its applications to influence analyses in terms of pruning, attribution and future predictions (free code issued). We describe some case studies on climatic applications which show reliable results and the potentialities of our method for medical studies. The discovery of the importance and role (linear, non-linear or threshold) of causal variables and the possibility of applying the relationships found to future scenarios could lead to very interesting applications in medical research and the study and treatment of cancer, which are proposed in this paper.

Keywords: neural networks; non-linearities; causality analyses; climate; medical applications

1. Introduction

When dealing with a complex system—for example, the human body in interaction with its environment—it is often difficult to understand what causes certain changes in the system itself. This is due to the very characteristics of complex systems, which do not have linear causal relationships among their 'components' but often have non-linear, threshold or even circular relationships, i.e., with feedback.

For complex systems studied by the so-called 'hard sciences', one often finds non-linear equations that link different variables dynamically and thus manage to algorithmically reduce the complexity. In the environmental sciences, doing this is already difficult, and in the medical sciences, it is probably even more so. In many of the latter cases, algorithmic reduction of this complexity must be achieved using data-driven methods.

In any case, once possible causal factors of a change in the system have been identified, these data-driven methods need to be able to capture the non-linearities and feedback that exist in the relationships between these variables. These non-linearities are obviously not 'seen' by a linear multiple regression but can be captured, at least implicitly, by non-linear multiple regressions, such as those that can be carried out by neural network (NN) models.

Given this context, much emphasis is now placed on so-called 'deep learning', whereby automated machine learning systems use huge available datasets to find regularities in the data and possible causal relationships [1]. This activity has even led to speculation of an 'end of theory' [2] and has also been largely applied in medical research (see, for instance [3,4] and references therein). In general, the first sector to see applications of deep learning was clinical image analysis, obviously due to the large amount of data available. Today, deep learning is still widely used with success for this sector in particular, along with the analysis of biosignals, i.e., the set of all the electrical, mechanical and thermal signals produced by a human body. Moreover, deep learning has recently been applied in biomedicine, the set of disciplines that study molecules involved in biological processes, and in the analysis of so-called 'electronic health records', the standard digital version of the patients' health records, although here with more difficulty due to the heterogeneity of the data. Obviously, by now, all areas of medical science where a large amount of data is available are involved in these deep learning analyses.

However, at least two problems arise here: Firstly, these huge systems (with many hidden layers) are certainly useful for discovering unsuspected relationships between apparently unconnected variables, but, usually, the stability of the systems requires quasi-linear transfer functions. Therefore, the relationships that are found are also quasi-linear (which can hide the real non-linear behaviour). Secondly, in environmental and medical sciences, there are often insufficient amounts of data available to make use of deep learning.

For all these reasons, a few years ago, one of us (A.P.) developed an NN modelling tool for small datasets [5], with an approach that can be considered complementary to that of deep learning: small NNs with just one hidden layer, highly non-linear transfer functions, and the possibility of highlighting non-linear links well. Furthermore, an ensemble strategy has given this tool the characteristics of reliability and robustness in its results.

In this paper, we present some methods of applying this tool (pruning, attribution and prediction), which have already been tried and tested in the climatic and environmental fields (see, e.g., [6–8]), and which make it possible to highlight the importance and roles (linear, non-linear or threshold) of certain causal variables in determining the behaviour of a target variable. This permits predictions of the target variable to be made for future scenarios of the causal variables, too. The tool has already been used in the biomedical field (see the many citations of paper [5], for instance, refs. [9–15]), but not with these specific applications, which can be very useful.

In short, the scope of this paper is to provide and discuss the application methods of a tool that can be used in all those fields in which our theoretical knowledge of the complex system of interest is insufficient for a detailed dynamical study of the causal relationships between different system variables. Obviously, the occurrence of diseases, including cancers, and their relationship to genetic, environmental or lifestyle causal variables is a topic to which this tool can certainly be applied and where it can yield interesting results.

The codes of the tool's applications are freely downloadable: see the Data Availability Statement in the Footnotes.

This paper is structured as follows: Section 2 briefly presents the NN tool in its basic features; in Section 3, the application methods for discovering the importance (linear, non-linear or threshold) of causal variables on climatic and environmental examples are explored; in Sections 4 and 5, respectively, application possibilities in the medical field are discussed and brief conclusions are drawn.

2. The NN Tool

When trying to achieve algorithmic reduction with a statistical model and small datasets, we often run the risk of finding unrealistic and unreliable relationships between causal variables and a variable representing the effect being studied. This is also the case with neural models, where we must avoid overfitting to obtain realistic relationships, and we must minimise the role of variability (due to the random choice of initial weights) to obtain reliable results. The tool presented here seeks precisely to avoid these problems. In the present paper, we describe NNs and this tool conceptually; for more technical details, see [5].

The NN models used in the tool are fairly standard, i.e., feedforward networks with backpropagation training; see [16,17] for the fundamentals of these kinds of networks (multi-layer perceptrons: MLPs). These networks possess just one hidden layer, as it is sufficient to approximate any continuous function [18,19]. The hidden neurons are endowed with hyperbolic tangent transfer functions, while the single output neuron is endowed with a linear one. In the latest applications of the tool, the training technique has been modified with respect to the original one described in [5]: a further improvement was made for the analysis of small datasets. We now use the Broyden–Fletcher–Golfarb–Shanno (BFGS) algorithm [20], which shows better performance than the standard backpropagation. The usual way to obtain a non-linear relationship between inputs and targets (to be approximated by outputs), which is generally valid, is to divide the total dataset into three subsets and apply a training–validation–testing procedure. The connection weights (i.e., the free parameters of the NNs) are fixed on the training set by stopping the training phase when the error on the validation set begins to increase; then, the model performance is measured on a third set, unknown to the NNs—the so-called test set. In our tool, developed for analysing small datasets, a generalised leave-one-out procedure is adopted for the phases of training, validation and testing.

This procedure is depicted in Figure 1. In our complete dataset, formed by a number of input–target pairs (patterns), we extract a single input–target pattern and consider it as the test set. Then, a validation set is randomly chosen, and the remaining patterns constitute the training set. At the end of all the epochs (iterations) of an NN run, the model is able to fix the connection weights, and a transfer function from inputs to output is obtained. But this result can be influenced by the specific random choices of the initial weights and of the members of the validation set. Thus, the NN tool performs multiple runs in an ensemble approach by choosing different random values for weights and members of the validation set. This allows us to calculate the ensemble mean of the outputs and 'average away' the intrinsic variability of the NN results.

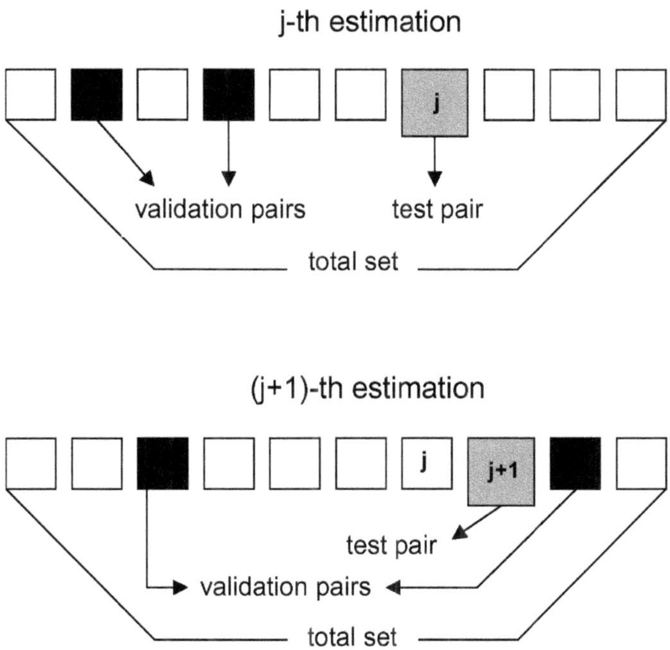

Figure 1. Sketch of the generalised leave-one-out procedure (from [7]).

After this reconstruction of one value of the target, the procedure is followed again for all the other patterns; each of them becomes, sequentially, the test set. As a final result, at the end of this generalised leave-one-out procedure, we are able to achieve the estimation of all output values and ensemble means.

Inside this tool, standard multilinear regressions are also performed to form a benchmark, which permits us to evaluate the specific value added by the use of NNs in the analyses. In these linear analyses, we adopt the same approach to training: for each single pattern, the coefficients of the linear regression are fixed on the other data (the union of the training and validation sets used in the NN method). Thus, the linear model can fix its coefficients on more data (this is an advantage with respect to the NN model); as a result, and as we show in the following, the better performance of the NNs is even more notable. Obviously, in the linear model, no ensemble strategy is required.

3. Environmental Applications of the Tool and Results

As mentioned earlier, neural network models are now widely used in the environmental sciences, and our tool in particular has been mainly applied in the climate field. Only three examples are given here to illustrate some of the application methods. These make it possible to identify the importance/role (linear, non-linear or threshold) of the causal variables in determining the behaviour of the target variable and to obtain predictions of the value of the target variable for future scenarios of the causal variables.

3.1. Importance and Roles of the Causal Variables (Pruning)

The first example we present follows the discussion in [7]. There, the problem was to understand the importance and role of climatic influences on human migration from the Sahel Belt to Italy in the period 1995–2009.

The data available for this analysis in our dataset were the annual flows of migrants from the ten Sahel countries to Italy (our target to be reconstructed by means of the NN model using climate data) and the data of direct and indirect climatic influences (our inputs). In particular, the latter were the annual mean temperature, annual mean cumulated precipitation, number of hours with a temperature higher than 30 °C during the growing season of crops, and, finally, cereal yields, which represent an indirect climate effect, as they are themselves influenced by the climate. We built a dataset composed of the annual patterns of four inputs and one output for each country.

The application of our tool led to several interesting results. Firstly, the reconstruction of migration data (using our non-linear neural model and climatic data as inputs) led to an explained variance close to 80% in terms of the ensemble mean performance, whereas the analogous linear multiple regression stopped at just over 60% (see Table 1 below). In Figure 2, we show a graphical view of the NN outputs in terms of the logarithm of the migration rate, defined as the annual migration flow from the origin country to Italy divided by the population of the country of origin in the same year. Given the lack of more social variables in our dataset that may have an influence on migration, the neural result surely looks good. Furthermore, the big difference in the explained variances of the NNs and multilinear regression already shows that the relationship between our inputs and the target is highly non-linear.

Table 1. Performance (in terms of R^2) of migration rate estimation by NNs (ensemble means) and multilinear regressions for the complete runs and for pruned models (from [7]).

Inputs	Target	NN (R^2)	Multilinear (R^2)
Prec.—temp.—# hours T > 30 °C—yield	ln(MigRate)	0.775	0.626
Prec.—temp.—# hours T > 30 °C	ln(MigRate)	0.671	0.611
Prec.—temp.—yield	ln(MigRate)	0.683	0.632
Prec.—# hours T > 30 °C—yield	ln(MigRate)	0.361	0.085
Temp.—# hours T > 30 °C—yield	ln(MigRate)	0.715	0.447

But is it possible to quantify the role of the individual input variables in the reconstruction of the target? In a linear model, their weight can be identified through the coefficients associated with the individual variables in the multiple regression. In a neural model, following this path—via the evaluation of the weights associated with the connections—is much more complicated and often does not lead to reliable results. Therefore, in our tool's applications, we follow a different path: that of pruning (or attribution, see later).

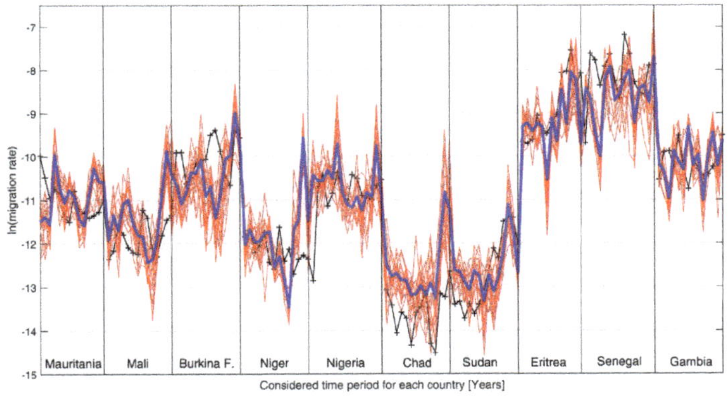

Figure 2. Modelling migration rates (black line) from ten countries of Sahel to Italy in the period 1995–2009 by NN models (red lines) and ensemble means (blue line) (from [7]).

Pruning means that we exclude the input variables in turn from the input layer and run the NN models again with more little networks, in order to test which inputs have a dominant role in achieving a correct estimate of the observed target data. The greater the decrease in performance when we extract a variable from the input, the more that variable 'drives' the behaviour of the target. In the meantime, by also pruning the linear model, we are able to investigate and identify specific linear and non-linear influences, too. If, when we remove a variable, the performances of the NNs and multilinear regressions become similar (and those of the multilinear model possibly change very little), then that variable plays an important non-linear role. Table 1 shows an example of the performance results of unpruned and pruned networks in the migration study (here, for simplicity, we adopted only R^2 as a measure of performance, but in the original papers, we also used others, e.g., the receiver operating characteristic—ROC—curve).

In this case, temperature is clearly the most influential variable on the migration rate, due to a strong decrease in the performance of both the NN and linear models when it was excluded from the input layer. The decrease in performance was less marked when other variables were extracted from the input layer. However, it is worthwhile to note that harvest yields and the number of hours with T > 30 °C have a clear non-linear role. In the case of their exclusion from the inputs, in fact, the performance of the multilinear model changed very little, and the performance of the NN model became very close to that of the linear one.

Of course, in each field of application, it is up to the researchers applying this tool to extract knowledge from these statistical results. In this case, for instance, it is clear that the average annual temperature strongly influences migration, but how? Another analysis of the same study shows that this mean temperature does not affect yields very much; therefore, its large observed increases could directly affect humans and animals. In this respect, it is very important to have noted the strong non-linear role of the hours of temperature exceeding 30 °C during the harvest period, because this variable is a proxy for the duration of a climatic phenomenon—the heat wave—so that there may be a threshold effect on crops, and also on the heat tolerance of humans and animals, induced by these heat waves.

Studies are now in progress to better identify the values of the threshold in variables showing non-linear relationships with the target.

3.2. *Importance and Roles of the Causal Variables (Attribution)*

We now describe an alternative way of understanding the role of the individual causal variables on the target variable, which also allows simulations of the latter's behaviour if the former have different values and trends. These simulations have been carried out for climate attribution studies, and we will use one of them here to exemplify the method; see [6] for further details.

A very important problem in recent climate research has been to understand what has caused the rapid rise in the global mean temperature over the last 60 years. To do this, dynamical models (global climate models—GCMs) have been used, which have shown that without the increase in CO_2 and other greenhouse gases (GHGs), recent global warming would not have occurred. But, given the complexity of these models, it was important to analyse this problem with very different (data-driven) models, such as neural networks and Granger causality models, to test the robustness of their results (see [21,22] and references therein).

As far as NN models are concerned, the concept with which we applied our tool to attribution studies is very simple. At the end of training, our networks found the best weights to reconstruct the trend of the target (over time) according to the input values that occurred in reality. Once these values have been fixed, we have thus found a 'law' that reconstructs the links between the inputs and the target, a law that we can consider valid in general. We can therefore apply it to values of the inputs other than those observed in historical reality, thus simulating different situations that could have occurred and obtaining the related values of the output variable. For instance, if we input to the network with fixed weights a constant or stationary value for one variable and real observed values for all the others, we will see the effect of real variations in the first variable on the target variable and will thus be able to understand its role in the evolution of the target (see the following example).

In the climate attribution example given in [6], the target was the global mean temperature, and the causal variables (expressed in terms of radiative forcings) were external natural influences (Sun and volcanoes) and anthropogenic ones (GHGs, black carbon (BC) and sulphate aerosols). In the latter forcings, GHGs and BC have a warming effect, while sulphates have a cooling one. Each of these causal variables has had a certain trend over time since 1850, and we estimated this from observations. But what would have happened if one of these trends had been different, e.g., constant or stationary? A first answer is in Figure 3, taken from [6].

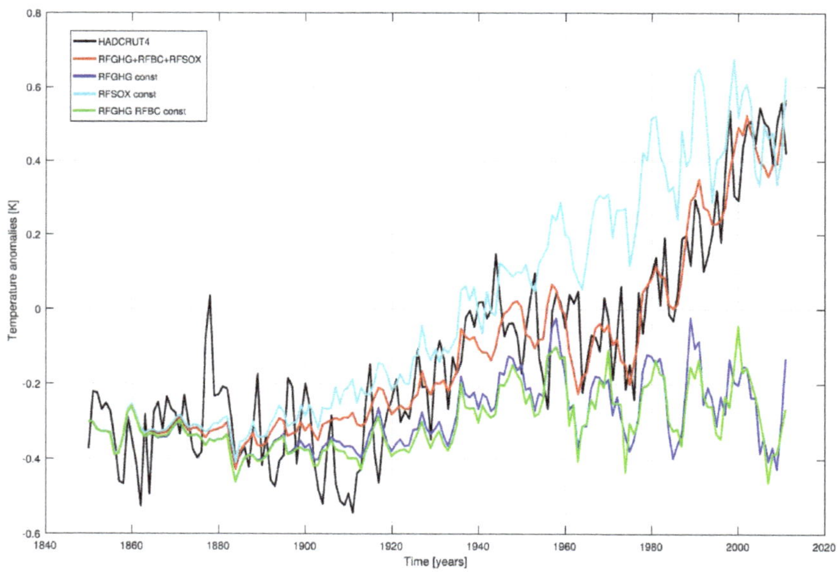

Figure 3. Warming and cooling roles of the distinct anthropogenic forcings by an NN attribution experiment. Black line = observed T; red line = reconstructed T by all inputs with actual values; blue, light blue and green lines = attribution runs with constant forcing(s) (from [6]).

In terms of the ensemble means of our NN runs, Figure 3 shows the very good performance of our NN models in reconstructing the real behaviour of temperature when the real trends of all forcings were considered (see how the black and red lines are close). The light blue line shows the further increase in temperature that would have occurred over the last century if sulphates had remained constant at their 1850 value. The blue and green lines come from runs where constant values for the inputs of GHGs and GHGs + BC radiative forcings, respectively, were propagated along the network with fixed weights. This last result shows that without the increase in anthropogenic warming factors, the recent global warming would not have occurred, so humans are responsible for this warming. This result corroborates the analogous one coming from GCMs.

But what about the influence of observed past changes in solar forcing on the global temperature? The solar forcing always showed its typical eleven-year cycle but with an additional increase in power in the first decades of the last century, which continued into the last decades. We can simulate what would have happened if there had not been this increase by feeding our fixed-weight neural networks with a synthetic series of solar forcing (RFSOLSTAT) that is stationary on the values of the first decades of our time series. The results can be seen in Figure 4. Here, the increasing trend in temperature during the years 1910–1945 was not caught with stationary power from the Sun, and during 1945–1975 the hiatus temperature was about 0.2 K lower than observed. The hypothesis of a 'stationary Sun' has no detectable influence on the value of the increasing temperature trend of the last period; this is a new proof that it has been more deeply influenced by anthropogenic forcings.

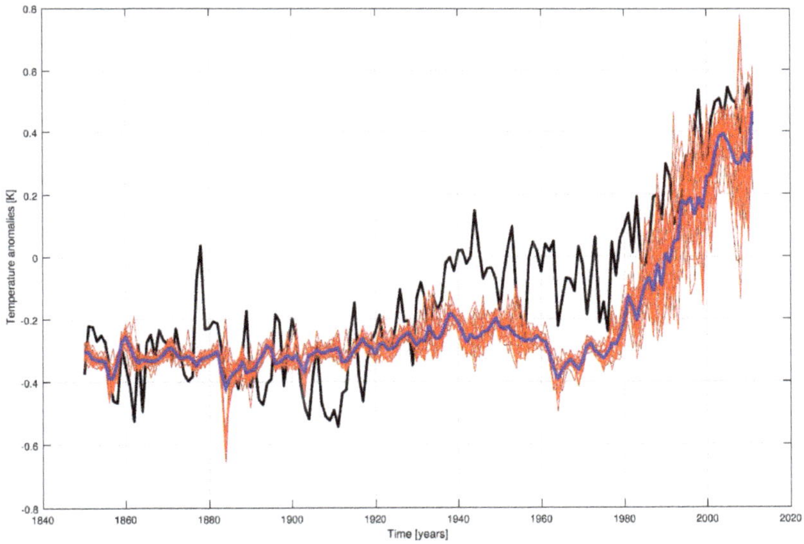

Figure 4. Attribution experiment for solar influence. Black line = observed T, red lines = results of ensemble runs, blue line = ensemble mean. We mimicked stationary solar forcing by using RFSOLSTAT as an input for the validated NN models (from [6]).

In short, attribution studies allow us to examine the role of a causal variable by decoupling it from the others in a non-linear model that is able to correctly reconstruct the observed trend of the target variable.

3.3. Predictions in Future Scenarios

Once we have found a general transfer function from the inputs to the target and fixed the network weights, we have seen in attribution studies how we can simulate the behaviour of the target variable for different values of the inputs, e.g., by placing a constant or stationary input together with the others with observed values.

At this point, however, nobody forbids exploiting the 'law' found through the neural model to simulate the behaviour of the target variable in very different situations, in 'scenarios' in which all input variables change their values. In particular, it is interesting to do this when one can hypothesise future changes in the trends of the input variables and wants to analyse what will happen to the values of the target variable.

This approach was recently followed in a climate application [8]. We will therefore refer to this example to briefly illustrate the potential of this method.

In addition to the finding that recent climate changes are largely driven by human influences, the climate also has an its own internal variability, due to natural cycles and oscillations. We are aware of many such examples of natural variability, and even the so-called Atlantic multidecadal oscillation (AMO) has long been considered a manifestation of natural variability. Recently, however, studies have shown how AMO may have been strongly influenced by certain anthropogenic forcings, such as sulphate aerosols.

These studies were always carried out using GCMs. In a recent study [6], however, we carried out an attribution analysis of AMO using our neural tool. This paper significantly contributed to the current debate on the natural or anthropogenic origin of AMO. The results showed how the AMO's behaviour from 1866 to the present has been strongly influenced by anthropogenic forcings, with a particular emphasis on the radiative forcing of human-origin sulphate aerosols.

Now, as is well known, there are future scenarios for anthropogenic forcings, such as the SSP scenarios of the Coupled Model Intercomparison Phase 6 (CMIP6). We used the scenarios from one of these models [23] to make future predictions of the AMO's behaviour by feeding these data into the networks that had best reconstructed the AMO's historical oscillations. Future data of natural forcings were statistically extrapolated, with a couple of different options for solar radiative forcing; see [8].

The key finding of this study revealed that in all future scenarios, the AMO is expected to lose its cyclical pattern (see Figure 5). It could only be preserved in a scenario with highly unrealistic values for sulphate aerosols.

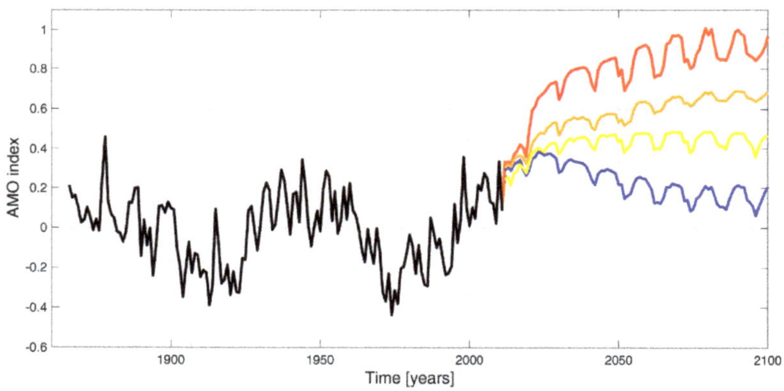

Figure 5. NN ensemble mean projections of the future behaviour of the AMO index under four SSP scenarios (SSP1-2.6, blue line; SSP2-4.5, yellow line; SSP3-7.0, brown line; SSP5-8.5, red line) in the case of high-power solar radiation hypothesised for the future (from [8]). Black line represents the historical behaviour of the AMO index.

This study showed how, by incorporating future scenarios for inputs, one can predict the behaviour of the target variable and come to very important conclusions. If these scenarios then depend on our actions, we can act to avoid the most damaging scenarios (in the context of climate, think of the so-called 'business as usual' scenarios for future global warming).

4. Possible Applications in the Medical Field

The main application of our tool in medical research is probably in the search for robust non-linear relationships between genetic, environmental or lifestyle factors and the development of a disease or cancer. The pruning or attribution methods described above could make it possible to highlight the roles of various factors and possible non-linearities, e.g., for phenomena affected by thresholds in inputs. Moreover, most of these factors are modifiable; thus, once a non-linear transfer function between the causes (inputs) and a disease index (target) has been found, we can also study what would happen in different scenarios that are possibly conceivable for the future in the case of changes in lifestyles or, for example, in different pollution or climate scenarios.

Another case where our tool could be very useful is in the study of drug–disease interaction, especially in the very critical cases of cancer treatments, the success of which is often measured in the years of survival after surgery. Cases observed in patients with certain physical characteristics and treatments actually given (as inputs) using our tool could lead to reliable reports for the reconstruction of their survival years (the possible target). At this point, numerical experimentation using NNs could be conducted to see which treatments (and doses) are preferable for other patients with different characteristics in the input data, in order to increase their survival time. This can be done by the application of our forecasting strategy.

In general, neural modelling can analyse complex interactions between genetic, environmental and lifestyle factors to predict an individual's cancer risk and estimate their prognosis. These models can capture non-linear relationships that traditional statistical methods may miss. At present, particular attention is paid to deep learning and its contribution to cancer research; see, for instance [24]. Here, however, we would like to briefly cite some research sectors in which our neural approach to small datasets can benefit cancer studies.

Neural modelling can assist in personalising cancer treatment by analysing patient-specific data, including genetic profiles and treatment responses. This approach can help to identify the most effective treatment strategies for individuals, for instance, in terms of personalised chemotherapy selection (see [25] for a problem of this type).

Neural networks can also analyse non-linear interactions within the tumour microenvironment, including interactions between cancer cells, immune cells and the extracellular matrix. This can shed light on tumour behaviour and immune responses, an important relationship which needs to be deepened; see [26] for a recent review on this topic.

Neural modelling can predict the non-linear responses of cancer cells to various drugs. Considering the complexity of drug–target interactions, these models can optimise drug selection for individual patients, including in cases of the use of "non-oncology drugs", such as in [27].

Another field in which neural modelling can be very useful is that of non-linear resistance mechanisms. For instance, our tool can help uncover non-linear resistance mechanisms affecting cancer therapies, including targeted therapies and immunotherapies, by considering the interplay between tumour cells and the immune system (see [28] for a review on this important topic).

Finally, our neural tool performs multiple non-linear regressions, but with a little modification, it could be adapted for classification problems. In this case, it could also help with diagnostic analyses (inputs) and their use for the early detection of cancer (the target). In particular, if databases that are not too small are available, the linear and non-linear influences of certain inputs on the target could be identified in the analysis values. And then, along with understanding the role of individual inputs, one could also apply the 'law' found to cases of new patients, identifying the eventual onset of cancer. In this manner, a neural network tool, such as our one, can also analyse multi-modal data, including imaging, genomic and clinical data, to improve the accuracy of early cancer detection and screening programs. Attempts have been made using deep learning (see, for instance [29]), but we are confident that an accurate preselection of inputs and the use of our robust tool may contribute to this field.

5. Conclusions

In this paper, we presented a neural network tool suitable for non-linear influence analyses in complex systems with small available datasets (as is often the case with environmental and health systems), together with its application methods. The latter were concretely exemplified in some climatic cases, but we believe that the methods discussed here of pruning, attribution and prediction can also be of great help for medical research and, in particular, cancer research, as we discussed in the previous section.

In particular, the discovery of the importance and role (linear, non-linear or threshold) of causal variables and the possibility of applying the relationships found to future scenarios could lead to very interesting applications in health sciences and the study and treatment of cancer.

We are, of course, aware that there are other methods, such as sensitivity analyses and generalised additive models (GAMs), that do similar things to our tool. However, what we consider 'innovative' here is the set of features of our tool, including ensemble runs, attribution analysis and forecasting activities for small available datasets. Obviously, we also know that the neural networks we used are quite simple (MLPs), and it is our intention in the future to include more powerful networks in this tool. In this perspective article, we only wanted to show the application potential of the current tool in the medical field.

Furthermore, our method should obviously be tested against the standard models used in medical research, and this will be done in our future works.

Finally, we hope that this perspective article can induce more researchers to adopt promising NN tools and their application methods in their influence analyses.

Author Contributions: Conceptualisation, A.P.; methodology, A.P. and S.A.; software, S.A.; validation, A.P. and S.A.; formal analysis, S.A.; investigation, A.P. and S.A.; data curation, S.A.; writing—original draft preparation, A.P.; writing—review and editing, A.P.; visualisation, A.P. and S.A.; supervision, A.P. All authors have read and agreed to the published version of the manuscript.

Funding: This research received no external funding.

Institutional Review Board Statement: Not applicable.

Informed Consent Statement: Not applicable.

Data Availability Statement: We have made the Matlab® codes of our tool for the 3 applications discussed in the text (pruning, attribution and prediction) freely available. The relevant program files, together with the 3 datasets used for the related climate applications and a function called in the main programs, can be found at https://cnrsc-my.sharepoint.com/:f:/g/personal/antonello_pasini_cnr_it/Eu4DxbFPD2dPu1pZINdct_IBxgkTLMRLHNTgeUAxVkf5dg?e=7a9kvN (accessed on 1 February 2024) (see the folder 'Free-codes&data').

Acknowledgments: We warmly acknowledge L. Bertolaccini for helpful discussions.

Conflicts of Interest: The authors declare no conflicts of interest.

References

1. Alzubaidi, L.; Zhang, J.; Humaidi, A.J.; Al-Dujaili, A.; Duan, Y.; Al-Shamma, O.; Santamaría, J.; Fadhel, M.A.; Al-Amidie, M.; Farhan, L. Review of deep learning: Concepts, CNN architectures, challenges, applications, future directions. *J. Big Data* **2021**, *8*, 53. [CrossRef]
2. Anderson, C. The End of Theory: The Data Deluge Makes the Scientific Method Obsolete. Wired. 23 June 2008, p. 16. Available online: https://www.wired.com/2008/06/pb-theory/ (accessed on 2 February 2024).
3. Egger, J.; Gsaxner, C.; Pepe, A.; Pomykala, K.L.; Jonske, F.; Kurz, M.; Li, J.; Kleesiek, J. Medical deep learning—A systematic meta-review. *Comput. Methods Prog. Biomed.* **2022**, *221*, 106874. [CrossRef]
4. Piccialli, F.; Di Somma, V.; Giampaolo, F.; Cuomo, S.; Fortino, G. A survey on deep learning in medicine: Why, how and when? *Inform. Fusion* **2021**, *66*, 111–137. [CrossRef]

5. Pasini, A. Artificial neural networks for small dataset analysis. *J. Thorac. Dis.* **2015**, *7*, 953–960.
6. Pasini, A.; Racca, P.; Amendola, S.; Cartocci, G.; Cassardo, C. Attribution of recent temperature behaviour reassessed by a neural-network method. *Sci. Rep.* **2017**, *7*, 17681. [CrossRef]
7. Pasini, A.; Amendola, S. Linear and nonlinear influences of climatic changes on migration flows: A case study for the 'Mediterranean bridge'. *Environ. Res. Commun.* **2019**, *1*, 011005. [CrossRef]
8. Pasini, A.; Amendola, S.; Federbusch, E. Is natural variability really natural? The case of Atlantic Multidecadal Oscillation investigated by a neural network model. *Theor. Appl. Clim.* **2022**, *150*, 881–892. [CrossRef]
9. Lualdi, M.; Cavalleri, A.; Battaglia, L.; Colombo, A.; Garrone, G.; Morelli, D.; Pignoli, E.; Sottotetti, E.; Leo, E. Early detection of colorectal adenocarcinoma: A clinical decision support tool based on plasma porphyrin accumulation and risk factors. *BMC Cancer* **2018**, *18*, 841. [CrossRef]
10. Bagher-Ebadian, H.; Janic, B.; Liu, C.; Pantelic, M.; Hearshen, D.; Elshaikh, M.; Movsas, B.; Chetty, I.J.; Wen, N. Detection of Dominant Intra-prostatic Lesions in Patients With Prostate Cancer Using an Artificial Neural Network and MR Multi-modal Radiomics Analysis. *Front. Oncol.* **2019**, *9*, 1313. [CrossRef]
11. Imai, S.; Takekuma, Y.; Kashiwagi, H.; Miyai, T.; Kobayashi, M.; Iseki, K.; Sugawara, M. Validation of the usefulness of artificial neural networks for risk prediction of adverse drug reactions used for individual patients in clinical practice. *PLoS ONE* **2020**, *15*, e0236789. [CrossRef]
12. Izonin, I.; Tkachenko, R.; Fedushko, S.; Koziy, D.; Zub, K.; Vovk, O. RBF-Based Input Doubling Method for Small Medical Data Processing. In *Advances in Artificial Systems for Logistics Engineering*; Hu, Z., Zhang, Q., Petoukhov, S., He, M., Eds.; Springer: Cham, Switzerland, 2021; pp. 23–31.
13. Sohn, J.; Jung, I.-Y.; Ku, Y.; Kim, Y. Machine-Learning-Based Rehabilitation Prognosis Predictionin Patients with Ischemic Stroke Using Brainstem Auditory Evoked Potential. *Diagnostics* **2021**, *11*, 673. [CrossRef]
14. Le, T.-D.; Noumeir, R.; Rambaud, J.; Sans, G.; Jouvet, P. Detecting of a Patient's Condition From Clinical Narratives Using Natural Language Representation. *IEEE Open J. Eng. Med. Biol.* **2022**, *3*, 142–149. [CrossRef]
15. Sebro, R.; De la Garza-Ramos, C.; Peterson, J.J. Detecting whether L1 or other lumbar levels would be excluded from DXA bone mineral density analysis during opportunistic CT screening for osteoporosis using machine learning. *Int. J. Comput. Assist. Radiol. Surg.* **2023**, *18*, 2261–2272. [CrossRef]
16. Hertz, J.; Krogh, A.; Palmer, R.G. *Introduction to the Theory of Neural Computation*; Addison-Wesley: New York, NY, USA, 1991.
17. Bishop, C.M. *Neural Networks for Pattern Recognition*; Oxford University Press: New York, NY, USA, 1995.
18. Cybenko, G. Approximation by superposition of a sigmoidal function. *Math. Control Signal Syst.* **1989**, *2*, 303–314. [CrossRef]
19. Hornik, K.; Stinchcombe, M.; White, H. Multilayer feedforward networks are universal approximators. *Neural Netw.* **1989**, *2*, 359–366. [CrossRef]
20. LeCun, Y.; Bottou, L.; Orr, G.B.; Müller, K.-R. Efficient BackProp. In *Neural Networks: Tricks of the Trade*; Orr, G.B., Müller, K.-R., Eds.; Springer: New York, NY, USA, 1998; pp. 9–50.
21. Knutti, R.; Baumberger, C.; Hirsch Hadorn, G. Uncertainty Quantification Using Multiple Models—Prospects and Challenges. In *Computer Simulation Validation. Simulation Foundations, Methods and Applications*; Beisbart, C., Saam, N., Eds.; Springer: Cham, Switzerland, 2019; pp. 835–855.
22. Walmsley, L.D. The strategy of model building in climate science. *Synthese* **2021**, *199*, 745–765. [CrossRef]
23. Leimbach, M.; Bauer, N.; Baumstark, L.; Edenhofer, O. Mitigation costs in a globalized world: Climate policy analysis with REMIND-R. *Environ. Model. Assess.* **2010**, *15*, 155–173. [CrossRef]
24. Howard, F.M.; Pearson, A.T. Prognosis and Treatment of Non–Small Cell Lung Cancer in the Age of Deep Learning. *JAMA Netw. Open* **2020**, *3*, e206368. [CrossRef]
25. Yu, K.; Sang, Q.-X.A.; Lung, P.-Y.; Tan, W.; Lively, T.; Sheffield, C.; Bou-Dargham, M.J.; Liu, J.S.; Zhang, J. Personalized chemotherapy selection for breast cancer using gene expression profiles. *Sci. Rep.* **2017**, *7*, 43294. [CrossRef]
26. Binnewies, M.; Roberts, E.W.; Kersten, K.; Chan, V.; Fearon, D.F.; Merad, M.; Coussens, L.M.; Gabrilovich, D.I.; Ostrand-Rosenberg, S.; Hedrick, C.C.; et al. Understanding the tumor immune microenvironment (TIME) for effective therapy. *Nat. Med.* **2018**, *24*, 541–550. [CrossRef]
27. Corsello, S.M.; Nagari, R.T.; Spangler, R.D.; Rossen, J.; Kocak, M.; Bryan, J.G.; Humeidi, R.; Peck, D.; Wu, X.; Tang, A.A.; et al. Discovering the anti-cancer potential of non-oncology drugs by systematic viability profiling. *Nat. Cancer* **2020**, *1*, 235–248. [CrossRef]
28. Sharma, P.; Allison, J.P. The future of immune checkpoint therapy. *Science* **2015**, *348*, 56–61. [CrossRef]
29. Esteva, A.; Kuprel, B.; Novoa, R.A.; Ko, J.; Swetter, S.M.; Blau, H.M.; Thrun, S. Dermatologist-level classification of skin cancer with deep neural networks. *Nature* **2017**, *542*, 115–118. [CrossRef]

Journal of
Clinical Medicine

MDPI

Review

AI in Cytopathology: A Narrative Umbrella Review on Innovations, Challenges, and Future Directions

Daniele Giansanti

Centro TISP, Istituto Superiore di Sanità, Via Regina Elena 299, 00161 Rome, Italy; daniele.giansanti@iss.it

Abstract: The integration of artificial intelligence (AI) in cytopathology is an emerging field with transformative potential, aiming to enhance diagnostic precision and operational efficiency. This umbrella review seeks to identify prevailing themes, opportunities, challenges, and recommendations related to AI in cytopathology. Utilizing a standardized checklist and quality control procedures, this review examines recent advancements and future implications of AI technologies in this domain. Twenty-one review studies were selected through a systematic process. AI has demonstrated promise in automating and refining diagnostic processes, potentially reducing errors and improving patient outcomes. However, several critical challenges need to be addressed to realize the benefits of AI fully. This review underscores the necessity for rigorous validation, ongoing empirical data on diagnostic accuracy, standardized protocols, and effective integration with existing clinical workflows. Ethical issues, including data privacy and algorithmic bias, must be managed to ensure responsible AI applications. Additionally, high costs and substantial training requirements present barriers to widespread AI adoption. Future directions highlight the importance of applying successful integration strategies from histopathology and radiology to cytopathology. Continuous research is needed to improve model interpretability, validation, and standardization. Developing effective strategies for incorporating AI into clinical practice and establishing comprehensive ethical and regulatory frameworks will be crucial for overcoming these challenges. In conclusion, while AI holds significant promise for advancing cytopathology, its full potential can only be achieved by addressing challenges related to validation, cost, and ethics. This review provides an overview of current advancements, identifies ongoing challenges, and offers a roadmap for the successful integration of AI into diagnostic cytopathology, informed by insights from related fields.

Keywords: cytopathology; artificial intelligence; AI; histopathology; radiology

1. Introduction

1.1. The Impact of Digitalization Cytopathology: Transforming Diagnostic Practices

Cytopathology is the branch of medicine and biology focused on studying cells to diagnose diseases, especially by analyzing cellular changes that could indicate conditions such as cancer. This involves using microscopes to examine cell samples from smears, aspirations, or biopsies to identify diseases and support clinical diagnoses [1–3].

In recent years, digital health technologies have shown the potential to transform cytopathology, with some improvements in the accuracy and efficiency of analyses. Digital imaging, for instance, enables the scanning of slides at high resolution, which can lead to more precise examinations and better diagnostic accuracy. However, the full extent of this improvement and its widespread impact remain subjects of ongoing study [4].

Digital tools also offer the possibility of remote consultations and second opinions, promoting global collaboration among specialists. While these advances could streamline workflows and boost productivity, their overall efficacy in supporting personalized patient care through detailed cytopathological data are still being evaluated. As of now, the integration of digital health in cytopathology presents promising, yet still evolving, benefits [5,6].

Key potential benefits include [5,6]:

Enhanced Diagnostic Accuracy: High-resolution imaging may improve the detection of subtle cellular abnormalities, though the level of precision in all cases is still under review [7].

Remote Consultations and Telepathology: Pathologists can conduct remote consultations and second opinions, though the reliability and accessibility of such methods vary [7,8].

Streamlined Workflow: While automating tasks such as slide management and data entry has the potential to enhance lab efficiency, its widespread adoption and real-world impact are still uncertain [9].

Long-term Data Storage: Digital storage of slides allows for secure, long-term management, but concerns about data integrity and retrieval over extended periods remain.

Integration with EHRs: The integration with electronic health records could improve care coordination, though seamless functionality across different systems remains a challenge.

Educational Tools: Virtual slides and interactive modules support training, yet their effectiveness compared with traditional methods is still being assessed.

Quality Assurance and Standardization: While standardized protocols and quality control measures could enhance consistency, there is ongoing discussion about the implementation of such measures across different laboratories.

Research and Data Analysis: Digital tools can help aggregate and analyze large datasets, but their utility in advancing research on disease patterns and new diagnostic methods requires further evidence.

The evolving nature of these technologies highlights both their potential and the need for continued evaluation.

The potential of digitalization and AI in cytopathology is significant, but several challenges need to be addressed to realize these advancements fully [10,11]. Cytopathology, dissimilar to radiology, has experienced a slower integration with the digital health landscape, which can be attributed to several factors [12,13]. One of the key issues is the complexity of cytopathological samples. Cytopathology requires the detailed and often intricate evaluation of individual cells, making it more challenging to automate compared with radiological images, which are generally more uniform and structural. For example, replicating the focus function in cytopathology is highly complex and demands substantial memory resources. Another contributing factor is the difference in imaging technologies. Radiology has benefited from rapid technological advancements, particularly with systems such as CT and MRI, which have facilitated swift digitalization and integration into clinical workflows, largely thanks to the rapid adoption of the DICOM standard [14]. In contrast, the development of a DICOM standard for cytopathology (DICOM WSI) has been slower and more complex [15,16]. Additionally, the diagnostic process in cytopathology involves finer and more interpretative work compared with radiology. The digitalization of cytopathology, therefore, faces specific technical and clinical challenges, including the need to interpret intricate cellular details and manage the variability of cell samples. Standardization presents yet another challenge. Radiology has benefited from well-established standards and protocols, while cytopathology remains more diversified and less standardized, which has contributed to the slower adoption of digital technologies in this field. However, despite these obstacles, cytopathology is progressively integrating digital technologies and advanced tools, and it is anticipated that this evolution will continue in the coming years.

1.2. Integrating Artificial Intelligence in Digital Cytopathology

Artificial intelligence (AI) is revolutionizing many areas of medicine, and cytopathology is no exception. Traditionally, cytopathology, which focuses on diagnosing diseases through cellular samples, has relied heavily on the expertise of pathologists examining slides under a microscope. However, the integration of AI into cytopathology is poised to bring significant advancements, aligning with broader objectives in digital pathology, such as enhancing diagnostic accuracy, improving workflow efficiency, and advancing patient care [17,18]. The insights provided in studies referenced by [17,18] underscore the transformative potential of AI technologies in cytopathology.

AI technologies, especially those based on machine learning (ML) and deep learning (DL), are increasingly being adopted in cytopathology. These advanced algorithms are capable of processing large volumes of cytological data swiftly and with high precision. By leveraging extensive datasets of annotated images, AI can assist in identifying cellular abnormalities, classifying cell types, and even predicting disease progression. This capability has the potential to complement and enhance the diagnostic process, allowing pathologists to detect subtle patterns and anomalies that may be missed in traditional evaluations.

According to the studies cited in [17,18], the adoption of AI in cytopathology offers several transformative benefits. First, AI tools can significantly improve diagnostic accuracy by providing consistent and objective analyses, thereby reducing variability and human error. Additionally, these tools can streamline diagnostic workflows by automating routine tasks such as image sorting and preliminary screening, which helps expedite the diagnostic process and alleviates the workload on cytopathologists. Moreover, AI supports the training and education of new cytopathologists by offering interactive learning modules and access to a broad range of case studies.

Furthermore, AI integration enhances access to cytopathology services by enabling remote consultations and fostering collaboration through digital platforms. This capability is particularly valuable in underserved areas or for institutions seeking expert second opinions from specialists located in other regions.

However, as noted in [17–19], the integration of AI into cytopathology also presents several challenges. Effective implementation requires seamless integration with existing diagnostic workflows and the establishment of standardized protocols to ensure compatibility across different systems. Additionally, important regulatory and ethical considerations need to be addressed, such as the rigorous validation of AI tools, concerns regarding data privacy, and the risk of over-reliance on machine-assisted diagnoses. Furthermore, there may be resistance from practitioners accustomed to traditional methods, who will need time to adapt to these new technologies.

1.3. Purpose of the Study

The integration of AI into the healthcare domain holds transformative potential with profound implications for cytopathology. AI has the capacity to revolutionize diagnostic processes, enhance accuracy, and streamline workflows while also presenting strategic challenges that must be addressed. An overview of reviews can provide a holistic view of how AI is reshaping cytopathology, revealing both the advancements and obstacles encountered in this integration.

The purpose of this study is to develop a narrative umbrella review to comprehensively explore the role of artificial intelligence (AI) in cytopathology. This review seeks to aggregate and synthesize findings from existing reviews to offer a consolidated understanding of how AI is being applied within the field. By identifying and analyzing the key themes and trends emerging from these studies, we aim to highlight significant advancements, such as improvements in diagnostic precision and workflow efficiency, as well as the challenges that have arisen, including issues related to implementation, standardization, and ethical considerations.

Specific aims:

1. Themes and categorization: Identify and organize the main themes emerging from existing studies, with a focus on how AI is being utilized to enhance cytopathological diagnosis.
2. Opportunities and challenges: Analyze the opportunities and challenges encountered in the field, examining benefits related to diagnostic precision and workflow optimization alongside the difficulties faced during implementation.
3. Emerging recommendations: Provide recommendations based on this review's findings, with a particular focus on critical issues such as practical implementation,

standardization of procedures, and ethical aspects related to the use of AI in cytopathology.

2. Methods

An umbrella review (narrative review of reviews) was conducted, focusing on the field of the intersection of cytopathology with AI. A standardized checklist for narrative reviews, the ANDJ Narrative Checklist available online [20] was used. The search was based on targeted searches on Google Scholar, PubMed, and Scopus.

2.1. Search Strategies

The search was performed both in the [Title/abstract] and in the full text.

The components of this overview were obtained by means of the combination of two groups of keywords also combined with AND/OR Boolean logic of a search:

- Machine Learning in Cytopathology
- Deep Learning Algorithms
- Digital Imaging in Cytopathology
- Automated Diagnostic Systems
- Cell Image Analysis
- AI-assisted Diagnosis
- Computer-Aided Diagnosis
- Predictive Analytics in Cytopathology
- Artificial Intelligence in Cellular Diagnostics
- Digital Pathology Tools
- Algorithmic Classification of Cells
- AI-based Cytological Screening
- Machine Learning for Cellular Abnormalities
- Image Recognition in Cytopathology
- AI-driven Cytopathological Innovation
- Diagnostic Precision with AI
- AI in Medical Imaging
- Remote Cytopathology Consultations
- Cytopathological Workflow Optimization
- AI and Pathologist Collaboration

Table 1 shows the research areas related to the application of artificial intelligence (AI) and machine learning (ML) in cytopathology, including key themes and their corresponding focused research queries. Each theme highlights the potential of AI in improving the accuracy and efficiency of cytopathological diagnostics, ranging from deep learning algorithms for cell analysis to the optimization of workflow in cytopathology.

Table 1. Research areas/focus and queries.

Theme	Research Focus	Query
Deep Learning Algorithms and Cell Image Analysis	Development of AI models for detailed cellular structure analysis	"Deep Learning Algorithms AND Cell Image Analysis in Cytopathology"
Digital Imaging & Digital Pathology Tools	Use of digital platforms and images for AI-assisted cytological analysis	"Digital Imaging OR Digital Pathology Tools for AI-based Cytology"
AI-assisted Diagnosis & Predictive Analytics	AI supporting diagnostic decisions and predicting clinical outcomes	"AI-assisted Diagnosis AND Predictive Analytics in Cytopathology"

Table 1. *Cont.*

Theme	Research Focus	Query
Automated Diagnostic Systems & Computer-Aided Diagnosis	Full or partial automation of cytology diagnostics using AI	"Automated Diagnostic Systems OR Computer-Aided Diagnosis with AI"
Algorithmic Classification of Cells & Image Recognition	Use of AI algorithms to classify cells based on image recognition	"Algorithmic Classification of Cells AND Image Recognition in Cytopathology"
Machine Learning & AI-based Cytological Screening	Application of ML algorithms for cytological screening processes	"Machine Learning AND AI-based Cytological Screening"
AI-driven Cytopathological Innovation & Diagnostic Precision	Innovations and precision improvements in cytopathology through AI	"AI-driven Cytopathological Innovation OR Diagnostic Precision with AI"
AI in Medical Imaging & Cytopathological Workflow Optimization	AI applied to medical imaging and optimizing the cytopathology diagnostic workflow	"AI in Medical Imaging AND Cytopathological Workflow Optimization"
Remote Cytopathology Consultations & AI-assisted Diagnosis	Use of AI for remote diagnosis and consultations in cytopathology	"Remote Cytopathology Consultations AND AI-assisted Diagnosis"
AI and Pathologist Collaboration & AI-based Cytological Screening	Research on the collaboration between AI systems and pathologists for screening and diagnosis	"AI and Pathologist Collaboration OR AI-based Cytological Screening"
General Search	Broad and focused research on AI, machine learning, deep learning, and neural networks in cytopathology	"(Cytopathology [Title/Abstract]) AND ((Artificial intelligence [Title/Abstract]) OR (machine learning [Title/Abstract]) OR (deep learning [Title/Abstract]) OR (neural network [Title/Abstract]))"

2.2. Assessment Criteria for Study Inclusion

To ensure a rigorous and high-quality narrative review, each selected study was assessed based on the following criteria:

Clarity of Rationale (N1): This criterion evaluates whether the study clearly articulates the reason for its investigation. The rationale should define the research problem, highlight its significance, and explain why the study is necessary. A well-defined rationale provides context and justifies the research effort.

Design Appropriateness (N2): This criterion assesses whether the study's design is suitable for answering the research question or hypothesis. The design should align with the objectives and scope of the study. Appropriate design includes selecting the right methodology, sample size, and data collection methods.

Methodological Clarity (N3): Methodological clarity refers to the extent to which the study's methods are described in detail and are replicable. This includes the transparency of procedures for data collection, analysis, and interpretation. The study should provide clear information on how data were gathered, the tools and techniques used, and how the analysis was conducted. This clarity ensures that the study can be reproduced or critiqued based on the methodology described.

Result Presentation (N4): This criterion evaluates how effectively the study presents its findings. Results should be clearly organized, accurately reported, and appropriately interpreted. The presentation should include relevant tables, figures, and statistical analyses that support the conclusions drawn. The clarity of the result presentation allows readers to understand and evaluate the study's outcomes.

Justification of Conclusions (N5): This criterion assesses whether the study's conclusions are supported by its results. The study should provide a logical link between presented data and the conclusions drawn. It should discuss the implications of the findings, address limitations, and suggest areas for future research. The justification of conclusions ensures that the study's outcomes are valid and that the conclusions are based on sound evidence.

Disclosure of Conflicts of Interest (N6): Disclosure of conflicts of interest is crucial for assessing the impartiality and credibility of the study. This criterion checks whether the authors have declared any financial, professional, or personal interests that could bias the research. Full disclosure helps in evaluating the objectivity of the study and ensures that the findings are not influenced by external pressures or biases.

The choice of the component elements of this overview was made taking into account the 5 parameters (N1–N5) evaluated with a score from 1 = minimum to 5 = maximum and one parameter (N6) with a binary assessment (Yes/No). These parameters have been identified into the following:

All the selected studies had to have the parameter N6 with "Yes" and the parameters N1-N5 with a score >3.

In addition to these parameters, in this umbrella review, we have also given weight to the publication date, prioritizing more recent reviews if the topic has been covered in later publications. In other words, we have established a sort of time-based priority to ensure that the most current and relevant findings are considered. This approach helps us capture the latest advancements and developments in the field while also maintaining a comprehensive overview of the existing literature.

The procedure ultimately identified 21 studies at the end of the selection process. Figure 1 outlines all the steps involved. This figure illustrates that the initial search yielded a total of 39 studies. From these, 13 studies were excluded because of their poor focus on AI. Following the evaluation according to the methodology described above, 21 studies were retained for further consideration, while 5 studies were excluded. See Section S1 for the narrative checklist.

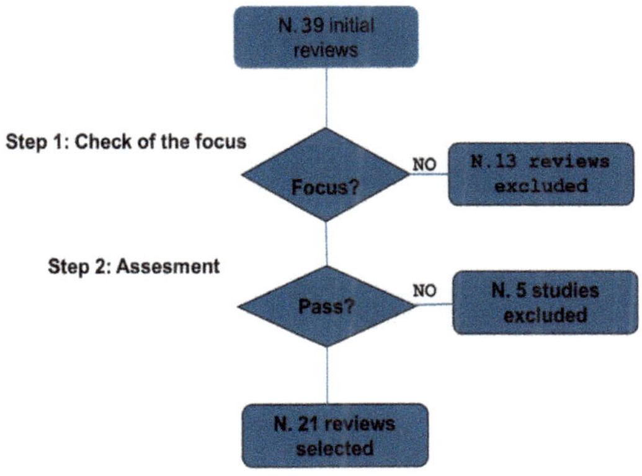

Figure 1. Details on the process of study selection.

3. Results

In total, 21 studies were selected [21–41], comprising all the relevant research identified on PubMed.

The results are systematically organized into multiple subsections to provide a comprehensive understanding of the findings.

Section 3.1 reports a synoptic diagram of the results.

Section 3.2 presents trends observed across the studies, enhanced by graphical representations that illustrate these data visually. This subsection aims to highlight overarching patterns and significant shifts within the field, offering a clear view of how the research landscape has evolved over time.

Section 3.3 aligns the outcomes with the specific objectives and is therefore divided into three subsections, each corresponding to a specific sub-aim.

Section 3.3.1 answers sub-aim (1: "*Themes and categorization: Identify and organize the main themes emerging from existing studies, with a focus on how AI is being utilized to enhance cytopathological diagnosis*"). This subsection explores:

(a) Extraction of common themes and interconnections among the studies, highlighting recurring messages and drawing correlations between research findings. This allows for a synthesis of insights that reflect broader implications within the literature.

(b) A detailed categorization of the studies, distinguishing fine-grained thematic areas as well as broader categories. This categorization organizes research into specific subfields and general domains, offering a comprehensive view of the diverse aspects covered by the studies and highlighting key areas of focus and specialization.

Section 3.3.2 answers sub-aim (2: "*Opportunities and challenges: Analyze the opportunities and challenges encountered in the field, examining benefits related to diagnostic precision and workflow optimization alongside the difficulties faced during implementation*"). This subsection discusses the potential for AI to enhance diagnostic precision and improve workflow efficiency while addressing challenges such as data variability, technical integration issues, and the need for resource investment during the implementation phase.

Section 3.3.3 addresses sub-aim (3: "*Emerging recommendations: Provide recommendations based on the review findings, with particular focus on critical issues such as practical implementation, standardization of procedures, and ethical aspects related to the use of AI in cytopathology*"). It synthesizes key recommendations from this review, emphasizing the need for standardized procedures to facilitate AI integration into clinical workflows. Additionally, it highlights practical challenges in implementation, such as data management and resource allocation, and underscores the importance of addressing ethical issues such as transparency, data privacy, and algorithmic biases in AI-driven cytopathology.

Analytical summaries of the overviewed reviews [21–41] are also reported in the Supplementary Materials.

3.1. Synoptic Diagram

The diagram in Figure 2 provides a highly concise sketch of the results organized into tabular connections and diagrams aligned with the overall aim and specific objectives.

Block 1 (from top to bottom) highlights trends supported by the diagrams in Figures 3–6.

Block 2 references both Table 2, which emphasizes the themes and the categorization emerging in the fields, and Table 3 reporting the main areas with the emerging diagnostic innovations. Block 3 focuses on the opportunities and challenges, as shown in Table 4.

Block 4 faces the emerging recommendations as presented in Table 5.

Blocks 5 and 6 deepen the analysis facing both the ethical and standardization issues emerging as cross-cutting recommendations form the analysis reported in Tables 6 and 7, respectively.

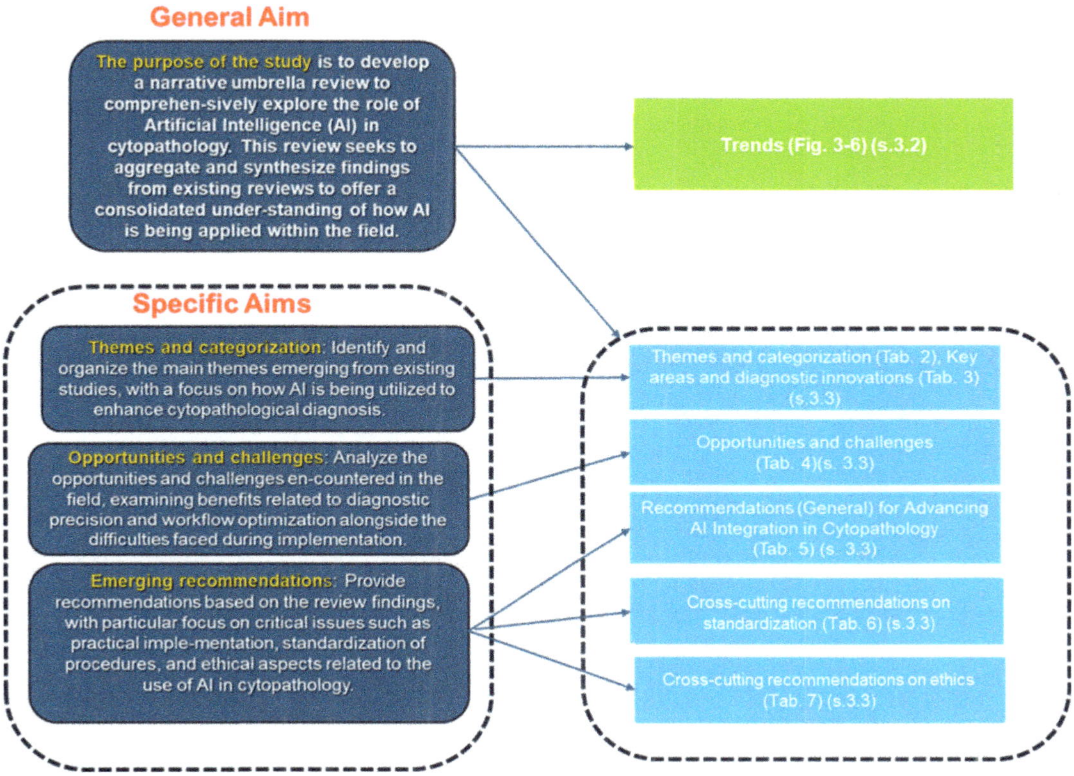

Figure 2. Synoptics diagram reporting a sketch of the the results.

3.2. The Trends in the Studies on AI in the Field of Cytopathology

A search conducted on PubMed on 15 July 2024 (when the overview started), using the composite keyword listed in position 1 of Box 1, returned 101 articles. It is intriguing to analyze both the temporal evolution of the scientific output and its proportion relative to the overall studies in cytopathology, as well as the types of studies produced.

The 101 articles were published starting in 1998, a period when discussions were more focused on neural networks rather than true artificial intelligence (AI). Notably, 98 of these studies, representing 97.0%, were published in the last decade. Furthermore, 86 of these studies, accounting for 85.1%, were published in the past five years, a period notably influenced by the COVID-19 pandemic.

The impact of the COVID-19 pandemic on research output in this period has been profound. The pandemic has accelerated the pace of research, particularly in fields where rapid technological advancements were crucial. The surge in AI-related studies within cytopathology reflects a broader trend driven by the urgent need for innovative solutions to manage the healthcare crisis. The pandemic has highlighted the critical role of AI in enhancing diagnostic capabilities, managing large volumes of data, and facilitating remote consultations. This heightened focus on digital health solutions has contributed to the significant increase in AI research output during the past five years.

In the broader context of cytopathology research, a total of 5669 studies have been produced (key in position 2, Box 1). Therefore, studies specifically addressing AI represent 1.79% of the total. Figure 3 reports the temporal trend of studies focusing on the integration of AI with digital cytopathology.

Figure 4 shows the number of studies in cytopathology not involving AI compared with the number of studies in cytopathology focused on AI.

It is noteworthy that a comparison limited to the past five years reveals a significant increase in studies conducted in cytopathology and AI. Specifically, a comparison between the total number of cytopathology studies over the last five years, which amounts to 1737, and those focused on AI, which total 86, results in a ratio of 4.95. Figure 5 illustrates, with reference to the past five years, the number of studies in cytopathology not involving AI compared with the number of studies centered on AI.

The COVID-19 pandemic has notably accelerated the focus on AI within the field of cytopathology. This is evidenced by the increased percentage of studies concentrating on AI, reflecting a surge in research and technological advancements prompted by the pandemic. The need for rapid, efficient diagnostics and remote consultation solutions drove this trend. The integration of AI technologies helped address the unprecedented challenges posed by COVID-19 by improving diagnostic accuracy, managing large volumes of patient data, and facilitating remote medical consultations.

The increased emphasis on AI during this period highlights its critical role in enhancing diagnostic capabilities and adapting to new healthcare demands. This shift not only underscores the growing importance of digital health innovations but also demonstrates how AI has become an essential component in advancing cytopathological practices in response to global health crises.

The types of studies produced are illustrated in Figure 6. This includes one systematic review and 30 reviews of various types, in addition to the remaining 70 primary studies. This distribution underscores the growing interest in AI applications within cytopathology and reflects the diverse nature of the research being conducted, influenced significantly by the pandemic-driven emphasis on technological innovation in healthcare.

Box 1. The proposed composite keys.

(Cytopathology [Title/Abstract]) AND ((Artificial intelligence [Title/Abstract]) OR (machine learning [Title/Abstract]) OR (deep learning [Title/Abstract]) OR (neural network [Title/Abstract]))
((Cytopathology [Title/Abstract])

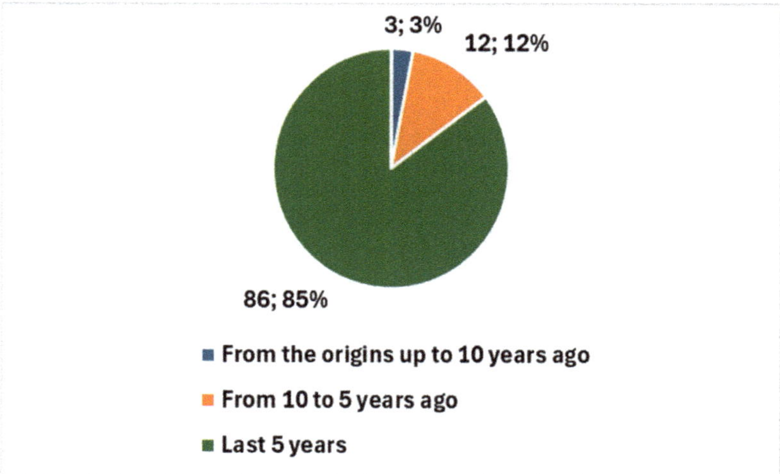

Figure 3. Temporal trend of studies focusing on the integration of AI with digital cytopathology.

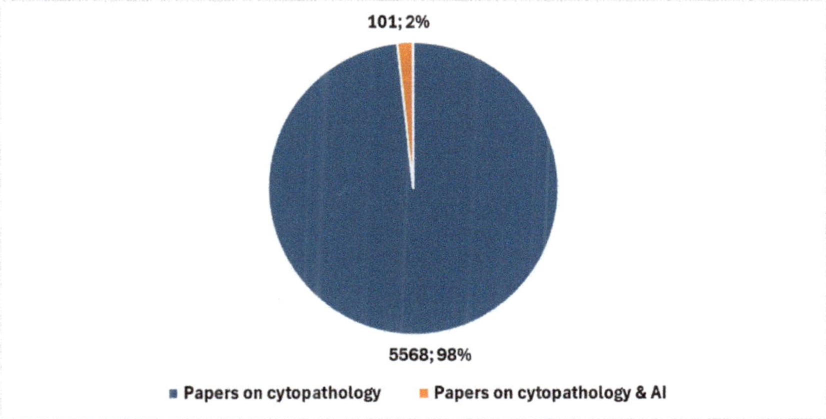

Figure 4. Studies in cytopathology that do not involve AI compared with studies in cytopathology focused on AI.

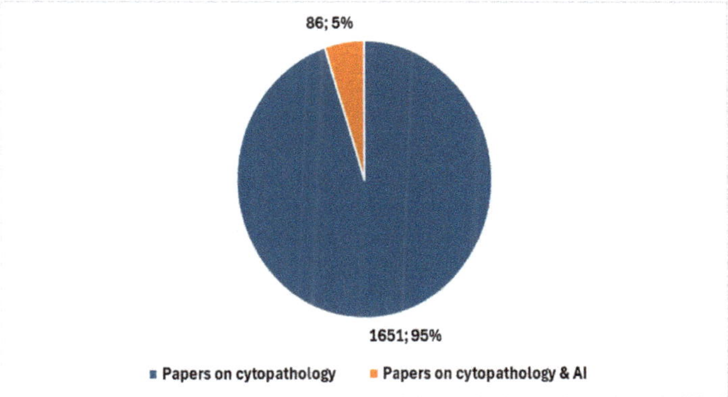

Figure 5. Studies in cytopathology that do not involve AI compared with studies in cytopathology focused on AI with reference to the last five years.

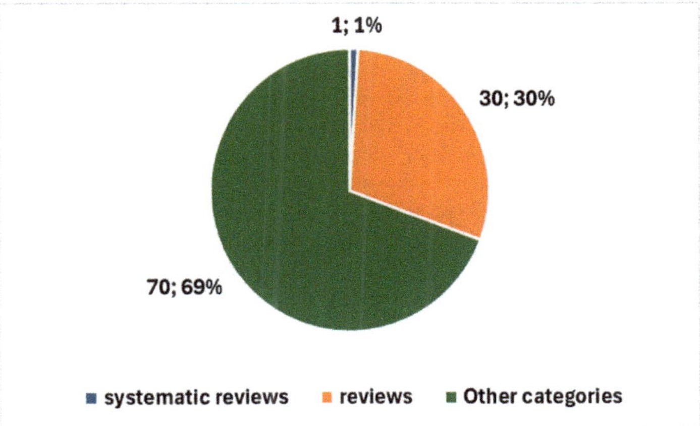

Figure 6. Proportion of studies in cytopathology and AI.

3.3. Outcome from the Umbrella Review Aligned with the Specific Aims

3.3.1. Themes and Categorization

Table 2 reports a categorization with a brief description of each contribution and the focus/role of the AI.

The integration of artificial intelligence (AI) into diagnostic medicine is profoundly transforming the field, as evidenced by recent studies [21–38]. The research collectively underscores how AI is enhancing diagnostic practices across various domains.

Studies such as those by Ciaparrone et al. [21] and Kim et al. [25,26] highlight the transformative role of AI in diagnostic automation and digital cytology. Ciaparrone et al. [21] focus on the impact of AI on urine cytology, demonstrating its potential to improve diagnostic speed, cost-efficiency, and accuracy by automating image analysis. Similarly, Kim et al. [25,26] provide comprehensive reviews on AI applications in digital cytology, offering guidelines for integrating AI technologies to enhance workflow and diagnostic precision.

The advancements in cancer diagnosis are notably reflected in the work of Zhang et al. [22] and Malik & Zaheer [27]. Zhang et al. [22] explore the potential of AI in detecting early markers of thyroid cancer, emphasizing its role in improving diagnostic accuracy and early detection. Malik & Zaheer [27] analyze the use of AI-driven tools such as ChatGPT to support cancer diagnosis, showcasing how conversational AI can integrate with traditional diagnostic processes.

The ability of AI to complement traditional diagnostic methods is also highlighted by Giovanella et al. [24] and Wong et al. [32]. Giovanella et al. [24] review how AI enhances the diagnostic accuracy and risk assessment of thyroid nodules when used alongside traditional methods such as ultrasound and fine needle aspiration (FNAC). Wong et al. [32] provide an overview of machine learning advancements in thyroid cytopathology, illustrating the integration of AI into established diagnostic practices. Furthermore, Ludwig et al. [33] update on recent advancements in AI for diagnosing and classifying thyroid nodules, reflecting how AI technologies are being incorporated into thyroid diagnostics.

In addition, Tessler et al. [35] review AI tools for thyroid nodule diagnosis with a particular focus on malignancy.

Specialized applications of AI are explored by Singla et al. [30] and Sunny et al. [31]. Singla et al. [30] focus on the role of AI in fungal cytology, highlighting its potential to improve the detection and classification of fungal infections. Sunny et al. [31] discuss the application of AI in analyzing CD44-SNA1 markers for identifying high-grade dysplastic and neoplastic oral lesions, demonstrating the ability of AI to enhance diagnostic precision in specific contexts.

In the realms of microbiological and pancreatic pathology, Marletta et al. [34,35] and Hameed & Krishnan [36] provide insights into the impact of AI. Marletta et al. [34]. Hameed & Krishnan [36] examine the effectiveness of AI in diagnosing pancreatic cancer, discussing both the benefits and challenges of AI-driven diagnostic tools.

Thakur et al. [37] offer a systematic review of AI applications in non-gynecological cancer cytopathology, while Alrafiah [38] assesses the overall performance and impact of AI technologies in cytopathology. These studies underscore the growing influence of AI in enhancing diagnostic accuracy, efficiency, and integration with traditional methods across various diagnostic fields. Finally, Vaickus et al. [39] review AI advancements in cytopathology and their integration with consensus rule sets, while Jorda et al. [40] discuss the role of AI in enhancing diagnostic accuracy in urinary tract cytopathology and Velez Torres et al. [41] examines the impact of AI on thyroid fine-needle aspiration cytology and risk assessment.

The body of research from [21] to [41] illustrates the transformative potential of AI in modern diagnostic medicine, showcasing its ability to refine diagnostic practices, enhance precision, and integrate with established methods.

Table 2. Summary of Recent Studies on AI Applications in Cytopathology: Focus, Impact, and Categorization.

Reference	Brief Description	Focus on AI	Categorization
Ciaparrone et al. (2024) [21]	This study evaluates computer-assisted urine cytology, emphasizing the role of AI in enhancing diagnostic speed, reducing costs, and improving accuracy. It examines how automation and AI-driven image analysis contribute to a more efficient diagnostic process.	Investigates AI in automating image analysis for urine cytology, aiming to speed up the diagnostic process and reduce costs.	AI in Diagnostic Automation
Zhang et al. (2024) [22]	Explores the role of AI in diagnosing early markers for thyroid cancer, focusing on how AI algorithms improve diagnostic precision. The paper highlights the potential of AI in identifying early cancer markers crucial for timely and accurate diagnosis.	Focuses on the role of AI in identifying and diagnosing early markers for thyroid cancer, improving accuracy and early detection.	AI in Cancer Diagnosis
Caputo et al. (2024) [23]	Discusses how AI and computational advancements are transforming cytopathology, with insights from emerging pathologists. The paper highlights the integration of AI in modern cytopathology practices, contributing to more precise diagnostics.	Highlights the integration of AI and computational methods in modern cytopathology, reflecting on their transformative effects on the field.	AI and Computational Integration
Giovanella et al. (2024) [24]	Reviews how AI integrates with traditional diagnostic methods for evaluating thyroid nodules, such as ultrasound and fine needle aspiration (FNAC). The study focuses on the role of AI in enhancing diagnostic accuracy and risk assessment.	Reviews the role of AI in integrating diagnostic tools such as ultrasound and FNAC, aiming to improve overall diagnostic accuracy and patient management.	AI in Integrated Diagnostics
Kim et al. (2024) [25]	Part two of a review on digital cytology focuses on AI applications in cytology practices. It offers guidelines and recommendations for incorporating AI technologies to enhance diagnostic workflows.	Examines AI technologies in digital cytology and offers recommendations for their implementation to improve diagnostic practices.	AI in Digital Cytology
Kim et al. (2024) [26]	The first part of a review series on digital cytology addresses the practical aspects of implementing AI tools in clinical settings. It discusses various AI tools and their benefits in enhancing cytology practices.	Discusses the implementation of AI tools in digital cytology, including practical considerations and potential benefits for clinical practice.	AI in Digital Cytology

Table 2. *Cont.*

Reference	Brief Description	Focus on AI	Categorization
Malik & Zaheer (2024) [27])	Analyze how ChatGPT and similar AI-driven tools can support cancer diagnosis. The study evaluates the integration of conversational AI into diagnostic processes, providing additional support for pathologists.	Evaluate the utility of ChatGPT in supporting cancer diagnosis through AI-driven conversational tools and diagnostic assistance.	AI in Diagnostic Support
Slabaugh et al. (2023) [28]	Reviews the application of machine learning and deep learning technologies in thyroid cytology and histopathology. The paper explores how these advanced AI methods enhance diagnostic accuracy and efficiency.	Focuses on the application of machine learning and deep learning in thyroid cytology and histopathology, highlighting improvements in diagnostic processes.	AI in Machine Learning and Deep Learning
Lebrun & Salmon (2024) [29]	Provides insights into recent advancements in classifying thyroid neoplasms according to the 2022 WHO classification. It highlights the contribution of AI to improving diagnostic accuracy in this field.	Examines how AI contributes to the diagnosis and classification of thyroid neoplasms, aligning with the updated WHO classification criteria.	AI in Thyroid Neoplasms
Singla et al. (2024) [30]	Investigates the role of AI in fungal cytology, focusing on improving the detection and classification of fungal infections. The study emphasizes the future potential of AI in this specialized diagnostic area.	Explores the role of AI in detecting and classifying fungal infections, emphasizing its potential impact on fungal cytology.	AI in Fungal Cytology
Sunny et al. (2023) [31]	Discusses the use of CD44-SNA1 markers in cytopathology for identifying high-grade dysplastic and neoplastic oral lesions. The paper evaluates the role of AI in analyzing these markers to enhance diagnostic precision.	Focuses on the application of AI in analyzing CD44-SNA1 markers for oral lesions, aiming to enhance diagnostic accuracy for high-grade dysplastic and neoplastic lesions.	AI in Oral Lesion Diagnosis
Wong et al. (2023) [32]	Reviews advancements and current applications of machine learning in thyroid cytopathology. The paper provides an overview of how machine learning improves diagnostic practices in this field.	Provides an overview of machine learning applications in thyroid cytopathology, highlighting advancements and current uses.	AI in Thyroid Cytopathology
Ludwig et al. (2023) [33]	Updates on the use of AI in diagnosing and classifying thyroid nodules. The study discusses recent advancements in AI technologies and their integration into diagnostic practices for thyroid conditions.	Highlights advancements in AI for diagnosing and classifying thyroid nodules, reflecting recent developments in the field.	AI in Thyroid Nodule Diagnosis

Table 2. *Cont.*

Reference	Brief Description	Focus on AI	Categorization
Marletta et al. (2023) [34]	Reviews AI-based tools for diagnosing microbiological diseases, discussing how these technologies improve diagnostic accuracy and efficiency. The paper highlights the impact of AI on pathological diagnoses in microbiology.	Investigates AI tools for diagnosing microbiological diseases, focusing on their impact on pathological diagnoses.	AI in Microbiological Pathology
Tessler et al. (2023) [35]	The study reviews the role of AI in diagnosing thyroid nodules, highlighting its potential for improving risk stratification and diagnostic accuracy. It does not cover microbiological diseases.	Reiterates the role of AI in thyroid cytopathology, highlighting advancements and current uses.	AI in thyroid Nodule Diagnosis
Hameed & Krishnan (2022) [36]	Examines the application of AI in diagnosing pancreatic cancer, highlighting its benefits, challenges, and the effectiveness of AI-driven diagnostic tools.	Discusses the potential of AI in enhancing pancreatic cancer diagnosis, including the benefits and challenges of AI-driven tools.	AI in Pancreatic Cancer Diagnosis
Thakur et al. (2022) [37]	Reviews AI applications in non-gynecological cancer cytopathology, focusing on recent advancements and their impact on diagnostic practices. The study provides a systematic review of the role of AI in this area.	Focuses on AI applications in non-gynecological cancer cytopathology, providing a systematic review of advancements and impacts.	AI in Non-Gynecological Cancer Diagnosis
Alrafiah (2022) [38]	Analyzes the application and performance of AI technologies in cytopathology. The study evaluates how different AI technologies enhance diagnostic accuracy and efficiency in the field.	Examines the effectiveness and impact of AI technologies in cytopathology, highlighting their role in improving diagnostic performance.	AI in Cytopathology Performance
Vaickus et al. (2024) [39]	Overview of AI advancements in cytopathology, including consensus rule sets such as Bethesda and Paris.	AI offers reproducible and objective diagnoses, addressing variability and biases in human interpretation.	AI in cytopathology standardization
Jorda et al. (2024) [40]	Current and future impacts of urinary tract cytopathology on patient care, including AI advancements.	AI enhances diagnostic accuracy and management strategies in urinary tract cytopathology.	AI in urinary tract cytopathology
Velez Torres et al. (2024) [41]	Review of AI applications in thyroid fine-needle aspiration (FNA) for improved diagnostic accuracy.	AI enhances diagnostic precision and risk stratification in thyroid FNA cytology.	AI in thyroid cytology

Table 3 presents the key areas of interest. It should be noted that some studies may cover multiple areas; thus, the areas where the contribution appears most dominant have been indicated. Therefore, the table categorizes studies based on their predominant focus areas, highlighting how AI technologies are integrated into various diagnostic processes to enhance accuracy, efficiency, and patient care.

AI in Diagnostic Automation and Digital Cytology

The integration of AI into diagnostic automation and digital cytology is transforming traditional methods by improving accuracy and workflow efficiency. Ciaparrone et al. (2024) [21] investigate the role of computer-assisted diagnosis (CAD) systems in urine cytopathology, focusing on their potential to enhance the diagnosis of urothelial carcinomas. Kim et al. (2024) [25,26] review the adoption of digital cytology and AI integration, discussing the benefits and challenges of incorporating these technologies into routine practice.

AI in Cancer Diagnosis and Prognosis

In cancer diagnosis and prognosis, AI technologies provide significant advancements by enhancing early detection and diagnostic support. Zhang et al. (2024) [22] explore AI applications in the early diagnosis of thyroid cancer, utilizing ultrasound images and cytopathology samples. Malik & Zaheer (2024) [27] examine the role of ChatGPT in aiding cancer diagnosis, while Slabaugh et al. (2023) [28] review the application of machine learning and deep learning in thyroid cytology and histopathology. Tessler et al. (2022) [35] focus on the role of AI in evaluating thyroid nodules, highlighting its impact on diagnostic accuracy. The application of AI in non-gynecological cancer cytopathology aims to improve diagnostic processes through advanced models. Thakur et al. (2022) [37] evaluate AI applications across various cancer types, focusing on the need for improved dataset quality and validation.

AI in Integrated Diagnostics

AI is increasingly integrated into established diagnostic frameworks, enhancing the precision of various diagnostic tools. Caputo et al. (2024) [23], for example, discuss how AI complements molecular and computational advancements in cytopathology. Giovanella et al. (2024) [24] review the integration of AI with multiple diagnostic tools for evaluating thyroid nodules, emphasizing a multimodal approach.

AI in Specialized Fields

AI applications are expanding into specialized diagnostic areas such as fungal infections [30] and oral lesions [31], providing innovative solutions for detecting and analyzing these conditions more accurately.

AI in Microbiological and Pancreatic Pathology

AI is transforming the diagnosis of microbiological and pancreatic diseases by enhancing diagnostic capabilities and addressing the unique challenges these fields present, leading to more precise and efficient diagnoses [34,36]

AI Performance and Challenges

Understanding the performance of AI and addressing its challenges is crucial for its successful implementation in diagnostic settings. Lebrun & Salmon (2024) [29] review updates from the WHO classification of thyroid neoplasms and the role of AI in refining diagnosis. Alrafiah (2022) [38] provides a comprehensive overview of AI advancements in cytopathology, addressing its challenges and future research directions. Vaikus et al. (2024) [39] discuss the integration of AI into cytopathology and its potential to enhance diagnostic consistency.

AI in Urinary Tract and Thyroid Cytopathology

In urinary tract cytopathology, AI is enhancing diagnostic accuracy and efficiency. Jorda et al. (2024) [40] discuss the role of AI in urine cytology, addressing challenges related to diagnostic accuracy and false results. AI technologies are making strides in thyroid cytology, improving diagnostic accuracy and risk assessment. Torres et al. (2024) [41] review the integration of AI in thyroid cytology, focusing on its impact on diagnosing thyroid nodules and stratifying risk.

Table 3. AI in Cytopathology: Key Areas and Diagnostic Innovations.

Broad Area	References	Overview
AI in Diagnostic Automation and Digital Cytology	[21] Ciaparrone et al. (2024) [25] Kim et al. (2024, Part 2) [26] Kim et al. (2024, Part 1).	AI is enhancing diagnostic efficiency by automating processes and advancing digital cytology, which offers significant improvements in diagnostic speed and cost-effectiveness.
AI in Cancer Diagnosis and Prognosis	[22] Zhang et al. (2024) [27] Malik & Zaheer (2024) [28] Slabaugh et al. (2023) [37] Thakur et al. (2022) [35] Tessler et al. (2022)	AI technologies are crucial for advancing cancer diagnosis and prognosis, providing sophisticated tools for early cancer detection, personalized diagnostic support, and better management of cancer cases.
AI in Integrated Diagnostics	[23] Caputo et al. (2024) [24] Giovanella et al. (2024) [32] Wong et al. (2023) [33] Ludwig et al. (2023)	AI is integrated into existing diagnostic frameworks to enhance the evaluation of thyroid conditions and other diagnoses, improving the precision of diagnostic results and comprehensive patient assessment.
AI in Specialized Fields	[30] Singla et al. (2024) [31] Sunny et al. (2023)	AI applications are expanding into specialized diagnostic areas such as fungal infections and oral lesions, providing innovative solutions for detecting and analyzing these conditions more accurately.
AI in Microbiological and Pancreatic Pathology	[34] Marletta et al. (2023) [36] Hameed & Krishnan (2022)	AI is transforming the diagnosis of microbiological and pancreatic diseases by enhancing diagnostic capabilities and tackling the unique challenges these fields present, leading to more precise and efficient diagnoses
AI Performance and Challenges	[38] Alrafiah (2022) [29] Lebrun & Salmon (2024) [39] Vaikus et al. (2024)	Analyzes the effectiveness and limitations of AI applications, focusing on how AI improves diagnostic performance while also addressing the challenges and areas needing further development and the perspectives of standardization
AI in Urinary Tract and Thyroid Cytopathology	[40] Jorda et al. (2024) [41] Torres et al. (2024)	Highlights the role of AI in urinary tract cytopathology, enhancing diagnostic accuracy. Reviews AI integration in thyroid FNA cytology for better diagnosis and risk stratification.

3.3.2. Opportunities and Areas Needing Broader Investigation

The application of artificial intelligence (AI) in diagnostic practices, particularly within cytopathology, is rapidly advancing, presenting significant opportunities to enhance diagnostic accuracy, efficiency, and workflow management. AI technologies, such as machine learning (ML) and deep learning (DL), are making substantial impacts across various diagnostic domains. For instance, Ciaparrone et al. (2024) [21] highlight the role of computer-assisted diagnosis (CAD) systems in improving the diagnosis of urothelial carcinomas by identifying subtle patterns that human reviewers might miss. Similarly, Zhang et al. (2024) [22] discuss the transformative potential of AI in the early diagnosis and risk stratification of thyroid cancer through the analysis of imaging and molecular data.

Opportunities are extensive, with AI tools enhancing diagnostic processes and offering new insights into complex cases. Kim et al. (2024) [25,26] provide a comprehensive review of the integration of digital cytology and AI, recommending best practices for improving diagnostic accuracy and laboratory workflows. Malik and Zaheer (2024) [27] explore how ChatGPT can support cancer diagnosis by processing large volumes of data and providing additional analytical perspectives.

Despite these advancements, several areas require further investigation. Slabaugh et al. (2023) [28] emphasize the need for prospective validation of ML and DL algorithms in thyroid cytology and histopathology, addressing issues related to algorithm interpretability and clinical integration. Giovanella et al. (2024) [24] call for more research to establish the clinical value of AI when combined with other diagnostic tools for thyroid nodules. Marletta et al. (2023) [34] stress the need for technological improvements and better datasets to expand the adoption of AI in microbiological diagnostics.

Challenges also persist, such as ensuring the practical usability and cost-effectiveness of AI tools. Wong et al. (2023) [32] highlight the necessity for diverse datasets and further validation to refine ML algorithms for thyroid cytopathology. Jorda et al. (2024) [40] note the importance of correlating urine cytology findings with tissue samples to minimize false results. Tessler et al. (2022) [35] discuss the need to address the practical usability and cost-effectiveness of AI tools in clinical settings.

The following table summarizes the key studies, outlining both the significant opportunities presented by AI in diagnostic practices and the areas that require further exploration to address existing challenges and ensure effective integration into clinical settings. Table 4 reports the emerging opportunities and the areas needing a broader investigation.

Table 4. Emerging opportunities and areas needing a broader investigation.

Study	Opportunities	Areas Needing Broader Investigation
Ciaparrone et al. (2024) [21]	Enhances diagnosis of urothelial carcinomas with CAD systems, improving diagnostic accuracy and workflow efficiency.	Requires rigorous validation and regulatory approval. Comprehensive training for pathologists is needed.
Zhang et al. (2024) [22]	Improves early diagnosis and risk stratification of thyroid cancer through AI analysis of ultrasound images and molecular markers.	Further development and clinical validation are necessary. Expansion of AI tools in routine practice is needed.
Caputo et al. (2024) [23]	Integrates digital pathology and molecular advancements for precise cancer risk stratification. Enhances diagnostic accuracy and cost-effectiveness.	Need for effective integration of digital and AI technologies in clinical settings. Perspectives on new tools from pathologists require exploration.
Giovanella et al. (2024) [24]	Combines ultrasound, FNAC, molecular imaging, and AI to refine the diagnosis of thyroid nodules and reduce unnecessary procedures.	Further research is needed to establish the clinical value of AI and its effectiveness in combination with other diagnostic tools.
Kim et al. (2024) [25,26]	Reviews and guides the integration of digital cytology and AI into cytology workflows, improving diagnostic accuracy and efficiency. Provides best practice recommendations.	Challenges include technology costs, workflow integration, standardized protocols, and the need for effective implementation strategies.
Malik and Zaheer (2024) [27]	Enhances cancer diagnosis by integrating ChatGPT and digital slides for additional analysis and knowledge synthesis.	Challenges include integrating AI with existing systems, addressing biases, and navigating legal issues.

Table 4. *Cont.*

Study	Opportunities	Areas Needing Broader Investigation
Slabaugh et al. (2023) [28]	ML and DL technologies address limitations in thyroid cytology and histopathology, improving the classification and diagnosis of thyroid lesions.	Need for prospective validation, improving algorithm interpretability, and integrating into clinical workflows.
Lebrun and Salmon (2024) [29]	Updates in thyroid neoplasm classification and molecular testing improve diagnosis and risk stratification.	Ongoing challenges in managing low-risk lesions and integrating AI into diagnostic strategies.
Singla et al. (2024) [30]	Transforms detection and typing of fungal infections using AI technologies, improving accuracy and real-time identification.	Requires further research to explore the full potential of AI in fungal cytology.
Sunny et al. (2023) [31]	Integrates biomarkers with AI to enhance diagnostic sensitivity and specificity for oral potentially malignant disorders.	Further research is needed to refine biomarker panels and automate image analysis for point-of-care diagnostics.
Wong et al. (2023) [32]	Promises improved diagnostic accuracy and efficiency in thyroid cytopathology through ML integration.	Need for larger, diverse datasets and further validation studies to refine ML algorithms and clinical integration.
Ludwig et al. (2023) [33]	AI improves the classification and management of thyroid nodules, potentially reducing unnecessary procedures.	Ongoing research is required to validate AI tools and enhance clinical applicability.
Marletta et al. (2023) [34]	Enhances microbiological disease diagnosis, particularly in resource-limited settings, by analyzing cytological images with AI.	Technological improvements and better datasets are needed to expand the adoption of AI in microbiological diagnostics.
Tessler et al. (2022) [35]	Utilizes AI for evaluating thyroid nodules, enhancing diagnostic accuracy and efficiency, particularly benefiting less experienced physicians.	Challenges include ensuring the practical usability and cost-effectiveness of AI tools in clinical settings.
Thakur et al. (2022) [37]	AI shows potential in enhancing non-gynecological cancer diagnostics, with promising results in various cancer types.	Requires larger, well-annotated datasets and external validation to improve AI models and their clinical application.
Alrafiah et al. (2022) [38]	Provides a comprehensive overview of AI advancements in cytopathology, highlighting improvements in diagnostic accuracy and workflow.	Emphasizes the need for transparency, robust validation, and practical integration into clinical workflows.
Vaikus et al. (2023) [39]	AI integration with consensus rule sets aims to reduce diagnostic variability and enhance accuracy.	Requires addressing biases and variability in AI systems to realize its potential in cytopathology fully.
Jorda et al. (2024) [40]	Enhances urinary tract cytopathology with AI, improving diagnostic accuracy and patient management.	Need for improved correlation between cytology findings and tissue samples to minimize false results.
Torres et al. (2024) [41]	Integrates AI with FNA and molecular testing in thyroid cytology, improving diagnostic accuracy and risk stratification.	Challenges include integrating AI with traditional methods and ensuring comprehensive validation in clinical settings.

3.3.3. Integrating AI into Cytopathology: Recommendations for Advancing Diagnostic Practices

The integration of artificial intelligence (AI) into cytopathology is transforming diagnostic practices by enhancing accuracy, efficiency, and workflow. To fully harness the benefits of AI, several key recommendations have emerged from the overview of reviews, as summarized in Table 4:

Further Research and Validation: It is crucial to continue refining AI algorithms, expanding datasets, and conducting prospective validation to address current limitations and improve AI performance [21,22,28].

Integration into Clinical Practice: Effective implementation of AI tools involves addressing practical challenges such as usability, system interoperability, and seamless incorporation into routine workflows [23,25,27].

Training and Education: Comprehensive training for pathologists and laboratory staff is essential to use AI tools effectively, understand their capabilities and limitations, and integrate them into daily practices [24,25,41].

Regulatory and Ethical Considerations: Rigorous validation and regulatory approval are necessary to ensure AI tools meet clinical standards and ethical guidelines, preventing biases and ensuring equitable diagnostic practices [21,27,38].

Combining AI with Existing Methods: Leveraging AI alongside traditional methods and molecular testing can enhance diagnostic accuracy and provide a more comprehensive assessment [23,24,33].

Addressing Cost and Infrastructure: Consideration of technology costs and the establishment of standardized protocols is vital for effective AI integration and widespread adoption [25,32,34].

These recommendations are detailed in Table 5, which provides a summary of the key findings and strategies for advancing AI integration into cytopathology.

Table 5. Recommendations for Advancing AI Integration in Cytopathology.

Recommendation	Description	References
Further Research and Validation	Continue refining algorithms, expand datasets, and conduct prospective validation to address limitations and improve performance.	[21,22,28]
Integration into Clinical Practice	Ensure AI tools complement existing methods by addressing usability, system interoperability, and workflow incorporation.	[23,25,27]
Training and Education	Provide comprehensive training for pathologists and laboratory staff to use AI tools and integrate them into practice effectively.	[24,25,41]
Regulatory and Ethical Considerations	Address regulatory approval, validation, and ethical guidelines to ensure AI tools meet clinical standards and prevent biases.	[21,27,38]
Combining AI with Existing Methods	Use AI alongside traditional methods and molecular testing to enhance diagnostic accuracy and provide comprehensive assessments.	[23,24,33]
Addressing Cost and Infrastructure	Consider technology costs and establish standardized protocols for effective AI integration and widespread adoption.	[25,32,34]

As can be seen in the table, ethics and standardization emerge as cross-cutting themes. For this reason, we have decided to further refine the analysis by focusing on specific recommendations related to these aspects.

Additionally, a fundamental aspect of optimal integration into the health domain is the ongoing effort to generate empirical data demonstrating the performance of AI in diagnostic cytopathology, particularly in terms of diagnostic precision. This is a theme to be addressed primarily in cutting-edge primary studies, as reviews often have a structural delay in forming conclusions because of their foundational data.

The integration of artificial intelligence (AI) into cytopathology presents significant opportunities for enhancing diagnostic accuracy and efficiency. However, to fully realize these benefits, it is essential to establish standardized practices that ensure the reliable and effective use of AI technologies.

This involves addressing several key areas, including validation, data quality, protocol integration, training, performance monitoring, and collaboration.

Validation and benchmarking are crucial for ensuring that AI tools perform consistently across different settings and populations. Standardized validation protocols help in assessing the reliability and accuracy of AI systems, making it possible to compare their performance with existing diagnostic methods and among various AI models [26,32].

Data consistency and quality play a vital role in the development and performance of AI models. Uniform data collection and preprocessing procedures are necessary to ensure that AI systems are trained on high-quality, consistent datasets. This consistency helps in achieving reliable diagnostic results and reducing biases [27,31].

Protocol integration involves incorporating AI tools seamlessly into existing diagnostic workflows. Standardized protocols for AI integration ensure that these tools complement traditional methods effectively, maintaining workflow efficiency and diagnostic accuracy [33,34].

Training and education are essential for pathologists and laboratory technicians to use and interpret AI tools effectively. Comprehensive training programs and educational resources should be developed to equip users with the skills needed to harness AI technologies effectively [30,31].

Performance monitoring is required to maintain the reliability of AI systems over time. Regular evaluations and quality control measures help in identifying and addressing performance issues, ensuring that AI tools continue to deliver accurate and reliable results [38,39].

Collaboration and communication among AI developers, healthcare professionals, and regulatory bodies are crucial for successful AI implementation. Effective communication channels and collaborative efforts help in addressing challenges and ensuring that AI technologies are integrated and regulated appropriately [26,27].

By focusing on these standardization aspects, the cytopathology field can ensure that AI technologies are used effectively, improving diagnostic outcomes and advancing patient care. The following Table 6 outlines specific recommendations for achieving these standards.

Table 6. Recommendations focused on the standardization.

Standardization Aspect	Description	Recommendations	References
Validation and Benchmarking	Ensuring AI tools meet consistent performance standards across diverse settings is crucial for reliable diagnostics.	Develop and adhere to standard validation protocols and actively participate in benchmarking studies to compare AI performance across different datasets and settings.	[26,32]
Data Consistency and Quality	High-quality, consistent data are essential for training effective AI models and ensuring accurate predictions.	Implement standardized procedures for data collection, annotation, and pre-processing to ensure data uniformity and enhance model training.	[27,31]

Table 6. *Cont.*

Standardization Aspect	Description	Recommendations	References
Protocol Integration	Seamless integration of AI tools into existing diagnostic workflows and protocols is necessary for efficient use.	Establish and follow standardized protocols for incorporating AI tools into clinical practice, ensuring they complement existing diagnostic methods.	[33,34]
Training and Education	Pathologists and laboratory technicians need proper training to use AI tools and interpret their outputs effectively.	Develop comprehensive training programs and educational resources to ensure that users of AI technologies are well-prepared to utilize and evaluate AI-assisted diagnostics.	[30,31]
Performance Monitoring	Continuous evaluation is necessary to maintain AI system performance and address any emerging issues.	Implement regular performance monitoring and quality control measures and update AI systems as needed to sustain reliability and accuracy over time.	[38,39]
Collaboration and Communication	Effective communication between AI developers, healthcare professionals, and regulatory bodies is crucial for successful AI implementation.	Foster communication channels and collaborative efforts among stakeholders to address challenges and ensure the successful integration and regulation of AI technologies.	[26,27]

The integration of artificial intelligence (AI) into cytopathology presents numerous ethical challenges and considerations. As AI technologies advance and become more prevalent in diagnostic processes, addressing these ethical issues is crucial to ensuring that AI applications are used responsibly and equitably. Here's an overview of the key ethical considerations and recommendations for AI in cytopathology:

Key ethical considerations in AI for cytopathology bias and fairness in AI systems are susceptible to biases present in training data. If data used to train AI models are not representative of diverse populations, the resulting models may exhibit biases that can lead to unequal diagnostic performance across different demographic groups. Ensuring fairness requires using diverse and representative datasets and regularly auditing AI systems for bias [27,34]. Transparency and explainability of the decision-making process of AI systems should be transparent and explainable to users. Pathologists and clinicians need to understand how AI systems arrive at their conclusions to trust and effectively use these tools. Developing AI systems with clear, interpretable models and providing explanations for AI-generated recommendations are essential for maintaining trust in AI-assisted diagnostics [26,27]. Data privacy and security handling of patient data responsibly is paramount. AI systems in cytopathology require access to sensitive patient information, which must be protected from unauthorized access and misuse. Implementing robust data security measures and complying with regulations such as GDPR or HIPAA are critical for safeguarding patient privacy [38,39]. Informed consent: patients should be informed about the use of AI in their diagnostic process. This includes understanding how their data will be used, the role of AI in their diagnosis, and any potential implications. Ensuring that patients provide informed consent before their data are used for AI applications is an important ethical requirement [30,33]. Accountability and responsibility for determining accountability when AI systems make errors or provide misleading results, is essential. It is necessary to establish clear guidelines on the responsibilities of AI developers, healthcare providers, and institutions in managing and addressing potential errors in AI-assisted diagnoses [31,32]. Regulatory compliance: AI systems must comply with relevant regulatory standards and guidelines to ensure their safety and effectiveness. Adhering to regulatory requirements and undergoing rigorous validation processes are vital for maintaining high standards in AI-assisted diagnostics [27,38].

Table 7 provides a comprehensive overview of ethical considerations and recommendations for integrating AI into cytopathology. Addressing these concerns is essential for the responsible and effective implementation of AI technologies in diagnostic practices.

Table 7. Ethical Recommendations for AI in Cytopathology.

Ethical Consideration	Description	Recommendations	References
Bias and Fairness	AI models may exhibit biases if trained on non-representative data.	Ensure diverse datasets, conduct regular audits for bias, and implement fairness metrics.	[27,34]
Transparency and Explainability	AI decision-making processes should be understandable to users.	Develop explainable AI models and provide clear explanations for AI-generated recommendations.	[26,27]
Data Privacy and Security	Protect sensitive patient data from unauthorized access and misuse.	Implement robust data security measures and comply with relevant privacy regulations.	[38,39]
Informed Consent	Patients must be aware of and consent to the use of AI in their diagnosis.	Obtain informed consent from patients, including details on AI usage and data handling.	[30,33]
Accountability and Responsibility	Define clear accountability for errors or misleading results from AI systems.	Establish guidelines for AI developers, healthcare providers, and institutions regarding AI errors.	[31,32]
Regulatory Compliance	Adhere to regulatory standards to ensure AI systems' safety and effectiveness.	Follow regulatory requirements and validation procedures for AI systems.	[27,38]

4. Discussion

The discussion is structured into the following sections:

Section 4.1 reports a synoptic diagram

Section 4.2 presents and discusses the added value of the umbrella review within the specific field.

Section 4.3, based on the recommendations emerging from the umbrella review results, focuses on specific aspects of standardization, ethics, and diagnostic accuracy (with the corresponding need for primary data). This section, organized into subsections, provides a deeper analysis through the additional exploration of primary studies in this area.

Section 4.4, organized into subsections, examines the integration of AI in cytopathology, comparing it with the experiences in histopathology and radiology. The experiences in these two fields, particularly in radiology, offer a potential roadmap for improving AI integration in cytopathology.

Section 4.5 concludes by outlining the limitations of the study.

4.1. Synoptic Diagram

The diagram in Figure 7 presents a concise overview of the discussion, organized into tabular connections and diagrams in alignment with the overall aim and specific objectives. Based on the findings from the analysis in the results of the umbrella review, specific focal points have emerged for discussion, highlighting recommendations and areas that require targeted exploration and complementation (see also Figure 2).

These focal points are displayed in Block 1 at the top right and address key aspects such as standardization, ethical considerations, and diagnostic accuracy. Additionally, the initial hypotheses have been confirmed, indicating that cytopathology lags histopathology and, particularly, radiology in integrating artificial intelligence (AI). This has underscored the need for a comparative analysis. Complementation in this regard has been pursued, as illustrated in Block 2 (descending from top to bottom). This part of the discussion has generated significant insights regarding primary studies on standardization and diagnostic accuracy, as summarized in Block 3 (moving down left) and Block 4 (moving right), which synthesize evidence from primary studies in these areas in Tables 7 and 8.

The group of blocks on the right (Blocks 5–7) conducts a comparison of the situations in radiology and histology, graphically presenting trends (Figures 7–14 in Block 5), a comparative analysis of scientific output volume (Table 9 in Block 6), and the recommendations emerging from the domains of radiology and histopathology aimed at cytopathology for better integration with AI.

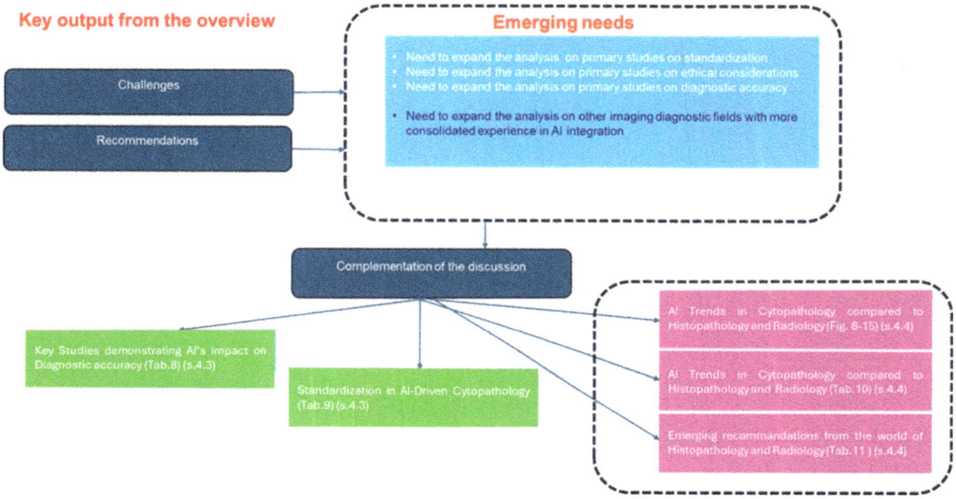

Figure 7. Synoptic diagram reporting a sketch of the discussion.

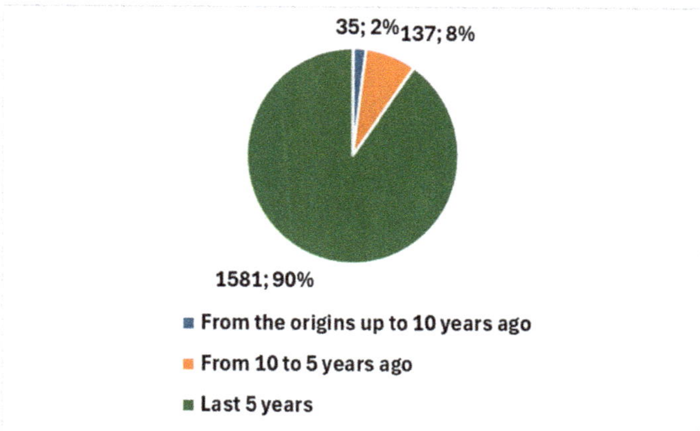

Figure 8. Temporal trends in scientific production in histopathology &AI with details for the last five and ten years.

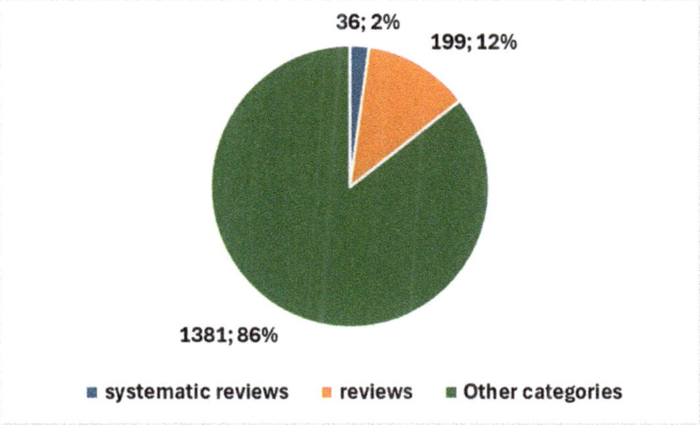

Figure 9. Scientific production in histopathology & AI (reviews and systematic reviews are illustrated separately.

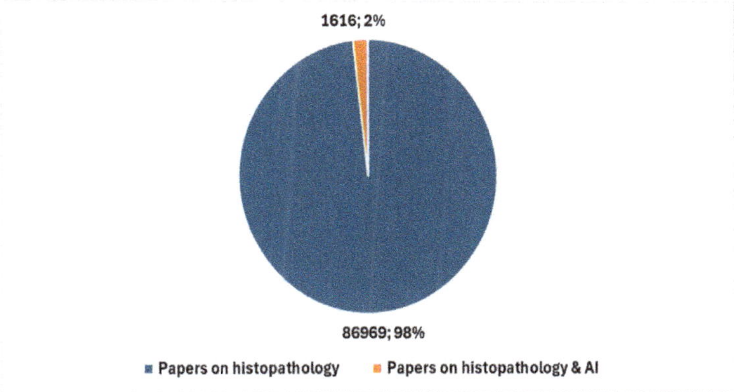

Figure 10. Ratio of AI-Focused to Non-AI-Focused Research in Histopathology.

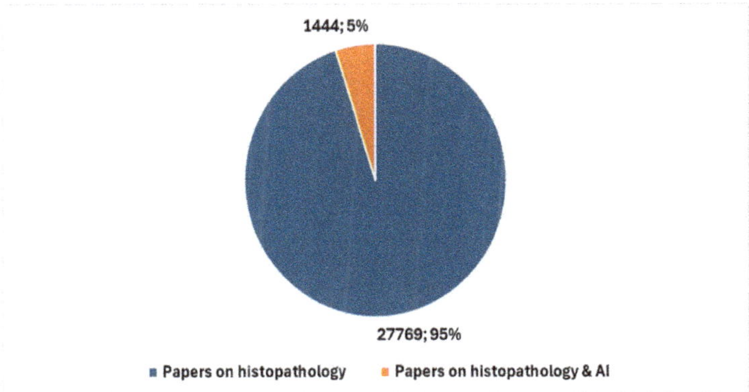

Figure 11. Ratio of AI-Focused to Non-AI-Focused Research in Histopathology in last five years.

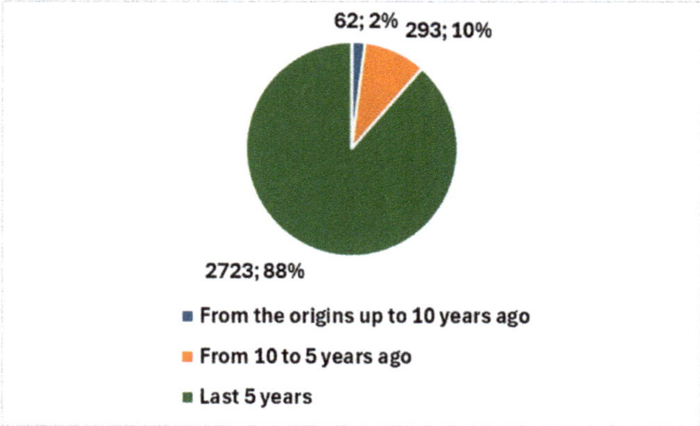

Figure 12. Temporal trends in scientific production in radiology & AI with details for the last five and ten years.

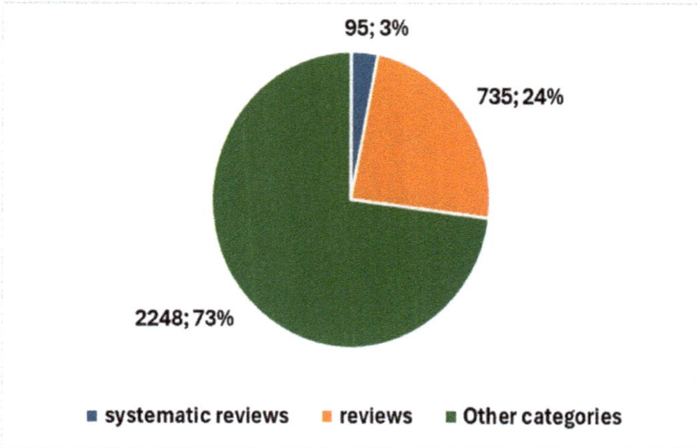

Figure 13. Scientific production in radiology & AI (reviews and systematic reviews are illustrated).

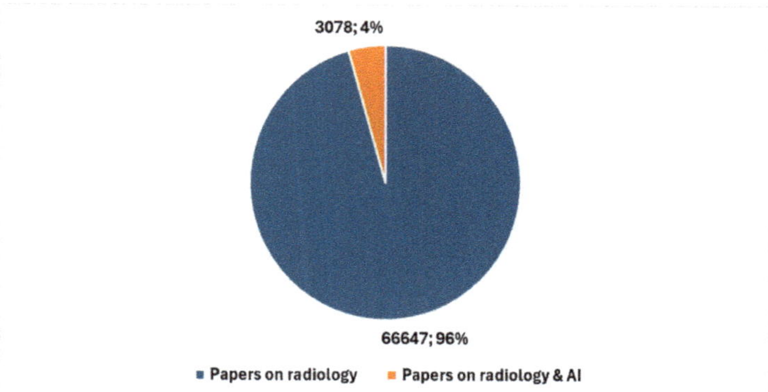

Figure 14. Ratio of AI-Focused to Non-AI-Focused Research in radiology.

4.2. The Umbrella Review: Added Value and Highlights

An increasing interest from professionals in the integration of AI in cytopathology is being observed [9].

An umbrella review in the realm of cytopathology and artificial intelligence (AI) is crucial for synthesizing the diverse and rapidly expanding body of research on this intersection. The significance of such a review lies in its ability to collate findings from various reviews, offering a comprehensive overview of the current advancements and challenges in this field.

As AI continues to enhance diagnostic accuracy and efficiency in cytopathology, it is vital to address emerging themes such as integration challenges, bias, and cost-effectiveness. By consolidating evidence from multiple studies, an umbrella review not only highlights the practical and theoretical gaps but also provides actionable insights for improving the implementation of AI technologies. This holistic perspective supports informed decision-making and fosters the development of best practices, ultimately guiding the effective integration of AI tools into clinical workflows and advancing the overall quality of diagnostic cytopathology. The umbrella review underscores the profound impact of artificial intelligence (AI) on diagnostic cytopathology, emphasizing its role in enhancing both the speed and accuracy of diagnostic processes. By integrating AI technologies, traditional methods of image analysis and diagnostic evaluation are significantly improved, leading to more efficient workflows and reduced diagnostic errors [21–26]. The ability of AI to automate and optimize image analysis is particularly notable in areas such as urine cytology and thyroid pathology, where it has demonstrated substantial benefits in early cancer detection and risk assessment [21,22,24,35].

Recent studies have shown that AI applications are not only accelerating diagnostic procedures but are also refining the precision of results through advanced machine learning models and digital cytology practices [27,32]. This is evidenced by the integration of AI into various diagnostic frameworks, such as those used for evaluating thyroid nodules and urinary tract conditions [24,40]. Despite these advancements, challenges related to standardization and the need for continuous validation of AI tools remain critical areas for ongoing research [38,39].

Overall, this review illustrates how AI can contribute to advancing diagnostic practices by enhancing accuracy and efficiency. It also highlights the ongoing need for further research to address the challenges and optimize AI integration in clinical settings [41].

The recommendations emerging from the umbrella review highlight key areas for advancing AI integration in cytopathology. Ethical considerations and the need for standardization are crucial, emphasizing the importance of ensuring that AI tools meet clinical standards and avoid biases. Establishing standardized practices, including uniform validation protocols, is essential to maintain diagnostic reliability across various settings [21,27,38]. Additionally, the generation of empirical data demonstrating the diagnostic accuracy of AI is fundamental. Ongoing research is required to validate AI performance in clinical environments, ensuring that tools are both effective and reliable [21,22,28].

This comprehensive analysis provides valuable insights, based on consolidated them, into the current state and future potential of AI in cytopathology, making a strong case for its continued development and application [21–41]

4.3. Deepening the Analysis: Exploring New Dimensions and Implications from Cutting-Edge Research

Among the cross-cutting recommendations emerging from the reviews across various studies are two primary areas of focus: (a) advancing towards specific and targeted research to produce empirical data, particularly in the promising area of diagnostic accuracy and AI related to cytopathology, and (b) concentrating on standardization, a crucial aspect for integrating methodologies into stable routines within the health domain.

Empirical data, which refer to information gathered through direct observation, experimentation, or measurement, are essential for validating the effectiveness and practical applicability of AI systems in cytopathology. Such data are derived from real-world studies that provide concrete evidence on the performance, reliability, and clinical integration of AI tools in diagnostic tasks.

To address these recommendations, the umbrella review specifically targeted these two topics, as reflected in primary studies (non-review studies but articles, comparative studies, etc.). These studies include:

Diagnostic Accuracy in AI for Cytopathology: Selected studies based on a composite key in Box 2, Position 1, include [42–49].

Standardization: As a critical component for integrating methodologies into routine health practices, we reviewed studies addressing this aspect using selected studies based on composite keys in Box 2, Position 2, including [50–55].

In the Supplementary Materials there is also a detailed analytical summary of each one of these studies [42–55].

By focusing on these studies, we aim to provide a comprehensive integrative and differential evaluation of the current state of diagnostic accuracy and standardization in AI applications for cytopathology. It is crucial to emphasize that many of the cross-cutting recommendations in the literature not only touch on technical and clinical aspects but also bring attention to the ethical considerations surrounding the use of AI in healthcare. Ethics plays a pivotal role, especially in areas where AI technologies intersect with sensitive decision-making processes, such as diagnostics, treatment planning, and patient privacy. Given the profound implications of AI-driven systems in medical settings, exploring ethical dimensions becomes indispensable.

However, a focused exploration of primary studies on ethics reveals a noticeable gap. Our search, based on a composite key (outlined in Box 2, Position 3), showed a surprising absence of primary studies explicitly directly focused on ethical issues in AI implementation, particularly within specific domains such as diagnostic cytopathology or patient data privacy in AI applications.

This result is significant, as it suggests that while ethical concerns are frequently highlighted in broader discussions or the recommendation sections of review articles, they are not receiving the focused empirical investigation they warrant. Most existing studies tend to address ethical concerns indirectly, subsuming them under general technological or clinical outcomes without placing them at the forefront of analysis. This indirect treatment leaves a gap in the development of specific ethical frameworks or guidelines that could help navigate the challenges AI poses in healthcare.

The absence of primary studies with a dedicated, ethical focus points to a need for research that not only outlines these concerns in theoretical terms but also grounds them in practical, real-world scenarios. With AI continuing to evolve and integrate into healthcare systems, the ethical implications—such as the transparency of AI decision-making, accountability, fairness, and patient consent—need to be explored through dedicated primary studies. These studies would provide concrete data and insights that could help shape more robust, ethically informed AI applications.

Box 2. The proposed composite keys in the analysis.

(Cytopathology [Title/Abstract]) AND ((Artificial intelligence [Title/Abstract]) OR (machine learning [Title/Abstract]) OR (deep learning [Title/Abstract]) OR (neural network [Title/Abstract])) AND (diagnostic accuracy [Title/Abstract])
(Cytopathology [Title/Abstract]) AND ((Artificial intelligence [Title/Abstract]) OR (machine learning [Title/Abstract]) OR (deep learning [Title/Abstract]) OR (neural network [Title/Abstract])) AND ((standard [Title/Abstract) OR (regulation [Title/Abstract))
(Cytopathology [Title/Abstract]) AND ((Artificial intelligence [Title/Abstract]) OR (machine learning [Title/Abstract]) OR (deep learning [Title/Abstract]) OR (neural network [Title/Abstract])) AND (ethics [Title/Abstract))

4.3.1. Deepening the Analysis: Exploring New Dimensions and Implications from Cutting-Edge Research on Diagnostic Accuracy in Cytopathology

Artificial intelligence (AI) is revolutionizing the field of cytopathology by offering advanced tools that significantly enhance diagnostic accuracy. Technologies such as deep learning models and convolutional neural networks have demonstrated considerable potential in various diagnostic domains, including urine cytology, thyroid cytology, and breast cancer diagnostics [42–49]. However, to fully realize these benefits, AI integration into clinical practice necessitates a robust foundation of empirical evidence to validate its efficacy across diverse clinical environments and patient populations.

The importance of fresh empirical data cannot be overstated. Many existing studies are retrospective or involve small, non-representative datasets, which may not fully capture clinical variability. Therefore, large-scale, prospective studies are essential for evaluating the performance of AI in real-world settings and its impact on diagnostic accuracy and patient outcomes. This is crucial for ensuring that AI tools are reliable and effective across different patient populations [42–49].

Recent research highlights the promising role of AI in improving diagnostic accuracy in cytopathology. For instance, Liu et al. [42] found that the AIxURO platform markedly improved sensitivity and efficiency in bladder cancer diagnosis through urine cytology. Zhao et al. [43] demonstrated that the ResNeSt model effectively differentiated between papillary thyroid carcinoma and benign nodules. Mhaske et al. [44] explored machine learning algorithms for analyzing nuclear features in oral exfoliative cytology, showcasing their potential to enhance diagnostic precision. Similarly, Kim et al. [45] and Park et al. [46] provided evidence of AI models significantly improving diagnostic accuracy for lung cancer and metastatic breast cancer, respectively.

Moreover, integrating AI into cytopathology presents both opportunities and challenges that require further investigation. Recent studies have shown the efficacy of advanced AI technologies in various contexts. For example, Ozer et al. [47] demonstrated that a deep neural network achieved 95% diagnostic accuracy for brain tumors in intraoperative cytology, while Saikia et al. [48] found that GoogLeNet-V3 achieved 96.25% accuracy in classifying breast FNAC images. Sanyal et al. [49] also highlighted the potential of AI in thyroid FNAC smears, showing 85.06% diagnostic accuracy for distinguishing between papillary and non-papillary carcinoma.

Table 8 provides a detailed summary of these empirical studies, illustrating the ongoing efforts to refine AI technologies to support diagnostic accuracy in cytopathology. This table underscores the need for additional empirical evidence and the importance of addressing challenges related to data quality, protocol integration, training, performance monitoring, and collaboration [47–49].

Table 8. Key Studies Demonstrating the Impact of AI on Diagnostic Accuracy.

Study	AI Tool/Model	Application Area	Key Findings	References
Liu TJ et al. [42]	AIxURO	Urine Cytology for Bladder Cancer	AIxURO improved sensitivity from 25.0–63.9%, positive predictive value (PPV) from 21.6–31.1%, and reduced screening time by 52.3–83.2%.	[42]
Zhao D et al. [43]	ResNeSt	Thyroid Nodules Diagnosed as AUS	Achieved 92.49% accuracy and improved sensitivity (95.79%) and specificity (88.46%) in differentiating papillary thyroid carcinoma from benign nodules.	[43]

Table 8. *Cont.*

Study	AI Tool/Model	Application Area	Key Findings	References
Mhaske S et al. [44]	CNN vs. SVM	Oral Exfoliative Cytology	The study found substantial variations between the study and control groups in nuclear size ($p < 0.05$), nuclear shape ($p < 0.01$), and chromatin distribution ($p < 0.001$). The Pearson correlation coefficient of SVM was 0.6472, and CNN was 0.7790, showing that SVM had more accuracy.	[44]
Kim T et al. [45]	Densenet121	Lung Cancer	Increased sensitivity to 95.9% and specificity to 98.2% compared with pathologists; enhanced interobserver agreement (Fleiss' Kappa from 0.553 to 0.908).	[45]
Park HS et al. [46]	Inception-ResNet-V2	Metastatic Breast Cancer in Pleural Fluid	Outperformed pathologists with an accuracy of 81.1%, sensitivity of 95.0%, and specificity of 98.6%; improved pathologists' diagnostic metrics after AI assistance.	[46]
Ozer E et al. [47]	Deep Neural Network	Brain Tumors (Intraoperative Cytology)	Achieved 95% diagnostic accuracy in patch-level classification and 97% at the patient-level classification for brain tumors.	[47]
Saikia AR et al. [48]	Various CNN Architectures	Breast FNAC Images	GoogLeNet-V3 achieved 96.25% accuracy in classifying benign and malignant breast FNAC images, showing improved diagnostic reliability.	[48]
Sanyal P et al. [49]	Properly proposed and customized Artificial Neural Network	Thyroid FNAC Smears	Demonstrated 85.06% diagnostic accuracy for distinguishing papillary carcinoma from non-papillary carcinoma thyroid lesions.	[49]

Overall, the table provides a summary sustained by a sketch of empirical data of significant studies that highlight the role of AI in improving diagnostic accuracy across various cytopathological contexts. These studies illustrate the effectiveness of AI tools in enhancing diagnostic precision, reducing interobserver variability, and improving overall efficiency.

In conclusion, while AI offers substantial advancements in cytopathology, ongoing empirical research is essential to validate its effectiveness. Such research will ensure that AI technologies not only perform well in controlled environments but also offer practical benefits in diverse clinical settings. As the field evolves, continued empirical validation will be crucial for achieving widespread, reliable integration of AI into routine cytopathological practice.

4.3.2. Deepening the Analysis: Exploring New Dimensions and Implications from Cutting-Edge Research on Standardization

In recent years, the rapid advancement of diagnostic technologies has underscored the importance of standardization to ensure accuracy and reproducibility across various applications. As new methodologies are introduced and refined, issues related to sample preparation, technology integration, and image processing become increasingly prominent. These challenges are central to achieving reliable and consistent diagnostic results.

The following Table 9 provides an overview of key studies that address different aspects of standardization in diagnostic technologies with AI in cytopathology. Each study highlights specific standardization issues and their implications, shedding light on how uniform procedures and protocols can enhance diagnostic practices. The studies included are reported in ref. [50–56]. In brief (an analytical summary is reported in the Supplementary Materials for each study). In brief:

Peñaranda et al. (2018) [50] explored the impact of sample preparation on Fourier transform infrared (FTIR) spectroscopy, emphasizing the need for consistency to achieve reliable spectral results.

Kumar et al. (2020) [51] reviewed whole-slide imaging (WSI) technologies, focusing on the integration of digital scanning, image visualization, and AI algorithms and the necessity of standardized protocols for effective implementation.

Liu et al. (2022) [52] investigated the effects of cell aspect ratio on deep learning model performance in cytopathology, discussing standardized preprocessing techniques to ensure consistent image dimensions.

Chen et al. (2021) [53] proposed a framework for automatic WSI diagnosis, highlighting the importance of standardized methods for unit selection and attention fusion to improve diagnostic accuracy.

Zhou et al. (2024) [54] compared the performance of AI diagnostic systems with traditional fine needle aspiration (FNA) cytopathology for thyroid nodules, stressing the need for standardized thresholds in AI systems to ensure comparable performance.

Sohn et al. (2023) [55] introduced a deep-learning model for pancreatic cancer diagnosis and discussed the importance of standardized training and evaluation procedures to enhance model reliability.

The table below summarizes these studies, illustrating the critical aspects of standardization and their impact on diagnostic technology:

Table 9. Standardization in AI-Driven Cytopathology: Insights from Emerging Diagnostic Technologies.

Study	Focus	Standardization Aspect	Description	Key Findings
Peñaranda et al. (2018) [50]	FTIR Spectroscopy	Sample Preparation	Focuses on the consistency of sample preparation across different batches. Variations in preparation methods can significantly impact spectral results and classification accuracy.	Variability in sample preparation affects classification accuracy. Standardizing sample preparation methods is crucial for reliable results.
Kumar et al. (2020) [51]	Whole-Slide Imaging (WSI)	Technology Integration and Protocols	Examines the integration of WSI technology into routine pathology practice, including digital scanning, image visualization, and AI algorithms. Addresses the need for standardized protocols for successful implementation.	Standardization in WSI technology and protocols could address high costs and technical challenges, facilitating broader adoption and consistency in diagnostic practices.
Liu et al. (2022) [52]	Deep Learning and Aspect Ratio	Image Preprocessing and Resizing	Investigates the impact of cell aspect ratio on deep learning model performance, focusing on preprocessing techniques to standardize image dimensions without compromising diagnostic quality.	Deep learning models are robust to changes in aspect ratio, suggesting that standardized preprocessing techniques can maintain model performance across varied images.

Table 9. *Cont.*

Study	Focus	Standardization Aspect	Description	Key Findings
Chen et al. (2021) [53]	Automatic WSI Diagnosis	Selection and Fusion Techniques	Develops a framework for selecting and fusing image units (e.g., patches or cells) for diagnosis. Emphasizes the need for standardized methods in unit selection and fusion to ensure consistent and accurate diagnoses.	Standardization in unit selection and attention fusion improves diagnostic consistency and accuracy across different types of slide images.
Zhou et al. (2024) [54]	AI vs. FNA for Thyroid Nodules	AI Diagnostic Systems and Thresholds	Compares AI diagnostic systems with traditional FNA cytopathology and mutation analysis, highlighting the importance of standardized thresholds for AI system performance.	Standardizing AI diagnostic tools can provide performance comparable to traditional methods, potentially enhancing efficiency and reducing the need for invasive procedures.
Sohn et al. (2023) [55]	Deep Learning for Pancreatic Cancer	Model Training and Evaluation	Proposes a deep learning model for pancreatic cancer diagnosis and evaluates its performance against existing models. Emphasizes the need for standardized training and evaluation procedures to improve accuracy.	Standardization in model training and evaluation enhances diagnostic performance and reliability of deep learning models in pancreatic cancer detection.

Overall, this table encapsulates the essential aspects of standardization as discussed in these studies, providing a clear perspective on how consistent methodologies contribute to advancements in diagnostic technology and practice.

4.4. Advancing Diagnostic Techniques: The Intersection of AI with Cytopathology, Histopathology, and Radiology

4.4.1. AI Trends in Cytopathology Compared with Histopathology and Radiology

It is insightful to examine the findings of this review in the context of other imaging domains, particularly digital pathology, which intersects with cytology and cytopathology. A comparative analysis with radiology is especially pertinent, given radiology's accelerated integration into digital health, primarily because of its early adoption of DICOM standards.

Radiology's swift digital adoption offers valuable lessons for digital pathology. The rapid and widespread implementation of standardized protocols in radiology has significantly facilitated the integration of advanced technologies, such as AI, into clinical practice. Emulating these standardization and interoperability measures could expedite similar advancements in digital pathology. Radiology's experience underscores the crucial role of well-defined standards in enhancing technology integration and optimizing clinical workflows. By adopting analogous strategies, digital pathology could experience substantial progress and smoother incorporation of new technologies.

In contrast, the scientific output in histopathology, which began in 1988—ten years earlier than cytopathology's start in 1998 [56,57]—reflects a more extensive body of research. For instance, there are (at the date of this review of 15 July 2024) 1616 publications related to histopathology and AI compared with just 101 in cytopathology and AI [56] based on a PubMed search (see keys in Box 2). This disparity likely arises from the greater challenges in managing digital cytology and cytopathology, where sophisticated solutions and significant memory resources are required due to the complexity of focus functions [58].

PubMed data further highlights this trend: there are 335 review articles in histopathology, including 36 systematic reviews, reflecting a proportion consistent with its larger research volume [57]. In the past five years, there has been a notable acceleration in AI-related publications in histopathology (Figures 8 and 9).

Historically, AI-related research in histopathology constitutes about 1.84% of its total publications, a figure that has risen to 4.84% in the last five years, aligning closely with cytopathology's rate (Figures 10 and 11).

In comparison, radiology's scientific output, which began 15 years earlier in 1983 [59], is significantly more extensive. Radiology has 3078 publications related to AI (Figure 12), compared with just 101 in cytopathology and AI [56,59] based on a PubMed search (see Box 3 for the used keys), This difference is attributable to the earlier and more rapid standardization and digital integration in radiology [58].

PubMed data shows 830 review articles in radiology, including 95 systematic reviews, maintaining a proportion that reflects its larger body of research [59] (Figure 13). Recent trends indicate a substantial increase in AI-related publications in radiology over the past five years (Figures 14 and 15).

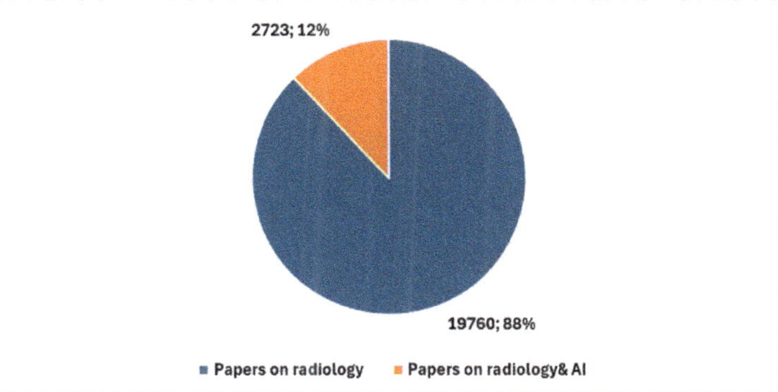

Figure 15. Ratio of AI-Focused to Non-AI-Focused Research in radiology in the last five years.

Historically, AI-related research in radiology represents 4.41% of the total publications, significantly higher than the sub-2% figures seen in both histopathology and cytopathology. In the past five years, this proportion has surged to 12.11%, nearly 2.5 times higher than the rates observed in cytopathology and histopathology, where it was below 5%. (Figures 14 and 15).

The rapid advancement and integration of AI in radiology provide a compelling model for other imaging domains, including cytopathology and histopathology. Radiology's success in adopting standardized protocols and embracing digital technologies serves as a valuable blueprint for accelerating similar progress in these fields. By drawing inspiration from radiology's approach to digital health, both cytopathology and histopathology can leverage these insights to overcome existing challenges, streamline workflows, and enhance the integration of AI technologies.

In conclusion, the table reported in the following and the figures presented before provide a comprehensive overview of scientific production in histopathology and radiology, focusing on the impact of artificial intelligence (AI). The table offers a comparative analysis of the total number of publications, review articles, and the proportion of AI-related research in both fields. This comparison highlights the significant differences in research volume and focus between histopathology and radiology. The figures below, anticipated in the text, illustrate key trends and ratios:

Figures 8 and 9 show the temporal trends and distribution of review and systematic review articles in histopathology.

Figures 10 and 11 present the ratio of AI-focused to non-AI-focused research in histopathology, including trends over the last five years.

Figures 12 and 13 detail the temporal trends and review article distribution in radiology&AI.

Figures 14 and 15 highlight the ratio of AI-focused research in radiology, emphasizing recent trends and allowing comparisons with histopathology.

These visualizations underscore the evolving focus on AI across these fields, revealing the rapid advancements and integration of AI technologies, particularly in radiology. Comparative data provide valuable insights into how AI is shaping research and clinical practices in medical imaging.

Table 10 reports a sketch of the Distribution and Trends of AI-Focused Scientific Publications in Histopathology, Cytopathology, and Radiology.

Table 10. Distribution and Trends of AI-Focused Scientific Publications in Histopathology, Cytopathology, and Radiology.

	Start Year	Total Publications	AI Publications	Percentage of AI Publications	Review Articles	Systematic Reviews Among the Review Articles	AI Research Ratio (Last 5 Years)
Histopathology	1988	88,585	1.616	1.84%	335	36	4.84%
Cytopathology	1998	5682	101	1.79%	31	1	4.95%
Radiology	1983	69,725	3.078	4.84%	830	95	12.11%

Box 3. Keys used for the Pubmed searches.

(Cytopathology [Title/Abstract]) AND ((Artificial intelligence [Title/Abstract]) OR (machine learning [Title/Abstract]) OR (deep learning [Title/Abstract]) OR (neural network [Title/Abstract]))
(histopathology [Title/Abstract]) AND ((Artificial intelligence [Title/Abstract]) OR (machine learning [Title/Abstract]) OR (deep learning [Title/Abstract]) OR (neural network [Title/Abstract]))
(radiology [Title/Abstract]) AND ((Artificial intelligence [Title/Abstract]) OR (machine learning [Title/Abstract]) OR (deep learning [Title/Abstract]) OR (neural network [Title/Abstract]))
(histopathology [Title/Abstract])
(Cytopathology [Title/Abstract])
(radiology [Title/Abstract])

4.4.2. Strategic Directions of Advancements in Cytopathology: Lessons from Histopathology and Radiology Comparisons

The integration of artificial intelligence (AI) into cytopathology is significantly hindered by challenges related to the specificity of the digitization process. These challenges render the integration complex and costly, particularly when compared with the more advanced integration seen in histopathology and digital radiology.

Cytopathology, similar to histopathology, is part of the broader digital pathology field, yet it lags in the incorporation of AI technologies. Histopathology has a more established pathway due to its shared focus on digital pathology, allowing it to navigate the integration process more smoothly. In contrast, digital radiology has experienced a more rapid evolution, achieving substantial milestones and advancements ahead of both cytopathology and histopathology.

This umbrella review aims to address not only the current challenges and trade-offs encountered in the integration of AI within cytopathology as emerged from the overview but also to explore valuable lessons and recommendations. By drawing insights from histopathology—an area with which cytopathology shares the digital pathology framework—and from digital radiology, which has progressed more swiftly, this review seeks to highlight effective strategies and potential solutions. These insights will be crucial for overcoming the barriers faced by cytopathology and aligning its progress with that of its counterparts in the digital health ecosystem.

Expanding Diagnostic Horizons: Insights from Histopathology for AI Integration in Cytopathology

As digital health evolves, integrating artificial intelligence (AI) into cytopathology poses unique challenges compared with advancements in histopathology. Traditional histopathology has faced barriers such as low throughput and interobserver variability, hampering progress in precision medicine. However, innovations in computational pathology, particularly through deep learning (DL) techniques, are overcoming these barriers [60–62].

Advancements in Histopathology and Computational Pathology

- DL models have significantly improved diagnostic tasks in histopathology, excelling in mutation prediction, large-scale pathomics analyses, and prognosis forecasting.
- The integration of multimodal data and the development of foundation models in computational pathology opens new diagnostic possibilities [60].
- **Implication for Cytopathology**: Similar advancements can enhance cytopathology, but a customized AI integration approach is essential to address its unique challenges.

The Role of Digital Pathology and AI Integration

- Digital pathology (DP) transforms clinical practice by converting glass slides into high-resolution whole-slide images (WSI), improving quality assurance and diagnostic accuracy.
- AI applications in DP, such as Immunoscore (IS) and Immunoscore-Immune Checkpoint (IS-IC), have shown great promise in cancer diagnostics [61].
- **Implication for Cytopathology**: AI tools similar to these can refine diagnostic processes in cytopathology, enhancing both precision and efficiency.

Challenges in AI Adoption and Utilization

- A study among Polish pathologists revealed a knowledge gap in AI applications, highlighting the need for improved awareness and education [62].
- **Implication for Cytopathology**: Targeted educational initiatives are crucial to promote AI adoption in cytopathology.

Lessons from Radiology for AI Integration in Cytopathology

AI is rapidly transforming radiology, offering valuable insights for cytopathology. Key lessons include [63–68]:

Enhancing Diagnostic Accuracy and Workflow

- AI has improved radiology's diagnostic accuracy and efficiency by automating tasks and aiding in detecting abnormalities [63,64].
- **Lesson for Cytopathology**: AI-driven image analysis can enhance the detection of typical cellular patterns, reducing false negatives and improving diagnostic precision.

Addressing Legal and Ethical Challenges

- The integration of AI into radiology presents legal and ethical issues, including liability and transparency concerns [63].
- **Lesson for Cytopathology**: Develop clear liability guidelines and transparent AI systems to facilitate responsible AI use in diagnostics.

Bridging Knowledge Gaps and Training Needs

- Radiologists face significant knowledge gaps in AI applications, making education and training crucial [67].
- **Lesson for Cytopathology**: Invest in comprehensive AI training programs to ensure effective AI integration and maximize diagnostic outcomes.

Understanding Cognitive and Contextual Challenges

- AI decision-making models differ from human processes, complicating clinical practice integration [65].

- **Lesson for Cytopathology**: Ensure AI tools complement human expertise by aligning them with the unique decision-making processes of cytopathology.

  Leveraging Advanced Technologies

- Technologies such as natural image captioning (NIC) have enhanced radiology report generation and documentation [66].
- **Lesson for Cytopathology**: Adapt similar technologies for cytopathology to streamline report generation and improve communication.

Suggestions for Advancing AI Integration in Cytopathology: Lessons from Histopathology and Radiology

Drawing from histopathology and radiology, several key strategies can be applied to cytopathology for enhanced AI adoption:

1. Conduct Comprehensive Acceptance and Utilization Studies
   - Studies in histopathology and radiology underscore the need for evaluating knowledge, attitudes, and practices regarding AI [62,67].
     - **Action**: Implement questionnaires to gauge cytopathologists' familiarity and attitudes towards AI. Identify gaps in education and training.
     - **Action**: Evaluate barriers to AI adoption in workflow, data management, and training to design effective strategies.
2. Foster Cross-Disciplinary Collaboration and Training
   - Collaboration between histopathology, radiology, and cytopathology drives AI tool development [63,64].
     - **Action:** Create interdisciplinary training programs and promote collaborative research across fields.
     - **Benefit:** Joint efforts can lead to integrated AI tools that enhance diagnostic accuracy and efficiency.
3. Explore Multidimensional Data Integration
   - Combining radiomic and pathognomic data has expanded disease understanding in radiology [68].
     - **Action:** Develop AI models integrating cytopathological data with radiographic and histopathological information.
     - **Benefit:** This multimodal approach can improve diagnostic precision and prognostic assessments.
4. Address Legal, Ethical, and Transparency Issues
   - Legal and ethical concerns in radiology highlight the need for clear guidelines and transparency in AI systems [63].
     - **Action:** Establish comprehensive legal and ethical guidelines for AI use in cytopathology.
     - **Action:** Ensure AI systems are transparent and explainable to build trust and facilitate clinical integration.
5. Enhance Reporting and Documentation
   - Radiology has improved report generation with advanced AI-driven tools [66].
     - **Action:** Implement AI-driven reporting tools to improve the clarity, consistency, and completeness of cytopathological reports.
     - **Action:** Utilize natural language processing (NLP) to automate report generation, ensuring comprehensive clinical decision-making support.
6. Expand Knowledge and Attitude Surveys
   - Expanding surveys can help identify gaps in knowledge and attitudes toward AI across medical fields [67].

- **Action:** Develop targeted questionnaires to assess cytopathologists' understanding of AI and their concerns regarding its integration.
- **Action:** Use survey data to design tailored educational programs and resources for cytopathologists.

By implementing these suggestions, cytopathology can effectively advance its AI integration efforts, drawing on lessons from histopathology and radiology. Comprehensive acceptance studies, interdisciplinary collaboration, and multimodal data integration will be critical for optimizing the potential of AI in cytopathology.

From Histopathology and Radiology to Cytopathology: Final Scheme for Enhancing AI Integration

To facilitate a comprehensive understanding of how advancements in histopathology and radiology can inform the integration of artificial intelligence (AI) in cytopathology, we present a detailed overview of the key lessons and strategies derived from these fields. The following Table 11 summarizes critical insights and recommendations based on recent studies and reviews. These insights highlight both the advancements achieved and the challenges faced in histopathology and radiology, which can be adapted to enhance AI integration in cytopathology.

Table 11. Emerging recommendations from histopathology and radiology domain for AI Integration in cytopathology.

Aspect	Histopathology Insights	Radiology Insights	Recommendations for Cytopathology	References
Acceptance and Utilization	- Evaluating knowledge, attitudes, and practices is crucial [62].	- Surveys show variable adoption and training needs [67].	- Conduct detailed surveys to assess cytopathologists' knowledge and attitudes towards AI. Address barriers to adoption.	[60–62,67]
Cross-Disciplinary Collaboration	- Collaboration enhances the development and implementation of AI tools [60].	- Interdisciplinary knowledge sharing improves AI integration [64].	- Develop joint training programs involving histopathologists, radiologists, and cytopathologists. Foster interdisciplinary research.	[60,64]
Multidimensional Data Integration	- Integration of multimodal data is advancing diagnostic capabilities [60].	- Combining radiomic and pathognomic features enhances diagnostic accuracy [68].	- Develop AI models that integrate cytopathological data with other diagnostic modalities. Explore advanced methodologies for data integration.	[60,68]
Legal and Ethical Issues	- AI use raises legal responsibility and transparency concerns [63].	- Legal responsibility and ethical considerations are complex [63].	- Establish clear guidelines for AI use in cytopathology, including liability, data privacy, and transparency.	[63]
Reporting and Documentation	- Advanced reporting tools enhance clarity and completeness [61].	- AI-driven reporting improves documentation quality [66].	- Implement AI-driven reporting tools to enhance the clarity and completeness of cytopathological reports. Utilize NLP for automation.	[61,66]
Knowledge and Attitude Surveys	- Increased awareness and education are needed for effective AI integration [62].	- Understanding knowledge gaps and attitudes is essential [67].	- Design and deploy targeted questionnaires to assess and improve cytopathologists' understanding and use of AI.	[62,67]

4.5. Limitations

The proposed study, described as a narrative review, has inherent limitations due to the methodology and inclusion/exclusion criteria applied. The absence of conference studies results in a potential lack of updates on ongoing research and recent advances, excluding preliminary data that may not have been officially published yet. Additionally, the exclusion of local studies and/or guidelines in local languages restricts the analysis to contributions published in English and international guidelines, potentially overlooking specific and relevant insights from particular cultural or clinical contexts. This limits the understanding of regional variations in clinical practices and treatment protocols.

5. Final Reflections: Broadening Ethical Considerations in AI Applications Cytopathology

The study highlighted that one of the key strategic aspects for the future of AI in cytopathology is the need to address ethical concerns coherently and appropriately. The umbrella review provided evidence from review articles, but complementary analyses of primary studies revealed that scholars have not yet conducted targeted research specifically focused on ethics in this field. However, it is clear that three emerging ethical polarities in AI within healthcare can be directly applied to cytopathology.

5.1. Emerging Ethical Polarities in AI and Their Implications for Cytopathology

5.1.1. Expansion of Algorethics in Healthcare

The first polarity concerns the growth of "algorethics"—the ethics of algorithms—which has expanded beyond the biomedical literature into national and international policy frameworks [69]. Organizations such as the World Health Organization (WHO), the European Union (EU), and various national regulatory bodies are establishing ethical standards that can influence AI applications, including in cytopathology.

In cytopathology, the application of AI-powered diagnostic tools, such as algorithms for automating the detection of abnormal cells, raises ethical issues regarding the transparency of algorithmic decisions and the accountability of automated systems. Ethical frameworks from WHO, the EU AI Act, and the U.S. FDA offer essential guidelines that can be adapted to ensure these technologies are developed in ways that safeguard patient rights, maintain accuracy, and promote equity in cytological diagnostics. In detail, the integration of AI into cytopathology brings profound ethical implications, which are increasingly being addressed through various global and national frameworks. These frameworks, although not always specifically focused on cytopathology, significantly impact the field by shaping ethical practices and standards for AI technologies. The following key areas illustrate this impact:

Ethical Standards and Equity: The WHO global AI ethics guidelines stress the importance of respecting human rights and promoting health equity [70]. These guidelines aim to ensure that AI applications in cytopathology are developed and utilized in ways that contribute positively to health outcomes while maintaining ethical standards.

Regulatory Frameworks: The EU AI Act represents a comprehensive effort to regulate AI usage across member states, focusing on ethical practices, transparency, and accountability [71]. This regulatory framework addresses how AI technologies should be implemented in cytopathology, striving for a balance between innovation and ethical responsibility.

Transparency and Safety: FDA guidelines on AI in medical research emphasize the need for transparency and safeguarding public health [72,73]. These guidelines are critical for ensuring that AI technologies in cytopathology are effective and ethically deployed, fostering trust in AI applications and protecting patient welfare.

Risk Management and Ethical Assurance: The NHS AI Ethics Initiative supports the ethical integration of AI within healthcare settings, including cytopathology, by providing assurance and managing associated risks [74]. This initiative focuses on maintaining high ethical standards in diagnostic practices, ensuring that AI systems are used responsibly and effectively.

Responsible Practices and Data Protection: The Public Health Agency of Canada has developed an ethical framework for AI applications in public health, which emphasizes responsible practices and personal data protection [75]. This framework guides the ethical deployment of AI technologies in cytopathology, ensuring that patient data privacy is safeguarded while enhancing diagnostic capabilities.

Ethical Norms and Enforcement: The CSET reports ethical norms for AI use in China, which cover the use and protection of personal information and human control over AI [76]. These norms can also influence the ethical deployment of AI in cytopathology, ensuring responsible practices are upheld.

Overall, while these documents are not exclusively focused on cytopathology, they profoundly influence the field by establishing ethical principles and standards for AI technologies. Ensuring that AI is developed and implemented in responsible, equitable, and ethically aligned ways is essential for addressing the complex challenges posed by AI in cytopathology.

5.1.2. Impact of Chatbots and Large Language Models (LLMs)

The second polarity involves the transformative impact of chatbots and large language models (LLMs) [27], which are already revolutionizing areas such as radiology and are poised to achieve the same in cytopathology. These technologies can automate diagnostic reporting, enhance communication, and support cytopathologists by providing real-time assistance in interpreting results.

In cytopathology, LLMs could assist with the initial screening of cytological samples or automate the communication of findings to clinicians. However, their implementation introduces ethical challenges, particularly around decision-making transparency, the potential for over-reliance on automated systems, and ensuring that patient data are handled responsibly. Clear ethical guidelines are necessary to ensure that AI-enhanced cytopathological diagnostics remain accurate and accountable while preserving trust in the healthcare system.

5.1.3. Role of Telemedicine and AI in Cytopathology

The third polarity is the increasing integration of telemedicine into various healthcare disciplines, including cytopathology [77]. Telemedicine is expanding access to diagnostic services by enabling remote analysis and consultations, but it also presents ethical issues, particularly regarding equitable access, the accuracy of remote diagnostics, and the secure transmission of patient data.

In cytopathology, the digital transmission of cytological images and patient data for remote analysis is becoming more common. While telemedicine can enhance diagnostic efficiency and accessibility, the integration of AI tools in this context requires stringent ethical oversight. Ensuring data privacy, maintaining diagnostic accuracy, and addressing disparities in access are key ethical concerns that must be managed as telemedicine becomes a standard practice in cytopathological workflows.

6. Conclusions

This umbrella review highlights the transformative potential of artificial intelligence (AI) in cytopathology, emphasizing the need to address a range of challenges for successful integration. The integration of AI technologies is poised to enhance diagnostic accuracy and operational efficiency within cytopathology significantly. By automating and refining diagnostic processes, AI has the potential to reduce errors and improve patient outcomes. The ongoing evolution of AI applications presents exciting opportunities to revolutionize diagnostic practices and patient management.

However, this review also identifies several critical challenges that must be overcome to leverage the benefits of AI in cytopathology fully. Key issues include:

Data Standardization: A significant barrier to AI integration is the lack of standardized data formats and terminology within cytopathology. Ensuring consistency in data collection and representation is essential for developing effective AI algorithms that can generalize across diverse datasets.

Integration with Existing Clinical Workflows: The successful implementation of AI tools requires seamless integration with existing clinical workflows. This necessitates collaboration between IT specialists, cytopathologists, and other healthcare professionals to ensure that AI applications fit naturally into routine practices without disrupting patient care.

Ethical and Legal Concerns: Addressing ethical dilemmas related to patient privacy, data security, and algorithmic biases is crucial. Establishing clear guidelines and governance frameworks will help navigate these complexities and ensure responsible AI deployment in clinical settings.

Validation and Quality Assurance: Rigorous validation of AI tools is essential to establish their reliability and accuracy. Continuous monitoring and quality assurance mechanisms should be implemented to evaluate AI performance over time, ensuring that these tools consistently meet clinical standards.

Key Insights:

Opportunities: AI demonstrates significant potential in enhancing diagnostic accuracy, improving workflow efficiency, and offering novel insights into cytopathology. Successful implementations in related fields such as histopathology and radiology provide valuable models for accelerating AI adoption in cytopathology.

Challenges: Major hurdles include the need for rigorous validation, data standardization, and addressing biases. Additionally, high costs and data quality issues must be managed to realize the benefits of AI fully.

Future Directions: To advance AI in cytopathology, it is crucial to apply lessons learned from histopathology and radiology while fostering focused research to tackle existing barriers. Addressing challenges related to data standardization, integration, and ethical considerations will be pivotal for effective AI integration, ultimately leading to improved diagnostic practices in cytopathology.

Supplementary Materials: The following supporting information can be downloaded at: https://www.mdpi.com/article/10.3390/jcm13226745/s1, Section S1: Analytical Summaries for reviews [21–41] in Section 3; Section S2: Analytical summaries for *primary studies* [42–55] in Section 4.

Funding: APC was funded by Daniele Giansanti.

Conflicts of Interest: The authors declare no conflict of interest.

References

1. Definition of Cytopathology. Available online: https://www.collinsdictionary.com/dictionary/english/cytopathology (accessed on 24 September 2024).
2. Definition of Cytopathology. Available online: https://www.dictionary.com/browse/cytopathology (accessed on 24 September 2024).
3. Definition of Cytopathology. Available online: https://www.merriam-webster.com/dictionary/cytopathology (accessed on 24 September 2024).
4. Nishat, R.; Ramachandra, S.; Behura, S.S.; Kumar, H. Digital cytopathology. *J. Oral. Maxillofac. Pathol.* **2017**, *21*, 99–106. [CrossRef]
5. Available online: https://cytojournal.com/the-impact-of-digital-imaging-in-the-field-of-cytopathology/ (accessed on 24 September 2024).
6. Pantanowitz, L.; Hornish, M.; Goulart, R.A. The impact of digital imaging in the field of cytopathology. *Cytojournal* **2009**, *6*, 6. [CrossRef] [PubMed] [PubMed Central]
7. Giansanti, D.; Castrichella, L.; Giovagnoli, M.R. Telepathology training in a master of cytology degree course. *J. Telemed. Telecare* **2008**, *14*, 338–341. [CrossRef] [PubMed]
8. Giansanti, D.; Castrichella, L.; Giovagnoli, M.R. The design of a health technology assessment system in telepathology. *Telemed. J. E Health* **2008**, *14*, 570–575. [CrossRef] [PubMed]
9. Kim, D.; Thrall, M.J.; Michelow, P.; Schmitt, F.C.; Vielh, P.R.; Siddiqui, M.T.; Sundling, K.E.; Virk, R.; Alperstein, S.; Bui, M.M.; et al. The current state of digital cytology and artificial intelligence (AI): Global survey results from the American Society of Cytopathology Digital Cytology Task Force. *J. Am. Soc. Cytopathol.* **2024**, *16*, 319–328. [CrossRef]

10. Capitanio, A.; Dina, R.E.; Treanor, D. Digital cytology: A short review of technical and methodological approaches and applications. *Cytopathology* **2018**, *29*, 317–325. [CrossRef] [PubMed]
11. Saini, T.; Bansal, B.; Dey, P. Digital cytology: Current status and future prospects. *Diagn. Cytopathol.* **2023**, *51*, 211–218. [CrossRef] [PubMed]
12. Available online: https://www.news-medical.net/life-sciences/Digital-Pathology-Challenges.aspx (accessed on 24 September 2024).
13. Jahn, S.W.; Plass, M.; Moinfar, F. Digital Pathology: Advantages, Limitations and Emerging Perspectives. *J. Clin. Med.* **2020**, *9*, 3697. [CrossRef]
14. Standard DICOM. Available online: https://www.dicomstandard.org/ (accessed on 24 September 2024).
15. Standard DICOM WSI. Available online: https://dicom.nema.org/dicom/dicomwsi/ (accessed on 24 September 2024).
16. Mastrosimini, M.G.; Eccher, A.; Nottegar, A.; Montin, U.; Scarpa, A.; Pantanowitz, L.; Girolami, I. WSI validation studies in breast and gynecological pathology. *Pathol. Res. Pract.* **2022**, *240*, 154191. [CrossRef] [PubMed]
17. Tizhoosh, H.R.; Pantanowitz, L. Artificial intelligence and digital pathology: Challenges and opportunities. *J. Pathol. Inform.* **2018**, *9*, 38. [CrossRef]
18. Go, H. Digital Pathology and Artificial Intelligence Applications in Pathology. *Brain Tumor Res. Treat.* **2022**, *10*, 76–82. [CrossRef] [PubMed] [PubMed Central]
19. Giovagnoli, M.R.; Giansanti, D. Artificial Intelligence in Digital Pathology: What Is the Future? Part 1: From the Digital Slide Onwards. *Healthcare* **2021**, *9*, 858. [CrossRef] [PubMed] [PubMed Central]
20. ANDJ Checklist. Available online: https://legacyfileshare.elsevier.com/promis_misc/ANDJ%20Narrative%20Review%20Checklist.pdf (accessed on 24 September 2024).
21. Ciaparrone, C.; Maffei, E.; L'Imperio, V.; Pisapia, P.; Eloy, C.; Fraggetta, F.; Zeppa, P.; Caputo, A. Computer-assisted urine cytology: Faster, cheaper, better? *Cytopathology* **2024**, *35*, 634–641. [CrossRef] [PubMed]
22. Zhang, L.; Wong, C.; Li, Y.; Huang, T.; Wang, J.; Lin, C. Artificial intelligence assisted diagnosis of early tc markers and its application. *Discov. Oncol.* **2024**, *15*, 172. [CrossRef] [PubMed] [PubMed Central]
23. Caputo, A.; Pisapia, P.; L'Imperio, V. Current role of cytopathology in the molecular and computational era: The perspective of young pathologists. *Cancer Cytopathol.* **2024**. *Epub ahead of print*. [CrossRef] [PubMed]
24. Giovanella, L.; Campennì, A.; Tuncel, M.; Petranović Ovčariček, P. Integrated Diagnostics of Thyroid Nodules. *Cancers* **2024**, *16*, 311. [CrossRef] [PubMed] [PubMed Central]
25. Kim, D.; Sundling, K.E.; Virk, R.; Thrall, M.J.; Alperstein, S.; Bui, M.M.; Chen-Yost, H.; Donnelly, A.D.; Lin, O.; Liu, X.; et al. Digital cytology part 2: Artificial intelligence in cytology: A concept paper with review and recommendations from the American Society of Cytopathology Digital Cytology Task Force. *J. Am. Soc. Cytopathol.* **2024**, *13*, 97–110. [CrossRef] [PubMed]
26. Kim, D.; Sundling, K.E.; Virk, R.; Thrall, M.J.; Alperstein, S.; Bui, M.M.; Chen-Yost, H.; Donnelly, A.D.; Lin, O.; Liu, X.; et al. Digital cytology part 1: Digital cytology implementation for practice: A concept paper with review and recommendations from the American Society of Cytopathology Digital Cytology Task Force. *J. Am. Soc. Cytopathol.* **2024**, *13*, 86–96. [CrossRef] [PubMed]
27. Malik, S.; Zaheer, S. ChatGPT as an aid for pathological diagnosis of cancer. *Pathol. Res. Pract.* **2024**, *253*, 154989. [CrossRef] [PubMed]
28. Slabaugh, G.; Beltran, L.; Rizvi, H.; Deloukas, P.; Marouli, E. Applications of machine and deep learning to thyroid cytology and histopathology: A review. *Front. Oncol.* **2023**, *13*, 958310. [CrossRef] [PubMed] [PubMed Central]
29. Lebrun, L.; Salmon, I. Pathology and new insights in thyroid neoplasms in the 2022 WHO classification. *Curr. Opin. Oncol.* **2024**, *36*, 13–21. [CrossRef] [PubMed] [PubMed Central]
30. Singla, N.; Kundu, R.; Dey, P. Artificial Intelligence: Exploring utility in detection and typing of fungus with futuristic application in fungal cytology. *Cytopathology* **2024**, *35*, 226–234. [CrossRef] [PubMed]
31. Sunny, S.P.; DR, R.; Hariharan, A.; Mukhia, N.; Gurudath, S.; Raghavan, S.; Kolur, T.; Shetty, V.; Surolia, A.; Chandrashekhar, P.; et al. CD44-SNA1 integrated cytopathology for delineation of high grade dysplastic and neoplastic oral lesions. *PLoS ONE* **2023**, *18*, e0291972. [CrossRef] [PubMed] [PubMed Central]
32. Wong, C.M.; Kezlarian, B.E.; Lin, O. Current status of machine learning in thyroid cytopathology. *J. Pathol. Inform.* **2023**, *14*, 100309. [CrossRef] [PubMed] [PubMed Central]
33. Ludwig, M.; Ludwig, B.; Mikuła, A.; Biernat, S.; Rudnicki, J.; Kaliszewski, K. The Use of Artificial Intelligence in the Diagnosis and Classification of Thyroid Nodules: An Update. *Cancers* **2023**, *15*, 708. [CrossRef] [PubMed] [PubMed Central]
34. Marletta, S.; L'Imperio, V.; Eccher, A.; Antonini, P.; Santonicco, N.; Girolami, I.; Dei Tos, A.P.; Sbaraglia, M.; Pagni, F.; Brunelli, M.; et al. Artificial intelligence-based tools applied to pathological diagnosis of microbiological diseases. *Pathol. Res. Pract.* **2023**, *243*, 154362. [CrossRef] [PubMed]
35. Tessler, F.N.; Thomas, J. Artificial Intelligence for Evaluation of Thyroid Nodules: A Primer. *Thyroid* **2023**, *33*, 150–158. [CrossRef] [PubMed]
36. Hameed, B.S.; Krishnan, U.M. Artificial Intelligence-Driven Diagnosis of Pancreatic Cancer. *Cancers* **2022**, *14*, 5382. [CrossRef] [PubMed] [PubMed Central]
37. Thakur, N.; Alam, M.R.; Abdul-Ghafar, J.; Chong, Y. Recent Application of Artificial Intelligence in Non-Gynecological Cancer Cytopathology: A Systematic Review. *Cancers* **2022**, *14*, 3529. [CrossRef] [PubMed] [PubMed Central]

38. Alrafiah, A.R. Application and performance of artificial intelligence technology in cytopathology. *Acta Histochem.* **2022**, *124*, 151890. [CrossRef] [PubMed]
39. Vaickus, L.J.; Kerr, D.A.; Velez Torres, J.M.; Levy, J. Artificial Intelligence Applications in Cytopathology: Current State of the Art. *Surg. Pathol. Clin.* **2024**, *17*, 521–531. [CrossRef] [PubMed]
40. Jorda, M.; Kryvenko, O.N.; Hanly, F.; Zuo, Y. Urinary Tract Cytopathology: Current and Future Impact on Patient Care. *Surg. Pathol. Clin.* **2024**, *17*, 383–394. [CrossRef] [PubMed]
41. Velez Torres, J.M.; Vaickus, L.J.; Kerr, D.A. Thyroid Fine-Needle Aspiration: The Current and Future Landscape of Cytopathology. *Surg. Pathol. Clin.* **2024**, *17*, 371–381. [CrossRef] [PubMed]
42. Liu, T.J.; Yang, W.C.; Huang, S.M.; Yang, W.L.; Wu, H.J.; Ho, H.W.; Hsu, S.W.; Yeh, C.H.; Lin, M.Y.; Hwang, Y.T.; et al. Evaluating artificial intelligence-enhanced digital urine cytology for bladder cancer diagnosis. *Cancer Cytopathol.* **2024**, *Epub ahead of print*. [CrossRef] [PubMed]
43. Zhao, D.; Luo, M.; Zeng, M.; Yang, Z.; Guan, Q.; Wan, X.; Wang, Y.; Zhang, H.; Wang, Y.; Lu, H.; et al. Deep convolutional neural network model ResNeSt for discrimination of papillary thyroid carcinomas and benign nodules in thyroid nodules diagnosed as atypia of undetermined significance. *Gland. Surg.* **2024**, *13*, 619–629. [CrossRef]
44. Mhaske, S.; Ramalingam, K.; Nair, P.; Patel, S.; Menon, P.A.; Malik, N.; Mhaske, S. Automated Analysis of Nuclear Parameters in Oral Exfoliative Cytology Using Machine Learning. *Cureus* **2024**, *16*, e58744. [CrossRef]
45. Kim, T.; Chang, H.; Kim, B.; Yang, J.; Koo, D.; Lee, J.; Chang, J.W.; Hwang, G.; Gong, G.; Cho, N.H.; et al. Deep learning-based diagnosis of lung cancer using a nationwide respiratory cytology image set: Improving accuracy and inter-observer variability. *Am. J. Cancer Res.* **2023**, *13*, 5493–5503. [PubMed] [PubMed Central]
46. Park, H.S.; Chong, Y.; Lee, Y.; Yim, K.; Seo, K.J.; Hwang, G.; Kim, D.; Gong, G.; Cho, N.H.; Yoo, C.W.; et al. Deep Learning-Based Computational Cytopathologic Diagnosis of Metastatic Breast Carcinoma in Pleural Fluid. *Cells* **2023**, *12*, 1847. [CrossRef] [PubMed] [PubMed Central]
47. Ozer, E.; Bilecen, A.E.; Ozer, N.B.; Yanikoglu, B. Intraoperative cytological diagnosis of brain tumours: A preliminary study using a deep learning model. *Cytopathology* **2023**, *34*, 113–119. [CrossRef] [PubMed]
48. Saikia, A.R.; Bora, K.; Mahanta, L.B.; Das, A.K. Comparative assessment of CNN architectures for classification of breast FNAC images. *Tissue Cell* **2019**, *57*, 8–14. [CrossRef] [PubMed]
49. Sanyal, P.; Mukherjee, T.; Barui, S.; Das, A.; Gangopadhyay, P. Artificial Intelligence in Cytopathology: A Neural Network to Identify Papillary Carcinoma on Thyroid Fine-Needle Aspiration Cytology Smears. *J. Pathol. Inform.* **2018**, *9*, 43. [CrossRef] [PubMed] [PubMed Central]
50. Peñaranda, F.; Naranjo, V.; Lloyd, G.R.; Kastl, L.; Kemper, B.; Schnekenburger, J.; Nallala, J.; Stone, N. Discrimination of skin cancer cells using Fourier transform infrared spectroscopy. *Comput. Biol. Med.* **2018**, *100*, 50–61. [CrossRef] [PubMed]
51. Kumar, N.; Gupta, R.; Gupta, S. Whole Slide Imaging (WSI) in Pathology: Current Perspectives and Future Directions. *J. Digit. Imaging* **2020**, *33*, 1034–1040. [CrossRef] [PubMed] [PubMed Central]
52. Liu, W.; Li, C.; Rahaman, M.M.; Jiang, T.; Sun, H.; Wu, X.; Hu, W.; Chen, H.; Sun, C.; Yao, Y.; et al. Is the aspect ratio of cells important in deep learning? A robust comparison of deep learning methods for multi-scale cytopathology cell image classification: From convolutional neural networks to visual transformers. *Comput. Biol. Med.* **2022**, *141*, 105026. [CrossRef] [PubMed]
53. Chen, P.; Liang, Y.; Shi, X.; Yang, L.; Gader, P. Automatic Whole Slide Pathology Image Diagnosis Framework via Unit Stochastic Selection and Attention Fusion. *Neurocomputing* **2021**, *453*, 312–325. [CrossRef] [PubMed] [PubMed Central]
54. Zhou, T.; Xu, L.; Shi, J.; Zhang, Y.; Lin, X.; Wang, Y.; Hu, T.; Xu, R.; Xie, L.; Sun, L.; et al. US of thyroid nodules: Can AI-assisted diagnostic system compete with fine needle aspiration? *Eur. Radiol.* **2024**, *34*, 1324–1333. [CrossRef] [PubMed]
55. Sohn, A.; Miller, D.; Ribeiro, E.; Shankar, N.; Ali, S.; Hruban, R.; Baras, A. A deep learning model to triage and predict adenocarcinoma on pancreas cytology whole slide imaging. *Sci. Rep.* **2023**, *13*, 16517. [CrossRef] [PubMed] [PubMed Central]
56. Pubmed Search. Available online: https://pubmed.ncbi.nlm.nih.gov/?term=(Cytopathology[Title/Abstract])+AND+((Artificial+intelligence[Title/Abstract])+OR+(machine+learning[Title/Abstract])+OR+(deep+learning[Title/Abstract])+OR+(neural+network[Title/Abstract]))&sort=date&size=200 (accessed on 24 September 2024).
57. Pubmed Search. Available online: https://pubmed.ncbi.nlm.nih.gov/?term=(histopathology[Title/Abstract])+AND+((Artificial+intelligence[Title/Abstract])+OR+(machine+learning[Title/Abstract])+OR+(deep+learning[Title/Abstract])+OR+(neural+network[Title/Abstract]))&sort=date&size=200 (accessed on 24 September 2024).
58. Giansanti, D.; Grigioni, M.; D'Avenio, G.; Morelli, S.; Maccioni, G.; Bondi, A.; Giovagnoli, M.R. Virtual microscopy and digital cytology: State of the art. *Ann. Dell'Istituto Super. Di Sanità* **2010**, *46*, 115–122. [CrossRef] [PubMed]
59. Pubmed Search. Available online: https://pubmed.ncbi.nlm.nih.gov/?term=(radiology[Title/Abstract])+AND+((Artificial+intelligence[Title/Abstract])+OR+(machine+learning[Title/Abstract])+OR+(deep+learning[Title/Abstract])+OR+(neural+network[Title/Abstract]))&sort=date&size=200 (accessed on 24 September 2024).
60. Hölscher, D.L.; Bülow, R.D. Decoding pathology: The role of computational pathology in research and diagnostics. *Pflugers Arch.* **2024**, *Epub ahead of print*. [CrossRef] [PubMed]
61. Hijazi, A.; Bifulco, C.; Baldin, P.; Galon, J. Digital Pathology for Better Clinical Practice. *Cancers* **2024**, *16*, 1686. [CrossRef] [PubMed] [PubMed Central]

62. Ahmed, A.A.; Brychcy, A.; Abouzid, M.; Witt, M.; Kaczmarek, E. Perception of Pathologists in Poland of Artificial Intelligence and Machine Learning in Medical Diagnosis-A Cross-Sectional Study. *J. Pers. Med.* **2023**, *13*, 962. [CrossRef] [PubMed] [PubMed Central]
63. Contaldo, M.T.; Pasceri, G.; Vignati, G.; Bracchi, L.; Triggiani, S.; Carrafiello, G. AI in Radiology: Navigating Medical Responsibility. *Diagnostics* **2024**, *14*, 1506. [CrossRef] [PubMed] [PubMed Central]
64. Pesapane, F.; Gnocchi, G.; Quarrella, C.; Sorce, A.; Nicosia, L.; Mariano, L.; Bozzini, A.C.; Marinucci, I.; Priolo, F.; Abbate, F.; et al. Errors in Radiology: A Standard Review. *J. Clin. Med.* **2024**, *13*, 4306. [CrossRef] [PubMed] [PubMed Central]
65. Tikhomirov, L.; Semmler, C.; McCradden, M.; Searston, R.; Ghassemi, M.; Oakden-Rayner, L. Medical artificial intelligence for clinicians: The lost cognitive perspective. *Lancet Digit. Health* **2024**, *6*, e589–e594. [CrossRef] [PubMed]
66. Reale-Nosei, G.; Amador-Domínguez, E.; Serrano, E. From vision to text: A comprehensive review of natural image captioning in medical diagnosis and radiology report generation. *Med. Image Anal.* **2024**, *97*, 103264. [CrossRef] [PubMed]
67. Huang, W.; Li, Y.; Bao, Z.; Ye, J.; Xia, W.; Lv, Y.; Lu, J.; Wang, C.; Zhu, X. Knowledge, Attitude and Practice of Radiologists Regarding Artificial Intelligence in Medical Imaging. *J. Multidiscip. Healthc.* **2024**, *17*, 3109–3119. [CrossRef] [PubMed] [PubMed Central]
68. Bourdillon, A.T. Computer Vision-Radiomics & Pathognomics. *Otolaryngol. Clin. N. Am.* **2024**, *22*, 719–751. [CrossRef] [PubMed]
69. Lastrucci, A.; Pirrera, A.; Lepri, G.; Giansanti, D. Algorethics in Healthcare: Balancing Innovation and Integrity in AI Development. *Algorithms* **2024**, *17*, 432. [CrossRef]
70. Available online: https://www.who.int/news/item/18-01-2024-who-releases-ai-ethics-and-governance-guidance-for-large-multi-modal-models (accessed on 20 July 2024).
71. Available online: https://www.modulos.ai/eu-ai-act/?utm_term=ai%20act%20european%20union&utm_campaign=EU+AI+Act+(December+2023)&utm_source=adwords&utm_medium=ppc&hsa_acc=9558976660&hsa_cam=20858946124&hsa_grp=159677877987&hsa_ad=705319461314&hsa_src=g&hsa_tgt=kwd-2178244031979&hsa_kw=ai%20act%20european%20union&hsa_mt=p&hsa_net=adwords&hsa_ver=3&gad_source=1&gclid=CjwKCAjw5Ky1BhAgEiwA5jGujik2Y5RZXOVwXSvUjE-1RARfMpPgen5q2S7-8FnFFLLIiF052SYAwxoC2oEQAvD_BwE (accessed on 20 July 2024).
72. Available online: https://www.dermatologytimes.com/view/fda-organizations-issue-joint-paper-on-responsible-and-ethical-use-of-artificial-intelligence-in-medical-research (accessed on 20 July 2024).
73. Available online: https://www.pharmacytimes.com/view/fda-issues-paper-on-the-responsible-use-of-artificial-intelligence-in-medical-research (accessed on 20 July 2024).
74. Available online: https://transform.england.nhs.uk/ai-lab/ai-lab-programmes/ethics/#:~:text=The%20AI%20Ethics%20Initiative%20supports,risk%20and%20providing%20ethical%20assurance (accessed on 20 July 2024).
75. Available online: https://www.canada.ca/en/public-health/services/reports-publications/canada-communicable-disease-report-ccdr/monthly-issue/2020-46/issue-6-june-4-2020/ethical-framework-artificial-intelligence-applications.html (accessed on 20 July 2024).
76. Available online: https://cset.georgetown.edu/publication/ethical-norms-for-new-generation-artificial-intelligence-released (accessed on 20 July 2024).
77. Battazza, A.; Brasileiro, F.C.D.S.; Tasaka, A.C.; Bulla, C.; Ximenes, P.P.; Hosomi, J.E.; da Silva, P.F.; da Silva, L.F.; de Moura, F.B.C.; Rocha, N.S. Integrating telepathology and digital pathology with artificial intelligence: An inevitable future. *Vet. World* **2024**, *17*, 1667–1671. [CrossRef] [PubMed] [PubMed Central]

bioengineering

MDPI

Review

Reimagining Radiology: A Comprehensive Overview of Reviews at the Intersection of Mobile and Domiciliary Radiology over the Last Five Years

Graziano Lepri [1], Francesco Oddi [2], Rosario Alfio Gulino [2] and Daniele Giansanti [3,*]

1 Azienda Unità Sanitaria Locale Umbria 1, Via Guerriero Guerra 21, 06127 Perugia, Italy; graziano.lepri@uslumbria1.it

2 Facoltà di Ingegneria, Università di Tor Vergata, Via del Politecnico, 1, 00133 Roma, Italy; francesco.oddi@alumni.uniroma2.eu (F.O.); gulino@disp.uniroma2.it (R.A.G.)

3 Centro Nazionale TISP, Istituto Superiore di Sanità, Viale Regina Elena 299, 00161 Roma, Italy

* Correspondence: daniele.giansanti@iss.it; Tel.: +39-0649902701

Abstract: (Background) Domiciliary radiology, which originated in pioneering studies in 1958, has transformed healthcare, particularly during the COVID-19 pandemic, through advancements such as miniaturization and digitization. This evolution, driven by the synergy of advanced technologies and robust data networks, reshapes the intersection of domiciliary radiology and mobile technology in healthcare delivery. (Objective) The objective of this study is to overview the reviews in this field with reference to the last five years to face the state of development and integration of this practice in the health domain. (Methods) A review was conducted on PubMed and Scopus, applying a standard checklist and a qualification process. The outcome detected 21 studies. (Key Content and Findings) The exploration of mobile and domiciliary radiology unveils a compelling and optimistic perspective. Notable strides in this dynamic field include the integration of Artificial Intelligence (AI), revolutionary applications in telemedicine, and the educational potential of mobile devices. Post-COVID-19, telemedicine advances and the influential role of AI in pediatric radiology signify significant progress. Mobile mammography units emerge as a solution for underserved women, highlighting the crucial importance of early breast cancer detection. The investigation into domiciliary radiology, especially with mobile X-ray equipment, points toward a promising frontier, prompting in-depth research for comprehensive insights into its potential benefits for diverse populations. The study also identifies limitations and suggests future exploration in various domains of mobile and domiciliary radiology. A key recommendation stresses the strategic prioritization of multi-domain technology assessment initiatives, with scientific societies' endorsement, emphasizing regulatory considerations for responsible and ethical technology integration in healthcare practices. The broader landscape of technology assessment should aim to be innovative, ethical, and aligned with societal needs and regulatory standards. (Conclusions) The dynamic state of the field is evident, with active exploration of new frontiers. This overview also provides a roadmap, urging scholars, industry players, and regulators to collectively contribute to the further integration of this technology in the health domain.

Keywords: domiciliary radiology; domiciliary radiography; mobile radiology; mobile radiography

1. Introduction

1.1. Background

Embarking on a historical journey, the roots of domiciliary radiology trace back to an era preceding the digitalization wave and the establishment of standardized DICOM protocols. In 1958 [1], we registered the first pioneering studies starting the revolutionary path regarding domiciliary radiology, a time when mobile technology and its associated contributions were conspicuously absent [1]. Domiciliary radiology, since its inception, has emerged as a modern convenience and a profound game-changer. It liberates individuals from the anguish of arduous journeys and shields them from potential contagion in hospital corridors. The impact extends beyond patients, offering assistance to families burdened with travel logistics [2]. Venturing into the realm of remote execution reveals a complex tapestry involving a meticulous choreography of activities. Reshaping roles, navigating stringent radiological safety protocols, complying with regulations, deciphering evolving technologies, and considering non-technological resources like transportation contribute to the intricate dance of domiciliary radiology [2]. While this avant-garde approach lightens the load on hospital resources, it introduces a distinct set of challenges, demanding recalibration of workflows and strategic reallocation of attention and resources. The ongoing discourse about its merits and challenges is a testament to the dynamic equilibrium it seeks to establish. The true crucible of domiciliary radiology, including the pivotal role of mobile radiology units, emerged during the COVID-19 pandemic [3]. Crafted to cater to unique patient needs, this practice became an indispensable lifeline, especially for individuals with fragilities and disabilities. Its role in crisis management not only elevated visibility but also kindled newfound appreciation, underscoring resilience and adaptability in adversity. Once a niche chapter, the narrative of domiciliary radiology now stands tall as a testament to transformative healthcare practices in the 21st century. The intersection of advancements in specific technologies, Information and Communication Technology (ICT), and mobile technology has collectively made a significant impact, marking a transformative period in this field [4–7]. The evolution of domiciliary radiology, driven by continuous innovation, is marked by the miniaturization of technology and the relentless progress of digitization. Since the 1960s, there has been a transformative shift in healthcare and radiology, with specific technologies becoming key drivers. Miniaturization has revolutionized the practicality and portability of radiological instruments, enabling healthcare professionals to extend services beyond traditional settings [4,5]. The digital revolution has played a pivotal role, enhancing the efficiency and accessibility of radiological data. The seamless transition from analog to digital imaging has improved precision and paved the way for integrating cutting-edge technologies. This digital shift, coupled with advancements in data networks, has ushered in a new era of domiciliary radiology. The interconnected world, characterized by fast and stable data networks, empowers healthcare providers to conduct remote radiological procedures with unprecedented ease. The synergy between advanced technologies and robust data networks has not only fostered the growth of home-based and mobile radiology but also amplified capabilities, resulting in a paradigm shift in healthcare delivery [5]. Diagnostic services can now be seamlessly extended to the comfort of the patient's home and to the mobile radiology interconnection. The journey from bulky technologies of the past to sleek, portable, and digitally empowered tools signifies a revolution in domiciliary radiology [6]. This evolution reflects a commitment to technological excellence and emphasizes a dedication to enhancing patient care through innovation and accessibility. The future of the intersection of domiciliary radiology and mobile technology following the COVID-19 pandemic appears poised for even greater strides, promising a continuum of advancements that will further redefine the healthcare delivery landscape [7].

1.2. Issues Emerging on the Horizon

In the evolving intersection of domiciliary and mobile radiology, a range of inquiries has propelled research into uncharted territories [2]. Artificial Intelligence and machine learning play a significant role in enhancing diagnostic precision. Simultaneously, the regulatory framework undergoes scrutiny alongside technological progress, exploring the intricate relationship between policies and the adoption of remote imaging. Patient outcomes, satisfaction, and the experiences of other involved actors become focal points, investigating the impact of remote imaging on well-being. Cybersecurity measures guarding data and infrastructure are crucial considerations. Economic aspects, including cost-effectiveness and accessibility, feature prominently in the discourse. Interdisciplinary collaboration optimizes domiciliary radiology services, emphasizing its impact on patient care. The roles of domiciliary radiology and mobile radiology in chronic disease management are explored, and attention shifts to challenges hindering adoption, with researchers seeking innovative solutions. Ethical considerations delicately address privacy and technology use, while patient empowerment and education emerge as vital components [6]. Together, these questions guide domiciliary radiology research, delving into technological advancements and broader human-centric considerations, shaping the dynamic healthcare landscape [7].

1.3. Defining the Grounds for Conducting a Review

The preceding introductory discussion not only raises crucial questions but also sheds light on the underlying reasons necessitating a thorough exploration of the developments and emerging issues surrounding this field of study of radiology. This need becomes particularly apparent in the wake of the technological revolution that unfolded in the second millennium, marked by miniaturization, digitization, and advancements in Information and Communication Technology (ICT), including the increasingly robust and stable capabilities of mobile connections. The overarching aim of this study is to conduct an exhaustive narrative review of existing reviews within the realm of the intersection of domiciliary radiology and mobile radiology over the past five years, including, therefore, also the advancements driven by the research during the COVID-19 pandemic. This comprehensive analysis seeks to delve into the multifaceted landscape of home-based radiology, considering technological advancements, evolving practices, and the broader implications for patient care.

Sub-Objectives Include the Following:

- Technological evolution: Examine the progression of technological innovations, such as miniaturization, digitization, and ICT, and their impact in this field related to radiology practices.
- Patient-centric implications: Explore the implications on patient experiences, outcomes, and overall satisfaction, with a focus on advancements in mobile connectivity.
- Interdisciplinary collaboration: Investigate the role of interdisciplinary collaboration in optimizing radiology services, considering the integration of various healthcare disciplines.
- Regulatory and ethical considerations: Analyze the regulatory and ethical considerations surrounding domiciliary and mobile radiology, particularly in the context of evolving technologies and practices.
- Comparative effectiveness: Assess the comparative effectiveness of mobile and domiciliary radiology against traditional in-hospital radiological procedures, considering factors like cost-effectiveness and diagnostic accuracy.

2. Methods

The narrative review of reviews used the ANDJ standardized checklist designed for narrative reviews [8]. The PubMed and Scopus databases were inserted in the overview. A qualification methodology was used to choose the studies based on the assessment of qualified parameters [9]. Based on [9], we evaluated each contribution based on key parameters:

- *N*1: *Clarity of study rationale in the introduction.*
- *N*2: *Appropriateness of work's design.*
- *N*3: *Clarity in describing methods.*
- *N*4: *Clear presentation of results.*
- *N*5: *Justification and alignment of conclusions with results.*
- *N*6: *Adequate disclosure of conflicts of interest by authors.*

We assigned a graded score (1 to 5) to *N*1–N5.

For $N6$, we provided a binary assessment (Yes/No) for disclosure of conflicts.

We preselect studies meeting the following criteria:

$N6$ must be "Yes" for conflict disclosure.

The cumulative score for $N1$–$N5$ must exceed 3.

Only peer-reviewed studies were considered (including congress proceedings if peer-reviewed). The defined search query * was the following: =

(mobile radiology[Title/Abstract]) OR (mobile radiography[Title/Abstract]) OR (domiciliary radiology[Title/Abstract]) OR (domiciliary radiography[Title/Abstract]) Filters: Review, Systematic Review, in the last 5 years Sort by: Most Recent

The procedure-based overview identified 21 reviews, all matching 100% of the PubMed query [10] and 94% of the Scopus query.

*Preliminary trials included the composite key at the second row of Box 1. Nevertheless, our observations revealed that the outcomes were primarily associated with distinct areas, such as radiologists operating remotely from home (especially during the COVID-19 pandemic) and the expansive realm of teleradiology. These aspects, while noteworthy, fall outside the specific scope of this overview and warrant a more specialized discussion.

3. Results

The results from the overview of the reviews are arranged into two paragraphs: Section 3.1 reports a detailed analysis, while Section 3.2 reports the key findings (supported by a summary table (Table 1).

Of the 21 selected review studies [11–31], a total of 14 studies specifically focused on the themes of the review [13–18,20,21,23,24,26–28,31], while the remaining [11,12,19,22,25,29,30] had a focus on different topics.

Table 1. Key elements/points emerging from the overview of these studies with the focus.

Reference	Focus	Key Points
[13]	*Musculoskeletal Ultrasound*	- *Radiation-free and dynamic imaging tool*
		- *Addresses increasing demand for training opportunities*
[14]	*Mobile Devices Integration in the Health Domain*	- *Challenges in the widespread adoption of mobile devices*
		- *Call for a universal mobile application in healthcare*
[15]	*Telemedicine and COVID-19 Impact*	- *Transformative impact on healthcare organizations*
		- *Evolution of telemedicine areas, complementing traditional medicine*
[16]	*AI Applications in Pediatric Radiology*	- *Dominance of deep convolutional neural networks*
		- *Necessity for further exploration of AI's value in optimizing doses*
[17]	*Mobile Mammography for Breast Cancer Screening*	- *Addresses disparities in breast cancer outcomes*
		- *Potential for earlier detection, especially in underserved women*
[18]	*Simulation-Based Training (SBT)*	- *Common use in allied health professions*
		- *Unclear impact on sustained skill enhancement, calls for further investigation*
[20]	*Focus on Diagnostic Radiology Standards in Low-Resource Settings*	- *Emphasis on the critical role of diagnostic imaging*
		- *Lack of evidence on standard quality control for mobile health units (MHUs)*

Table 1. *Cont.*

Reference	Focus	Key Points
[21]	*Augmented Reality in Anatomy Education*	- *Identification and assessment of various AR modalities* - *Need for sufficiently powered studies and validated assessment tools*
[23]	*Domiciliary Radiology with Mobile X-ray Equipment*	- *Exploration of mobile X-ray equipment outside the hospital* - *Need for further research, considering limitations in language, databases, and grey literature*
[24]	*Trends in Ultrasound Imaging*	- *Emphasis on widespread use and portability of mobile devices* - *Developments in miniaturization and improved imaging performance*
[26]	*Quality Improvement Interventions in Radiology*	- *Improvements in operational efficiency, report turnaround time, and teamwork* - *Positive outcomes associated with the introduction of mobile radiography*
[27]	*Integration of Internet-Based Technology in Radiology*	- *Integral connection between radiology and the Internet* - *Seamless integration of Internet-based applications, including mobile devices and wearables*
[28]	*Mobile Diagnostic Imaging Device*	- *Review of Mobile MIM diagnostic imaging device on iOS mobile devices* - *Emphasis on features and usability, especially in radiation treatment plans and medical image analysis*
[31]	*Workflow Optimization with Mobile Tools*	- *Addressing challenges in communication and workflow efficiency* - *Development of a mobile tool to optimize workflow efficiency in academic radiology departments*

3.1. In-Depth Analysis of the Detected Reviews: A Comprehensive Overview

In Neubauer et al.'s research [13], the focus is on musculoskeletal ultrasound as a radiation-free and dynamic imaging tool that enhances diagnostic and therapeutic safety. The study aims to map the current state of musculoskeletal ultrasonography education, highlighting the increasing demand for training opportunities. The systematic literature search conducted in January 2022 reveals a diverse range of course concepts and programs in various disciplines, with a particular emphasis on residents in rheumatology, radiology, and physical medicine and rehabilitation. International institutions have proposed guidelines and curricula to standardize ultrasound training. The important role of the mobile devices is recognized. The study concludes that standardized musculoskeletal ultrasound curricula would enhance training and facilitate the implementation of new programs.

Kufel et al. [14] explore the utilization of mobile devices in medicine, emphasizing the challenges in their widespread adoption. The study compares the usability of mobile applications for diagnostic image evaluation with stationary descriptive stations. Despite differences in procedures, device availability, and regulatory frameworks, the research identifies both positive and negative features of portable methods for analyzing radiological images. The authors stress the need for a universal mobile application with convenient and simple usage in hospital infrastructure. Future research will focus on advancements in using mobile devices and applications in the medical sector.

Perrone et al.'s study [15] delves into the impact of the COVID-19 pandemic on healthcare organizations and the evolution of telemedicine areas. The review highlights the role of electronic health records, teleradiology (including mobile/domiciliary radiology), telecardiology, teledermatology, and other telemedicine applications in managing the challenges posed by the pandemic. The authors stress the importance of telemedicine as complementary to traditional medicine and discuss its significant applications in radiology and dermatology.

Ng et al. [16] address the crucial aspect of radiation dose optimization in pediatric radiology. The systematic review focuses on Artificial Intelligence (AI) techniques and architectures for dose optimization, highlighting the dominance of deep convolutional neural networks in reducing radiation dose without compromising diagnostic information. Mobile radiography devices were included in the study. The study emphasizes the necessity for further explorations of AI's value in dose optimization for various modalities in pediatric radiology.

Trivedi et al. [17] examine the disparities in breast cancer outcomes among different populations and highlight the role of mobile mammography units in providing convenient screening services. The review discusses the history and benefits of mobile mammography, especially for underserved women, emphasizing its potential to enable earlier detection of breast cancer and alleviate the impact of missed screenings during the COVID-19 pandemic.

Heuer et al. [18] conducted a systematic review of the utilization of simulation-based training (SBT) in allied health professions. The study identifies the common use of SBT in paramedics, emergency medical technicians, and respiratory therapists. Almost half of the studies were conducted in a stationary or mobile simulation lab. While SBT proves effective in enhancing short-term measures like post-training skill improvement and participant confidence, its impact on sustained skill enhancement and patient outcomes remains unclear.

Dinar et al. [20] focus on diagnostic radiology standards in low-resource settings, conducting a systematic review of the quality control for mobile health units (MHUs). The study notes a lack of evidence on standard quality control for MHUs and emphasizes the critical role of diagnostic imaging in ensuring successful patient management in crisis situations. The authors call for investigations to assess the feasibility of different quality control standards in MHUs.

McBain et al. [21] conducted a scoping review to identify augmented reality (AR) modalities used in anatomy education and examined assessment tools for their performance. Four AR modalities were identified, including head-mounted display, projection, instrument and screen, and mobile devices. The assessment focused on usability, feasibility, and acceptability, with a recent interest in visuospatial ability, cognitive load, time on task, and academic achievement outcomes. The authors emphasized the need for sufficiently powered studies using validated assessment tools to better understand AR's role in anatomical education.

Toppemberg et al. [23] center their scoping review on domiciliary radiology, exploring the use of mobile X-ray equipment outside the hospital. The review included 12 studies published between 2009 and 2020 and highlighted the potential benefits for various populations, such as hospice patients, those with intellectual disabilities, and psychiatric patients. The results suggested improvements in population health, image quality, and potential cost-effectiveness. However, the authors noted limitations in language, databases, and grey literature, emphasizing the need for further research.

Wang et al. [24] provide a comprehensive review of current trends in ultrasound imaging, emphasizing its widespread use, portability of mobile devices, and recent advancements. The review highlights developments in ultrasound systems, including their miniaturization, improved imaging performance, and lower costs. The authors discuss ultrasound's expanded applications, such as molecular imaging, super-resolution imaging, and focused treatments with intravascular microbubbles. The article projects a promising future for ultrasound in solving various medical challenges.

Jabin et al. [26] conducted a review of quality improvement interventions in radiology, focusing on both staff and patient perspectives. The study includes 18 selected studies covering interventions such as health information technology, training and education, immediate and critical reporting, safety programs, and the introduction of mobile radiography. The results demonstrate improvements in operational efficiency, reported turnaround time, teamwork, communication, and patient safety. The introduction of mobile radiography demonstrated improvements in outcomes, such as improved operational and workflow efficiency, report turnaround time, and teamwork and communication.

The authors called for further research to explore additional dimensions of quality, cost, and risk versus benefit.

Gupta et al. [27] discuss the integral connection between radiology and the Internet, emphasizing the rapid rise of Internet-based technology in healthcare. The article highlighted the seamless integration of Internet-based applications in radiology, including the use of mobile devices and wearables. The authors explore the impact of the Internet of Things (IoT) on radiology workflows, resident and medical student education, research, and patient engagement.

Adusumilli et al. [28] reviewed the Mobile MIM diagnostic imaging device, which is available on the Apple App Store. The FDA-approved app allows physicians to visualize scans from multiple modalities on iOS mobile devices, focusing on radiation treatment plans and medical image analysis. The review discusses the app's features and usability, emphasizing its strengths and limitations, including incompatibility with mammography.

Makary et al. [31] address the challenges of communication and workflow efficiency in radiology operations. They shared their experience developing a mobile tool to optimize workflow efficiency and streamline access to relevant information in academic radiology departments. The mobile tool aims to enhance communication among care team members, provide access to guidelines and schedules, and keep users informed about local and international news.

3.2. *Common Findings and Key Findings*

From these studies, we can identify more general common findings and more specific emerging themes.

The analyzed reviews cover a diverse range of topics related to mobile/domiciliary radiology, including the use of AR in anatomy education, [21] domiciliary radiology with mobile X-ray equipment [23], advancements in ultrasound imaging [24], quality improvement interventions [26], the integration of Internet-based technology, mobile diagnostic imaging apps, and the development of a mobile tool for workflow optimization in academic radiology departments [27,28,31]. Furthermore, interesting perspectives are detected, such as musculoskeletal ultrasonography education with radiology training [13], the development and integration of innovative mobile devices in medicine [14,20], AI integration in pediatric radiology [16], the development and use of mobile mammography units in breast cancer screening [17], applications in simulation training [18], the development of models (including standards and quality control) in low resource settings [20], and integration in telemedicine models [15]. An important boost in all areas was given by the COVID-19 epidemic, such as in the integration with telemedicine [15]. In relation to telemedicine and the impact of COVID-19, this overview highlights how the intersection between mobile and domiciliary radiology has undergone significant transformations, driven by technological innovations and a growing emphasis on patient-centered care. A synthesis of various research themes sheds light on key trends and breakthroughs, providing a comprehensive understanding of the current landscape.

3.2.1. Musculoskeletal Ultrasound

The exploration of musculoskeletal ultrasound as a radiation-free and dynamic imaging tool is a focal point in Neubauer et al.'s research [13]. This modality not only enhances diagnostic and therapeutic safety but also addresses the increasing demand for training opportunities. The recognition of mobile devices' important role underscores the potential for standardized musculoskeletal ultrasound curricula to drive advancements in training and program implementation.

3.2.2. Mobile Devices Integration in the Health Domain

Kufel et al. [14] delve into the challenges surrounding the widespread adoption of mobile devices in medicine. The study compares the usability of mobile applications for diagnostic image evaluation with stationary stations, highlighting both positive and negative features. The call for a universal mobile application underscores the need for seamless integration into hospital infrastructure, fostering future research on advancements in mobile devices in the medical sector.

3.2.3. Telemedicine and COVID-19 Impact

Perrone et al.'s study [15] explores the transformative impact of the COVID-19 pandemic on healthcare organizations, emphasizing the evolution of telemedicine areas. Electronic health records, teleradiology, and mobile radiology emerge as crucial components, with telemedicine seen as complementary to traditional medicine, especially in radiology and dermatology applications.

3.2.4. AI Applications in Pediatric Radiology

Addressing the critical aspect of radiation dose optimization in pediatric radiology, Ng et al. [16] focus on the dominance of deep convolutional neural networks in reducing radiation dose without compromising diagnostic information. The inclusion of mobile radiography devices in the study emphasizes the necessity for further exploration of AI's value in optimizing doses for various modalities in pediatric radiology.

3.2.5. Mobile Mammography for Breast Cancer Screening

Trivedi et al. [17] highlight disparities in breast cancer outcomes among different populations and stress the role of mobile mammography units in providing convenient screening services. The study underscores the potential of mobile mammography to enable earlier detection, particularly in underserved women, and to mitigate the impact of missed screenings during the COVID-19 pandemic.

3.2.6. Simulation-Based Training (SBT)

Conducting a systematic review, Heuer et al. [18] identify the common use of simulation-based training in allied health professions. While SBT proves effective in enhancing short-term measures, its impact on sustained skill enhancement and patient outcomes remains unclear, suggesting a need for further investigation.

3.2.7. Focus on Diagnostic Radiology Standards in Low-Resource Settings

Dinar et al. [20] focus on diagnostic radiology standards in low-resource settings, emphasizing the critical role of diagnostic imaging in crisis situations. The lack of evidence on standard quality control for mobile health units (MHUs) calls for investigations to assess the feasibility of different quality control standards in MHUs.

3.2.8. Augmented Reality in Anatomy Education

McBain et al. [21] identify and assess various AR modalities used in anatomy education, emphasizing the need for sufficiently powered studies using validated assessment tools. The exploration of AR's role in anatomical education extends to considerations of usability, feasibility, and acceptability.

3.2.9. Domiciliary Radiology with Mobile X-ray Equipment

Toppemberg et al.'s [23] scoping review on domiciliary radiology explores the use of mobile X-ray equipment outside the hospital. While suggesting potential benefits for various populations, the authors emphasize the need for further research, noting limitations in language, databases, and grey literature.

3.2.10. Trends in Ultrasound Imaging

Wang et al. [24] provide a comprehensive review of current trends in ultrasound imaging. The emphasis on widespread use, portability of mobile devices, and recent advancements, including developments in miniaturization and improved imaging performance, point towards a promising future for ultrasound in addressing various medical challenges.

3.2.11. Quality Improvement Interventions in Radiology

Jabin et al. [26] review quality improvement interventions in radiology, showcasing improvements in operational efficiency, reported turnaround time, teamwork, communication, and patient safety. The positive outcomes associated with the introduction of mobile radiography underscore its potential to enhance overall workflow efficiency.

3.2.12. Integration of Internet-Based Technology in Radiology

Gupta et al. [27] discuss the integral connection between radiology and the Internet, emphasizing the rapid rise of Internet-based technology. The seamless integration of Internet-based applications, including mobile devices and wearables, highlights the transformative impact on radiology workflows, education, research, and patient engagement.

3.2.13. Mobile Diagnostic Imaging Device

Adusumilli et al. [28] review the Mobile MIM diagnostic imaging device, emphasizing its features and usability on iOS mobile devices. The focus on radiation treatment plans and medical image analysis highlights the potential of mobile applications in enhancing specific aspects of diagnostic imaging.

3.2.14. Workflow Optimization with Mobile Tools

Makary et al. [31] address the challenges of communication and workflow efficiency in radiology operations. The development of a mobile tool to optimize workflow efficiency in academic radiology departments underscores the potential for mobile technologies to enhance communication, provide access to guidelines, and keep users informed.

In conclusion, this comprehensive overview of recent research in medical imaging demonstrates a rich tapestry of advancements, challenges, and potential avenues for future exploration. From musculoskeletal ultrasound to AI applications, telemedicine, and mobile technologies, the collective findings underscore the dynamic evolution of medical imaging and its pivotal role in advancing healthcare. As technology continues to shape the landscape, the intersection of innovation and patient-centered care remains at the forefront of the field's progression. Table 1 reports the focus and the key points emerging for each study.

4. Discussion

The discussion is organized into five sections, each carefully rendered into distinct paragraphs. The *first opening paragraph* establishes the context by exploring the prevailing trends in the dissemination of knowledge within this domain. The subsequent *second paragraph* then unfolds in two facets: (I) a meticulous examination of the pivotal findings arising from the study results, with a keen focus on discerning emerging opportunities, and (II) an analysis of the limitations and areas demanding a more extensive investigation, aiming to provide a comprehensive perspective. The *third paragraph* discusses the key issue of *mobile radiology as a tool taking services directly to patients*, also integrating the overview with comparisons. The *fourth paragraph* provides the takeaway and emerging considerations. The *fifth and last paragraph* discusses the limitations of the study.

4.1. Numerical Trends

Exploring the evolving landscape of scientific publications in this domain using the first composite keywords in Box 1 yields valuable insights. We applied the research on the PubMed platform [32]. The initial references to these technologies date back to 1947 [1], marking the first time they came under discussion. However, it was not until 1958 that their mention gained prominence, particularly in the context of their applications within communities [1]. The cumulative count of publications since 1947 has surged to 433 [10], as depicted in Figure 1. Notably, 16% of these publications, totalling 70, are reviews (including systematic reviews). If we focus on the last decade (Figure 2), we observe that 68% of the studies have been produced during this period.

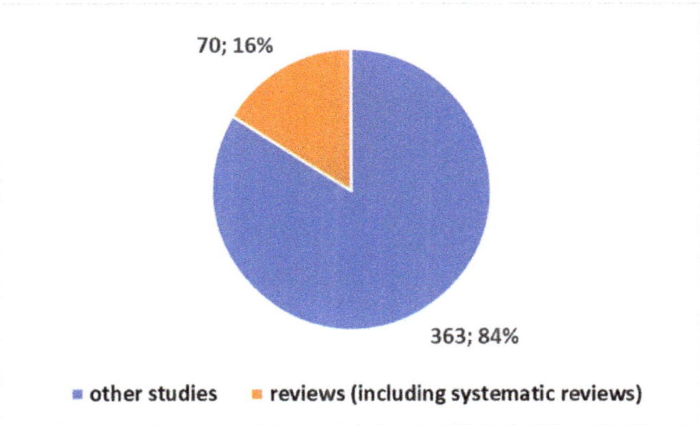

Figure 1. Trends in the studies since 1960.

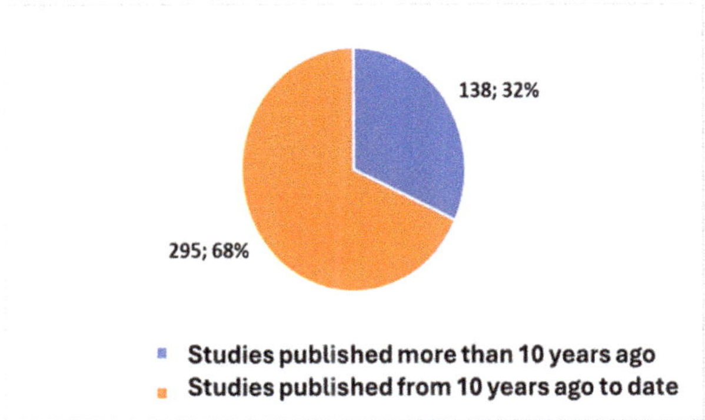

Figure 2. Trends in the studies with reference to the last ten years.

Upon scrutinizing the body of work generated in response to the COVID-19 pandemic to date, we uncovered a total of 149 studies, constituting a noteworthy 34% more than 1/3 of the total published papers. This revelation underscores that nearly one-third (as illustrated in Figure 3) of all studies conducted since 1947 have remarkably converged within the last four years. This trend serves as a compelling indication of how COVID-19 has not only accelerated advancements in this domain but has also acted as a driving force in various sectors linked to the integration of digital technologies within the patient's domicile. This shift is particularly pronounced in efforts aimed at safeguarding the well-being of individuals who are frail or living with disabilities.

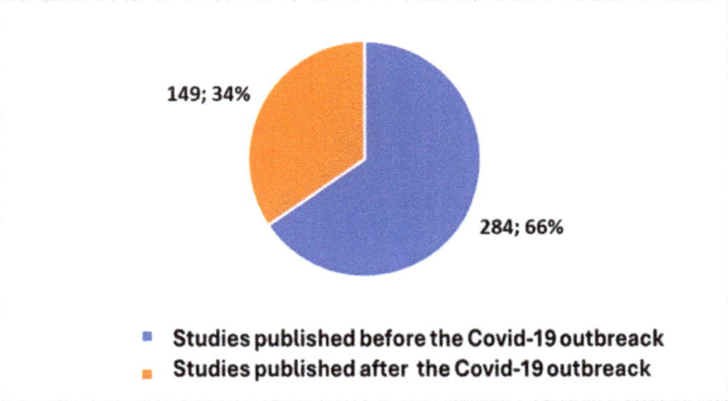

Figure 3. Trends of studies before and after the COVID-19 pandemic.

Box 1. The proposed composite keys.

((“mobile”[All Fields] OR “mobiles”[All Fields]) AND “radiology”[Title/Abstract]) OR “mobile radiography”[Title/Abstract] OR ((“domiciliaries”[All Fields] OR “domiciliary”[All Fields]) AND “radiology”[Title/Abstract]) OR “domiciliary radiography”[Title/Abstract]   *(Home radiology[Title/Abstract]) OR (Home radiography [Title/Abstract]) OR (Remote radiography[Title/Abstract]) OR (remote radiology[Title/Abstract]) OR (remote radiography[Title/Abstract])*

4.2. Interpretation of Results: Opportunities, Limitations, and Suggestions for a Broader Investigation

The explored reviews delve into a myriad of captivating realms within mobile/domiciliary radiology, encompassing a rich tapestry of subjects. These include the dynamic incorporation of augmented reality (AR) in anatomy education [21], the intricate domain of domiciliary radiology utilizing mobile X-ray equipment [23], cutting-edge advancements in ultrasound imaging [24], transformative quality improvement interventions [26], the seamless integration of Internet-based technology, mobile diagnostic imaging applications, and the development of a mobile tool for workflow optimization in academic radiology departments [27,28,31]. Amidst this vast landscape, intriguing perspectives surface, demanding focused attention on opportunities, limitations, and the identification of areas warrant a more comprehensive investigation. Noteworthy findings include the profound impact of musculoskeletal ultrasonography education on radiology training [13], the dynamic evolution of innovative mobile devices in medicine [14,20], the integration of Artificial Intelligence (AI) in pediatric settings [16], the pioneering development and utilization of mobile mammography units for breast cancer screening [17], the revolutionary applications in simulation training [18], the imperative need for model development (including standards and quality control) in resource-limited settings [20], and the integration of these technologies into evolving telemedicine models [15].

The catalyzing force of the COVID-19 epidemic has served as a transformative catalyst across all these domains, which is especially evident in the enhanced integration with telemedicine [15]. This pivotal moment underscores the urgency of not only acknowledging but also meticulously examining the opportunities, limitations, and potential avenues for broader investigation that have unfurled within the intricate intersections of mobile/domiciliary radiology and the evolving healthcare landscape.

4.2.1. Emerging Opportunities

In the rapidly evolving landscape of the investigated field, a tapestry of emerging opportunities unfolds, promising to reshape the way we approach diagnostics, training, and patient care. Technological advancements stand at the forefront, offering a dual promise of precision and accessibility.

One notable opportunity lies in the realm of musculoskeletal ultrasound education, as illuminated by Neubauer et al. [13]. The emphasis on a radiation-free and dynamic imaging tool not only enhances diagnostic and therapeutic safety but also addresses the escalating demand for training. The recognition of mobile devices as pivotal in this landscape underscores the potential for standardized curricula, ushering in a new era of proficiency and program implementation. In tandem, the integration of mobile devices in medicine, as explored by Kufel et al. [14], presents a dynamic frontier. The challenges associated with widespread adoption become a call to action, emphasizing the need for a universal mobile application seamlessly integrated into the hospital infrastructure. This not only addresses current hurdles but also paves the way for future advancements in the utilization of mobile devices within the medical sector. The transformative impact of the COVID-19 pandemic has opened vistas for the evolution of telemedicine, as uncovered by Perrone et al. [15]. Electronic health records, teleradiology, and mobile radiology emerge as key players, synergizing with traditional medicine, particularly in the domains of radiology and dermatology. The pandemic, while challenging, acted as a catalyst for telemedicine's complementary role. AI took center stage in pediatric radiology, as elucidated by Ng et al. [16]. The dominance of deep convolutional neural networks in reducing radiation dose without compromising diagnostic information heralds a new era. The study's inclusion of mobile radiography devices underlines the necessity for further exploration, suggesting AI's pivotal role in optimizing doses across diverse modalities.

Breast cancer screening, a perennial concern, finds an ally in mobile mammography units, as highlighted by Trivedi et al. [17]. The disparities in outcomes between different populations become a focal point, and mobile mammography emerges as a solution, particularly for underserved women. Its potential to enable earlier detection and mitigate the impact of missed screenings, especially in the wake of the COVID-19 pandemic, marks a significant stride forward. Simulation-based training (SBT) in allied health professions, per Heuer et al. [18], presents a dual narrative. While proving effective in enhancing short-term measures, the sustained impact on skill enhancement and patient outcomes remains elusive. This ambiguity becomes a clarion call for further investigations, opening the door for refining training methodologies. The global discourse expands to encompass diagnostic radiology standards in low-resource settings, as investigated by Dinar et al. [20]. The emphasis on the critical role of diagnostic imaging in crisis situations unveils an urgent need for standard quality control for mobile health units (MHUs). This beckons investigations to assess the feasibility of different quality control standards, laying the groundwork for successful patient management in challenging environments. AR in anatomy education, as explored by McBain et al. [21], offers a visionary perspective. The identification and assessment of AR modalities lay the groundwork for an immersive educational experience. The call for sufficiently powered studies becomes a clarion call, offering the potential for a paradigm shift in anatomical education methodologies. Domiciliary radiology, with a focus on mobile X-ray equipment, unfolds as a promising frontier, as revealed by Toppemberg et al. [23]. While potential benefits for diverse populations surface, the need for further research becomes apparent. This highlights the nascent nature of this avenue, urging researchers to delve deeper into language, databases, and grey literature.

The discourse broadens to encompass trends in ultrasound imaging, a domain meticulously reviewed by Wang et al. [24]. The emphasis on widespread use, portability of mobile devices, and recent advancements becomes a harbinger of progress. Developments in miniaturization and improved imaging performance set the stage for ultrasound's promising future, extending its applications into molecular imaging and focused treatments. Quality improvement interventions in radiology, as reviewed by Jabin et al. [26], form a nexus of positive outcomes. The integration of mobile radiography demonstrates improvements in operational efficiency, report turnaround time, and teamwork. The call for further research becomes an invitation to explore additional dimensions of quality, cost, and risk versus benefit, sculpting a roadmap for enhanced outcomes. The integral connection between radiology and the Internet, as discussed by Gupta et al. [27], opens up a new frontier. The seamless integration of Internet-based applications, including mobile devices and wearables, sets the stage for transformative changes. The impact of the Internet of Things (IoT) on radiology workflows, education, research, and patient engagement becomes a realm ripe for exploration. The discourse turns towards a review of the Mobile MIM diagnostic imaging device by Adusumilli et al. [28]. The emphasis on features and usability, particularly on iOS mobile devices, heralds a niche in enhancing specific aspects of diagnostic imaging. The focus on radiation treatment plans and medical image analysis uncovers a realm where mobile applications can become indispensable tools. Challenges in communication and workflow efficiency within radiology operations find a solution in the development of mobile tools, as shared by Makary et al. [31]. The optimization of workflow efficiency in academic radiology departments becomes a testament to the transformative power of mobile technologies. The tool's development, aimed at enhancing communication, providing access to guidelines, and keeping users informed, marks a pivotal moment in radiology operations.

4.2.2. Emerging Limitations and Suggestions for a Broader Investigation

From the analysis of the reviews, important limitations emerge, and indirectly, suggestions for a broader investigation are included in Table 2.

Table 2. Focus and suggestions for a broader investigatio.

Focus [Reference ID]	Suggestion
Musculoskeletal Ultrasound Education [13]	Undertake a comprehensive, cross-disciplinary investigation to understand the nuanced training needs in musculoskeletal ultrasound across diverse medical specialties. This broader exploration could inform the development of educational frameworks tailored to the specific requirements of each field.
Mobile Devices Integration in Medicine [14]	Engage in an interdisciplinary examination of the impediments to the widespread adoption of mobile devices in medical settings. Broader investigations involving the collaboration between healthcare professionals, technology experts, and policymakers can pave the way for comprehensive guidelines for seamless integration.
Telemedicine and COVID-19 Impact [15]	Initiate longitudinal studies to assess the enduring impact of telemedicine on patient outcomes, healthcare costs, and the quality of physician-patient interactions. A broader investigation can delve into the integration of telemedicine into routine medical practices, ensuring its sustainability and effectiveness beyond crisis situations.
AI Applications in Pediatric Radiology [16]	Expand the scope of AI applications in pediatric radiology by exploring the intricacies of different imaging modalities and clinical scenarios. Collaborate with pediatric specialists to tailor AI algorithms to diverse patient populations and medical conditions.
Mobile Mammography for Breast Cancer Screening [17]	Conduct in-depth studies to identify and address logistical, financial, and infrastructural barriers in implementing mobile mammography units. Broader investigations could involve partnerships with community organizations to develop targeted strategies for reaching underserved populations.
Simulation-Based Training (SBT) in Allied Health Professions [18]	Undertake longitudinal studies to assess the sustained impact of simulation-based training on skill enhancement and patient outcomes. Broader investigations might involve exploring innovative approaches within SBT, such as incorporating virtual reality or gamification elements.
Diagnostic Radiology Standards in Low-Resource Settings [20]	Collaborate with international organizations and healthcare providers to establish evidence-based standards for quality control in mobile health units (MHUs) in low-resource settings. Broader investigations could involve assessing the feasibility of different quality control standards and adapting them to the specific challenges of crisis situations.
Augmented Reality in Anatomy Education [21]	Extend the scope of AR applications in anatomy education by exploring their effectiveness in diverse educational settings. Broader investigations might involve collaborations with educational institutions to implement AR-enhanced curricula and assess their impact on student learning outcomes.

Table 2. *Cont.*

Focus [Reference ID]	Suggestion
Domiciliary Radiology with Mobile X-ray Equipment [23]	Collaborate with diverse healthcare providers and communities to identify potential benefits and challenges in the use of mobile X-ray equipment outside the hospital. Broader investigations could contribute to optimizing the implementation of such technology for various populations.
Trends in Ultrasound Imaging [24]	Explore evolving trends in ultrasound imaging, emphasizing not only technological advancements but also the societal and economic factors influencing its widespread use. Broader investigations could shed light on the transformative potential of ultrasound in addressing broader healthcare challenges.
Quality Improvement Interventions in Radiology [26]	Investigate additional dimensions of quality improvement interventions in radiology, including cost-effectiveness and a comprehensive risk versus benefit analysis. Broader investigations could contribute to a more holistic understanding of the impact of interventions on various aspects of healthcare delivery.
Integration of Internet-Based Technology in Radiology [27]	Delve into the evolving landscape of Internet-based technology in radiology, with a focus on its impact on medical education and patient engagement. Broader investigations could explore the intersection of technology, education, and patient care, shaping the future of radiology workflows.
Mobile Diagnostic Imaging Device [28]	Explore the potential applications of mobile diagnostic imaging devices in diverse medical scenarios. Broader investigations could focus on expanding the functionalities and compatibility of such devices, addressing current limitations and enhancing their overall utility.
Workflow Optimization with Mobile Tools [31]	Investigate the broader implications of workflow optimization with mobile tools in radiology operations. Broader investigations could explore innovative approaches to enhance communication, streamline access to information, and improve overall efficiency in academic radiology departments.

Musculoskeletal ultrasound education, as illuminated by Neubauer et al. [13], grapples with its own set of limitations. Despite its potential as a radiation-free and dynamic imaging tool, the challenge lies in developing standardized curricula. The diversity in course concepts and programs across disciplines, coupled with the emphasis on mobile devices, highlights the need for careful consideration of educational frameworks that cater to the unique demands of different specialties. The integration of mobile devices in medicine, as explored by Kufel et al. [14], faces hurdles in widespread adoption. Usability comparisons between mobile applications and stationary stations reveal a dichotomy in procedures, device availability, and regulatory frameworks. The envisioned universal mobile application, while promising, must contend with the intricate nuances of hospital infrastructure, calling for meticulous development and integration strategies.

The transformative impact of the COVID-19 pandemic on telemedicine, as discussed by Perrone et al. [15], also unravels limitations. While electronic health records, teleradiology, and telemedicine applications emerged as crucial during the pandemic, challenges in fully replacing traditional medicine persist. The integration of telemedicine into certain specialties, particularly radiology and dermatology, requires a delicate balance to ensure comprehensive patient care. AI optimization in pediatric radiology, per Ng et al. [16], encounters limitations despite its promise in dose optimization. The dominance of deep convolutional neural networks is not without challenges, and the study emphasizes the necessity for further exploration. The nuanced considerations of AI's value in optimizing doses for various modalities in pediatric radiology underscore the intricate balance needed to ensure both diagnostic accuracy and radiation safety. Mobile mammography for breast cancer screening, as explored by Trivedi et al. [17], grapples with challenges in addressing disparities. While mobile mammography units hold promise, reaching underserved populations and mitigating the impact of missed screenings during the COVID-19 pandemic is no small feat. The effectiveness of these units hinges on overcoming logistical, financial, and infrastructural barriers. Simulation-based training (SBT) in allied health professions, per Heuer et al. [18], demonstrates effectiveness in short-term measures but reveals uncertainties in long-term impacts. The sustained enhancement of skills and its translation into improved patient outcomes remain elusive, necessitating further investigations to decipher the nuanced dynamics of SBT. Diagnostic radiology standards in low-resource settings, according to Dinar et al. [20], confront the challenge of a lack of evidence on standard quality control for mobile health units (MHUs). The call for investigations to assess the feasibility of different quality control standards in MHUs highlights the inherent complexities in maintaining diagnostic imaging standards in crisis situations. AR, in anatomy education, as explored by McBain et al. [21], grapples with the need for sufficiently powered studies. While AR modalities hold promise in enhancing anatomical education, the current discourse stresses the importance of validated assessment tools and comprehensive studies to understand the full scope of AR's impact. Domiciliary radiology with mobile X-ray equipment, as outlined by Toppemberg et al. [23], unveils limitations in language, databases, and grey literature. The potential benefits suggested by the studies need to be interpreted within the confines of these limitations, calling for a cautious approach to generalize findings and a comprehensive exploration of the existing gaps. Future trends in ultrasound imaging, as reviewed by Wang et al. [24], encounter limitations in the breadth of their projections. While the emphasis on widespread use, portability of mobile devices, and recent advancements paints a promising picture, the feasibility and applicability of these trends in diverse healthcare settings warrant careful consideration. Quality improvement interventions in radiology, per Jabin et al. [26], underscore the need for further research to explore additional dimensions of quality, cost, and risk versus benefit. While the introduction of mobile radiography demonstrates improvements in various aspects, a nuanced understanding of its limitations is crucial to refine and optimize its integration into radiology workflows. The integral connection between radiology and the Internet, as discussed by Gupta et al. [27], faces challenges in the rapid rise of Internet-based technology. The transformative impact of the Internet of Things (IoT) on radiology workflows, education, research, and patient engagement necessitates a thorough understanding of the potential risks and ethical considerations associated with such integration. The review of the Mobile MIM diagnostic imaging device by Adusumilli et al. [28] brings to light limitations in compatibility, particularly with mammography. The strengths and limitations of the app, while notable, call for a nuanced approach to its usage, acknowledging its role while considering alternative solutions for specific diagnostic needs. Addressing challenges in communication and workflow efficiency within radiology operations, as shared by Makary et al. [31], while optimizing workflow efficiency with mobile tools underscores the need for comprehensive solutions. While mobile tools show promise in enhancing communication and providing access to guidelines, their broader integration into complex healthcare systems demands meticulous planning and continuous refinement.

4.3. Mobile Radiology: Taking Services Directly to Patients

The dynamic interplay between mobile radiology and domiciliary radiology, explored through insightful reviews, unveils nuanced themes and intricacies, shedding light on both emerging opportunities and challenges within this intersection. This vibrant convergence exposes a kaleidoscope of diverse interests, yet the true amalgamation dedicated to delivering radiology services to patients at home or in alternative locations like protected residences or service dispensing kiosks has received comparatively limited attention in existing studies. Amidst this landscape, a solitary review study identified in our research [23] delves into this specific facet, prompting a call for a deeper exploration to address the identified limitations. Our comprehensive overview underscores a significant gap: despite the inception of domiciliary radiology as a discipline in 1958 [1], there remains a conspicuous dearth of substantial reviews in this domain. As a consequence, a shift toward recent, specific studies (not only reviews overviewed by us), not captured by our search keywords, becomes imperative, facilitating more in-depth comparative analyses. In an effort to delve further into this targeted exploration, the discourse on domiciliary radiology unfolds as a narrative spanning decades. This narrative not only captures historical landmarks but also integrates contemporary research, providing a comprehensive understanding of the evolutionary trajectory of domiciliary radiology. This multifaceted approach allows for a more nuanced exploration of the discipline, paving the way for a deeper comprehension of its complexities, challenges, and potential avenues for advancement in the realm of healthcare delivery. Originating in 1958, Losev's pioneering work aimed at enhancing roentgenological services in villages through improved mobile X-ray units sets the stage for subsequent developments [1]. Examining General Practitioners' attitudes toward domiciliary radiography in 1995, Sawyer et al.'s survey [2] unveils the perceived significance of the service. The findings indicate a consensus among practitioners regarding its importance, with potential implications highlighted if the service were to be discontinued. However, the nuanced variations in opinions on different examinations underscore the intricate challenges associated with integrating domiciliary radiology into routine healthcare practices [2]. In recent times, Mark et al.'s (2022) [3] establishment of a domiciliary-based X-ray response team marks a practical advancement. This initiative not only garnered positive feedback from patients but also demonstrated a substantial reduction in avoidable conveyance, offering a promising avenue for improving patient care and experiences. While advancements in domiciliary radiology showcase promising outcomes, the research by Toppenberg et al. (2020) [6] in the form of a randomized controlled trial reveals the inherent complexities involved. Challenges such as doctor withdrawal and randomization issues underscore the need for careful consideration in designing and executing studies within this domain. Operational challenges are brought to light by Andersen et al. (2023) [33], shedding insights into the intricacies of setting up a mobile X-ray unit. This study emphasizes the dual impact of increased physicality for radiographers and positive outcomes for vulnerable patients who can undergo examinations in familiar surroundings. Exploring the patient's perspective, Dollard et al. (2022) [34] delve into residents' views on mobile X-ray services in aged care facilities. The positive reception among residents, coupled with the emphasis on equivalent quality services in familiar surroundings, reinforces the patient-centric nature of domiciliary radiology [34]. In economic terms, Kjelle et al.'s (2019) [35] cost analysis showcases a 30% reduction in costs with the implementation of mobile radiography services for nursing home residents. Aldridge et al.'s study [36] assesses the impact of volunteer peer educators on the uptake of mobile X-ray tuberculosis screening at homeless hostels. Conducted as a cluster randomized controlled trial in London, the research involved 46 hostels and 2342 residents. Despite the intervention's meticulous design, results revealed no substantial evidence that volunteer peer educators significantly increased screening uptake. The study emphasizes the need for further qualitative investigations to explore potential ancillary benefits associated with the involvement of peer volunteers. In essence, the research underscores the challenges in leveraging peer educators to enhance tuberculosis screening participation in homeless populations.

This economic viability underscores the potential for domiciliary radiology to not only enhance patient care but also offer a pragmatic solution in terms of cost-effectiveness. Kjelle and Lysdahl (2017) [37] consolidate evidence on the benefits of mobile radiography services, emphasizing reduced hospital transfers and timely diagnosis. This broad analysis reaffirms the potential advantages that domiciliary radiology can bring to the healthcare landscape. In a broader societal context, public–private partnerships, as exemplified by Datta et al. (2017) [38], illustrate the potential impact of collaborative efforts in addressing healthcare gaps. The success of this specific initiative in detecting pulmonary TB highlights the broader role such partnerships can play in scaling up and designing impactful interventions.

It is also crucial to take into account that the realm of radiology is currently undergoing profound transformations driven by technological innovations, and these advancements shed light on crucial considerations that demand careful attention, particularly when discussing domiciliary radiology. It becomes imperative to factor in both the existing social disparities and the emerging technological potentials. Geographic and ethnic variations can introduce significant inequalities in access to the healthcare system, especially in the realm of radiological services [39]. Hence, a thorough examination is necessary to deliberate and implement solutions that not only acknowledge but actively work toward enhancing inclusivity.

Moreover, a comprehensive evaluation of solutions is required to facilitate broader access to emerging opportunities facilitated by technological innovations. Cloud technology, for instance, is increasingly playing a pivotal role in radiology, making substantial contributions to both environmental and economic aspects [40]. Decision-makers in the field of domiciliary radiology must conduct a meticulous analysis, weighing the benefits against the costs to make informed decisions that harmonize with both economic and environmental sustainability.

In addition, the novel imaging solutions brought forth by cutting-edge technologies, encompassing advancements in imaging techniques and detectors [41,42], ought to be intricately considered by all stakeholders involved in domiciliary radiology services. This is crucial given the transformative potential these innovations hold and the opportunities they can offer in advancing the landscape of domiciliary radiology.

In addition, there are specific challenges in domiciliary radiology, particularly given that digital healthcare is brought into homes along with the necessary equipment. This introduces new paradigms. Therefore, studies should also address potential challenges associated with the logistics of transporting radiological equipment to patients' homes. This endeavor involves more than only technical considerations; it should encompass the need for infrastructural support, such as the presence of elevators and the availability of dedicated technicians. Furthermore, factors related to the application context, such as the complexities of providing services in large and congested cities, including issues of timely service delivery due to traffic, parking difficulties, and other logistical constraints, should be carefully addressed. Additionally, a thorough analysis is needed regarding the requirements for an appropriate reporting workstation. Essential questions arise, such as determining the minimum characteristics necessary for accurate reporting and identifying the type of screen required. This becomes especially crucial when dealing with mammography reporting, where precision is paramount. Another critical aspect to consider is the communication of the report to patients, given that they may not have easy access to hospitals. All these aspects could be the subject of targeted studies, also based on surveys involving relevant stakeholders. Surveys are indeed valuable for collecting experiences, constructive feedback, identifying challenges, and proposing solutions. Such surveys could be conducted through convenient tools like Computer-Aided Web Interviewing, as seen in other experiences [43].

Currently, a rapid overview of recent surveys in teleradiology, apart from not focusing on domiciliary radiology, does not highlight a focus on these strategic issues.

The topics covered in these studies include: the examinations of teleradiology practices in Turkey [44], the perceptions of clinical medical students towards radiology careers in Ghana [45], patient-reported outcomes after fracture treatment in primary healthcare [46], usability and efficiency evaluations of an application in orthopedics [47], the socio-economic and psychological impacts of the COVID-19 outbreak on radiologists [48], work-style reform and technology utilization among diagnostic radiologists in Japan [49], skepticism about artificial intelligence in the radiology field [50], patient satisfaction with teleradiology services in Italy [51], patient satisfaction with teleradiology services in general practice [52], on-call service of neurosurgeons in Germany [53], attitudes of Korean primary care family physicians toward telehealth [54], Factors influencing clinician satisfaction with radiology services [55], and positive aspects found in healthcare information and communication technology implementation in Finland [56].

In light of the absence of the above-mentioned themes in these studies [44–56], *it is recommended that researchers address these issues promptly.*

Overall, the narrative on domiciliary radiology, weaving through historical foundations, practitioner and patient perspectives, operational challenges, economic considerations, and collaborative models, paints a vivid picture of an evolving field. As we navigate these intricacies, the synthesis of these facets not only guides future research and implementation strategies but also underscores the potential of domiciliary radiology in transforming healthcare delivery.

Collectively, these studies underscore the imperative need for a comprehensive approach to technology assessment that can effectively navigate diverse domains. Foremost among these domains is the technological realm, where advancements and innovations play a pivotal role. Equally critical is the economic domain, where a thorough cost–benefit analysis becomes a linchpin for informed decision-making.

Of particular interest is the identification of application domains, extending the impact of technology assessment from fragile patient populations to those experiencing homelessness. This inclusive approach speaks to the broader societal implications and potential benefits that can be derived from a well-executed technology assessment strategy.

Noteworthy is the emphasis on monitoring, a dynamic process encompassing both social aspects and general outcomes. The integration of targeted surveys adds depth to the evaluative process, offering insights into the nuanced intersections of technology with human experiences.

A salient recommendation emanating clearly from these studies is the strategic focus on multi-domain technology assessment initiatives. The endorsement and sponsorship of such initiatives by scientific societies could serve as a catalyst for their effectiveness. Additionally, in the realm of monitoring tools, the utilization of computer-aided web interviewing tools [43] emerges as a valuable resource, contributing to the robust evaluation of technological interventions.

Within the ambit of technology assessment, regulatory considerations assume paramount importance. This extends to encompassing the regulatory landscape for both Medical Devices and radiation protection, addressing critical aspects that ensure the responsible and ethical integration of technology into healthcare practices.

In essence, these studies advocate for a holistic and interdisciplinary approach to technology assessment, urging the inclusion of regulatory frameworks and endorsing collaborative efforts supported by scientific societies. The landscape of technology assessment should not only be innovative but also ethical, ensuring that technological advancements align with societal needs and well-defined regulatory standards.

4.4. Final Takeaway Message

In navigating mobile and domiciliary radiology research, a key takeaway emerges: ongoing advancements, including AI integration and telemedicine applications, present opportunities for reshaping healthcare diagnostics. However, challenges exist, emphasizing the need for a vigilant recognition of the limitations. To propel the field forward, a dedicated focus on multi-domain technology assessment is crucial, especially when providing mobile radiology at patients' homes or point-of-care settings. This involves assessing technological, economic, social, and regulatory aspects for a comprehensive understanding. Through conscientious exploration and commitment to precision, we unlock the true potential of mobile/domiciliary radiology, fostering advancements across healthcare.

4.5. Limitations

The study conducted a comprehensive analysis by scrutinizing two prominent databases, PubMed and Scopus. It deliberately excluded other databases primarily concentrated on technological advancements, irrespective of their medical implications. This deliberate choice in database selection was made with the specific aim of honing in on a thorough examination of both the technological developments and their direct applicability to the medical domain. In doing so, the study aimed to provide a nuanced and detailed insight into the current state of the art at the intersection of technology and medicine.

5. Conclusions

In conclusion, the overview of mobile and domiciliary radiology, derived from a comprehensive study review, reveals an intriguing and promising outlook. Noteworthy advancements in this dynamic field include the integration of AI, groundbreaking applications in telemedicine, and the educational potential of mobile devices. The post-COVID-19 landscape witnesses significant progress in telemedicine evolution and the impactful role of AI in pediatric radiology. Mobile mammography units emerge as a solution for underserved women, underscoring the critical importance of early detection in breast cancer screening. Exploring domiciliary radiology, particularly with mobile X-ray equipment, signals a promising frontier, urging in-depth research for comprehensive insights into its potential benefits for diverse populations. Limitations have been identified, along with suggestions for future exploration. Various domains within mobile and domiciliary radiology, encompassing musculoskeletal ultrasound education, mobile device integration in medicine, telemedicine, AI applications in pediatric radiology, and mobile mammography for breast cancer screening, present specific challenges. Addressing these challenges requires thorough investigations and tailored approaches. Additional areas like simulation-based training, diagnostic radiology standards in low-resource settings, augmented reality in anatomy education, domiciliary radiology with mobile X-ray equipment, trends in ultrasound imaging, quality improvement interventions, Internet-based technology integration, mobile diagnostic imaging devices, and workflow optimization with mobile tools each pose unique considerations, emphasizing the need for extensive research efforts and specialized approaches in their respective domains. A crucial recommendation underscores the importance of strategically prioritizing multi-domain technology assessment initiatives, with the endorsement and sponsorship of scientific societies playing a pivotal role. Furthermore, regulatory considerations, an integral facet of technology assessment, are emphasized as paramount. These considerations span both Medical Devices and radiation protection, aiming to guarantee responsible and ethical technology integration in healthcare practices. The broader landscape of technology assessment should strive to be innovative, ethical, and in alignment with societal needs and regulatory standards.

Author Contributions: Conceptualization, D.G.; methodology, D.G; software, All.; validation, All; formal analysis, G.L., F.O. and D.G.; investigation, D.G.; resources, All; data curation, G.L., F.O. and D.G.; writing—original draft preparation, D.G.; writing—review and editing, G.L., F.O., D.G. and R.A.G.; visualization, All; supervision, D.G.; project administration, G.L. and D.G.; funding acquisition, G.L. and D.G. All authors have read and agreed to the published version of the manuscript.

Funding: This research received no external funding.

Data Availability Statement: Not applicable.

Conflicts of Interest: The authors declare no conflicts of interest.

References

1. Losev, I. Improvement of quality of roentgenological work in villages by improvement of mobile x-ray units. *Vestn. Rentgenol. Radiol.* **1958**, *33*, 86–87. (In Russian)
2. Sawyer, R.H.; Patel, U.; Horrocks, A.W. Domiciliary radiography: An important service? *Clin. Radiol.* **1995**, *50*, 51–55. [CrossRef] [PubMed]
3. Mark, S.; Henderson, D.; Brealey, J. Taking acute medical imaging to the patient, the domiciliary based X-ray response team. *Radiography* **2022**, *28*, 550–552. [CrossRef] [PubMed]
4. Ossola, C.; Piacentino, F.; Fontana, F.; Curti, M.; Zorzetto, G.; Coppola, A.; Carcano, G.; Venturini, M. Pocket-sized, wireless-Bluetooth ultrasound system to perform diagnostic and low-complexity interventional procedures in bedridden patients during the COVID-19 pandemic: From intensive care unit to domiciliary service? *Eur. Radiol. Exp.* **2022**, *6*, 20. [CrossRef] [PubMed]
5. Henderson, D.; Mark, S.; Rawlings, D.; Robson, K. Portable X-rays–A new era? *IPEM-Transl.* **2022**, *3–4*, 100005. [CrossRef]
6. Toppenberg, M.; Christiansen, T.; Rasmussen, F.; Nielsen, C.; Damsgaard, E.M. Mobile X-ray Outside the Hospital vs. X-ray at the Hospital Challenges Exposed in an Explorative RCT Study. *Healthcare* **2020**, *8*, 118. [CrossRef] [PubMed]
7. Lock, H.S.; Teng, X.L.; Low, Z.X.; Ooi, J. Success criteria and challenges of mobile radiography in the era of COVID-19 pandemic: A Singapore perspective. *J. Med. Imaging Radiat. Sci.* **2022**, *53*, 404–411. [CrossRef]

8. ANDJ Checklist. Available online: https://www.elsevier.com/__data/promis_misc/ANDJ%20Narrative%20Review%20Checklist.pdf (accessed on 3 June 2023).
9. Iannone, A.; Giansanti, D. Breaking Barriers—The Intersection of AI and Assistive Technology in Autism Care: A Narrative Review. *J. Pers. Med.* **2023**, *14*, 41. [CrossRef]
10. Available online: https://pubmed.ncbi.nlm.nih.gov/?term=(mobile+radiology[Title/Abstract])+OR+(mobile+radiography[Title/Abstract])+OR+(domiciliary+radiology[Title/Abstract])+OR+(domiciliary+radiography[Title/Abstract])&filter=pubt.review&filter=pubt.systematicreview&filter=datesearch.y_5&sort=date&size=50 (accessed on 2 February 2024).
11. Taylor, B.; McLean, G. Exploring the use of mobile translation applications for culturally and linguistically diverse patients during medical imaging examinations in Australia—A systematic review. *J. Med. Radiat. Sci.* **2024**. [CrossRef]
12. Ravindran, B. Innovations in the Management of the Difficult Airway: A Narrative Review. *Cureus* **2023**, *15*, e35117. [CrossRef]
13. Neubauer, R.; Recker, F.; Bauer, C.J.; Brossart, P.; Schäfer, V.S. The Current Situation of Musculoskeletal Ultrasound Education: A Systematic Literature Review. *Ultrasound Med. Biol.* **2023**, *49*, 1363–1374. [CrossRef]
14. Kufel, J.; Bargieł, K.; Koźlik, M.; Czogalik, Ł.; Dudek, P.; Jaworski, A.; Magiera, M.; Bartnikowska, W.; Cebula, M.; Nawrat, Z.; et al. Usability of Mobile Solutions Intended for Diagnostic Images—A Systematic Review. *Healthcare* **2022**, *10*, 2040. [CrossRef] [PubMed]
15. Perrone, G.; Bilotta, C.; Tullio, V.; Pirrone, R.; Argo, A.; Zerbo, S. Telehealth modulation and new proposals during the Covid-19 pandemic: A literature review. *Clin. Ter.* **2022**, *173*, 489–495. [CrossRef] [PubMed]
16. Ng, C.K.C. Artificial Intelligence for Radiation Dose Optimization in Pediatric Radiology: A Systematic Review. *Children* **2022**, *9*, 1044. [CrossRef] [PubMed]
17. Trivedi, U.; Omofoye, T.S.; Marquez, C.; Sullivan, C.R.; Benson, D.M.; Whitman, G.J. Mobile Mammography Services and Underserved Women. *Diagnostics* **2022**, *12*, 902. [CrossRef] [PubMed]
18. Heuer, A.; Bienstock, J.; Zhang, Y. Simulation-Based Training Within Selected Allied Health Professions: An Evidence-Based Systematic Review. *J. Allied Health* **2022**, *51*, 59–71. [PubMed]
19. Patel, B.; Makaryus, A.N. Artificial Intelligence Advances in the World of Cardiovascular Imaging. *Healthcare* **2022**, *10*, 154. [CrossRef] [PubMed]
20. Dinar, H.A.; Hassan Alzain, A.F. Field hospitals' diagnostic radiology standards in low-resource settings. *Am. J. Disaster Med.* **2022**, *17*, 197–205. [CrossRef] [PubMed]
21. McBain, K.A.; Habib, R.; Laggis, G.; Quaiattini, A.; Ventura, N.M.; Noel, G.P.J.C. Scoping review: The use of augmented reality in clinical anatomical education and its assessment tools. *Anat. Sci. Educ.* **2022**, *15*, 765–796. [CrossRef]
22. Ondruš, D.; Chorvath, M.; Piňáková, Z. Personalities and their contribution to the development of radiation oncology. *Klin. Onkol.* **2021**, *34*, 374–381. [CrossRef]
23. Toppenberg, M.D.; Christiansen, T.E.M.; Rasmussen, F.; Nielsen, C.P.; Damsgaard, E.M. Mobile X-ray outside the hospital: A scoping review. *BMC Health Serv. Res.* **2020**, *20*, 767. [CrossRef] [PubMed]
24. Wang, S.; Hossack, J.A.; Klibanov, A.L. From Anatomy to Functional and Molecular Biomarker Imaging and Therapy: Ultrasound Is Safe, Ultrafast, Portable, and Inexpensive. *Investig. Radiol.* **2020**, *55*, 559–572. [CrossRef] [PubMed]
25. Makary, M.S.; da Silva, A.; Kingsbury, J.; Bozer, J.; Dowell, J.D.; Nguyen, X.V. Noninvasive Approaches for Anxiety Reduction during Interventional Radiology Procedures. *Top. Magn. Reson. Imaging* **2020**, *29*, 197–201. [CrossRef]
26. Jabin, M.S.R.; Schultz, T.; Mandel, C.; Bessen, T.; Hibbert, P.; Wiles, L.; Runciman, W. A Mixed-Methods Systematic Review of the Effectiveness and Experiences of Quality Improvement Interventions in Radiology. *J. Patient Saf.* **2022**, *18*, e97–e107. [CrossRef]
27. Gupta, S.; Johnson, E.M.; Peacock, J.G.; Jiang, L.; McBee, M.P.; Sneider, M.B.; Krupinski, E.A. Radiology, Mobile Devices, and Internet of Things (IoT). *J. Digit. Imaging* **2020**, *33*, 735–746. [CrossRef]
28. Adusumilli, N. Mobile MIM: A Portable Solution in Imaging. *J. Digit. Imaging* **2020**, *33*, 722–725. [CrossRef]
29. Herr, A.; Collins, D.; White, M.; Mandato, K.; Keating, L.; Stark, C.; Lee, H.; Siskin, G. Percutaneous Biliary Endoscopy for Stones. *Tech. Vasc. Interv. Radiol.* **2019**, *22*, 127–134. [CrossRef] [PubMed]
30. Kauffman, L.; Weisberg, E.M.; Fishman, E.K. What Can Pinterest Do for Radiology? *J. Digit. Imaging* **2019**, *32*, 1062–1070. [CrossRef]
31. Makary, M.S.; Hartwell, C.; Egbert, N.K.; Prevedello, L.M. Streamlining Communications and Enabling Point-of-care Education in Radiology through a Mobile Application Solution. *Curr. Probl. Diagn. Radiol.* **2020**, *49*, 150–153. [CrossRef]
32. Ronneaux, G.G. About reflections on mobile radiography installations. *Concours Med.* **1947**, *69*, 1624. (In French)
33. Andersen, P.A.B.; Precht, H.; McEntee, M.F.; Pedersen, M.R.V. How to set up a mobile X-ray unit in the community—Implementation initiatives for patient-centred care. *Radiography* **2023**, *29* (Suppl. S1), S148–S151. [CrossRef]
34. Dollard, J.; Edwards, J.; Yadav, L.; Gaget, V.; Tivey, D.; Inacio, M.; Maddern, G.; Visvanathan, R. Residents' perspectives of mobile X-ray services in support of healthcare-in-place in residential aged care facilities: A qualitative study. *BMC Geriatr.* **2022**, *22*, 525. [CrossRef] [PubMed]
35. Kjelle, E.; Kleven, L.; Olerud, H.M.; Melberg, H.O. Cost analysis of mobile radiography services for nursing home residents in Southeast Norway. *J. Eval. Clin. Pract.* **2019**, *25*, 275–281. [CrossRef]
36. Aldridge, R.W.; Hayward, A.C.; Hemming, S.; Possas, L.; Ferenando, G.; Garber, E.; Lipman, M.; McHugh, T.D.; Story, A. Effectiveness of peer educators on the uptake of mobile X-ray tuberculosis screening at homeless hostels: A cluster randomised controlled trial. *BMJ Open* **2015**, *5*, e008050. [CrossRef] [PubMed]

37. Kjelle, E.; Lysdahl, K.B. Mobile radiography services in nursing homes: A systematic review of residents' and societal outcomes. *BMC Health Serv. Res.* **2017**, *17*, 231. [CrossRef] [PubMed]
38. Datta, B.; Hazarika, A.; Shewade, H.D.; Ayyagari, K.; Kumar, A.M. Digital chest X-ray through a mobile van: Public private partnership to detect sputum negative pulmonary TB. *BMC Res. Notes* **2017**, *10*, 96. [CrossRef]
39. De Benedectis, C.M.; Spalluto, L.B.; Americo, L.; Bishop, C.; Mian, A.; Sarkany, D.; Kagetsu, N.J.; Slanetz, J.P. Health Care Disparities in Radiology—A Review of the Current Literature. *J. Am. Coll. Radiol.* **2022**, *19*, 101–111. [CrossRef]
40. Doo, F.X.; Kulkarni, P.; Siegel, E.L.; Toland, M.; Yi, P.H.; Carlos, R.C.; Parekh, V.S. Economic and Environmental Costs of Cloud Technologies for Medical Imaging and Radiology Artificial Intelligence. *J. Am. Coll. Radiol.* **2024**, *21*, 248–256. [CrossRef] [PubMed]
41. Pfeiffer, D.; Pfeiffer, F.; Rummeny, E. Advanced X-ray Imaging Technology. In *Molecular Imaging in Oncology*; Recent Results in Cancer Research; Springer: Cham, Swizerland, 2020; Volume 216, pp. 3–30. [CrossRef]
42. Datta, A.; Zhong, Z.; Motakef, S. A new generation of direct X-ray detectors for medical and synchrotron imaging applications. *Sci. Rep.* **2020**, *10*, 20097. [CrossRef]
43. Di Basilio, F.; Esposisto, G.; Monoscalco, L.; Giansanti, D. The Artificial Intelligence in Digital Radiology: Part 2: Towards an Investigation of acceptance and consensus on the Insiders. *Healthcare* **2022**, *10*, 153. [CrossRef]
44. Dicle, O.; Şenol, U.; Özmen, M.N.; Aydıngöz, Ü. A snapshot of teleradiology practice in Turkey: The results of a survey among radiologists. *Diagn. Interv. Radiol.* **2023**, *29*, 46–52. [CrossRef]
45. Dzefi-Tettey, K.; Edzie, E.K.M.; Brakohiapa, E.K.; Gorleku, P.N.; Amankwa, A.T.; Abdulai, A.B.; Yabasin, I.B.; Kekessie, K.K.; Idun, E.A.; Ntiamoah-Koufie, C.E.; et al. Career in radiology; the Ghanaian clinical medical Student's perception. *Heliyon* **2022**, *8*, e12603. [CrossRef]
46. Vabo, S.; Steen, K.; Brudvik, C.; Hunskaar, S.; Morken, T. Patient-reported outcomes after initial conservative fracture treatment in primary healthcare—A survey study. *BMC Prim. Care* **2022**, *23*, 191. [CrossRef]
47. Macedo, F.S.; Silva, P.G.B.; Marçal, E.B.F.; Rolim, J.P.M.L. Evaluation of Usability, Perception of Usefulness, and Efficiency of an Application in Interpreting Imaging Examinations and Supporting Decision-Making in Orthopedics. *Telemed. J. e-Health* **2021**, *27*, 561–567. [CrossRef]
48. Florin, M.; Pinar, U.; Chavigny, E.; Bouaboula, M.; Jarboui, L.; Coulibaly, A.; Lemogne, C.; Fournier, L. Socio-economic and psychological impact of the COVID-19 outbreak on private practice and public hospital radiologists. *Eur. J. Radiol.* **2020**, *132*, 109285. [CrossRef]
49. Yamashiro, T.; Kumamaru, K.K.; Kido, A.; Matsubayashi, R.N.; Ota, H.; Ida, M.; Aoki, S. Work-style reform and use of information and communication technology among diagnostic radiologists in Japan: Results of the 2018 JRS/JCR joint survey. *Jpn. J. Radiol.* **2020**, *38*, 636–642. [CrossRef] [PubMed]
50. van Hoek, J.; Huber, A.; Leichtle, A.; Härmä, K.; Hilt, D.; von Tengg-Kobligk, H.; Heverhagen, J.; Poellinger, A. A survey on the future of radiology among radiologists, medical students and surgeons: Students and surgeons tend to be more skeptical about artificial intelligence and radiologists may fear that other disciplines take over. *Eur. J. Radiol.* **2019**, *121*, 108742. [CrossRef] [PubMed]
51. Coppola, F.; Bibbolino, C.; Grassi, R.; Pierotti, L.; Silverio, R.; Lassandro, F.; Neri, E.; Regge, D. Results of an Italian survey on teleradiology. *Radiol. Med.* **2016**, *121*, 652–659. [CrossRef] [PubMed]
52. Jacobs, J.J.W.M.; Ekkelboom, R.; Jacobs, J.P.A.M.; van der Molen, T.; Sanderman, R. Patient satisfaction with a teleradiology service in general practice. *BMC Fam. Pract.* **2016**, *17*, 17. [CrossRef] [PubMed]
53. Brenke, C.; Lassel, E.A.; Terris, D.; Kurt, A.; Schmieder, K.; Schoenberg, S.O.; Weisser, G. On-call service of neurosurgeons in Germany: Organization, use of communication services, and personal acceptance of modern technologies. *J. Neurol. Surg. Part A Cent. Eur. Neurosurg.* **2014**, *75*, 217–223. [CrossRef]
54. Kim, J.E.; Song, Y.M.; Park, J.H.; Lee, J.R. Attitude of korean primary care family physicians towards telehealth. *Korean J. Fam. Med.* **2011**, *32*, 341–351. [CrossRef] [PubMed]
55. Lindsay, R.; McKinstry, S.; Vallely, S.; Thornbury, G. What influences clinician's satisfaction with radiology services? *Insights Imaging* **2011**, *2*, 425–430. [CrossRef] [PubMed]
56. Winblad, I.; Hämäläinen, P.; Reponen, J. What is found positive in healthcare information and communication technology implementation?—The results of a nationwide survey in Finland. *Telemed. e-Health* **2011**, *17*, 118–123. [CrossRef] [PubMed]

healthcare

MDPI

Review

The Effects of Artificial Intelligence Chatbots on Women's Health: A Systematic Review and Meta-Analysis

Hyun-Kyoung Kim

Department of Nursing, Kongju National University, 56 Gongjudaehak-ro, Gongju 32588, Republic of Korea; hkk@kongju.ac.kr

Abstract: Purpose: This systematic review and meta-analysis aimed to investigate the effects of artificial intelligence chatbot interventions on health outcomes in women. Methods: Ten relevant studies published between 2019 and 2023 were extracted from the PubMed, Cochrane Library, EMBASE, CINAHL, and RISS databases in accordance with the Preferred Reporting Items for Systematic Reviews and Meta-Analyses guidelines. This review focused on experimental studies concerning chatbot interventions in women's health. The literature was assessed using the ROB 2 quality appraisal checklist, and the results were visualized with a risk-of-bias visualization program. Results: This review encompassed seven randomized controlled trials and three single-group experimental studies. Chatbots were effective in addressing anxiety, depression, distress, healthy relationships, cancer self-care behavior, preconception intentions, risk perception in eating disorders, and gender attitudes. Chatbot users experienced benefits in terms of internalization, acceptability, feasibility, and interaction. A meta-analysis of three studies revealed significant effects in reducing anxiety ($I^2 = 0\%$, $Q = 8.10$, $p < 0.017$), with an effect size of -0.30 (95% CI, -0.42 to -0.18). Conclusions: Artificial intelligence chatbot interventions had positive effects on physical, physiological, and cognitive health outcomes. Using chatbots may represent pivotal nursing interventions for female populations to improve health status and support women socially as a form of digital therapy.

Keywords: anxiety; artificial intelligence; meta-analysis; systematic review; women's health

1. Introduction

Artificial intelligence (AI) refers to the capability of a computer to exhibit human-like intelligence. An AI chatbot is a natural-language processing system that can independently engage in conversation with humans using artificial intelligence technology. Chatbots are software programs designed to interact in a manner similar to humans. They are distinguished by their use of machine learning and deep learning, which enable them to process data more efficiently and improve the quality of their responses through repeated learning [1]. Digital intervention platforms are taking various forms, such as mobile applications, telehealth, and web-based interventions. AI chatbots represent the latest innovation being employed in health interventions. These chatbots automatically generate knowledge from extensive language models and respond in a manner akin to humans, but with a greater volume and quality of information. This makes them an effective tool for delivering health education and interventions in the field of nursing [2].

Chatbots offer a range of advantages: they are engaging, entertaining, easy to use, informal, convenient, and interactive, without imposing an emotional burden on the user [3]. Additionally, they are cost-effective, foster a sense of social connection, provide aesthetic and hedonic pleasure, and possess a human-like tone, demeanor, and identity, all of which contribute to their potential to deliver digital therapy and mental health care [4]. Users tend to readily accept chatbots because they provide easy access to information, encourage ongoing use, are scalable, and have the capacity to store and retrieve knowledge [5]. However, there are potential drawbacks to using chatbots. These include the inability to verify the reliability of the information they provide, a human-like yet sometimes awkward interaction experience, varied outcomes based on the user's skill in crafting prompts, and the risk of receiving simplistic, basic, or even misleading information. Moreover, chatbots lack an understanding of human complexity, which sets them apart from genuine human interactions [6]. An AI chatbot's interaction with a user starts with an input, either text or spoken language, which is then analyzed using natural-language processing (NLP) to understand the intent and context. The chatbot determines the user's intent through NLP analysis and generates a response either through rule-based methods for simple queries or machine learning for more complex interactions, improving over time with feedback [7]. It is anticipated that with NLP training, chatbots achieve capabilities that are nearly human-like or even surpass human quality. However, AI chatbots may lack the nuanced understanding and empathy of human healthcare providers. This limitation can be particularly significant in sensitive areas of women's health, where emotional support and understanding are crucial [8]. They are expected to play a transformative role in the fields of health and education, serving as a new model for interaction between nurses and patients, as well as educators and learners [9].

The use of chatbots in health interventions has been explored in numerous recent studies. A thematic analysis of 37 papers focusing on chatbots in mental health revealed that these tools provide high-quality responses, characterized by their usability, responsiveness, understandability, acceptability, attractiveness, reliability, pleasantness, and content fidelity. Chatbots have demonstrated some effectiveness in interventions for conditions such as depression, anxiety, autism, addiction, post-traumatic stress disorder, schizophrenia, and stress [9]. Additionally, chatbots have been employed in interventions aimed at improving physical activity, diet, and weight loss. A systematic review of nine studies concluded that chatbots were effective in increasing physical activity, suggesting their potential as a physical health intervention [10]. Recent research has begun to explore chatbot interventions for specific populations, including pregnant women [4] and in the context of sex education [3]. The World Health Organization (WHO) identified cancer, infertility, reproductive health, violence, and mental health as crucial areas for improving women's health globally. In 2023, the WHO reported that every two minutes, a woman still dies from complications related to pregnancy or childbirth [11]. AI chatbots can address specific challenges in women's health by offering personalized health education, timely reminders for health-related tasks, and confidential consultations on sensitive issues [12]. However, there is a lack of systematic reviews focusing on chatbot interventions for women's health. It is crucial to comprehensively investigate the impact of chatbot interventions on various aspects of reproductive health, such as pregnancy, childbirth, sexual health, female cancers, and women's mental health. This would help determine the effectiveness of chatbots in these areas and inform future interventions. This paper provides the following major contributions:

- It systematically reviews the impact of AI chatbot interventions on women's health outcomes, providing a comprehensive analysis of current research.
- It summarizes and synthesizes evidence on the effectiveness of chatbots in addressing key areas such as mental health, reproductive health, and chronic disease management among women.
- It calls for further research into the development of culturally sensitive, user-friendly chatbot interventions to meet diverse health needs.

The aim of this study was to systematically review experimental studies analyzing the effects of AI chatbot interventions on women's health. This review synthesized information on the topics addressed by chatbot interventions, the methods employed, and the outcomes of these interventions, presenting an integrated overview of the field. The systematic review synthesizes the literature on the impact of AI chatbots on women's health, and the meta-analysis analyzes the effect size of the impact on women's health outcomes.

2. Methods

2.1. Study Design

This study is a meta-analysis that systematically reviews experimental studies analyzing the impact of AI chatbot interventions on women's health and analyzes the effect sizes of the interventions. The research question is "What is the impact of AI chatbot interventions on women's health?" This study was conducted in accordance with the reporting guidelines for systematic reviews, as outlined in PRISMA [13] and the Cochrane Handbook for Systematic Reviews of Interventions version 6.3 [14].

2.2. Search Strategy

The researcher carried out a literature search from 30 September to 15 October 2023, using electronic information retrieval systems. Searches were conducted in the PubMed, Cochrane Library, EMBASE, CINAHL, and RISS databases, employing MeSH terms, Emtree terms, and natural language. The literature was identified based on inclusion criteria that followed the participant, intervention, comparison, outcome, setting, time-study design (PICOST-SD) framework [14]. The search strategy encompassed core databases and adhered to the guidelines of the Center for Occupational Safety and Health at the National Library of Medicine [15]. The inclusion criteria specified that studies must be (1) AI chatbot intervention studies applied to female users; (2) experimental studies designed as before-and-after studies, interrupted time series, non-randomized controlled trials, and randomized controlled trials; (3) studies that employed random, stratified, cluster, convenient, quota, or systematic sampling of participants; (4) studies that focused on women's health, including cancer and reproductive, sexual, mental, and behavioral health; (5) studies published in either English or Korean; and (6) articles from peer-reviewed journals. The exclusion criteria ruled out (1) dissertations or conference presentations, (2) gray literature, (3) study protocols, (4) institutional reports or books, and (5) studies lacking statistical results. For the search, an advanced strategy was employed: (("Text Messaging"[Mesh] OR "Instant Messaging"[Mesh]) OR ("Artificial Intelligence"[Mesh] OR "Chat*")), (("Text Messaging"[Mesh] OR "Instant Messaging"[Mesh]) OR ("Artificial Intelligence"[Mesh] OR "Chat*")) AND "Nursing", 'chatbot women health' OR (('chatbot'/exp OR chatbot) AND ('women'/exp OR women) AND ('health'/exp OR health)).

2.3. Literature Extraction

Literature extraction was performed using five databases: PubMed, Cochrane Library, EMBASE, CINAHL, and RISS. In total, 1592 articles were identified (899, 201, 427, 65, and 0, respectively) from 2011 to 2023. An additional 19 articles were sourced from reference lists and Google Scholar, bringing the total to 1611. After removing 257 duplicates, the researcher excluded 1314 articles based on their titles, resulting in 40 articles for further review. Upon reading the abstracts, the researcher selected three full-text articles for closer examination. Following a full-text review, the researcher excluded seven articles that did not focus on women's health outcomes, five that were not experimental studies, eight that did not include female participants, and seven that did not involve chatbot interventions. Ultimately, 10 articles met the study criteria and were included in the review (Figure 1).

2.4. Quality Appraisal

The researcher assessed the quality of six out of the ten randomized controlled trials using the Cochrane Risk of Bias 2 (ROB-2) tool [16], which is designed to assess the quality of randomized controlled trials. This assessment was conducted independently by the researcher and a specialist in systematic reviews, with checks in place to ensure agreement. Inter-rater consistency was measured using the kappa coefficient; a coefficient of 0.80 or higher was considered acceptable, while a lower value prompted a consensus meeting for resolution [17]. The outcomes of the quality assessment were presented using traffic light charts and summary plots, generated by the Risk-of-bias VISualization (robvis) tool [18] (Figure 2).

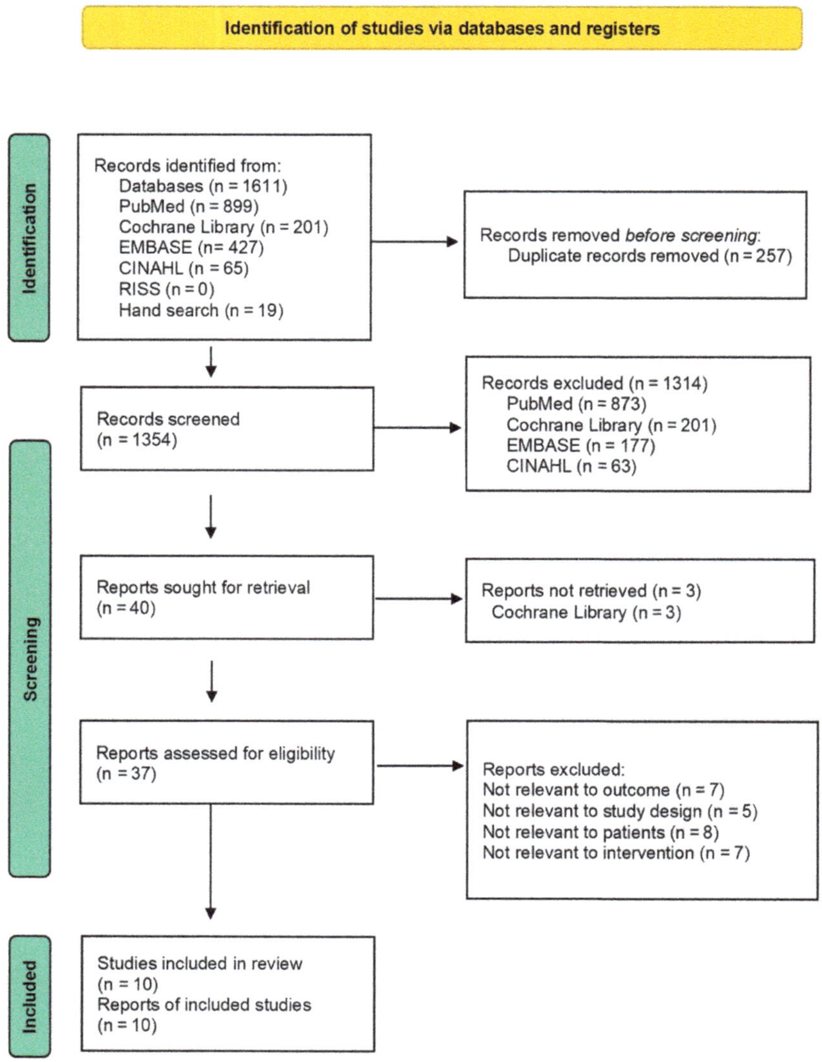

Figure 1. PRISMA flow diagram.

2.5. Data Analysis

For a total of 10 papers, the researcher summarized (1) the topic of chatbot intervention, (2) the method of chatbot intervention, and (3) the effect of chatbot intervention, as detailed in a case report for each study tailored to the study's objectives (Table A1). The case reports include the first author, publication year, country, chatbot title, intervention duration, setting, study design, participants, number of participants analyzed, and inclusion criteria (Table 1). Utilizing the study results, the researcher presents the primary and secondary outcomes, measurement scales, mean and standard deviation for both the experimental and control groups, effect size, and statistical significance (Table 2).

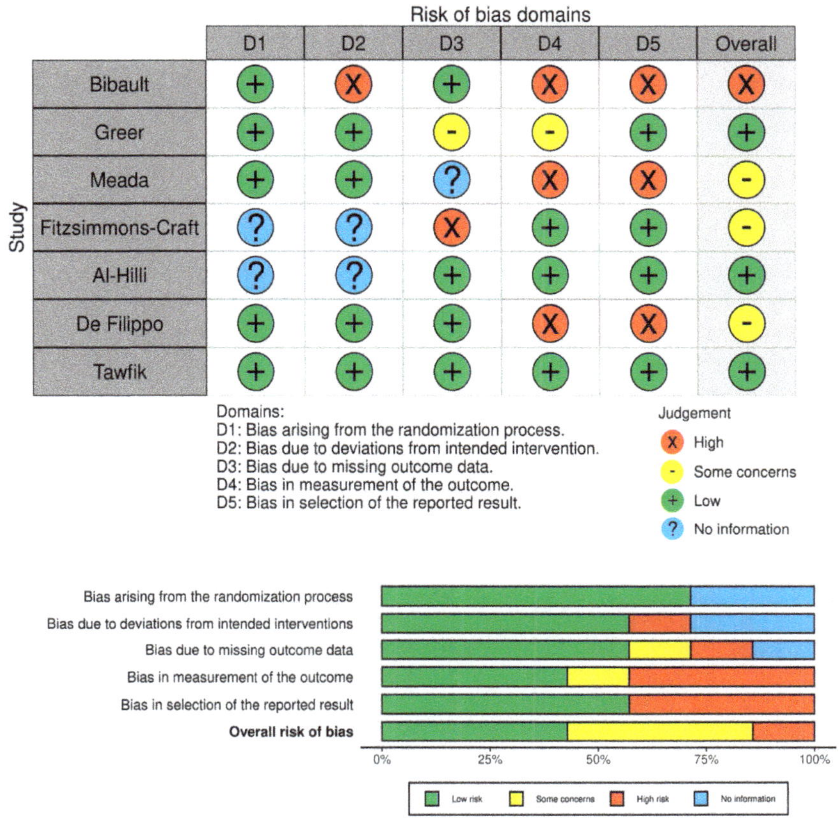

Figure 2. Risk of bias for the randomized controlled trials.

Table 1. Characteristics of the selected studies.

No	First Author	Publication Year	Country	Name of Chatbot	Theme	Intervention Time	Setting	Study Design	Participants	Number of Participants (Exp.–Cont.)	Inclusion Criteria
A1	Bibault [19]	2019	France	Vik	Breast cancer information	Four weeks	Hospital	Randomized controlled trial	Patients	142 (71–71)	Breast cancer patients
A2	Greer [20]	2019	USA	Vivibot	Psychological skill	Four weeks	Hospital	Randomized controlled trial	Patients	45 (25–20)	Young women aged 18–29 after cancer
A3	Maeda [3]	2020	Japan	Education Chatbot	Preconception health	Ten days, 574 sessions	Community	Three-armed randomized controlled trial	Young women	927 (309–309–309)	Young women aged 20–34
A4	Fitzsimmons-Craft [21]	2021	Zambia	Student Bodies	Eating disorder prevention	One month	Community	Randomized controlled trial	Young women	439 (207–232)	Young women aged 18–30
A5	Chung [4]	2021	South Korea	Dr. Joy	Prenatal mental health	13 days	Hospital	Single-group pre-post-test design	Pregnant women	15	Pregnant women with spouses
A6	Yam [5]	2022	USA	HIV Chatbot	HIV education and family planning	20–30 min	Community	Single-group pre-post-test design	Reproductive-age women	30	Women aged 15–49 in Zambia
A7	Al-Hilli [22]	2023	USA	Gia	Cancer genetic counseling	No information	Hospital	Randomized controlled trial	Patients	37 (19–18)	Breast cancer patients who received genetic counseling
A8	De Filippo [23]	2023	South Africa	Chatty Cuz	Intimate partner violence attitude	31 days	Community	Four-armed randomized controlled trial	Young women	19,643 (5891–5893–3930–3929)	Women aged 18–24 suffering intimate partner violence in South Africa

Table 1. *Cont.*

No	First Author	Publication Year	Country	Name of Chatbot	Theme	Intervention Time	Setting	Study Design	Participants	Number of Participants (Exp.–Cont.)	Inclusion Criteria
A9	Mane [24]	2023	USA	Rosie	Prenatal health education	No information	Hospital	Single-group pre-post-test design	Pregnant women	109	Primi-pregnant women aged over 14
A10	Tawfik [6]	2023	Egypt	Chemofree Bot	Chemotherapy self-care	45 min, 7–10 sessions	Hospital	Three-armed randomized controlled trial	Patients	150 (50–50–50)	Breast cancer patients undergoing chemotherapy

Cont = Control group; Exp = Experimental group; HIV = Human immunodeficiency virus; USA = United States of America.

Table 2. Outcomes of selected studies.

No	Author	Primary Outcomes	Secondary Outcomes	Measurement Scales	Exp. Group M (SD) or *n* (%)	Con. Group M (SD) or *n* (%)	t or F or r	*p*
A1	Bibault [19]	① Quality of information	② Answer rate	① EORTCQLQ ② *n* (%)	① 2.89 ② 49 (69%)	① 2.82 ② 46 (64%)	① - ② -	① <0.001 ② -
A2	Greer [20]	① Anxiety ② Depression	③ Negative emotion ④ Positive emotion ⑤ Usage time	①–④ PROMIS ⑤ Minute	① 61.9 ± 7.7 ② 59.1 ± 9.2 ③ 1.5 ± 0.9 ④ 2.5 ± 1.0 ⑤ 12.1 ± 7.1	① 63.3 ± 5.5 ② 57.7 ± 6.1 ③ 1.6 ± 0.6 ④ 2.3 ± 0.8 ⑤ 18.1 ± 8.6	① 0.41 ② 0.09 ③ 0.01 ④ 0.07 ⑤ -	① 0.09 ② 0.77 ③ 0.97 ④ 0.82 ⑤ -
A3	Maeda [3]	① Anxiety	② Fertility knowledge ③ Intention of preconception	① STAI ② CFKS-J ③ Survey	① 43.2 ± 9.5 ② - ③ 68.7 ± 23.0	① 47.5 ± 9.5 ② - ③ 76.4 ± 18.4	① - ② - ③ -	① <0.001 ② 0.001~0.005 ③ <0.001
A4	Fitzsimmons-Craft [21]	① Eating disorder risk	② Internalization ③ Eating disorder ④ Depression ⑤ Anxiety	① WCS ② SATAQ-4R ③ EDE-Q ④ PHQ-8 ⑤ GAD-7	① 60.80 ± 20.55 ② 15.35 ± 3.94 ③ 2.77 ± 1.34 ④ 11.09 ± 6.42 ⑤ 10.40 ± 6.14	① 63.99 ± 17.30 ② 16.11 ± 3.84 ③ 3.03 ± 1.24 ④ 11.67 ± 5.55 ⑤ 10.96 ± 5.51	① −0.45 ② −0.21 ③ −0.38 ④ −0.26 ⑤ −0.11	① <0.001 ② 0.001 ③ <0.001 ④ <0.001 ⑤ 0.09

Table 2. *Cont.*

No	Author	Primary Outcomes	Secondary Outcomes	Measurement Scales	Exp. Group M (SD) or *n* (%)	Con. Group M (SD) or *n* (%)	t or F or r	*p*
A5	Chung [4]	① Satisfaction	② Usability ③ Ese of use ④ Ease of learning	① SAT ② USE ③ EOU ④ EOL	① - ② - ③ - ④ -	① - ② - ③ - ④ -	① r = 0.97 ② r = 0.89 ③ r = 0.32 ④ r = 0.95	① <0.001 ② <0.001 ③ 0.24 ④ <0.001
A6	Yam [5]	① Acceptability	② Feasibility ③ Knowledge ④ Interaction	① - ② - ③ -	① 100% ② 97% ③ 83% ④ 96%	① - ② - ③ - ④ -	① - ② - ③ - ④ -	① - ② - ③ - ④ -
A7	Al-Hilli [22]	① Satisfaction	② Knowledge	① Median ② Median	① 30 (6–30) ② 11 (8–13)	① 30 (24–30) ② 12 (8–14)	① - ② -	① 0.19 ② 0.09
A8	De Filippo [23]	① Depression	② Gender attitudes ③ IPV exposure ④ Unhealthy relationships	① PHQ-2 ② GRS ③ WHO ④ VAS	① 17% ② 20.06 ③ 62% ④ 0.62	① 6.9% ② 19.56 ③ 55% ④ 0.55	① - ② - ③ - ④ -	① <0.01 ② <0.01 ③ >0.05 ④ <0.001
A9	Mane [24]	① Usability	② Use rate	① % ② %	① 61.76% ② 24.27%	① - ② -	① - ② -	① - ② -
A10	Tawfik [6]	① Physical effect ② Psychological effect ③ Distress	④ Effectiveness of self-care behavior ⑤ Usability	①–③ MSAS ④ SCBD ⑤ CUQ	① 1.37 ± 0.30 ② 1.42 ± 0.30 ③ 1.80 ± 0.93 ④ 2.42 ± 0.49 ⑤ 49.94 ± 5.64	① 2.77 ± 0.21 ② 2.79 ± 0.21 ③ 3.00 ± 0.30 ④ 1.81 ± 0.44 ⑤ -	① 97.0 ② 62.13 ③ 80.26 ④ 20.03 ⑤ -	① <0.001 ② <0.001 ③ <0.001 ④ <0.001 ⑤ -

CFKS-J = Japanese version of the Cardiff Fertility Knowledge Scale; Cont = control group; CUQ = Chatbot Usability Questionnaire; EDE-Q = Eating Disorder Examination Questionnaire; EOL = ease of learning; EORTCQLQ = questionnaire developed to assess the quality of life of cancer patients; EOU = ease of use; Exp = experimental group; GAD = generalized anxiety disorder; GRS = Gender Relation Scale; MSAS = Memorial Symptoms Assessment Scale; PHQ = Patient Health Questionnaire; PROMIS = Patient-Reported Outcome Measurement Information System; SATAQ-4R = Sociocultural Attitudes Toward Appearance Questionnaire—4; SAT = satisfaction; SCBD = self-care behavior diary; STAI = State–Trait Anxiety Inventory; USE = usability; VAS = Violence Assessment Scale; WCS = Weight and Shape Concern; WHO = World Health Organization multi-country study instrument.

3. Results

3.1. Themes of Chatbot Interventions

The publication years of the articles were 2019 (A1, A2), 2020 (A3), 2021 (A4, A5), 2022 (A6), and 2023 (A7, A8, A9, A10). The countries of the articles were the United States (A2, A4, A7, A9), France (A1), Japan (A3), South Korea (A5), Zambia (A6), South Africa (A8), and Egypt (A10). The chatbot was given a proper name in nine articles (A1, A2, A4, A5, A6, A7, A8, A9, A10). The topics of the chatbots were as follows: breast cancer information (A1), psychological skills for young women (A2), preconception health (A3), eating disorders (A4), prenatal mental health (A5), HIV education and family planning (A6), genetic counseling for diagnosed breast cancer (A7), attitudes toward intimate partner violence (A8), prenatal health education for first-time mothers (A9), and self-care for chemotherapy side effects (A10) (Table 1).

3.2. Methods of Chatbot Interventions

The duration of the interventions varied, with the shortest being 20–30 min (A6) and the longest lasting up to 31 days (A8). Interventions took place in hospitals for six of the studies (A1, A2, A5, A7, A9, A10) and in community settings for the remaining four (A3, A4, A6, A8). Seven studies were randomized controlled trials (A1, A2, A3, A4, A7, A8, A10), and three had single-arm pre-post-test designs (A5, A6, A9). The participant demographics varied across studies: four targeted patients (A1, A2, A7, A10), three focused on young women (A3, A4, A7), two involved pregnant women (A5, A9), and one study included women of childbearing age (A6). The sample sizes also ranged widely, from as few as 15 participants (A5) to as many as 19,643 (A8) (Table 1).

3.3. Effects of Chatbot Interventions

The outcome variables were anxiety (A2, A3, A4), depression (A2, A4, A8), knowledge (A3, A6), satisfaction (A5, A7), answer or use rate (A1, A9), quality of information (A1), usage time (A2), emotion (A2), preconception intention (A3), eating disorder risk (A4), eating disorders (A4), internalization (A4), ease of learning (A5), acceptability (A6), feasibility (A6), interaction (A6), gender attitude (A8), intimate partner violence exposure (A8), unhealthy relationships (A8), physical effect (A10), psychological effect (A10), distress (A10), effectiveness of self-care behavior (A10), and usability (A10). The Patient Health Questionnaire was used to measure depression in two studies (A4, A8), and all other studies used their own instruments.

The effects of the outcome variables showed that anxiety levels varied across studies ($p = 0.09$ and $p < 0.001$) (A2, A3, A4), and depression levels also varied ($p = 0.07$, < 0.001, and 0.01) (A2, A4, A8). Knowledge was found to be effective in both studies ($p < 0.001$) (A3,6), while satisfaction levels differed ($p < 0.001$ and 0.19) (A5, A7). The answer or use rate also differed, with values of 69% and 24.27%, respectively (A1, A9). Other effective outcome variables included the quality of information ($p < 0.001$) (A1), preconception intention ($p < 0.001$) (A3), risk of eating disorders ($p < 0.001$) (A4), eating disorders ($p < 0.001$) (A4), internalization ($p = 0.001$) (A4), ease of learning ($p < 0.001$) (A5), gender attitudes ($p < 0.01$) (A8), unhealthy relationships ($p < 0.01$) (A8), physical effects of unhealthy relationships ($p < 0.001$) (A10), psychological effects ($p < 0.001$) (A10), distress ($p < 0.001$) (A10), and the effectiveness of self-care behavior ($p < 0.001$) (A10). Outcome variables that were not found to be effective included ease of use ($p = 0.24$) (A5), positive and negative emotions ($p = 0.97$ and 0.82) (A2), and exposure to intimate partner violence ($p > 0.05$) (A8) (Table 2).

3.4. Results of Quality Appraisal

Seven randomized controlled trials (RCTs) (A1, A2, A3, A4, A7, A8, A10) were assessed for quality using the ROB 2 and robvis tools. In the first category, "bias arising from the randomization process", bias was low except in two studies (A4, A7). In the second domain, "bias due to deviations from the intended interventions", one study was rated as high (A1), while the others showed either no information or low bias. In the third domain, "bias due to missing outcome data", all but three studies (A2, A3, A4) exhibited low bias. The fourth domain, "bias in measurement of the outcome", presented high bias in three studies (A1, A3, A8). Similarly, the fifth domain, "bias due to the selection of reported outcomes", indicated high bias in three studies (A1, A3, A8). In the overall evaluation, there was one study with a high risk of bias (A1), three with some concerns (A3, A4, A8), and three with a low risk of bias (A2, A7, A10) (Figure 2).

3.5. Effects of Chatbot Interventions on Anxiety

For the meta-analysis, the researcher utilized the Comprehensive Meta-Analysis V4 program to assess the effect size of three studies (A2, A3, A4) that examined the impact of chatbot intervention on anxiety. The researcher chose a fixed-effect model due to the limited number of studies, which precluded a reliable estimation of study variation [25]. The combined effect size was found to be −0.30, with a 95% confidence interval ranging from −0.42 to −0.18 ($z = -4.91$, $p < 0.001$) [26]. The heterogeneity analysis indicated no significant variation across the studies ($I^2 = 0\%$, $Q = 8.10$, $p < 0.017$) (Figure 3).

Study name	Statistics for each study						
	Std diff in means	Standard error	Variance	Lower limit	Upper limit	Z-Value	p-Value
Greer (2019): cancer patients	-0.210	0.349	0.122	-0.895	0.474	-0.602	0.547
Meada (2020): preconception	-0.453	0.081	0.007	-0.612	-0.293	-5.555	0.000
Fitzsimmons-Craft (2021): eating disorder	-0.096	0.096	0.009	-0.284	0.091	-1.007	0.314
Pooled	-0.270	0.150	0.022	-0.563	0.024	-1.799	0.072
Prediction Interval	-0.270			-3.546	3.007		

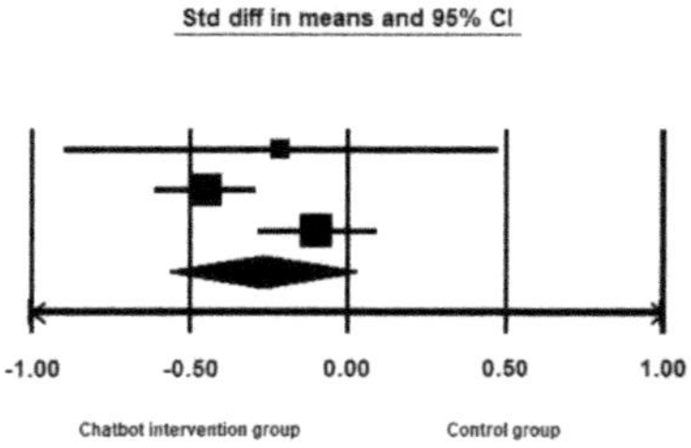

Figure 3. Forest plot of anxiety as an outcome [3,20,21].

4. Discussion

This study conducted a systematic review of 10 articles examining the effects of AI chatbot interventions on women's health and performed a meta-analysis on their impact on depression. The findings indicate that AI chatbot interventions are being utilized across a range of women's health areas, although the number of such interventions remains limited and is still in the initial stages of development. The meta-analysis revealed a medium effect size for depression, suggesting that AI chatbot interventions can significantly influence women's health. This study identified that AI chatbot interventions are being implemented in various domains of women's health, including cancer care (A1, A7, A10), contraception (A3), violence (A8), sexually transmitted diseases (A6), dietary issues (A4), and pregnancy preparation (A5, A9). Overall, the results demonstrate that AI chatbot interventions are effective in enhancing both physical and mental health outcomes in the context of women's health.

The studies reviewed were published from 2019 onward, indicating that the subject has seen active interest over the past five years, with the United States contributing four (A2, A4, A7, A9) out of the ten articles. Generative AI as we understand it today—particularly in the context of generating text, images, music, and other forms of media—began to gain prominence with the advent of more sophisticated machine learning models in the 2010s [27]. Breast cancer care emerged as the most frequently addressed topic in women's health, represented in three out of the ten studies (A1, A7, A10). These studies explored the suitability of knowledge-generating chatbots for various functions: answering women's questions about breast cancer (A1), providing genetic counseling for breast cancer (A7), and offering self-care strategies for managing chemotherapy side effects (A10). Chatbot interventions in cancer care offered the possibility for seamless integration into healthcare settings, complementing healthcare providers to improve patient care, streamline operations, and cut expenses [28].

The second most common intervention identified was prenatal education, covering topics such as mental health (A5) and general education (A9). The other five interventions each had distinct themes and targeted specific demographics: adolescents (A2, A4), women of childbearing age in need of contraceptive education (A3, A6), pregnant women (A5, A9), and women with partners (A8). The health conditions addressed included HIV (A6), breast cancer (A1, A7, A10), eating disorders (A4), and issues affecting women without other specific diseases. The findings suggest that chatbot interventions, which have traditionally focused on breast cancer and prenatal education, hold the potential to broaden their scope to encompass various aspects of women's health throughout their life cycle. Privacy, security, and culturally sensitive approaches are essential for all women's health topics. In the field of women's health, the private nature of certain subjects, such as infertility, abstinence, and sexually transmitted diseases [24], may lead women to prefer the discretion of digital interventions over face-to-face interactions, which can be perceived as judgmental [3].

Physical health outcomes encompassed eating disorders (A4), intimate partner violence exposure (A8), and the effectiveness of self-care behavior (A10). Within these, interventions for eating disorders and breast cancer self-care proved to be effective. These interventions provided personalized education and improved access to real-time, high-quality information, showing usefulness and cost-effectiveness compared to traditional nurse-led education. This suggests that chatbots can play a significant role in physical self-care, particularly in managing chemotherapy-related side effects, by offering tailored support and information (A10). Another study presented the use of a teleassessment nursing chatbot application that enabled patients and families to assess general conditions, identify danger signs, and make informed decisions on utilizing health services during the COVID-19 pandemic [29]. Emotional health outcomes included anxiety (A2, A3, A4), depression (A2, A4, A8), satisfaction (A5, A7), emotion (A2), distress (A10), gender attitude (A8), and unhealthy relationships (A8). Of these, interventions addressing distress (A10), gender attitude (A8), and unhealthy relationships (A8) were found to be effective. Psychotherapy administered through a chatbot has been shown to significantly alleviate depressive symptoms, with a notable effect size ($g = 0.54$), indicating its effectiveness for adults dealing with depression or anxiety [30].

Cognitive health outcomes covered a range of areas such as knowledge (A3, A6), answer or use rate (A1, A9), quality of information (A1), usage time (A2), preconception intention (A3), ease of learning (A5), acceptability (A6), feasibility (A6), interaction (A6), internalization (A4), and usability (A10). Effective outcomes were observed in knowledge (A3, A6), quality of information (A1), preconception intention (A3), internalization (A4), ease of learning (A5), acceptability (A6), feasibility (A6), interaction (A6), and usability (A10). An AI chatbot was effective in encouraging healthy behaviors, with significant success in areas such as enhancing healthy living habits (40%), aiding in smoking cessation efforts (27%), supporting treatment and medication compliance (13%), and helping to decrease substance abuse (7%) [31].

The relatively small number of physical health outcome domains suggests that conversational AI chatbots may offer counseling comparable to that of health professionals, but may also provide inappropriate advice relative to human healthcare providers [19]. A significant limitation of AI, particularly when generated using large-scale language models, is the phenomenon of hallucination, which means it can complement but not surpass human interventions [19]. AI hallucinations could adversely affect decision making and pose ethical and legal concerns [32]. Chatbots currently lack the capability to fully grasp human complexity and do not match the level of human interaction. This was highlighted by a study showing that individuals still preferred to consult a doctor or nurse after interacting with a chatbot [6]. The proposed functional features of chatbots include functionality, efficiency, technical satisfaction, humanity, effectiveness, and ethics [7]. Consequently, while chatbots cannot substitute human involvement in physical health promotion, they can improve the efficiency of treatment when their use is validated by an expert.

Chatbot interventions have demonstrated effectiveness in improving cognitive outcomes in women's health. The process of knowledge acquisition is intrinsically linked to individual perceptual experiences, highlighting the need for personalized educational strategies to enhance health outcomes for women. The results showed that chatbot technology has a medium-to-high impact on overall learning outcomes. In particular, chatbots significantly improved explicit reasoning, learning achievement, knowledge retention, and learning interest. However, some negative effects were observed in areas such as critical thinking, learning engagement, and motivation [33]. A review of 32 empirical studies on chatbot intervention revealed that chatbot technology had a medium-to-high effect on overall learning outcomes [33]. The cognitive benefits may stem from the fact that chatbot users experienced less cognitive load, were more productive, had lower frustration levels, and performed better overall, despite slightly longer task completion times [34]. Altogether, this meta-analysis determined that chatbot interventions had a moderate-sized effect on reducing anxiety in women's health [17].

Another meta-analysis investigated the efficacy of digital interventions for all types of anxiety disorders. It reported a substantial pooled effect size ($g = 0.80$) in favor of digital interventions [35]. A chatbot designed to assess symptoms of depression and anxiety among university students was evaluated. The study revealed no significant differences in symptoms of depression or anxiety between the experimental group and the control group. However, there was a notable reduction in anxiety symptoms within the experimental group [36]. In another study, a psychoeducational chatbot aimed at helping university students manage stress and anxiety was interacted with an average of 78 times over the course of the study. This interaction led to a significant reduction in symptoms of anxiety and stress [37]. Chatbots are beneficial in mental health interventions for several reasons. One is that social support provided through conversation elicits positive emotions [20]. Another is that chatbots disseminate knowledge, thereby increasing the information available to users, enhancing their understanding, and reducing health-related anxiety. Additionally, the interactive feedback from chatbots can reduce stress because it is accessible, convenient, informal, and free from embarrassment. Chatbots engage in a human-like manner, offering empathy without human judgment and creating a sense of safety [3].

No chatbot interventions were found that studied the long-term effects of women's health, but mental health, HIV, and cancer management are issues that warrant long-term interventions. The acceptability of an autonomous virtual agent designed to support self-management for patients with chronic diseases, which are long-term conditions that often co-occur with mental health problems such as anxiety and depression, remains to be determined. AI chatbots overcome the physical limitations of human therapists, such as the ability to operate without fatigue and to be available almost anywhere and anytime [38]. Schmidhuber et al.'s suggested improvement to reduce physical workload and cognitive demand was the implementation of text prediction features, which could help lower the effort required for typing [34]. The integration of AI-powered chatbots into the healthcare system promises to improve patient engagement, streamline administrative processes, and increase access to care, particularly in mental health support. However, realizing their full potential requires addressing challenges related to data privacy, accuracy, and the ethical implications of AI in healthcare [39]. Further research is needed to directly compare the effectiveness of AI chatbots with traditional healthcare interventions like face-to-face counseling, telehealth, and mobile applications, to better understand their potential and limitations in enhancing healthcare delivery.

AI chatbots are at the forefront of technology in behavior change interventions [34]. Understanding how human intervention can effectively induce behavior changes is crucial, especially in reducing anxiety. There is a need to explore the relationship between chatbot intervention strategies and their impact on women's perceived barriers and social support for health outcomes [40]. Despite the rapid user growth of chatbots and their utility for health interventions, concerns have been raised about their decision-making accuracy, precision, and the ethical and legal implications [32]. AI and robotics are starting to be deployed in women's health globally, emphasizing the disparity between developed and underdeveloped regions. This study advocates for an inclusive approach in technology design and implementation to ensure equitable healthcare access, highlighting the importance of multi-sectoral collaborations to foster innovation while mitigating risks [41]. Not all women may have equal access to the technology needed to interact with AI chatbots, especially in low-resource settings or among older populations. This digital divide can exacerbate existing health disparities. Outcome variables that were not found to be effective included ease of use (A5). AI chatbots developed without considering diverse cultural and linguistic contexts may not be effective for all women. Tailoring interventions to fit different cultural backgrounds and languages is essential but challenging [42]. These interventions must be applied to various women's health issues through more interdisciplinary work to circumvent ethical problems [43].

Limitations

This study has a few limitations. First, articles published after October 2023 were not included as they fell outside the search period. Despite the recent surge in chatbot interventions, this may have resulted in the exclusion of a significant body of research. Second, limiting the article search to English and Korean publications may have resulted in a geographical and cultural bias, excluding potentially valuable studies conducted in other languages. Third, the wide variety of outcome variables presented challenges for meta-analysis, which led to the decision to only conduct a meta-analysis of data related to anxiety. Fourth, the rapid development of AI technologies means that significant contributions to the literature could have been made just after the cutoff, potentially leaving out innovative approaches or critical evaluations of chatbot interventions. Fifth, the small sample sizes of the included studies may not provide sufficient power to detect significant differences or to ensure the representativeness of the results.

5. Conclusions

Thus systematic review and meta-analysis of AI chatbot interventions in women's health has illuminated the significant potential of these technologies to enhance healthcare outcomes. Chatbots have shown considerable promise in delivering health education, supporting mental health, managing chronic diseases, and providing targeted interventions across a spectrum of women's health issues, including reproductive health, cancer care, and prenatal education. Notably, these interventions have been effective in improving both physical and mental health outcomes, with a particular emphasis on reducing anxiety, underscoring the value of integrating AI chatbots into healthcare strategies. Consequently, the use of chatbot interventions is recommended in mental health programs due to their proven effectiveness in alleviating anxiety. Given that chatbot interventions have demonstrated high feasibility, usability, and acceptability, they hold significant potential to become scalable interventions.

Funding: This research was funded by the National Research Foundation of Korea (RS-2023-00239284).

Institutional Review Board Statement: Not applicable.

Informed Consent Statement: Not applicable.

Data Availability Statement: Not applicable.

Conflicts of Interest: The author declares no conflict of interest.

Appendix A

Table A1. Analysis articles.

A1 [19]	Bibault, J.E.; Chaix, B.; Guillemassé, A.; Cousin, S.; Escande, A.; Perrin, M.; Pienkowski, A.; Delamon, G.; Nectoux, P.; Brouard, B. A Chatbot Versus Physicians to Provide Information for Patients with Breast Cancer: Blind, Randomized Controlled Noninferiority Trial. *J. Med. Internet Res.* **2019**, *21*, e15787. https://doi.org/10.2196/15787.
A2 [20]	Greer, S.; Ramo, D.; Chang, Y.J.; Fu, M.; Moskowitz, J.; Haritatos, J. Use of the Chatbot "Vivibot" to Deliver Positive Psychology Skills and Promote Well-Being Among Young People After Cancer Treatment: Randomized Controlled Feasibility Trial. *JMIR Mhealth Uhealth* **2019**, *7*, e15018. https://doi.org/10.2196/15018.
A3 [3]	Maeda, E.; Miyata, A.; Boivin, J.; Nomura, K.; Kumazawa, Y.; Shirasawa, H.; Saito, H.; Terada, Y. Promoting fertility awareness and preconception health using a chatbot: A randomized controlled trial. *Reprod. Biomed. Online* **2020**, *41*, 1133–1143. https://doi.org/10.1016/j.rbmo.2020.09.006.
A4 [21]	Fitzsimmons-Craft, E.E.; Chan, W.W.; Smith, A.C.; Firebaugh, M.L.; Fowler, L.A.; Topooco, N.; DePietro, B.; Wilfley, D.E.; Taylor, C.B.; Jacobson, N.C. Effectiveness of a chatbot for eating disorders prevention: A randomized clinical trial. *Int. J. Eat. Disord.* **2022**, *55*, 343–353. https://doi.org/10.1002/eat.23662.
A5 [4]	Chung, K.; Cho, H.Y.; Park, J.Y. A Chatbot for Perinatal Women's and Partners' Obstetric and Mental Health Care: Development and Usability Evaluation Study. *JMIR Med. Inform.* **2021**, *9*, e18607. https://doi.org/10.2196/18607.
A6 [5]	Yam, E.A.; Namukonda, E.; McClair, T.; Souidi, S.; Chelwa, N.; Muntalima, N.; Mbizvo, M.; Bellows, B. Developing and Testing a Chatbot to Integrate HIV Education Into Family Planning Clinic Waiting Areas in Lusaka, Zambia. *Glob. Health Sci. Pract.* **2022**, *10*, e2100721. https://doi.org/10.9745/GHSP-D-21-00721.
A7 [22]	Al-Hilli, Z.; Noss, R.; Dickard, J.; Wei, W.; Chichura, A.; Wu, V.; Renicker, K.; Pederson, H.J.; Eng, C. A Randomized Trial Comparing the Effectiveness of Pre-test Genetic Counseling Using an Artificial Intelligence Automated Chatbot and Traditional In-person Genetic Counseling in Women Newly Diagnosed with Breast Cancer. *Ann. Surg. Oncol.* **2023**, *30*, 5990–5996. https://doi.org/10.1245/s10434-023-13888-4.
A8 [23]	De Filippo, A.; Bellatin, P.; Tietz, N.; Grant, E.; Whitefield, A.; Nkopane, P.; Devereux, C.; Crawford, K.; Vermeulen, B.; Hatcher, A.M. Effects of digital chatbot on gender attitudes and exposure to intimate partner violence among young women in South Africa. *PLoS Digit. Health* **2023**, *2*, e0000358. https://doi.org/10.1371/journal.pdig.0000358.
A9 [24]	Mane, H.Y.; Channell Doig, A.; Marin Gutierrez, F.X.; Jasczynski, M.; Yue, X.; Srikanth, N.P.; Mane, S.; Sun, A.; Moats, R.A.; Patel, P.; et al. Practical Guidance for the Development of Rosie, a Health Education Question-and-Answer Chatbot for New Mothers. *J. Public. Health Manag. Pract.* **2023**, *29*, 663–670. https://doi.org/10.1097/PHH.0000000000001781.
A10 [6]	Tawfik, E.; Ghallab, E.; Moustafa, A. A nurse versus a chatbot—The effect of an empowerment program on chemotherapy-related side effects and the self-care behaviors of women living with breast Cancer: A randomized controlled trial. BMC Nurs. **2023**, *22*, 102. https://doi.org/10.1186/s12912-023-01243-7.

References

1. Wilson, L.; Marasoiu, M. The Development and Use of Chatbots in Public Health: Scoping Review. *JMIR Hum. Factors* **2022**, *9*, e35882. [CrossRef]
2. Archibald, M.M.; Clark, A.M. ChatGTP: What is it and how can nursing and health science education use it? *J. Adv. Nurs.* **2023**, *79*, 3648–3651. [CrossRef] [PubMed]
3. Maeda, E.; Miyata, A.; Boivin, J.; Nomura, K.; Kumazawa, Y.; Shirasawa, H.; Saito, H.; Terada, Y. Promoting fertility awareness and preconception health using a chatbot: A randomized controlled trial. *Reprod. Biomed. Online* **2020**, *41*, 1133–1143. [CrossRef]
4. Chung, K.; Cho, H.Y.; Park, J.Y. A Chatbot for Perinatal Women's and Partners' Obstetric and Mental Health Care: Development and Usability Evaluation Study. *JMIR Med. Inform.* **2021**, *9*, e18607. [CrossRef] [PubMed]
5. Yam, E.A.; Namukonda, E.; McClair, T.; Souidi, S.; Chelwa, N.; Muntalima, N.; Mbizvo, M.; Bellows, B. Developing and Testing a Chatbot to Integrate HIV Education into Family Planning Clinic Waiting Areas in Lusaka, Zambia. *Glob. Health Sci. Pract.* **2022**, *10*, e2100721. [CrossRef]
6. Tawfik, E.; Ghallab, E.; Moustafa, A. A nurse versus a chatbot—The effect of an empowerment program on chemotherapy-related side effects and the self-care behaviors of women living with breast Cancer: A randomized controlled trial. *BMC Nurs.* **2023**, *22*, 102. [CrossRef] [PubMed]
7. Johari, N.M.; Nohuddin, P.N.; Baharin, A.H.A.; Yakob, N.A.; Ebadi, M.J. Features requirement elicitation process for designing a chatbot application. *IET Netw.* **2022**, 1–15. [CrossRef]
8. Luxton, D.D. Artificial Intelligence in Psychological Practice: Current and Future Applications and Implications. *Prof. Psychol. Res. Pract.* **2014**, *45*, 332–339. [CrossRef]

9. Abd-Alrazaq, A.A.; Alajlani, M.; Ali, N.; Denecke, K.; Bewick, B.M.; Househ, M. Perceptions and Opinions of Patients About Mental Health Chatbots: Scoping Review. *J. Med. Internet Res.* **2021**, *23*, e17828. [CrossRef]
10. Oh, Y.J.; Zhang, J.; Fang, M.L.; Fukuoka, Y. A systematic review of artificial intelligence chatbots for promoting physical activity, healthy diet, and weight loss. *Int. J. Behav. Nutr. Phys. Act.* **2021**, *18*, 160. [CrossRef]
11. World Health Organization. *A Woman Dies Every Two Minutes Due to Pregnancy or Childbirth: UN Agencies*; World Health Organization: Geneva, Switzerland, 23 February 2023; Available online: https://www.who.int/news/item/23-02-2023-a-woman-dies-every-two-minutes-due-to-pregnancy-or-childbirth--un-agencies (accessed on 12 February 2024).
12. World Health Organization. *WHO Launches Women's Health Chatbot with Messaging on Breast Cancer*; World Health Organization: Geneva, Switzerland, 20 October 2021; Available online: https://www.who.int/news/item/20-10-2021-who-launches-women-s-health-chatbot-with-messaging-on-breast-cancer (accessed on 12 February 2024).
13. Page, M.J.; Moher, D.; Bossuyt, P.M.; Boutron, I.; Hoffmann, T.C.; Mulrow, C.D.; Shamseer, L.; Tetzlaff, J.M.; Akl, E.A.; Brennan, S.E.; et al. PRISMA 2020 explanation and elaboration: Updated guidance and exemplars for reporting systematic reviews. *BMJ* **2021**, *372*, n160. [CrossRef]
14. Higgins, J.P.T.; Thomas, J.; Chandler, J.; Cumpston, M.; Li, T.; Page, M.J.; Welch, V.A. (Eds.) *Cochrane Handbook for Systematic Reviews of Interventions Version 6.3 (Updated February 2022)*; Cochrane: London, UK, 2022; Available online: www.training.cochrane.org/handbook (accessed on 18 February 2023).
15. Bidwell, S.; Jensen, M.F. *Etext on Health Technology Assessment (HTA) Information Resources. Chapter 3: Using a Search Protocol to Identify Sources of Information: The COSI Model*; U.S. National Library of Medicine: Bethesda, MD, USA, 2003; [Updated 14 June 2003]. Available online: https://www.nlm.nih.gov/archive/20060905/nichsr/ehta/chapter3.html#COSI (accessed on 20 August 2019).
16. Sterne, J.A.C.; Savović, J.; Page, M.J.; Elbers, R.G.; Blencowe, N.S.; Boutron, I.; Cates, C.J.; Cheng, H.Y.; Corbett, M.S.; Eldridge, S.M.; et al. RoB 2: A revised tool for assessing risk of bias in randomised trials. *BMJ* **2019**, *366*, l4898. [CrossRef]
17. Cohen, J. *Statistical Power for the Behavioral Sciences*; Lawrence Erlbaum Associates: Hillsdale, NJ, USA, 1988.
18. McGuinness, L.A.; Higgins, J.P.T. Risk-of-bias VISualization (robvis): An R package and Shiny web app for visualizing risk-of-bias assessments. *Res. Synth. Methods* **2020**, *12*, 55–61. [CrossRef]
19. Bibault, J.E.; Chaix, B.; Guillemassé, A.; Cousin, S.; Escande, A.; Perrin, M.; Pienkowski, A.; Delamon, G.; Nectoux, P.; Brouard, B. A Chatbot Versus Physicians to Provide Information for Patients with Breast Cancer: Blind, Randomized Controlled Noninferiority Trial. *J. Med. Internet Res.* **2019**, *21*, e15787. [CrossRef]
20. Greer, S.; Ramo, D.; Chang, Y.J.; Fu, M.; Moskowitz, J.; Haritatos, J. Use of the Chatbot "Vivibot" to Deliver Positive Psychology Skills and Promote Well-Being among Young People after Cancer Treatment: Randomized Controlled Feasibility Trial. *JMIR Mhealth Uhealth* **2019**, *7*, e15018. [CrossRef] [PubMed]
21. Fitzsimmons-Craft, E.E.; Chan, W.W.; Smith, A.C.; Firebaugh, M.L.; Fowler, L.A.; Topooco, N.; DePietro, B.; Wilfley, D.E.; Taylor, C.B.; Jacobson, N.C. Effectiveness of a chatbot for eating disorders prevention: A randomized clinical trial. *Int. J. Eat. Disord.* **2022**, *55*, 343–353. [CrossRef] [PubMed]
22. Al-Hilli, Z.; Noss, R.; Dickard, J.; Wei, W.; Chichura, A.; Wu, V.; Renicker, K.; Pederson, H.J.; Eng, C. A Randomized Trial Comparing the Effectiveness of Pre-test Genetic Counseling Using an Artificial Intelligence Automated Chatbot and Traditional In-person Genetic Counseling in Women Newly Diagnosed with Breast Cancer. *Ann. Surg. Oncol.* **2023**, *30*, 5990–5996. [CrossRef] [PubMed]
23. De Filippo, A.; Bellatin, P.; Tietz, N.; Grant, E.; Whitefield, A.; Nkopane, P.; Devereux, C.; Crawford, K.; Vermeulen, B.; Hatcher, A.M. Effects of digital chatbot on gender attitudes and exposure to intimate partner violence among young women in South Africa. *PLoS Digit. Health* **2023**, *2*, e0000358. [CrossRef] [PubMed]
24. Mane, H.Y.; Channell Doig, A.; Marin Gutierrez, F.X.; Jasczynski, M.; Yue, X.; Srikanth, N.P.; Mane, S.; Sun, A.; Moats, R.A.; Patel, P.; et al. Practical Guidance for the Development of Rosie, a Health Education Question-and-Answer Chatbot for New Mothers. *J. Public Health Manag. Pract.* **2023**, *29*, 663–670. [CrossRef]
25. Borenstein, M.; Hedges, L.V.; Higgins, J.P.; Rothstein, H.R. A basic introduction to fixed-effect and random-effects models for meta-analysis. *Res. Synth. Methods* **2010**, *1*, 97–111. [CrossRef]
26. Hedges, L.V.; Vevea, J.L. Fixed and random-effects models in meta-analysis. *Psychol. Methods* **1998**, *3*, 486–504. [CrossRef]
27. Patil, S.S.; Shelke, S.; Velankar, M.; Koul, T.; Rani, V. A systematic survey of approaches used in computer music generation. *J. Intell. Data Syst. Bus. Data Manag.* **2023**, *2*, 6–23. [CrossRef]
28. Xu, L.; Sanders, L.; Li, K.; Chow, J.C.L. Chatbot for Health Care and Oncology Applications Using Artificial Intelligence and Machine Learning: Systematic Review. *JMIR Cancer* **2021**, *7*, e27850. [CrossRef]
29. Ariga, R.A.; Amelia, R.; Astuti, S.B.; Fajar, F.A.A.; Ariga, S.; Ariga, H.P.S.; Pane, N.K. Self Care Nursing: Teleassessment Nursing with Chatbot Application the Coronavirus Disease-19 Pandemic Period in North Sumatra. *Open Access Maced. J. Med. Sci.* **2021**, *9*, 306–310. [CrossRef]
30. Lim, S.M.; Shiau, C.W.C.; Cheng, L.J.; Lau, Y. Chatbot-Delivered Psychotherapy for Adults with Depressive and Anxiety Symptoms: A Systematic Review and Meta-Regression. *Behav. Ther.* **2022**, *53*, 334–347. [CrossRef] [PubMed]
31. Aggarwal, A.; Tam, C.C.; Wu, D.; Li, X.; Qiao, S. Artificial Intelligence-Based Chatbots for Promoting Health Behavioral Changes: Systematic Review. *J. Med. Internet Res.* **2023**, *25*, e40789. [CrossRef]
32. Thomas-Tran, E.P.; Thomas-Tran, J.; Tran, I.P.; Hu, R.J. Exploring the Boundaries of Reality: Investigating the Phenomenon of Artificial Intelligence Hallucination in Scientific Writing through ChatGPT References. *Cureus* **2023**, *15*, e37432. [CrossRef]

33. Deng, X.; Yu, Z. A Meta-Analysis and Systematic Review of the Effect of Chatbot Technology Use in Sustainable Education. *Sustainability* **2023**, *15*, 2940. [CrossRef]
34. Schmidhuber, J.; Schlögl, S.; Ploder, C. Cognitive Load and Productivity Implications in Human-Chatbot Interaction. In Proceedings of the 2021 IEEE International Conference on Human-Machine Systems (ICHMS), Magdeburg, Germany, 8–10 September 2021; IEEE: New York, NY, USA, 2021; pp. 1–6. [CrossRef]
35. Pauley, D.; Cuijpers, P.; Papola, D.; Miguel, C.; Karyotaki, E. Two decades of digital interventions for anxiety disorders: A systematic review and meta-analysis of treatment effectiveness. *Psychol. Med.* **2021**, *53*, 567–579. [CrossRef]
36. Klos, M.C.; Escoredo, M.; Joerin, A.; Lemos, V.; Rauws, M.; Bunge, E. Artificial Intelligence–Based Chatbot for Anxiety and Depression in University Students: Pilot Randomized Controlled Trial. *JMIR Form. Res.* **2021**, *5*, e20678. [CrossRef]
37. Gabrielli, S.; Rizzi, S.; Bassi, G.; Carbone, S.; Maimone, R.; Marchesoni, M.; Forti, S. Engagement and Effectiveness of a Healthy-Coping Intervention via Chatbot for University Students during the COVID-19 Pandemic: Mixed Methods Proof-of-Concept Study. *JMIR Mhealth Uhealth* **2021**, *9*, e27965. [CrossRef] [PubMed]
38. Easton, K.; Potter, S.; Bec, R.; Bennion, M.; Christensen, H.; Grindell, C.; Mirheidari, B.; Weich, S.; de Witte, L.D.; Wolstenholme, D.; et al. A virtual agent to support individuals living with physical and mental comorbidities: Co-design and acceptability testing. *J. Med. Internet Res.* **2019**, *21*, e12996. [CrossRef]
39. Sun, G.; Zhou, Y.H. AI in healthcare: Navigating opportunities and challenges in digital communication. *Front. Digit. Health* **2023**, *5*, 1291132. [CrossRef] [PubMed]
40. Liang, K.H.; Lange, P.; Oh, Y.; Zhang, J.; Fukuoka, Y.; Yu, Z. Evaluation of in-Person Counseling Strategies to Develop Physical Activity Chatbot for Women. In Proceedings of the 22nd Annual Meeting of the Special Interest Group on Discourse and Dialogue, Singapore, 29–31 July 2021; Association for Computational Linguistics: Kerrville, TX, USA, 2021; pp. 38–47. [CrossRef]
41. Afaq, M.; Abraham, D.E.; Patel, S.H.; Al-Dhoon, A.D.; Arshad, Z.; Abraham, D.E. Empowering Women's Health: A Global Perspective on Artificial Intelligence and Robotics. *Cureus* **2023**, *15*, e49611. [CrossRef] [PubMed]
42. Miner, A.; Laranjo, L.; Kocaballi, A.B. Chatbots in the Fight Against the COVID-19 Pandemic. *npj Digit. Med.* **2020**, *3*, 65. [CrossRef]
43. Zhang, J.; Oh, Y.J.; Lange, P.; Yu, Z.; Fukuoka, Y. Artificial Intelligence Chatbot Behavior Change Model for Designing Artificial Intelligence Chatbots to Promote Physical Activity and a Healthy Diet: Viewpoint. *J. Med. Internet Res.* **2020**, *22*, e22845. [CrossRef]

International Journal of
Environmental Research and Public Health

MDPI

Review

The Utility of Language Models in Cardiology: A Narrative Review of the Benefits and Concerns of ChatGPT-4

Dhir Gala [1] and Amgad N. Makaryus [2,3,*]

1 Department of Clinical Science, American University of the Caribbean School of Medicine, Cupecoy, Sint Maarten, The Netherlands; dhirgala@gmail.com
2 Donald and Barbara Zucker School of Medicine at Hofstra/Northwell, Hofstra University, 500 Hofstra Blvd., Hempstead, NY 11549, USA
3 Department of Cardiology, Nassau University Medical Center, Hempstead, NY 11554, USA
* Correspondence: amakaryu@numc.edu; Tel.: +1-516-296-2567

Abstract: Artificial intelligence (AI) and language models such as ChatGPT-4 (Generative Pretrained Transformer) have made tremendous advances recently and are rapidly transforming the landscape of medicine. Cardiology is among many of the specialties that utilize AI with the intention of improving patient care. Generative AI, with the use of its advanced machine learning algorithms, has the potential to diagnose heart disease and recommend management options suitable for the patient. This may lead to improved patient outcomes not only by recommending the best treatment plan but also by increasing physician efficiency. Language models could assist physicians with administrative tasks, allowing them to spend more time on patient care. However, there are several concerns with the use of AI and language models in the field of medicine. These technologies may not be the most up-to-date with the latest research and could provide outdated information, which may lead to an adverse event. Secondly, AI tools can be expensive, leading to increased healthcare costs and reduced accessibility to the general population. There is also concern about the loss of the human touch and empathy as AI becomes more mainstream. Healthcare professionals would need to be adequately trained to utilize these tools. While AI and language models have many beneficial traits, all healthcare providers need to be involved and aware of generative AI so as to assure its optimal use and mitigate any potential risks and challenges associated with its implementation. In this review, we discuss the various uses of language models in the field of cardiology.

Keywords: language models; artificial intelligence; ChatGPT; generative artificial intelligence; generative language models; cardiology; medical education; patient outcomes

1. Introduction

Artificial intelligence (AI) is changing the way medicine is practiced. AI refers to the capability of machines to do tasks that require human intelligence, such as recognizing speech, making decisions, and learning [1]. This is accomplished through the use of algorithms, computer programs that can process data and make predictions based on patterns in that data. One of the most intriguing applications of AI in natural language processing has resulted in the creation of complex language models [2]. Language models are AI systems that use machine learning algorithms to comprehend and produce text like a human. Their sophisticated design enables them to create logical and contextually appropriate text by learning language structure and patterns from vast amounts of text data that is used to train the language models [3].

Language models are created using a process called machine learning, which involves training a computer program to recognize patterns in data. In the case of language models, the program is trained on a large dataset of text, such as books, online articles, or social media posts. The program uses sophisticated statistical methods to identify patterns in the language, such as the probability of certain words appearing together or the likelihood of a particular sentence structure. Once the program is trained, it can be used for a variety of tasks. One common use of language models is in natural language processing (NLP), which involves analyzing and understanding human language [4]. For example, a language model can be used to automatically summarize a long text document or to extract key information from a customer support chat conversation. Another use of language models is in speech recognition, where they are used to convert spoken language into text [5]. This is particularly useful for virtual assistants like Siri or Alexa, which rely on language models to understand and respond to user requests. Language models can also be used for machine translation, where they are used to automatically translate text from one language to another [6]. This is a particularly challenging task, as languages have different grammatical structures and idioms that can be difficult to translate accurately. However, recent advances in language models have led to significant improvements in machine translation accuracy. Finally, language models are increasingly being used in research to analyze text data and to generate new insights [7,8].

A number of uses for language models exist, such as chatbots, sentiment analysis, and language translation [9]. One of the most well-known language models is OpenAI's ChatGPT-4 (Generative Pre-trained Transformer 4), which is capable of writing various texts such as poetry, essays, and even computer code [10]. BERT (Bidirectional Encoder Representations from Transformers) is another language model created by Google and is capable of comprehending the context and meaning of words in a sentence [11].

Language models have recently entered the medical field and have the potential to completely change how healthcare providers communicate with patients. Language models can be used to automate administrative tasks, enhance patient outcomes, and even help with medical diagnosis [2]. Medical records and other types of healthcare data can be analyzed using language models, which can reveal information about patient outcomes and available treatments. Accurately diagnosing and foreseeing the progression of cardiovascular diseases (CVDs) is one of cardiology's biggest challenges. To gain insights into the diagnosis and treatment of CVDs, AI-powered language models have the capacity to analyze vast amounts of patient data, including medical records, test results, and clinical observations. This review aims to identify the various uses of language models in the field of cardiology.

2. Language Models in Cardiology

2.1. Medical Diagnosis and Decision Support

AI and language models have the potential to revolutionize medical diagnosis and decision support in cardiology by analyzing vast amounts of medical data and assisting healthcare professionals in making more accurate diagnoses and treatment decisions. Analyzing medical images like echocardiograms, angiograms, and electrocardiograms (ECGs) is one way that AI and language models can assist in cardiology. It is possible to train AI algorithms to recognize patterns in these images that may be challenging for human clinicians. AI can be used, for instance, to identify abnormalities in ECGs that may be a sign of heart failure, ischemic heart disease, or arrhythmias [12].

Language models can also help in cardiology by analyzing patient medical records and other relevant data, such as family history and lifestyle factors [13,14]. Language models can identify patterns in this data that may be indicative of certain cardiovascular conditions or risk factors, enabling clinicians to make more accurate diagnoses and treatment recommendations. For example, language models can analyze patient data to predict the risk of developing cardiovascular disease and recommend appropriate lifestyle modifications or medications to reduce that risk. They can aid in early diagnosis and treatment by identifying patients who are most at risk of contracting specific cardiac diseases. Language models can guide healthcare providers on the appropriate questions to ask patients. Figure 1 gives an example of the follow-up questions necessary to appropriately diagnose a patient presenting with symptoms of shortness of breath and orthopnea from ChatGPT-4. Secondly, language models can assist in identifying potential red-flag symptoms that may require urgent treatment. ChatGPT-4 was able to appropriately identify potential red flag symptoms in patients presenting with shortness of breath and orthopnea (Figure 2). The responses provided by ChatGPT-4 are appropriate starting points for healthcare providers.

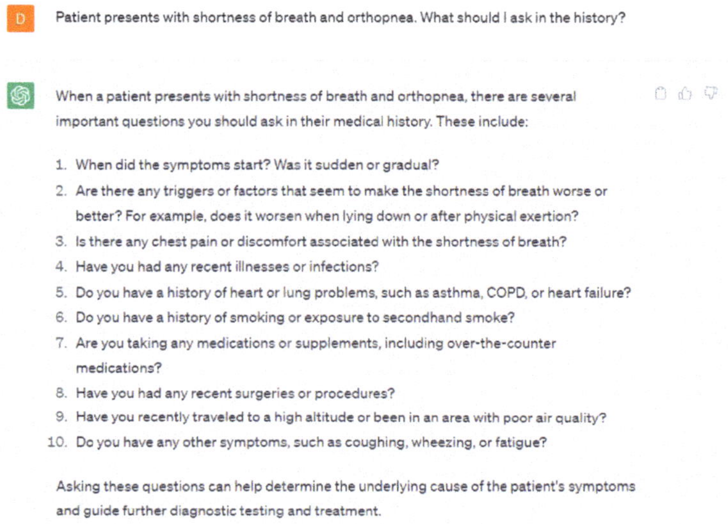
D Patient presents with shortness of breath and orthopnea. What should I ask in the history?

When a patient presents with shortness of breath and orthopnea, there are several important questions you should ask in their medical history. These include:

1. When did the symptoms start? Was it sudden or gradual?
2. Are there any triggers or factors that seem to make the shortness of breath worse or better? For example, does it worsen when lying down or after physical exertion?
3. Is there any chest pain or discomfort associated with the shortness of breath?
4. Have you had any recent illnesses or infections?
5. Do you have a history of heart or lung problems, such as asthma, COPD, or heart failure?
6. Do you have a history of smoking or exposure to secondhand smoke?
7. Are you taking any medications or supplements, including over-the-counter medications?
8. Have you had any recent surgeries or procedures?
9. Have you recently traveled to a high altitude or been in an area with poor air quality?
10. Do you have any other symptoms, such as coughing, wheezing, or fatigue?

Asking these questions can help determine the underlying cause of the patient's symptoms and guide further diagnostic testing and treatment.

Figure 1. A response from ChatGPT-4 for the question "Patient presents with shortness of breath and orthopnea. What should I ask in the history?" [15].

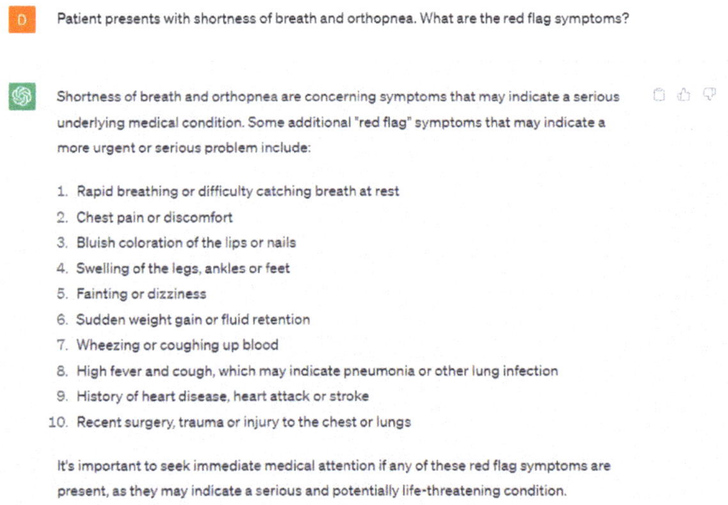
D Patient presents with shortness of breath and orthopnea. What are the red flag symptoms?

Shortness of breath and orthopnea are concerning symptoms that may indicate a serious underlying medical condition. Some additional "red flag" symptoms that may indicate a more urgent or serious problem include:

1. Rapid breathing or difficulty catching breath at rest
2. Chest pain or discomfort
3. Bluish coloration of the lips or nails
4. Swelling of the legs, ankles or feet
5. Fainting or dizziness
6. Sudden weight gain or fluid retention
7. Wheezing or coughing up blood
8. High fever and cough, which may indicate pneumonia or other lung infection
9. History of heart disease, heart attack or stroke
10. Recent surgery, trauma or injury to the chest or lungs

It's important to seek immediate medical attention if any of these red flag symptoms are present, as they may indicate a serious and potentially life-threatening condition.

Figure 2. A response from ChatGPT-4 for the question "Patient presents with shortness of breath and orthopnea. What are some red flag symptoms?" [15].

In addition to diagnosis, AI and language models can also assist in decision support by analyzing medical data and providing personalized treatment recommendations in cardiology. For example, AI can be used to analyze patient data and identify the most effective treatment options for a particular cardiovascular condition, based on factors such as the patient's age, medical history, and genetic profile. AI can also help monitor patients with implanted devices such as pacemakers or defibrillators and alert clinicians to potential issues or malfunctions.

A potential concern about language models is patients self-diagnosing and treating their symptoms. Interestingly, ChatGPT-4 did not suggest any medications or treatments when asked about it but instead recommended visiting a healthcare provider (Figure 3). From a healthcare provider's perspective, ChatGPT-4 was able to suggest medications used to treat heart failure but did not provide a specific medication or prescription (Figure 4). These responses from ChatGPT-4 are appropriate as there is always a concern about patients self-treating their symptoms or conditions without consulting healthcare providers. From the healthcare provider's perspective, although the responses were correct, they were not the gold-standard goal-directed medical therapy. This could have been due to the lack of training of ChatGPT-4 on the various guidelines or the lack of a specific prompt. It is crucial to make sure that the training data used to create language models is not only correct but also up-to-date to provide the most accurate response.

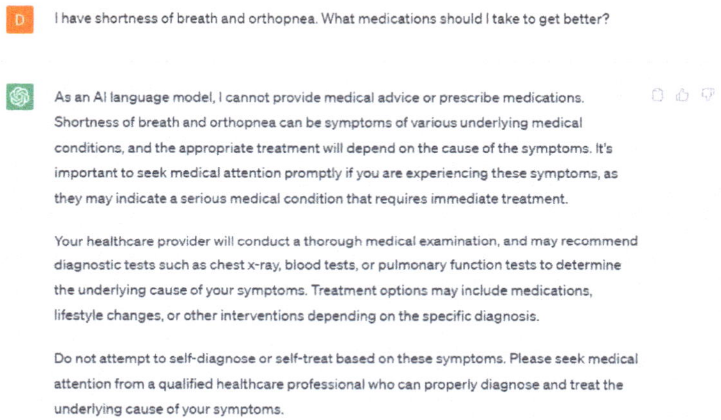

Figure 3. A response from ChatGPT-4 for the question "I have shortness of breath and orthopnea. What medications should I take to get better?" [15].

Language models can guide healthcare providers on the appropriate questions to ask patients during consultations, in addition to identifying at-risk patients. Language models can help healthcare providers narrow down potential diagnoses and suggest appropriate treatment plans by analyzing the patient's symptoms, medical history, and other relevant information.

Despite these benefits, there are some important considerations to keep in mind while utilizing language models. The language models are limited to the quality and quantity of data used to train them, which may limit their ability to make accurate predictions or recommendations. Secondly, as language models rely only on information provided, they may be biased and fail to account for all relevant factors that may influence a patient's diagnosis or treatment plan. Lastly, language models may be incapable of accounting for the nuances and complexities of individual patient cases especially rare pathologies or uncommon presentations, leading to incorrect recommendations or diagnoses.

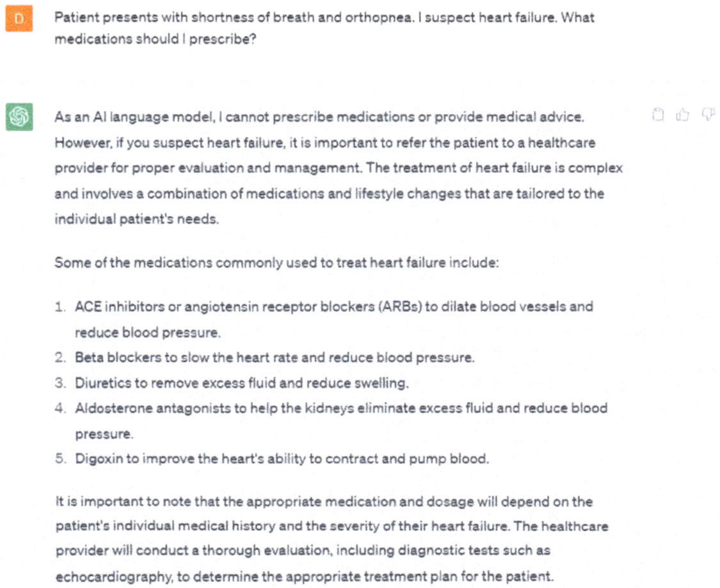

Figure 4. A response from ChatGPT-4 for the question "Patient presents with shortness of breath and orthopnea. I suspect heart failure. What medications should I prescribe?" [15].

2.2. *Patient Communication and Education*

AI and language models can also help in patient communication and education in the field of cardiology. By analyzing patient data, these technologies can provide personalized recommendations to patients, help them understand their medical conditions, and improve their adherence to treatment plans.

One way that AI and language models can help in patient communication and education in cardiology is by providing tailored education materials for patients [16,17]. For example, a language model could analyze a patient's medical records and generate personalized educational content that explains their specific condition, treatment options, and potential risks and benefits. This can help patients better understand their diagnosis and treatment, which may lead to increased adherence to treatment plans and improved outcomes. By using language models, it is possible to produce patient education materials that are easy to comprehend and accessible to a range of patients. They can be used to generate individualized health recommendations and provide patients with real-time feedback on their health based on patient data. An example of educational material about heart failure is seen in Figure 5. These responses can be tailored to patients' specific education levels, interests, and prognoses. By utilizing language models, healthcare providers can provide patients with appropriate personalized explanations and written materials compared to utilizing a general text for all patients.

AI can also be used to develop chatbots or other conversational interfaces that can interact with patients and answer their questions in real time. For example, a patient with a heart condition could interact with a chatbot that provides information about their specific condition, medication, and lifestyle recommendations. The chatbot could also offer reminders for medications or appointments, which could help patients adhere to their treatment plans and manage their condition more effectively.

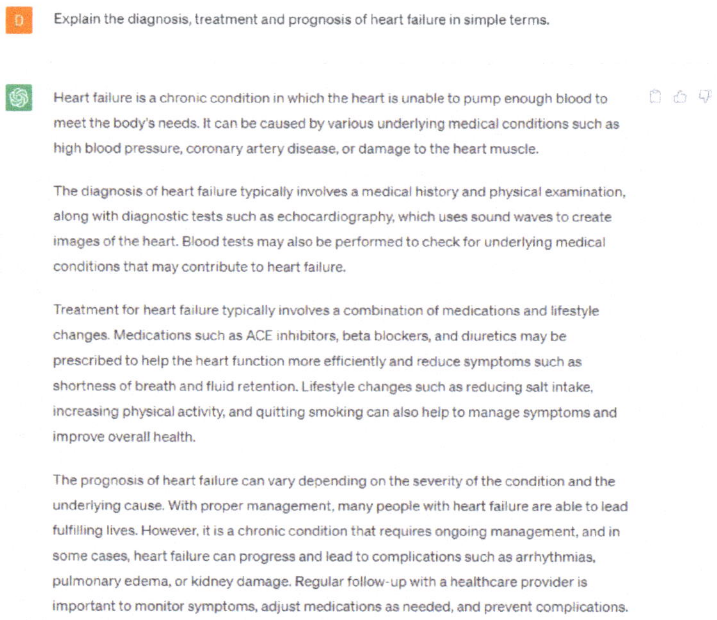

Figure 5. A response from ChatGPT-4 for the question "Explain the diagnosis, treatment, and prognosis of heart failure in simple terms" [15].

In addition, AI and language models can analyze patient data to identify patterns and provide proactive recommendations for lifestyle modifications [18]. For example, a language model could analyze a patient's medical records and lifestyle data to identify factors that contribute to their cardiovascular disease risk, such as smoking, obesity, or lack of exercise. The model could then provide personalized recommendations for diet and exercise modifications, which could help patients improve their cardiovascular health.

There are some pitfalls that healthcare providers need to understand when using language models. There is a chance that language models may provide inaccurate or irrelevant information which can lead to misunderstanding or misinterpretation of medical information. Language models may also struggle to provide information in different languages, and these will need to be verified by a medical translator before providing it to the patient. Lastly, language models may also be limited by their inability to account for an individual patient's unique needs and preferences. It is essential that any material generated through the use of AI be reviewed by an appropriately credentialed provider to assure accuracy.

2.3. Medical Education and Training

AI and language models can also help in medical education and training in the field of cardiology. These technologies can analyze large amounts of medical data and provide insights and recommendations to healthcare professionals, enabling them to make more accurate diagnoses and treatment decisions. One way that AI and language models can help in medical education and training in cardiology is by providing access to educational materials and resources. For example, a language model could analyze medical textbooks, research papers, and other resources to provide healthcare professionals with the latest information about cardiovascular conditions and treatment options. This could help clinicians stay up-to-date on the latest advances in cardiology and provide the best possible care to their patients.

AI can also be used to develop virtual training tools and simulations for healthcare professionals. For example, a virtual training tool could simulate a patient with a cardiac condition and allow healthcare professionals to practice diagnosing and treating the condition in a realistic setting. This could help clinicians develop their skills and improve their confidence in managing cardiovascular conditions. Language models can be used to create educational materials for medical students and healthcare professionals. By simulating real-world clinical scenarios, they can help train medical professionals to make more accurate diagnoses and treatment decisions. Language models are able to create simulated cases and questions for varying levels of training in the healthcare field. An example case created by ChatGPT-4 is shown in Figure 6. Additionally, ChatGPT-4 was able to generate three questions about the case for different levels of training such as medical students, residents, and cardiology fellows. ChatGPT-4 also provided answers for all of those questions (Figure 7). The case and the follow-up questions generated by ChatGPT-4 were appropriate in terms of context and the various levels of training.

In addition, AI and language models can analyze patient data to identify patterns and provide insights into the most effective treatment options for specific cardiovascular conditions. This could help healthcare professionals develop more effective treatment plans and improve patient outcomes. For example, a language model could analyze patient data to identify the most effective medications and dosages for a patient with heart failure.

There are limitations to the use of language models in education. Language models may not be able to provide the same level of hands-on experience and exposure to real-world clinical scenarios compared to traditional teaching models. Language models may also have difficulty accounting for cultural or contextual factors that may influence medical practice and patient outcomes.

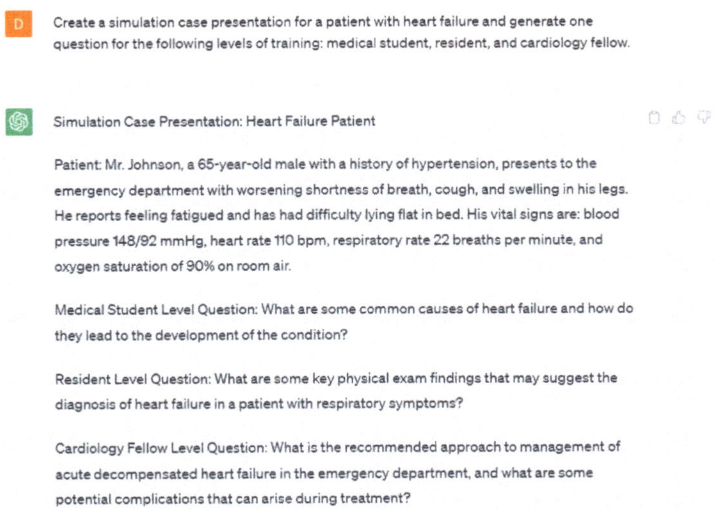
D
Create a simulation case presentation for a patient with heart failure and generate one question for the following levels of training: medical student, resident, and cardiology fellow.

Simulation Case Presentation: Heart Failure Patient

Patient: Mr. Johnson, a 65-year-old male with a history of hypertension, presents to the emergency department with worsening shortness of breath, cough, and swelling in his legs. He reports feeling fatigued and has had difficulty lying flat in bed. His vital signs are: blood pressure 148/92 mmHg, heart rate 110 bpm, respiratory rate 22 breaths per minute, and oxygen saturation of 90% on room air.

Medical Student Level Question: What are some common causes of heart failure and how do they lead to the development of the condition?

Resident Level Question: What are some key physical exam findings that may suggest the diagnosis of heart failure in a patient with respiratory symptoms?

Cardiology Fellow Level Question: What is the recommended approach to management of acute decompensated heart failure in the emergency department, and what are some potential complications that can arise during treatment?

Figure 6. A response from ChatGPT-4 for the question "Create a simulation case presentation for a patient with heart failure and generate one question for the following levels of training: medical student, resident, and cardiology fellow" [15].

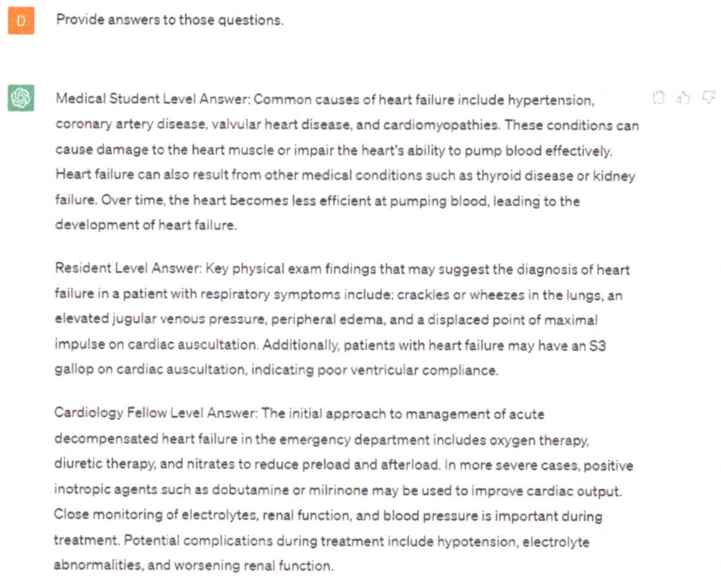

Figure 7. A response from ChatGPT-4 for the question "Provide answers to those questions" [15].

2.4. *Streamlining Administrative Tasks*

AI and language models can also help streamline administrative tasks in the field of cardiology. By automating routine administrative tasks, these technologies can free up time for healthcare professionals to focus on patient care and improve efficiency in healthcare operations.

One way that AI and language models can help streamline administrative tasks in cardiology is by automating documentation and record-keeping. For example, a language model could be used to automatically transcribe physician notes and patient medical records, reducing the need for manual data entry and allowing healthcare professionals to spend more time with their patients. This could also improve accuracy and reduce the risk of errors in patient records.

Generative AI will be able to offload many medical provider tasks that have robbed healthcare providers of their central role of interacting with our patients on a humanistic level [19]. The never-ending task of composition and completion of medical records for appropriate documentation is an essential endeavor and will be augmented and improved by utilizing AI. AI can be utilized to update progress notes, summarize the results of various tests, and write discharge summaries. An example discharge summary written by ChatGPT-4 is in Figure 8. Although, the discharge summary was appropriate, ChatGPT-4 added additional information that was not provided in the input. This may lead to misleading information and healthcare providers need to be aware of these flaws. This can potentially be prevented by providing in-depth input that includes all the essential information and training ChatGPT-4 to avoid adding additional information.

Additionally, other regulatory and required tasks such as obtaining pre-approvals and filing appeals for medical care will be made easier for providers by utilizing generative AI. The automation of these tasks will allow physicians to spend more time caring for patients and improving patient outcomes.

Another great area of benefit will be in the gathering, synthesis, and summarization of ever-increasing amounts of data for each patient to make sure nothing is missed in the consideration of the differential diagnosis [20,21]. By freeing up providers from these and many more time-consuming and low-value tasks, care providers will be able to focus more attention on patient interaction through the ideal gathering of an appropriate history and performance of a complete physical exam. By focusing on this, maintenance of the emotional intelligence central to the humanistic approach in medicine is assured. Additionally, assuring a collaborative healthcare environment for interprofessional teams requires optimal communication, role clarification, and optimal relationships between team members [22,23]. These qualities require time to develop.

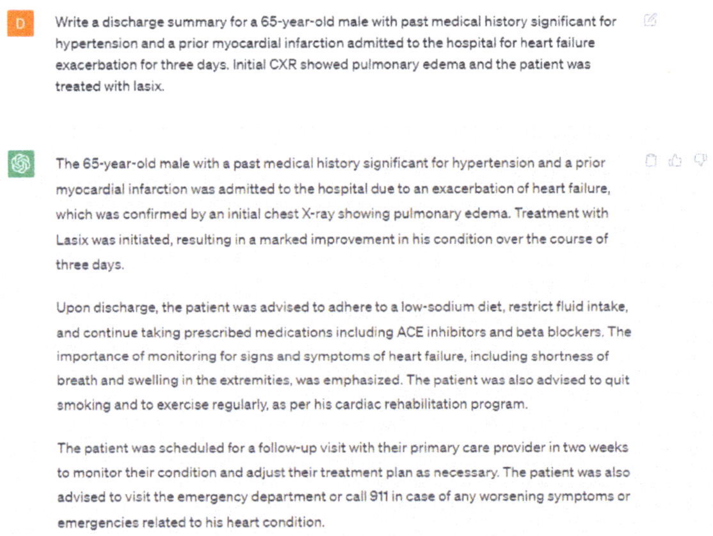

Figure 8. A response from ChatGPT-4 for the question "Write a discharge summary for a 65-year-old male with a past medical history significant for hypertension and a prior myocardial infarction admitted to the hospital for heart failure exacerbation for three days. Initial CXR showed pulmonary edema and the patient was treated with Lasix" [15].

AI can also be used to develop predictive analytics tools that can help healthcare organizations better manage patient populations. For example, a predictive analytics tool could analyze patient data and identify those who are at high risk of developing cardiovascular disease. Healthcare organizations can then proactively reach out to these patients with preventative care measures, such as lifestyle recommendations and early interventions, before their conditions worsen. In addition, AI and language models can help improve communication and collaboration between healthcare professionals. For example, a language model could be used to automatically schedule appointments, coordinate patient care between different healthcare providers, and manage electronic health records. This could improve efficiency and reduce the risk of miscommunication between healthcare professionals.

3. Discussion

ChatGPT-4, especially when used with chatbots, is the perfect tool for human-machine conversations because of its ability to generate meaningful text. In this manuscript, we demonstrate how ChatGPT-4 can be used within the field of cardiology [15]. The use of language models and AI in medicine has the potential to enhance physician productivity and improve patient outcomes. The diagnosis and management of various cardiovascular diseases could be aided by AI and language models in the field of cardiology. To gain insights into the diagnosis and treatment of conditions, language models can analyze enormous amounts of patient data, including medical records, test results, and clinical observations [24]. By identifying patients who are most likely to develop particular cardiac diseases, language models can help medical professionals in the early diagnosis and treatment of cardiac conditions [25,26]. They can assist in identifying potential red flag symptoms that may require urgent treatment and instruct healthcare professionals on the right questions to ask patients during consultations.

In cardiology, the use of language models can help with medical diagnosis and decision-making [27,28]. By examining the patient's symptoms, medical history, and other pertinent data, they can aid healthcare professionals in reducing the number of potential diagnoses and making suitable treatment recommendations. AI can also assure that the diagnostic imaging performed on cardiology patients is scrutinized and evaluated appropriately [29]. Additionally, language models can be used to create patient education materials that are simple to understand and useful for a variety of patients.

Although AI and language models have several benefits in clinical practice, it is important to acknowledge and address the limitations of their use. One concern is that these technologies might not always reflect the most up-to-date scientific information and may offer out-of-date information. Secondly, the cost of AI tools may result in higher healthcare expenditures and less accessibility for the general public [30]. Since some patients might feel uncomfortable if their care is solely determined by computer-driven recommendations, it's also crucial to take the doctor-patient relationship into account. Additionally, due to inadequate representation in the training data, language models may not have the necessary knowledge in cases involving uncommon pathologies or presentations [31,32]. As a result, healthcare professionals must be cautious when utilizing AI, use their clinical judgment, and interpret the language model's recommendations in light of the particular circumstances surrounding each patient.

It is important to acknowledge both the strengths and weaknesses of AI in cardiology. By reducing the number of possible diagnoses and offering suggested treatments, language models like ChatGPT-4 can help medical professionals in diagnosing and treating patients [16]. Large patient data sets are processed efficiently and expertly by language models, allowing them to identify associations and provide insightful information. Healthcare providers can increase productivity and improve decision-making by making use of AI capabilities [33]. However, it is imperative to keep in mind that AI should not replace the role of healthcare professionals. In order to provide patients with the best care possible, clinical judgment and the human touch are still crucial. While language models are capable of data analysis, they might ignore the contextual factors that affect treatment choices. A balance must be struck between using AI as a tool to support clinical expertise and providing healthcare professionals with insightful information while ensuring that final decisions are made jointly by healthcare providers and patients. Maintaining trust and preserving the doctor-patient relationship are facilitated by open discussions about the role of AI in healthcare and transparency with patients, which ultimately results in safe, efficient, and individualized care.

Language models are powerful tools that have been trained using vast amounts of data to understand and generate human language. The quality and quantity of the data they are trained on, however, have a limit on how accurate and useful their predictions or recommendations can be. In the case of language models used in healthcare, the data used to train them is frequently restricted to electronic health records (EHRs) or medical literature, which may not accurately capture the entire scope of clinical practice or the complexity of individual patients. These restrictions could lead to bias in language models or a failure to consider all relevant factors that might influence a patient's diagnosis or course of treatment. For example, language models may not have access to all relevant lab results, imaging studies, or other diagnostic tests, which can be critical in making an accurate diagnosis. Additionally, language models may not be able to consider the context of a patient's individual circumstances, such as their medical history, lifestyle, or social determinants of health. Furthermore, language models may be particularly prone to inaccuracies in cases where patients have rare pathologies or unusual presentations. This is because these cases may not be well-represented in the training data, meaning that the language model may not have sufficient knowledge to make accurate predictions or suggestions. In such cases, healthcare providers must use their clinical judgment and expertise to evaluate the language model's recommendations and adjust them accordingly.

The selection of appropriate training data is of utmost importance in generating optimal outputs. In the context of language models, using high-quality and diverse training data can significantly enhance the accuracy and relevance of the generated text. Making sure to use relevant and trustworthy medical data is essential for producing trustworthy and medically sound information when it comes to applications of language models in the medical field, like ChatGPT. The quality and relevance of the training data used have a significant impact on the accuracy and reliability of AI-generated insights. The use of comprehensive and high-quality medical data must be given top priority in the healthcare industry for patient safety. Data from EHRs, peer-reviewed medical journals, and only other reliable sources should be included. AI models like ChatGPT can produce more accurate and trustworthy information by utilizing substantial and comprehensive datasets, empowering healthcare professionals to make wise decisions and give patients the best care possible. The meticulous selection and curation of training data play a vital role in maintaining the integrity and trustworthiness of AI applications in the medical field. It is worth noting that ChatGPT has demonstrated impressive capabilities, including passing medical board exams, which highlights the potential of language models to assist and augment healthcare professionals [34].

It is essential to understand that language models are not a replacement for human healthcare providers. While they can be powerful tools to augment clinical decision-making, they should be used in conjunction with a provider's clinical judgment and expertise. Ultimately, it is the responsibility of the healthcare provider to ensure that the care they provide is safe, effective, and personalized to the individual needs of each patient.

As AI and language models become more prevalent in healthcare, it is crucial that healthcare professionals receive adequate training to use these tools effectively. This training should cover not only the technical aspects of using AI but also the ethical and legal implications of its use. The healthcare professionals who use AI tools must understand the strengths and limitations of the technology, the importance of verifying its accuracy, and how to interpret the results generated by the tool. This training should also include discussions on the potential biases and limitations of AI and how these could impact patient care. Proper training is especially important because improper use of AI technology could have negative consequences for patient outcomes. For example, relying solely on a language model's recommendation could lead to misdiagnosis or incorrect treatment decisions, potentially harming patients. Additionally, if the AI model is not properly trained or verified, it may produce inaccurate or misleading results that could lead to unintended consequences. Another potential risk is the impact of AI on the doctor-patient relationship. Patients may become concerned if they feel that their care is being determined solely by a machine, rather than by a human healthcare professional who can provide a personalized approach. It is essential to note that while AI can be a powerful tool in healthcare, it is not a replacement for healthcare professionals. The use of AI should be viewed as an augmentation of clinical decision-making rather than a replacement for it. Ultimately, the healthcare professional is responsible for the care and well-being of their patients, and they must use their clinical judgment to interpret the results generated by AI tools and provide individualized care to each patient.

The major limitation of this study is that many of the ideas presented are hypothetical and reflect the perspectives of the authors. This is partly because language AI is still in its early stages in terms of its application to cardiology aspects. While ChatGPT-4, particularly when used with chatbots, is a valuable tool for human-machine conversations and generating meaningful text, its specific application to the field of cardiology may still require further development and validation.

4. Conclusions

In summary, language models have a range of uses and benefits in cardiology, including medical diagnosis and decision support, patient communication and education, and medical education and training. These benefits can improve patient outcomes, enhance medical education, and advance clinical research in the field of cardiology. While language models have these positives, there are also several pitfalls and limitations. These limitations should be carefully considered and addressed to ensure the safe and effective use of language models in cardiology.

5. Future Directions

Although language models like ChatGPT-4 have a lot of potential in the field of cardiology, a lot of work needs to be completed to create more precise and customized language models. Future research should focus on enhancing the quantity and quality of training data as well as adding more diverse types of data to language models, such as social determinants of health, wearable device data, and genomic data. This might aid in addressing some of the shortcomings and biases present in language models currently used in healthcare.

The incorporation of language models into clinical decision-making workflow is a crucial area for future research. This would entail creating intuitive dashboards and user interfaces that facilitate access to and interpretation of language model results by healthcare professionals. Further work needs to be conducted on creating more complex algorithms that can produce predictions or recommendations as well as explain their justification. This would promote transparency and trust in language models used in the healthcare industry.

Last but not least, future studies should focus on addressing some of the moral and legal issues that come up when using language models in healthcare. This might entail establishing uniform protocols for the application of language models in clinical settings as well as dealing with concerns about patient privacy and consent. Research also needs to be conducted on creating more thorough methods for assessing the security and effectiveness of language models in healthcare.

In conclusion, even though there are still many obstacles to be overcome, the application of language models in cardiology has the potential to completely alter how medical care is provided. With continued research and development, language models could help improve patient outcomes and enhance physician productivity.

Author Contributions: Conceptualization, A.N.M.; methodology, investigation, writing—original draft preparation, writing—review and editing, and visualization, D.G. and A.N.M. All authors have read and agreed to the published version of the manuscript.

Funding: This research received no external funding.

Institutional Review Board Statement: Not applicable.

Informed Consent Statement: Not applicable.

Data Availability Statement: Not applicable.

Acknowledgments: We acknowledge the use of OpenAI's GPT-4 in the preparation of this manuscript. All work has been cited appropriately.

Conflicts of Interest: The authors declare no conflict of interest.

Declaration of Generative AI and AI-assisted technologies in the writing process: During the preparation of this work the authors used ChatGPT-4 in order to provide insight into language models utilities and responses. After using ChatGPT-4, the authors reviewed and edited the content as needed and take full responsibility for the content of the publication.

References

1. McGrow, K. Artificial intelligence: Essentials for nursing. *Nursing* **2019**, *49*, 46–49. [CrossRef] [PubMed]
2. Davenport, T.; Kalakota, R. The potential for artificial intelligence in healthcare. *Futur. Health J.* **2019**, *6*, 94–98. [CrossRef] [PubMed]
3. Janssen, B.V.; Kazemier, G.; Besselink, M.G. The use of ChatGPT and other large language models in surgical science. *BJS Open* **2023**, *7*, zrad032. [CrossRef] [PubMed]
4. Nadkarni, P.M.; Ohno-Machado, L.; Chapman, W.W. Natural language processing: An introduction. *J. Am. Med. Inform. Assoc.* **2011**, *18*, 544–551. [CrossRef] [PubMed]
5. Madahana, M.C.; Khoza-Shangase, K.; Moroe, N.; Mayombo, D.; Nyandoro, O.; Ekoru, J. A proposed artificial intelligence-based real-time speech-to-text to sign language translator for South African official languages for the COVID-19 era and beyond: In pursuit of solutions for the hearing impaired. *S. Afr. J. Commun. Disord.* **2022**, *69*, e1–e11. [CrossRef] [PubMed]
6. Popel, M.; Tomkova, M.; Tomek, J.; Kaiser, Ł.; Uszkoreit, J.; Bojar, O.; Žabokrtský, Z. Transforming machine translation: A deep learning system reaches news translation quality comparable to human professionals. *Nat. Commun.* **2020**, *11*, 4381. [CrossRef]
7. Lahat, A.; Shachar, E.; Avidan, B.; Shatz, Z.; Glicksberg, B.S.; Klang, E. Evaluating the use of large language model in identifying top research questions in gastroenterology. *Sci. Rep.* **2023**, *13*, 4164. [CrossRef]
8. Zhang, R.; Pakhomov, S.V.; Lee, J.T.; Melton, G.B. Using language models to identify relevant new information in inpatient clinical notes. *AMIA Annu. Symp. Proc.* **2014**, *2014*, 1268–1276.
9. Linardatos, P.; Papastefanopoulos, V.; Kotsiantis, S. Explainable AI: A Review of Machine Learning Interpretability Methods. *Entropy* **2020**, *23*, 18. [CrossRef]
10. Sezgin, E.; Sirrianni, J.; Linwood, S.L. Operationalizing and Implementing Pretrained, Large Artificial Intelligence Linguistic Models in the US Health Care System: Outlook of Generative Pretrained Transformer 3 (GPT-3) as a Service Model. *JMIR Med. Inform.* **2022**, *10*, e32875. [CrossRef]
11. Kades, K.; Sellner, J.; Koehler, G.; Full, P.M.; Lai, T.Y.E.; Kleesiek, J.; Maier-Hein, K.H. Adapting Bidirectional Encoder Representations from Transformers (BERT) to Assess Clinical Semantic Textual Similarity: Algorithm Development and Validation Study. *JMIR Med. Inform.* **2021**, *9*, e22795. [CrossRef]
12. Siontis, K.C.; Noseworthy, P.A.; Attia, Z.I.; Friedman, P.A. Artificial intelligence-enhanced electrocardiography in cardiovascular disease management. *Nat. Rev. Cardiol.* **2021**, *18*, 465–478. [CrossRef]
13. Houssein, E.H.; Mohamed, R.E.; Ali, A.A. Heart disease risk factors detection from electronic health records using advanced NLP and deep learning techniques. *Sci. Rep.* **2023**, *13*, 7173. [CrossRef]
14. Sheikhalishahi, S.; Miotto, R.; Dudley, J.T.; Lavelli, A.; Rinaldi, F.; Osmani, V. Natural Language Processing of Clinical Notes on Chronic Diseases: Systematic Review. *JMIR Med. Inform.* **2019**, *7*, e12239. [CrossRef]
15. Chat Generative Pre-Trained Transformer-4. 2023. Available online: https://chat.openai.com/chat (accessed on 28 April 2023).
16. Eysenbach, G. The Role of ChatGPT, Generative Language Models, and Artificial Intelligence in Medical Education: A Conversation With ChatGPT and a Call for Papers. *JMIR Med. Educ.* **2023**, *9*, e46885. [CrossRef]
17. Ricci, L.; Villegente, J.; Loyal, D.; Ayav, C.; Kivits, J.; Rat, A. Tailored patient therapeutic educational interventions: A patient-centred communication model. *Health Expect.* **2022**, *25*, 276–289. [CrossRef]
18. Shoenbill, K.; Song, Y.; Craven, M.; Johnson, H.; Smith, M.; Mendonca, E.A. Identifying patterns and predictors of lifestyle modification in electronic health record documentation using statistical and machine learning methods. *Prev. Med.* **2020**, *136*, 106061. [CrossRef]
19. Tortez, L.M.; Quinlan, P.S.; Makaryus, A.N.; George, C.; Caruso, V.; Gilman, S.; Ricardo, A.; Fornari, A. The long-term impact of an interprofessional humanistic faculty development programme: A qualitative investigation. *J. Eval. Clin. Pract.* **2020**, *26*, 738–746. [CrossRef]
20. Gupta, M.D.; Kunal, S.; Girish, M.; Gupta, A.; Yadav, R. Artificial intelligence in cardiology: The past, present and future. *Indian Heart J.* **2022**, *74*, 265–269. [CrossRef]
21. D'Costa, A.; Zatale, A. AI and the cardiologist: When mind, heart and machine unite. *Open Hear.* **2021**, *8*, e001874. [CrossRef]
22. Wei, H.; Corbett, R.W.; Ray, J.; Wei, T.L. A culture of caring: The essence of healthcare interprofessional collaboration. *J. Interpro. Care* **2020**, *34*, 324–331. [CrossRef] [PubMed]
23. Rider, A.E.; Chou, C.; Abraham, C.; Weissmann, P.; Litzelman, D.K.; Hatem, D.; Branch, W. Longitudinal faculty development to improve interprofessional collaboration and practice: A multisite qualitative study at five US academic health centres. *BMJ Open* **2023**, *13*, e069466. [CrossRef] [PubMed]
24. Yang, X.; Chen, A.; PourNejatian, N.; Shin, H.C.; Smith, K.E.; Parisien, C.; Compas, C.; Martin, C.; Costa, A.B.; Flores, M.G.; et al. A large language model for electronic health records. *NPJ Digit. Med.* **2022**, *5*, 194. [CrossRef] [PubMed]
25. Ulloa-Cerna, A.E.; Jing, L.; Pfeifer, J.M.; Raghunath, S.; Ruhl, J.A.; Rocha, D.B.; Leader, J.B.; Zimmerman, N.; Lee, G.; Steinhubl, S.R.; et al. rECHOmmend: An ECG-Based Machine Learning Approach for Identifying Patients at Increased Risk of Undiagnosed Structural Heart Disease Detectable by Echocardiography. *Circulation* **2022**, *146*, 36–47. [CrossRef] [PubMed]
26. Kumar, Y.; Koul, A.; Singla, R.; Ijaz, M.F. Artificial intelligence in disease diagnosis: A systematic literature review, synthesizing framework and future research agenda. *J. Ambient. Intell. Humaniz. Comput.* **2022**, *14*, 8459–8486. [CrossRef]
27. Alabdaljabar, M.S.; Hasan, B.; Noseworthy, A.P.; Maalouf, J.F.; Ammash, N.M.; Hashmi, S.K. Machine Learning in Cardiology: A Potential Real-World Solution in Low- and Middle-Income Countries. *J. Multidiscip. Health* **2023**, *16*, 285–295. [CrossRef]

28. Sanchez-Martinez, S.; Camara, O.; Piella, G.; Cikes, M.; González-Ballester, M.; Miron, M.; Vellido, A.; Gómez, E.; Fraser, A.G.; Bijnens, B. Machine Learning for Clinical Decision-Making: Challenges and Opportunities in Cardiovascular Imaging. *Front. Cardiovasc. Med.* **2021**, *8*, 765693. [CrossRef]
29. Patel, B.; Makaryus, A.N. Artificial Intelligence Advances in the World of Cardiovascular Imaging. *Healthcare* **2022**, *10*, 154. [CrossRef]
30. Esmaeilzadeh, P. Use of AI-based tools for healthcare purposes: A survey study from consumers' perspectives. *BMC Med. Inform. Decis. Mak.* **2020**, *20*, 170. [CrossRef]
31. Morrow, E.; Zidaru, T.; Ross, F.; Mason, C.; Patel, K.D.; Ream, M.; Stockley, R. Artificial intelligence technologies and compassion in healthcare: A systematic scoping review. *Front. Psychol.* **2022**, *13*, 971044. [CrossRef]
32. Kerasidou, A. Artificial intelligence and the ongoing need for empathy, compassion and trust in healthcare. *Bull. World Health Organ.* **2020**, *98*, 245–250. [CrossRef]
33. Hazarika, I. Artificial intelligence: Opportunities and implications for the health workforce. *Int. Health* **2020**, *12*, 241–245. [CrossRef]
34. Kung, T.H.; Cheatham, M.; Medenilla, A.; Sillos, C.; De Leon, L.; Elepaño, C.; Madriaga, M.; Aggabao, R.; Diaz-Candido, G.; Maningo, J.; et al. Performance of ChatGPT on USMLE: Potential for AI-assisted medical education using large language models. *PLoS Digit. Health* **2023**, *2*, e0000198. [CrossRef]

International Journal of
Environmental Research and Public Health

MDPI

Review

The Artificial Intelligence in Teledermatology: A Narrative Review on Opportunities, Perspectives, and Bottlenecks

Daniele Giansanti

Centre Tisp, Istituto Superiore di Sanità, 00161 Rome, Italy; daniele.giansanti@iss.it; Tel.: +39-06-49902701

Abstract: Artificial intelligence (AI) is recently seeing significant advances in teledermatology (TD), also thanks to the developments that have taken place during the COVID-19 pandemic. In the last two years, there was an important development of studies that focused on opportunities, perspectives, and problems in this field. The topic is very important because the telemedicine and AI applied to dermatology have the opportunity to improve both the quality of healthcare for citizens and the workflow of healthcare professionals. This study conducted an overview on the opportunities, the perspectives, and the problems related to the integration of TD with AI. The methodology of this review, following a standardized checklist, was based on: (I) a search of PubMed and Scopus and (II) an eligibility assessment, using parameters with five levels of score. The outcome highlighted that applications of this integration have been identified in various skin pathologies and in quality control, both in *eHealth* and *mHealth*. Many of these applications are based on Apps used by citizens in *mHealth* for self-care with new opportunities but also open questions. A generalized enthusiasm has been registered regarding the opportunities and general perspectives on improving the quality of care, optimizing the healthcare processes, minimizing costs, reducing the stress in the healthcare facilities, and in making citizens, now at the center, more satisfied. However, critical issues have emerged related to: (a) the need to improve the process of diffusion of the Apps in the hands of citizens, with better design, validation, standardization, and cybersecurity; (b) the need for better attention paid to medico-legal and ethical issues; and (c) the need for the stabilization of international and national regulations. Targeted agreement initiatives, such as position statements, guidelines, and/or consensus initiatives, are needed to ensure a better result for all, along with the design of both specific plans and shared workflows.

Keywords: telemedicine; mobile health; remote monitoring digital solutions; dermatology; medical device; teledermatology; App; self-care; artificial intelligence; survey

1. Introduction

1.1. Background

The application of the principles of telemedicine to dermatology is referred to as teledermatology. Historically, teledermatology (TD) has been classified into *real-time* (RT) TD and *store-and-forward* (SaF) TD [1]. SaF TD allows a patient to contact the dermatologists through asynchronous consultations; this reduces the wait time to have a meeting. RT TD is also frequently used in dermatology, using video channels for the interaction between the patient and the doctors.

Since 1995, there has been a pseudo-exponential growth in the use of TD. It is documented by the very high scientific production trend in this area. The number of publications is well over one thousand to date [2]. Its use has an important impact on the perceived quality of the service delivery. It has the potential to improve the relationship between the patient and the *health domain* in terms of monitoring, treatment, and the process itself. This can lead to an increase in the satisfaction of both the patient [3] and of the other actors involved (e.g., general practitioners, specialists, assistants [4]). The COVID-19 pandemic demonstrated that TD could be an accessible, accurate, and cost-effective substitute for conventional *face-to-face* dermatological consultations [5]. Artificial intelligence (AI) has also proven to be, together with other technologies, a far-reaching technological solution during the pandemic [6]. In particular, AI has shown to be of great support in the dermatological field during the pandemic [7].

The combination of AI with TD can bring a synergistic benefit to the practice of dermatology.

TD, on the one hand, thanks to digital health solutions (e.g., *eHealth* and *mHealth*), can reduce distances, avoid travel, and bring treatment directly to the patient's home.

AI, on the other hand, is using increasingly performing algorithms, developed by data science experts. Both AI and TD have advantages from the availability of Big Data. They are useful both for training and for large volumes of digital data access. AI is presenting itself as a technological opportunity with the potential to improve the clinical process, the decision making, and the workflow in dermatology practice.

These considerations lead us to believe that among the challenges and perspectives of dermatology we precisely find the embedding of AI into TD [8]. This is why it is important to focus efforts and initiatives in this area.

Other studies on the introduction of AI in the digital sharing processes of diagnostic imaging in other sectors of the *health domain* have shown a very recent scientific interest. They focused both on the development opportunities and prospects and on the bottlenecks [9,10]. In fact, in addition to the development of algorithms, when facing integration into healthcare, it is necessary to address a series of issues (e.g., acceptance, regulations, standardization, safety, workflows) involving different professional figures. This is happening also in other fields of imaging.

In digital radiology, for example, challenges and opportunities of integration with AI have been highlighted in several studies [11,12], together with important emerging problems [13,14].

Further, in digital pathology, similar studies are also facing the opportunities and problems [14–18].

In view of the rapid technological innovations in the *health domain*, it is strategic to address the same issue in TD as well.

1.2. Problems, Research Question, and Purpose of the Study

The scientific dissemination of TD and AI is available starting from 2018 [19]. Two papers have been published in the years 2018 and 2019, while the other ones are from the year 2020 up to the present. The interest in this topic is therefore quite recent [19]. The topic is very important because applying telemedicine and AI to dermatology could improve both the quality of healthcare of citizens and the workflow of healthcare professionals. This introduction in the *health domain* must address many issues, ranging from the development of algorithms to the regulations implemented. A *narrative review* has been proposed in this study as a practical tool to face this relatively young sector.

The aim of the *narrative review* is to provide a comprehensive overview of the current state of the field, identify opportunities and challenges for integration, and provide guidance for clinicians, researchers, and policymakers interested in advancing this area of healthcare.

The specific aims are, in detail:

- To assess the trends and the evolution of the studies in this field;
- To assess the current state of the art methods in teledermatology and artificial intelligence, including their strengths and limitations;
- To identify the potential benefits of integrating teledermatology with artificial intelligence, such as increased accuracy and efficiency in diagnosing skin conditions, to improve patient outcomes and prioritize cost savings;
- To explore the challenges of and barriers to integrating teledermatology with artificial intelligence, such as data privacy concerns, regulatory issues, and the need for specialized expertise;

- To provide guidance on best practices for implementing and using teledermatology and artificial intelligence in dermatology, including recommendations for data collection and management, model development and validation, and clinical decision-making.

Overall, the subjects addressed in the studies provide a useful idea for both future research directions and, indirectly, to address the current gaps and bottleneck.

2. Methods

The study was based on a *narrative review*. In this *narrative review*, after having defined the research question and sub-questions in the aims, we decided to follow: (a) a standardized checklist for narrative reviews and (b) a properly defined process of review.

The process of review, reported in the algorithm below, comprehended the development of a search strategy.

- The definition of a process of selection;
- The assessment of the study quality;
- A data analysis/synthesis identifying the emerging patterns.

This *narrative review* used a standardized checklist designed for the category of narrative reviews (ANDJ Narrative Checklist).

It is available online at [20]. The algorithm was the following:

Algorithm

1. Set the search query to: "(teledermatology [Title/Abstract]) AND (artificial intelligence [Title/Abstract])";
2. Conduct a targeted search on PubMed and Scopus using the search query from step 1;
3. Exclude conference papers from the search results;
4. Select studies published in peer-reviewed journals that focus on experiences of integration of artificial intelligence with teledermatology;
5. For each study, evaluate the following parameters:
    - N1: Is the rationale for the study in the introduction clear?
    - N2: Is the design of the work appropriate?
    - N3: Are the methods described clearly?
    - N4: Are the results presented clearly?
    - N5: Are the conclusions based and justified by results?
    - N6: Did the authors disclose all the conflicts of interest?
6. Assign a graded score to parameters N1–N5, ranging from 1 (minimum) to 5 (maximum);
7. For parameter N6, assign a binary assessment of "Yes" or "No" to indicate if the authors disclosed all the conflicts of interest;
8. Preselect studies that meet the following criteria:
    - Parameter N6 must be "Yes";
    - Parameters N1–N5 must have a score greater than 3;
9. Include the preselected studies in the overview.

3. Results

3.1. Preliminary Considerations on the Results

All the studies returned by the algorithm had the parameter N6 with "*Yes*" and the parameters N1–N5 with a score > 3.

The search [19] provided 36 components [8,21–54] at the date of this study.

In detail, the components were arranged into four groups:

(1) Twenty-two scientific papers [8,21–40];
(2) One randomized controlled trial [41];
(3) Twelve reviews [42–45,47–54];
(4) One systematic review [46].

The scientific dissemination is available starting from year 2018. Two papers have been published in the years 2018 and 2019; 34 papers (94.45%) have been published from the year 2020 up to the present. It is notable that the increase in the number of publications started with the outbreak of the COVID-19 pandemic. All this highlights that this is a very young scientific sector.

All this shows that the topic is very recent and is receiving significant attention, and that TD and AI, integrated, are offering themselves as an important resource in dermatology, in a wide range diagnosis applications, from skin cancer lesions to sun damage perilesions [23,41].

We decided to analyze *papers* and *reviews* separately.

Separating the analysis of scientific papers from the reviews is a logical and sensible approach. The reason behind this is that scientific papers and reviews serve different purposes and have distinct characteristics. Scientific papers are typically written by researchers who conduct specific experiments or studies to generate new data or medical knowledge (MK). The analysis of scientific papers, therefore, tends to be more focused on the specific research question, methodology, and data analysis, with a strict angle and focus on the research problem being investigated. On the other hand, reviews are broader and consolidate fields by analyzing and synthesizing a large body of the literature to identify patterns, trends, and gaps in the MK. Reviews may cover multiple studies, experiments, or research areas and draw conclusions based on the analysis of the collective evidence. Authors of reviews may also critique the research methods and findings of individual studies, but their main focus is on providing an overview of the field as a whole. Therefore, by separating the analysis of scientific papers from reviews, it is easier to maintain a clear and concise focus on the specific research question being investigated in the scientific papers, while also providing a comprehensive overview of the field as a whole through the reviews. This approach can help ensure that both the specific details and the broader context of the research are properly addressed and understood, especially in this relatively young sector.

3.2. Data Syntesys of the Overview of Scientific Papers

The analysis suggests a possible categorization according to the following emerging fields of interest detected in the scientific papers:

- *The opportunities and the perspectives.* Those studies that have mostly focused on the horizons of the application of TD and AI are included here;
- *The role of the tool and the devices.* The studies that have addressed the topic by focusing, in particular, on the tool dedicated to AI are included here;
- *The applications in quality control.* The studies that have addressed the applications of AI in quality control in diagnostic imaging are included here;
- *The integration in mHealth.* The studies that have addressed the integration in *mHealth* (where recently self-diagnosis applied to telemonitoring is gaining ground) are included here;
- *The integration in the health domain: the acceptance, the standardization, and the management issues.* All the studies that have somehow dealt with the aspects related to the integration of the health domain are included here (i.e., those studies that have offered a look at the problems of integration in stable healthcare processes). This topic is broad and includes, for example, studies on accuracy, acceptance, and regulatory and organizational aspects.
- Some studies, in addition to having primarily dealt with one of the issues identified above, have also dealt with other issues that overlap in a secondary way.

Table 1 reports a sketch of the data synthesis of the overview of scientific papers.

Table 1. Table supporting the data synthesis of overview of scientific papers.

	Brief Summary of the Research
[8]	Great opportunities in using TD and AI for remote diagnosis of skin lesions have been highlighted.
[21]	Three key elements in TD and AI have been identified: the role and expectations of AI, the applicability of imaging techniques, and the developments in many applications. These elements offer great help in health and define routine models.
[22]	Important prospects for TD and AI have been identified in virtual diagnosis, research, and development of advanced machine learning models for prognosticating dermatoses and classification, detection, and diagnosis.
[23]	A proposed unified CAD model approach using AI showed to provide both lesion segmenting and classifying at the skin level with high performance and accuracy in imaging parameters.
[24]	External testing was demonstrated essential for regulating the development of machine learning models in primary care settings.
[25]	Important steps in the evolution of the tools that can be used in TD and AI have resumed. In this area, together with new technologies, new approaches and methodologies must coexist with historically consolidated methods.
[26]	An automatic TD and AI tool improved the diagnosis of skin lesions by non-dermatologists, such as nurse practitioners or primary care specialists, with high potential for improving healthcare quality in dermatology.
[27]	Quality assessment tools based on AI could identify criticalities in image quality, demonstrating performance similar to that of dermatologists and improving the TD process.
[28]	A tool demonstrated a quality detection performance like that of dermatologists, allowing an improvement of the TD process.
[29]	AI showed a leading role in ensuring the usefulness of a certain image in TD, and that different solutions for quality assessment require tuning for specific TD applications.
[30]	The use of mobile applications demonstrated the potential to improve the participation in research projects during the pandemic. *Pros* and *cons* have been highlighted.
[31]	A study on the assessment of user satisfaction with a smartphone-compatible application using an AI algorithm was proposed. The results highlighted both a high satisfaction and that the Apps were promising for all the actors of the *health domain*.
[32]	A study in two parts was proposed. The first part highlighted that image postprocessing capabilities varied greatly based on the user and the intended function. Second, technology standards were not always implemented or reported. Critical issues were also detected on the consent procedure and on other aspects of privacy and data confidentiality.
[33]	The second part of the study (se immediately above) highlighted that: the choices of different technical applications of image acquisition were hardly ever proposed in the tools, and users of these applications should consider which tools had standardized functionalities capable of improving the image quality.
[34]	The problem of standards was addressed in a study with specific reference to the reality of the Canadian nation.
[35]	A survey highlighted the belief that after COVID-19 this technology: could be of aid; will not replace but support professionals; and needed specific regulatory measures.
[36]	A survey concluded that the technological innovations, including the use of AI and TD, could contribute to improving and enlarging the use of dermoscopy among general practitioners.
[37]	An AI algorithm was evaluated in a telemedicine setting configured for TD where patients provided images via telemedicine. The study demonstrated that this configuration of the healthcare process was promising both in triage and in the assessment of skin lesions.
[38]	An applied specific tool had very high specificity and sensitivity in TD and AI applications, showing potential to assist the clinical decision-making process.
[39]	The accuracy of two countries in the national screenings in a certain dermatological field was compared. It was deduced that TD and AI could aid in speeding up the early diagnosis of melanoma, making the process easier and more economical without stressing the structures of the health systems.
[40]	A project in progress was summarized. The aim was to: compare the decision taken by an AI-based classifier with that of the teledermatologist, the histopathologist, and other key professional figures. Consequently, to assess the impact on diagnostic and process management decisions including time, costs, personnel, and activities.

Table 1. *Cont.*

	Brief Summary of the Research
[28]	Applications of AI in Dermatology Image Quality Assessment was discussed. AI was was find useful to ensure the clinical utility of images for remote consultations and clinical trials.
[41]	Applications and perspectives on sun damage perilesions were reported, showing strengths and weakness of the applications.

3.2.1. The Opportunities and the Perspectives

This theme has been touched upon, albeit sometimes in a nuanced way, by all 23 papers [8,21–41]. Generally, all the studies converge on the opportunities and general perspectives of the TD and AI in improving the quality of one or more services/applications in the *health domain*.

Three studies have focused on identifying in a specific way the opportunities and perspectives that TD and AI seem to have in the middle and long term [8,21,22].

Liopoys et al. [8], highlighted the important prospects of AI in this area, noting that thanks to the characteristics of learning from imaging obtained in dermoscopy, great opportunities are expected in the field of diagnosis of skin lesions, which thanks to TD can even be performed remotely. In this direction, we also find the studies by Li et al. [21] and by Mahmood [22]. According to Li et al. [21], recently, there are three key elements to consider in TD and AI: there has been a clarification of the role and expectations of AI in TD; there has been an expansion of the applicability of imaging techniques; and the developments of TD have been completed in many applications. According to their predictions, these three elements will have the ability both to offer great help in the *health domain* and to define routine models. Mahmood et al. [22] recognized important developments in this sector with a leading role in prognosticating dermatoses and, of course, in the three stages of analysis articulated in *classification, detection and diagnosis*. The authors foresaw important prospects in *mHealth* in virtual diagnosis and in the research and development of increasingly advanced machine learning models.

3.2.2. The Role of the Tools and Devices

According to six studies, an important role in this area is played by the tools and devices [23–26,30,31]. Four studies investigated this in a specific way [23–26].

Maqsood and Damaševičius [23] proposed a unified CAD model approach using a proposed AI structure capable of providing both the lesion segmenting and classifying at the level of the skin. They showed that their tool achieved high performance with regard to several imaging parameters, including comprehending the accuracy. Escalé-Besa et al. [24] proposed a project addressing the use of AI as a support tool, with the aim of providing an outcome on the AI effectiveness and limitations, highlighting that external testing is essential for regulating the tools in the development of machine learning models in the settings of primary care. Lee et al. [25] revisited the important steps in the evolution of the tools that can be used in TD and AI, highlighting how, in this area, together with new technologies, new approaches and methodologies must coexist with historically consolidated methods. Jain A et al. [26] remarked that many cases in dermatology are often initially valued by non-dermatologists, as with, for example, nurse practitioners or primary care specialists. They proposed an automatic tool based on TD and AI that demonstrated an improvement of the diagnosis by these professionals with a high potential for improving the quality of healthcare in dermatology.

Two studies, which focused on the category dedicated to *mHealth* [30,31], indirectly addressed the importance of wearable devices based on smartphones and Apps installed therein as a secondary aspect.

3.2.3. The Applications in Quality Control

Aspects related to the application of AI in the quality control of the images have been specifically addressed in four studies [27–29]. Quality is a crucial parameter for an effective and efficient TD consultation. The application of AI seems to be, in these studies, promising.

Jaloboi et al. [27] introduced a tool based on AI implementing a quality assessment based on a convolutional neural network approach capable of identifying criticalities in the image quality. The tool demonstrated quality detection performances similar to that of dermatologists allowing for the improvement of the TD process. Montilla et al. [28], in line with the previous study, focused on the topic of quality assessment in TD and demonstrated that AI has a leading role in ensuring the usefulness of a certain image in TD. Mayer et al. [29], also facing the field of quality assessment in TD, proposed a comparative analysis among different AI solutions for the quality assessment, highlighting the importance to tune an AI model for a specific TD application. In addition, Henandez Montilla et al. [28] faced the field of the Dermatology Image Quality Assessment and discussed how AI could be useful to ensure the clinical utility of images for remote consultations and clinical trials.

3.2.4. The Applications in mHealth

Two studies particularly focused on the application of TD and AI in *mHealth*. The study by Hadeler et al. [30] was entirely focused on this topic with reference to clinical research. The study highlighted that, thanks to the boost of research during the pandemic, there has been a great boom in this sector. According to the authors, the use of mobile applications demonstrated the potential to improve the experience of study subjects and physicians and to increase the pool of individuals willing to participate in research beyond the pandemic. However, there were *pros* and *cons* that must be taken into consideration together with system components that are essential. Po et al. [31] also focused entirely on *mHealth* and addressed user satisfaction in the *health domain*. They proposed a study on the assessment of user satisfaction with a smartphone-compatible application using an AI algorithm designed for the assessment of pigmented lesions. The results highlighted both that the parameters related to user satisfaction were high and that these Apps based on AI solutions were promising and have potential for all the actors within the *health domain*. However, it should be noted that all the other 21 studies [8,21–29,32–41] unanimously consider the application in mHealth of TD and AI as a promising future.

3.2.5. Towards the Integration in the Health Domain: The Acceptance, the Standardization, and the Management Issues

Nine studies have specifically focused on particular aspects of the *integration in the health domain*, a core aspect to comprehending the issues of *standardization, acceptance, performance analysis, management aspects* and any other related ones [32–40].

Sun et al. [32,33] proposed a study divided into two parts which addressed the critical issues of the use of TD and AI with reference also to standardization. Taken together, the two studies delivered two important and strategic scientific messages:

(a) Ref. [32] Image post-processing capabilities vary greatly based on the user and the intended function. Technology standards are not always implemented or reported. Critical issues are also detected on the consent procedure and on other aspects of privacy and data confidentiality;
(b) Ref. [33] The choices of different technical applications of image acquisition are hardly ever proposed in the tools. Users of these applications should consider which tools have standardized functionalities capable of improving the image quality.

The problem of the use of standards was also addressed in a study conducted by Lewinson et al. [34] with specific reference to the reality of the Canadian nation.

Some studies have evaluated *acceptance* through surveys [35,36]. The survey reported in [35] highlighted the belief that, after COVID-19, these methods could be of aid, though it did not replace but instead supported professionals; thus, specific regulatory measures were needed. Jones et al. [36] based on a survey concluded that the technological innovations, including the use of AI and TD, could contribute to improving and enlarging the use of dermoscopy among general practitioners.

The accuracy and performance in relation to TD and AI under different perspectives have been investigated in [37–39]. In the study by Muñoz-López et al. [37], an AI algorithm was evaluated in a telemedicine setting configured for TD where patients provided images via telemedicine. The study demonstrated that this configuration of the healthcare process was promising both in the triage and in the assessment of skin lesions. MacLellan et al. [38] demonstrated that a specific tool had very high specificity and sensitivity in TD and AI applications, showing potential to assist the clinical decision-making process. From another perspective, Papachristou and Bosanquet, by carrying out a study comparing the accuracy of two countries in the national screenings within a certain dermatological field [39], deduced that TD and AI could aid in speeding up the early diagnosis of melanoma, making the process easier and more economical without stressing the structures of the health systems.

The issue of process improvements in management terms has also been addressed in a project proposed by Felmingham et al. [40].

Felmingham et al. [40] have proposed a study, now in progress, with the aim to: (a) compare the decision taken by an AI-based classifier with that of the teledermatologist, the histopathologist, and other key professional figures. (b) Consequently, the study aims to assess the impact on diagnostic and process management decisions including time, costs, personnel, and activities.

Two studies, which focused on the category dedicated to mHealth [30,31], indirectly addressed the aspects of integration in the health domain, in terms of problems to overcome [30] and acceptance [31].

3.3. *Data Syntesys of the Overview of the Reviews*

It is important to analyze the point of view of the reviews in this area, as in all the relatively young research areas, in order to also have a measure of progress of the specific research, together with the development of related topics.

In this specific case, it can be observed that the selected reviews did not have the specific task of addressing the development of the integration of TD and AI jointly, which we find were handled as a non-primary sub-research topic. Taking this into account, it is reported that: four reviews addressed the issue by relating it to the impact of the COVID-19 epidemic [42–44,46], also with specific reference to some national realities [46]. Some studies have focused on specific pathologies, such as melanoma [47], psoriasis [45], or occupational medicine [54]. Other studies have addressed the perspectives and issues of incorporating TD and/or AI into the *health domain* [48–53], also with reference to mHealth [51] and to opportunities in disadvantaged countries [50].

Table 2 reports a sketch of the data synthesis of the overview of the reviews.

Table 2. Table supporting the data synthesis of the *overview of the reviews*.

	Brief Summary of the Research
[42]	The use of mobile teledermoscopy (mTD) as a tool to improve communication and diagnosis between physicians, general practitioners, and patients was described. Patients could monitor suspicious skin lesions and send images for teleconsultation with the help of various AI-based Apps. It was highlighted that while this technology offered a promising solution in the post-COVID era, it should be noted that AI algorithms used in these Apps were not specific to dermoscopy, which could lead to problems with diagnostic accuracy.
[43]	The role of technological innovation in various sectors of healthcare during the COVID-19 pandemic, including dermatology, was highlighted. The review reported that technology had enabled the sharing and rapid detection of cutaneous signs and symptoms of COVID-19, resulting in reduced face-to-face visits and cost and time savings
[44]	The development of AI during the COVID-19 pandemic with reference to dermatology was addressed. Research showed that the use of TD and AI was strategic to discern six clinical dermatological patterns with a probable prognostic connection to COVID-19.

Table 2. *Cont.*

	Brief Summary of the Research
[45]	The application of the TD and AI in psoriasis was investigated highlighting: the presence of a high number of Apps designed to help and guide to discern and/or monitor the pathology, and criticalities due to scarce App testing, validation, and publication data.
[46]	The technological efforts to face COVID-19 in South Africa were remarked on in the review. It was reported that, among all the technologies, TD and AI provided an important contribution to the battle against COVID-19.
[47]	The application of TD and AI in melanoma was investigated, highlighting that the novel noninvasive melanoma detection techniques were useful in the early detection of the pathology, as well as several useful pieces of advice on the use of different noninvasive techniques in clinical practice.
[48]	It was reported a map point on the state of the art advances in TD and AI from both technological and clinical perspectives, including the role of AI and web platforms. The review highlighted the benefits of TD and AI, but also identified three limits to its implementation: the absence of clear regulations for TD and AI practice, the need for efficient workflows and plans to better interact with different actors, and the absence of agreement initiatives such as position statements and guidelines.
[49]	The review focused on mobile TD (mTD) and its advantages in the *health domain*, such as low cost, practicality, and user-friendliness. mTD was considered not useful for monitoring chronic conditions that required continuous follow up and therapy tuning. Recommendations include expanding the applications of mTD in other fields and focusing more on the investigation of the role of AI and image assessment in TD.
[50]	The review discussed the advantages of TD and AI in countries with limited resources and complex territories such as in Africa. It highlighted the importance of increasing the volume of medical data to improve the performance of AI models and systems.
[51]	The review faced the potential disadvantages and risks of using AI in TD, particularly in the context of mHealth. The study recommended that satisfactory use of AI in mHealth required high-quality images, easy patient data upload, data exchange for both image upload and results download, as well as robust cybersecurity, and full disclosure of medical reimbursement and medico-legal aspects.
[52]	The study reviewed dermatological applications of deep learning and categorized them into three fields: TD, clinical assessment augmentation, and dermatopathology. It stressed the importance of using standardized metrics for performance assessment of deep learning models and for addressing equity and ethical issues when applying these tools in clinical use.
[53]	The review highlighted the importance of TD as a valid alternative to *face-to-face* visits and a useful tool for tele-consultation, tele-education, second opinions, and remote monitoring. It was also discussed the potential of combining artificial intelligence with TD techniques and medical imaging theory and the legal and ethical issues surrounding these applications.
[54]	The potential of both store and forward TD and real-time TD in supporting specialists in occupational medicine for preventive care and cancer screening was reported. The study concluded that TD could play an important role in the prevention and monitoring of occupational skin pathologies and that Apps, including AI software, could have a strategic role in the self-monitoring of workers in high-risk job positions.

3.3.1. The Impact of the COVID-19 Pandemic

It is recognized that the COVID-19 pandemic has represented a real driving force for AI and TD, as reported in five reviews [42–44,46]. Lee et al. [42] reported how the mobile teledermoscopy (mTD) may represent a strategic tool between the physicians, the general practitioners, and the citizen patients. People can monitor a suspicious skin lesion previously detected at a visit or self-detect suspicious lesions and transmit images for the medical tele-consulting. Authors reported that several Apps based on AI allow this. The authors concluded that this represents an important perspective in the post COVID-19 era; however, it must be taken into account that these Apps apply AI to assess medical images, but the AI algorithms are not specific for dermoscopy, creating problems of diagnostic accuracy. Perrone et al. [43] recalled the contribution of technological innovation during the COVID-19 pandemic in different sectors of the *health domain*. They remembered that, among these sectors there is also that of dermatology, where technological innovation has allowed for the sharing and rapid detection of presumptive cutaneous signs and symptoms of COVID-19 in the context of a drastic reduction of face-to-face visits and with the saving of costs, time, and resources. In line with the two previous studies, there is the review by Goldust et al. [44] focused on the development of AI during the COVID-19 pandemic, with reference to dermatology. They showed that TD and AI were used strategically to discern six clinical dermatological patterns with a probable prognostic connection to COVID-19: (1) the livedo reticularis racemosa-like; (2) the purpuric vasculitic pattern; (3) the chilblain-like acral pattern; (4) the confluent erythematous/maculopapular/morbilliform rash; (5) the urticarial rash; and (6) the papulovesicular exanthem. The authors remarked that there is support of the scientific societies, both in the use of and in generating further medical knowledge around this. Mbunge et al. [46] focused on the technological efforts to face COVID-19 in South Africa. They remarked that among all the technologies, TD and AI also made an important contribution to the battle against COVID-19.

3.3.2. Opportunities in the Field of the Melanoma, Psoriasis, and Occupational Care

Three studies specifically focused on three particular sectors regarding pathologies [45,47,54].

Havelin et al. [45] focused on psoriasis care with three points of view: applications with mobile phones, TD, and AI. They also searched for specific Apps for "psoriasis" on the website www.appannie.com (accessed on 25 April 2023). This review highlighted the presence of a high number of Apps designed to help and guide to discern and/or monitor the pathology. Authors also highlighted some criticalities: only one App had followed a validation testing; very few Apps were clinically tested; and very few Apps made published data available.

Skudalky et al. [47] focused on melanoma in response to rising rates of melanoma worldwide. They reported the novel noninvasive melanoma detection techniques useful in the early detection of the pathology and provided guided advice on the use of the different noninvasive techniques in clinical practice related to melanoma including AI.

Elsner et al. [54] remarked that both the SaF TD and the RT TD could support specialists in occupational medicine, both in the preventive care and in the cancer screening. They concluded that: TD might provide important support both in the prevention and monitoring of occupational skin pathologies and a strategic role could be played by the Apps, including AI software in the self-monitoring of workers with a high-risk job position.

3.3.3. Perspectives in the Health Domain

It is strategic to consider the aspects of integration in the *health domain* in terms of perspectives, opportunities, and problems.

This theme has been touched upon, albeit sometimes in a nuanced way, by all 13 review papers [45–54].

Six studies have addressed this [48–53] from different perspectives with a wide angle of view.

Young et al. [52] reviewed dermatological applications of deep learning and analyzed the current opportunities and problems of the related applications. They categorized the applications into three fields: (i) TD, with the inclusion of triage; (ii) the augmentation of the clinical assessment in the visits in presence; and (iii) dermatopathology. The authors also remarked on the importance of the use of specific standardized metrics for the assessment of the performance of the models, as well as the need to face both equity and ethical issues when applying these tools in clinical use.

Pasquali et al. [53] highlighted the importance of TD as a valid alternative to face-to-face visits, and, in general, as a valid tool for tele-consultation, tele-education, second opinions, and remote monitoring. They also discussed the potential of artificial intelligence combined with TD techniques and medical imaging theory. It has also opened up potential legal and ethical issues.

Greis et al. [50] highlighted the advantages of TD use in countries with limited resources and with complex territories, such as those in Africa. They reported that currently there are several projects on TD active in Africa with an increasing use of AI to provide support for doctors. The authors remarked on the importance of increasing the volume of medical data to improve the performance of AI models and systems. The participation of local healthcare providers and of the global dermatological field is, according to the authors, strategic to reach this point.

Blum et al. [51] remarked on the well-known advantages of TD and AI and particularly focused on the potential disadvantages and risks of AI use, as well as on the perspectives on mHealth. They categorized the disadvantages and risks of AI use into: (1) the lack of mutual trust generated by the diminished patient–physician direct relationship. (2) The additional time needed to assess the benign lesions. (3) Absence of enough medical knowledge to detect incorrectly classified AI decisions. (4) The need to contact again the patient rapidly in the case of not correct AI classification. (5) Medico-legal issues due to lack of regulation in this field. (6) The problem of the reimbursement. (7) The Apps based on AI are currently not able to provide adequate assistance based on an image of a positive test for a cancer skin lesion.

They reported the requirements for user satisfaction for *mHealth*: Apps can be applied correctly if the quality of images is adequate, the patient's data can be uploaded easily, data exchange allows for both the image upload and the results download, and medical reimbursement and medico-legal aspects have been disclosed.

Uppal et al. [49] particularly focused on TD. They reported the well-known advantages while also remarking that TD is not useful in monitoring chronic conditions, as this requires a continuous follow up and tuning of the therapy. They also highlighted that mTD has an increasing potential in the *health domain*. It is low cost, practicable, and user-friendly. They concluded with the recommendation to expand the applications in more fields and to focus more on the investigation of the role of AI and in the expertise in the assessment of the images exchanged by means of TD.

Tognetti et al. [48] made a map point of the state of the art advances in TD, both from a technological and clinical point of view, including the role of AI and of the web platforms. They highlighted the enormous advantages. The map point also showed the current limits of the employment of the technology. The first limit is the absence of clear regulations for TD practice. They reported the current lack of a common and clear European regulation for practicing TD, while also comprehending issues of cybersecurity. The second limit is represented by the need to design efficient workflows and plans allowing for better spread and interaction among the different actors. The third limit is a consequence of the previous two; it is the absence of agreement initiatives, with particular reference to position statements and guidelines.

4. Discussion

The topic investigated in the overview, relating to the integration of TD with AI, is particularly complex. In fact, the two technologies historically show, also separated, important complexities in the integration with the *health domain*. *First*, TD inherits the problems of *telemedicine*, *e-Health*, and *mHealth*. These problems, such as the regulation, were only patchily overcome during the COVID-19 pandemic [55,56]. *Second*, AI has a very recent history connected to its integration with digital health imaging (see, for example, the AI in digital radiology and in digital pathology [10]) and with dermatology itself [20,21]. Like any new technology, AI needs to be accepted and standardized in the scope of the applications [32–34,48,51–53].

AI is a large container of technological solutions that aims to make machines learn from their experiences, adapt to new inputs and changes quickly, and perform tasks with human logic. Surely dermatology can benefit from all the components of AI. Many promising solutions applied in a standalone way can be integrated with telemedicine, expanding the potential. In this way, many applications of dermatology will be able to have a wider extension on the territory, incorporating disadvantaged areas, and improving the aspects of service equity in the *health domain*. Many promising uses of AI, ranging from monitoring the efficacy of drugs to even the impact of diet in dermatology, will benefit from an integration with telemedicine [57–60]. For reasons of clarity, it is appropriate to report some of these experiences to make it clear how AI is integrating at 360 degrees with dermatology and how telemedicine could play a further driving role [57–60]. For example, important perspectives have been glimpsed in the use of AI to predict drug efficacy in dermatology [57], applying, for example, two different approaches based on artificial neural networks (ANN)s: the auto-contractive map (Auto-CM) and an unsupervised ANN to study how these variables cluster, and a supervised ANN and Training with Input Selection and Testing (TWIST), to build the predictive model. The use of an artificial neural network to identify patient clusters in a large cohort of patients with melanoma was proposed in [58]. It allowed for a simultaneous analysis of costs and clinical characteristics, both relevant aspects for the health service in the *health domain*. The study reported in [59] is very significant, as it is also linked to aspects of therapy, specifically, to aspects of radiotherapy. This study highlighted how ANNs allow for response prediction in squamous cell carcinoma of the scalp treated with radiotherapy [59]. A very important example of the use of AI in relation to acne (a very common problem affecting young people) is reported in [60]. This study confirmed the link between several dietetic items and acne, highlighting the complex interconnection between dietetic factors and acne, which must be taken into serious consideration by dermatologists [60].

4.1. Added Value of the Review

Several studies based on scientific articles and reviews have separately addressed the introduction of AI and TD into dermatological practice. The narrative reviews are particularly useful in relatively young sectors in the processes of MK construction. In fact, they are flexible in terms of the search strategy and selection criteria, and do not require the inclusion of a formal quality assessment, in comparison to the systematic reviews. Systematic reviews are an important tool, but sometimes they are ineffective to apply in very young scientific fields where there is still little MK. This narrative review intended to make a contribution by investigating the introduction of the two technologies jointly. In particular, the proposed overview aimed to provide added value by acting as a connector between all the specific issues addressed in this field to date.

4.2. Interpretation of Results

The research conducted has revealed how this line of studies is particularly recent [19]. Furthermore, an important driving force was represented by the technological innovations that occurred during COVID-19 [42–44,46]. TD and AI contributed to maintaining both a high quality of care during the pandemic and in the monitoring and detection of some skin pathologies with prognostic probabilities of the COVID-19 disease [48]. This initiated the diffusion of technology which affects all the actors involved in dermatology, including the citizen, and presents opportunities, perspectives, peculiarities, and bottlenecks.

4.2.1. Opportunities and Perspectives

The overview showed various opportunities and perspectives in this area. Generally, all the studies converged on the opportunities and general perspectives of TD and AI in improving the quality of service overall. Specifically, they showed that TD and AI could improve: the quality of care, healthcare processes, the cost savings, the stress in healthcare facilities, citizens' satisfaction, and the care, even in disadvantaged realities (as shown, for example, in a study conducted in Africa [50]). Several studies have documented opportunities in different sectors of dermatology. One of TD and AI 's greatest strengths may be its utility as a triage and monitoring tool. This is critical in the early detection of skin cancer, as it can reduce the number of unnecessary referrals, the wait times, and the cost of providing and receiving dermatological care [23,47,54]. Other sectors of interest in the application of AI have also been highlighted, such as that for sun perilesions [41] and in occupational medicine [54]. In the latter sector of occupational medicine, the authors highlighted how TD and AI might provide important support both in the prevention and monitoring of occupational skin pathologies. They recognized a strategic role of the Apps including AI software in the self-monitoring of workers with a high-risk job position. It is precisely the Apps and their integration into *mHealth* that present great opportunities for the self-care of a citizen who can remotely integrate with the health system [30,31,45,49,51] with high satisfaction, as per the specific survey [31].

The opportunities and prospects for integration into the *health domain* are promising based on acceptance studies conducted through surveys [35,36]. In these studies, conducted through specific surveys, emerged a balanced view on the use of AI (which is considered complementary to human decision making) and an interesting, positive opinion on the opportunity. Important opportunities for TD and AI are also perceived in image quality control. Here, it has been seen that through appropriate tools and models [27–29], it is possible to carry out targeted assessments to guarantee images with parameters suitable for diagnostics.

The integration of the TD and AI has many elements in common with digital radiology and digital pathology. Among these elements, as highlighted in this overview, we find: the improvement of the quality of the service (in all its components), the quality control of the images [27–29], the revision of the workflows, and the need to tackle in a decisive and incisive way the medico-legal, ethical and regulatory issues [48,52,53]. We also find these fields of investigation in digital radiology and digital pathology [18,61]. Even the way of proposing specific and non-standardized surveys in the literature to evaluate acceptance [35,36] is something in common between these three disciplines [61,62]. However, we should consider that dermatology is more patient oriented. In other words, the patient (citizen) is more involved with providing a picture of a lesion/wound. With pathology and radiology, physicians are looking at images provided by a lab, clinic, imaging center, etc.

The real peculiarity of TD and AI, inherited by the dermatology is the possibility of citizens directly using Apps in *mHealth* to access virtual or remote diagnosis and self-care [30,31,45,49,51], in a decidedly stimulating way [31]. This certainly opens many opportunities for TD and AI but also new problems. In both digital radiology and digital pathology, the virtual interaction is, in fact, reserved exclusively for the professionals in a working network connection environment. Table 3 reports in brief the emerging advantages and opportunities of the TD and AI in dermatology.

Table 3. Advantages and opportunities of TD and AI in dermatology.

	Advantages/Opportunities
1	Improved quality of care, healthcare processes, and cost savings.
2	Reduced stress in healthcare facilities.
3	Increased citizen satisfaction and care, also in disadvantaged realities.
4	Early detection of skin cancer, leading to a reduction in unnecessary referrals, wait times, and cost of care.
5	Opportunities in specific sectors, such as the skin cancer, the sun perilesions, and the occupational medicine.
6	Utility as a triage and monitoring tool.
7	Integration with mHealth for self-care and remote diagnosis.
8	Balanced view on the use of AI and positive opinions on the opportunities.
9	Image quality control through appropriate tools and models.
10	Similar elements of process improvement, quality control, workflow revision as in digital radiology and digital pathology.

4.2.2. Emerging Problems and Bottlenecks

The overview also showed some important problems and bottlenecks to overcome.

First, these rapid developments to ensure a better fruition by all should be accompanied by [48]:

(a) targeted agreement initiatives, with reference to position statements and guidelines;
(b) the design of both efficient workflows and plans, allowing for better spread and interaction among the different actors.

Second, synergistic regulatory initiatives at an international and local level are indispensable for these complex systems, which suffer in this area from the same shortcomings of other systems in other sectors [61].

Third, it is necessary to focus on the peculiarities of the use of Apps in TD and AI in the hands of citizens. It is important to: clarify the validation processes [45], pay attention to the aspect of cybersecurity, and carefully focus on the system design, standards, and the completeness of the features proposed to citizens [32,33,48,51].

Fourth, in both *eHealth* and *mHealth* applications, before applying TD and AI, it is necessary to provide for the disclosure of all medico-legal (including reimbursement) and ethical aspects.

Fifth, with reference to Apps for citizens, it is necessary to avoid the risks of so-called self-care (i.e., the citizen controls/monitors themselves in a pathological way and/or does everything by themselves without consulting experts). Table 4 outlines, in brief, the emerging problems and the bottlenecks.

Table 4. Problems and bottlenecks of TD and AI in dermatology.

	Problem/Bottlenecks
1	Targeted agreement initiatives, with reference to position statements and guidelines (including regulations and ethics), to accompany the rapid developments of TD and AI (especially in mHealth) are strongly needed
2	Efficient workflows and plans are necessary to allow for better spread and interaction among the different actors involved in the use of TD and AI.
3	Synergistic regulatory initiatives are indispensable, both at an international and local level, to address the shortcomings of complex systems in TD and AI, as well as in other sectors.
4	It is crucial to focus on the peculiarities of the use of Apps in TD and AI in the hands of citizens. This includes clarifying validation processes, paying attention to cybersecurity aspects, and carefully focusing on system design, standards, and completeness of features proposed to citizens.
5	Before applying TD and AI in eHealth and mHealth applications, it is necessary to provide for the disclosure of all medico-legal (including reimbursement) and ethical aspects.
6	The risks of self-care, where citizens control/monitor themselves in a pathological way or without consulting experts, must be avoided when designing Apps for citizens.

4.3. Limitations

This narrative overview has limitations. This review considered papers written in English and two in German (available via PubMed). The reviews in different languages not available in these databases were not considered. PubMed and Scopus databases were consulted, and only peer-reviewed papers were considered in this review. Databases at a local/national level were not consulted.

5. Conclusions

There is great enthusiasm for the introduction of AI in the healthcare field and, in particular, in TD.

The pandemic provided an important impetus for the integration of AI in TD, as in other fields. The study conducted a narrative review investigating the opportunities, the perspectives, and the bottlenecks of this integration.

Applications of this integration have been identified in various pathologies and in quality control, both in *eHealth* and *mHealth*. Many of these applications are based on Apps used by citizens for self-care in *mHealth*. This is an important peculiarity of TD that differentiates it from other imaging applications (such as digital radiology and digital pathology) with new opportunities but also open questions.

A generalized enthusiasm has been registered which converges on the opportunities and general perspectives of the TD and AI in improving the quality of the service overall, and, specifically, in the quality of care, in optimizing the healthcare processes, in minimizing costs, in reducing stress in healthcare facilities, and in making citizens, now at the center, more satisfied.

However, critical issues have emerged. Particular attention must always be paid on the Apps in the hands of the citizen, in the validation, the design, the proposal of functions, and in the safety requirements for completing the flow image detection up to the diagnosis, in terms of standardization and cybersecurity. International and national regulations have not yet been stabilized. It is always necessary to proceed with clarifications of the medico-legal and ethical aspects, before using a specific tool in a connection. In general, to ensure a better fruition by all, the following should accompany TD and AI: targeted agreement initiatives, with particular reference to position statements, guidelines, and consensus initiatives, and the design of both efficient workflows and plans, allowing for better spread and interaction.

Funding: The APC was funded by Daniele Giansanti.

Institutional Review Board Statement: Not applicable.

Informed Consent Statement: Not applicable.

Data Availability Statement: Not applicable.

Conflicts of Interest: The author declares no conflict of interest.

References

1. Kaliyadan, F.; Ramsey, M.L. Teledermatology. In *StatPearls*; StatPearls Publishing: Treasure Island, FL, USA, 2022.
2. Pubmed Search. Available online: https://pubmed.ncbi.nlm.nih.gov/?term=teledermatology%5BTitle%2FAbstract%5D&sort=date (accessed on 25 April 2023).
3. Santiago, S.; Lu, J. Patient Satisfaction in Teledermatology: An Updated Review. *Curr. Dermatol. Rep.* **2023**. *ahead of print*. [CrossRef]
4. Kriwy, P.; Nötzold, A.; Seitz, A.T.; Berger, R. Akzeptanz der Teledermatologie Ergebnisseeiner Befragung sächsischer Haus und HautärztInnen (Acceptance of Teledermatology: Results of a Survey of General Practitioners and Dermatologists in Saxony (Germany)). *Gesundheitswesen* **2023**. *ahead of print* (In German)
5. Ibrahim, A.E.; Magdy, M.; Khalaf, E.M.; Mostafa, A.; Arafa, A. Teledermatology in the time of COVID-19. *Int. J. Clin. Pract.* **2021**, *75*, e15000. [CrossRef] [PubMed]
6. Mondal, S.; Mitra, P. The Role of Emerging Technologies to Fight Against COVID-19 Pandemic: An Exploratory Review. *Trans. Indian Natl. Acad. Eng.* **2022**, *7*, 157–174. [CrossRef] [PubMed]
7. Ahuja, G.; Tahmazian, S.; Atoba, S.; Nelson, K. Exploring the Utility of Artificial Intelligence During COVID-19 in Dermatology Practice. *Cutis* **2021**, *108*, 71–72. [CrossRef]
8. Liopyris, K.; Gregoriou, S.; Dias, J.; Stratigos, A.J. Artificial Intelligence in Dermatology: Challenges and Perspectives. *Dermatol. Ther.* **2022**, *12*, 2637–2651. [CrossRef] [PubMed]
9. Giansanti, D. The Artificial Intelligence in Digital Pathology and Digital Radiology: Where Are We? *Healthcare* **2020**, *9*, 30. [CrossRef]
10. Giansanti, D. (Ed.) *The Artificial Intelligence in Digital Pathology and Digital Radiology: Where Are We?*; MDPI: Basel, Switzerland, 2022; ISBN 9783036543109.
11. Majumder, A.; Sen, D. Artificial intelligence in cancer diagnostics and therapy: Current perspectives. *Indian J. Cancer* **2021**, *58*, 481–492. [CrossRef]
12. Le, E.P.V.; Wang, Y.; Huang, Y.; Hickman, S.; Gilbert, F.J. Artificial intelligence in breast imaging. *Clin. Radiol.* **2019**, *74*, 357–366. [CrossRef]
13. van Assen, M.; Banerjee, I.; De Cecco, C.N. Beyond the Artificial Intelligence Hype: What Lies Behind the Algorithms and What We Can Achieve. *J. Thorac. Imaging* **2020**, *35* (Suppl. S1), S3–S10. [CrossRef]
14. Giansanti, D. The Regulation of Artificial Intelligence in Digital Radiology in the Scientific Literature: A Narrative Review of Reviews. *Healthcare* **2022**, *10*, 1824. [CrossRef] [PubMed]
15. Niazi, M.K.K.; Parwani, A.V.; Gurcan, M.N. Digital pathology and artificial intelligence. *Lancet Oncol.* **2019**, *20*, e253–e261. [CrossRef] [PubMed]

16. Jurmeister, P.; Müller, K.R.; Klauschen, F. Künstliche Intelligenz als Lösung des PathologInnenmangels? (Artificial intelligence: A solution for the lack of pathologists?). *Pathologe* **2022**, *43*, 218–221. (In German) [CrossRef] [PubMed]
17. Viswanathan, V.S.; Toro, P.; Corredor, G.; Mukhopadhyay, S.; Madabhushi, A. The state of the art for artificial intelligence in lung digital pathology. *J. Pathol.* **2022**, *257*, 413–429. [CrossRef] [PubMed]
18. Giovagnoli, M.R.; Giansanti, D. Artificial Intelligence in Digital Pathology: What Is the Future? Part 1: From the Digital Slide Onwards. *Healthcare* **2021**, *9*, 858. [CrossRef] [PubMed]
19. Pubmed Search. Available online: https://pubmed.ncbi.nlm.nih.gov/?term=%22teledermatology%22%5BTitle%2FAbstract%5D+AND+%22artificial+intelligence%22%5BTitle%2FAbstract%5D%E2%80%9D&sort=date&size=200 (accessed on 25 April 2023).
20. Narative Review Checklist. Available online: https://www.elsevier.com/__data/promis_misc/ANDJ%20Narrative%20Review%20Checklist.pdf (accessed on 25 April 2023).
21. Li, C.; Mun, J.H.; Pasquali, P.; Li, H.; Soyer, H.P.; Cui, Y. Editorial: Progress and Prospects on Skin Imaging Technology, Teledermatology and Artificial Intelligence in Dermatology. *Front. Med.* **2021**, *8*, 757538. [CrossRef]
22. Mahmood, F.; Bendayan, S.; Ghazawi, F.M.; Litvinov, I.V. Editorial: The Emerging Role of Artificial Intelligence in Dermatology. *Front. Med.* **2021**, *8*, 751649. [CrossRef]
23. Maqsood, S.; Damaševičius, R. Multiclass skin lesion localization and classification using deep learning based features fusion and selection framework for smart healthcare. *Neural. Netw.* **2023**, *160*, 238–258. [CrossRef]
24. Escalé-Besa, A.; Fuster-Casanovas, A.; Börve, A.; Yélamos, O.; Fustà-Novell, X.; Esquius Rafat, M.; Marin-Gomez, F.X.; Vidal-Alaball, J. Using Artificial Intelligence as a Diagnostic Decision Support Tool in Skin Disease: Protocol for an Observational Prospective Cohort Study. *JMIR Res. Protoc.* **2022**, *11*, e37531. [CrossRef]
25. Lee, H.; Ramani, L.T.; Parish, L.C.; Lee, J.B. Tools of dermatology: A historical perspective. *Clin. Dermatol.* **2021**, *39*, 555–562. [CrossRef]
26. Jain, A.; Way, D.; Gupta, V.; Gao, Y.; de Oliveira Marinho, G.; Hartford, J.; Sayres, R.; Kanada, K.; Eng, C.; Nagpal, K.; et al. Development and Assessment of an Artificial Intelligence-Based Tool for Skin Condition Diagnosis by Primary Care Physicians and Nurse Practitioners in Teledermatology Practices. *JAMA Netw. Open* **2021**, *4*, e217249. [CrossRef]
27. Jalaboi, R.; Winther, O.; Galimzianova, A. Explainable Image Quality Assessments in Teledermatological Photography. *Telemed. J. e-Health* **2023**. *ahead of print*. [CrossRef] [PubMed]
28. Hernández Montilla, I.; Mac Carthy, T.; Aguilar, A.; Medela, A. Dermatology Image Quality Assessment (DIQA): Artificial intelligence to ensure the clinical utility of images for remote consultations and clinical trials. *J. Am. Acad. Dermatol.* **2023**, *88*, 927–928. [CrossRef] [PubMed]
29. Maier, K.; Zaniolo, L.; Marques, O. Image quality issues in teledermatology: A comparative analysis of artificial intelligence solutions. *J. Am. Acad. Dermatol.* **2022**, *87*, 240–242. [CrossRef]
30. Hadeler, E.; Hong, J.; Mosca, M.; Hakimi, M.; Brownstone, N.; Bhutani, T.; Liao, W. Perspectives on the Future Development of Mobile Applications for Dermatology Clinical Research. *Dermatol. Ther.* **2021**, *11*, 1451–1456. [CrossRef] [PubMed]
31. Po (Harvey) Chin, Y.; Hsin Huang, I.; Yu Hou, Z.; Yu Chen, P.; Bassir, F.; Han Wang, H.; Ting Lin, Y.; Chuan (Jack) Li, Y. User satisfaction with a smartphone-compatible, artificial intelligence-based cutaneous pigmented lesion evaluator. *Comput. Methods Programs Biomed.* **2020**, *195*, 105649. [CrossRef]
32. Sun, M.D.; Kentley, J.; Wilson, B.W.; Soyer, H.P.; Curiel-Lewandrowski, C.N.; Rotemberg, V.M.; Halpern, A.C.; ISIC Technique Working Group. Digital skin imaging applications, part II: A comprehensive survey of post-acquisition image utilization features and technology standards. *Skin Res. Technol.* **2022**, *28*, 771–779. [CrossRef]
33. Sun, M.D.; Kentley, J.; Wilson, B.W.; Soyer, H.P.; Curiel-Lewandrowski, C.N.; Rotemberg, V.; Halpern, A.C.; ISIC Technique Working Group. Digital skin imaging applications, part I: Assessment of image acquisition technique features. *Skin Res. Technol.* **2022**, *28*, 623–632. [CrossRef]
34. Lewinson, R.T.; Vallerand, I.A. The Need for a National Strategy on Artificial Intelligence in Canadian Dermatology. *J. Cutan. Med. Surg.* **2020**, *24*, 428–429. [CrossRef]
35. Sharma, A.; Jindal, V.; Singla, P.; Goldust, M.; Mhatre, M. Will teledermatology be the silver lining during and after COVID-19? *Dermatol. Ther.* **2020**, *33*, e13643. [CrossRef]
36. Jones, O.T.; Jurascheck, L.C.; Utukuri, M.; Pannebakker, M.M.; Emery, J.; Walter, F.M. Dermoscopy use in UK primary care: A survey of GPs with a special interest in dermatology. *J. Eur. Acad. Dermatol. Venereol.* **2019**, *33*, 1706–1712. [CrossRef] [PubMed]
37. Muñoz-López, C.; Ramírez-Cornejo, C.; Marchetti, M.A.; Han, S.S.; Del Barrio-Díaz, P.; Jaque, A.; Uribe, P.; Majerson, D.; Curi, M.; Del Puerto, C.; et al. Performance of a deep neural network in teledermatology: A single-centre prospective diagnostic study. *J. Eur. Acad. Dermatol. Venereol.* **2021**, *35*, 546–553. [CrossRef] [PubMed]
38. MacLellan, A.N.; Price, E.L.; Publicover-Brouwer, P.; Matheson, K.; Ly, T.Y.; Pasternak, S.; Walsh, N.M.; Gallant, C.J.; Oakley, A.; Hull, P.R.; et al. The use of noninvasive imaging techniques in the diagnosis of melanoma: A prospective diagnostic accuracy study. *J. Am. Acad. Dermatol.* **2021**, *85*, 353–359. [CrossRef]
39. Papachristou, I.; Bosanquet, N. Improving the prevention and diagnosis of melanoma on a national scale: A comparative study of performance in the United Kingdom and Australia. *J. Public Health Policy* **2020**, *41*, 28–38. [CrossRef] [PubMed]

40. Felmingham, C.; MacNamara, S.; Cranwell, W.; Williams, N.; Wada, M.; Adler, N.R.; Ge, Z.; Sharfe, A.; Bowling, A.; Haskett, M.; et al. Improving Skin cancer Management with ARTificial Intelligence (SMARTI): Protocol for a preintervention/postintervention trial of an artificial intelligence system used as a diagnostic aid for skin cancer management in a specialist dermatology setting. *BMJ Open* **2022**, *12*, e050203. [CrossRef] [PubMed]
41. Weber, P.; Sinz, C.; Rinner, C.; Kittler, H.; Tschandl, P. Perilesional sun damage as a diagnostic clue for pigmented actinic keratosis and Bowen's disease. *J. Eur. Acad. Dermatol. Venereol.* **2021**, *35*, 2022–2026. [CrossRef] [PubMed]
42. Lee, C.; Witkowski, A.; Żychowska, M.; Ludzik, J. The role of mobile teledermoscopy in skin cancer triage and management during the COVID-19 pandemic. *Indian J. Dermatol. Venereol. Leprol.* **2022**. *ahead of print*. [CrossRef] [PubMed]
43. Perrone, G.; Bilotta, C.; Tullio, V.; Pirrone, R.; Argo, A.; Zerbo, S. Telehealth modulation and new proposals during the Covid-19 pandemic: A literature review. *Clin. Ter.* **2022**, *173*, 489–495. [CrossRef]
44. Goldust, Y.; Sameem, F.; Mearaj, S.; Gupta, A.; Patil, A.; Goldust, M. COVID-19 and artificial intelligence: Experts and dermatologists perspective. *J. Cosmet. Dermatol.* **2023**, *22*, 11–15. [CrossRef]
45. Havelin, A.; Hampton, P. Telemedicine and e-Health in the Management of Psoriasis: Improving Patient Outcomes—A Narrative Review. *Psoriasis* **2022**, *12*, 15–24. [CrossRef]
46. Mbunge, E.; Batani, J.; Gaobotse, G.; Muchemwa, B. Virtual healthcare services and digital health technologies deployed during coronavirus disease 2019 (COVID-19) pandemic in South Africa: A systematic review. *Glob. Health J.* **2022**, *6*, 102–113. [CrossRef] [PubMed]
47. Skudalski, L.; Waldman, R.; Kerr, P.E.; Grant-Kels, J.M. Melanoma: How and when to consider clinical diagnostic technologies. *J. Am. Acad. Dermatol.* **2022**, *86*, 503–512. [CrossRef] [PubMed]
48. Tognetti, L.; Fiorani, D.; Russo, F.; Lazzeri, L.; Trovato, E.; Flori, M.L.; Moscarella, E.; Cinotti, E.; Rubegni, P. Teledermatology in 2020: Past, present and future perspectives. *Ital. J. Dermatol. Venerol.* **2021**, *156*, 198–212. [CrossRef] [PubMed]
49. Uppal, S.K.; Beer, J.; Hadeler, E.; Gitlow, H.; Nouri, K. The clinical utility of teledermoscopy in the era of telemedicine. *Dermatol. Ther.* **2021**, *34*, e14766. [CrossRef]
50. Greis, C.; Maul, L.V.; Hsu, C.; Djamei, V.; Schmid-Grendelmeier, P.; Navarini, A.A. Künstliche Intelligenz zur Unterstützung der Telemedizin am Beispiel Afrikas (Artificial intelligence to support telemedicine in Africa). *Hautarzt* **2020**, *71*, 686–690. (In German) [CrossRef]
51. Blum, A.; Bosch, S.; Haenssle, H.A.; Fink, C.; Hofmann-Wellenhof, R.; Zalaudek, I.; Kittler, H.; Tschandl, P. Künstliche Intelligenz und Smartphone-Programm—Applikationen (Apps): Bedeutung für die dermatologische Praxis (Artificial intelligence and smartphone program applications (Apps): Relevance for dermatological practice). *Hautarzt* **2020**, *71*, 691–698. (In German) [CrossRef]
52. Young, A.T.; Xiong, M.; Pfau, J.; Keiser, M.J.; Wei, M.L. Artificial Intelligence in Dermatology: A Primer. *J. Investig. Dermatol.* **2020**, *140*, 1504–1512. [CrossRef]
53. Pasquali, P.; Sonthalia, S.; Moreno-Ramirez, D.; Sharma, P.; Agrawal, M.; Gupta, S.; Kumar, D.; Arora, D. Teledermatology and its Current Perspective. *Indian Dermatol. Online J.* **2020**, *11*, 12–20. [CrossRef]
54. Elsner, P.; Bauer, A.; Diepgen, T.L.; Drexler, H.; Fartasch, M.; John, S.M.; Schliemann, S.; Wehrmann, W.; Tittelbach, J. Position paper: Telemedicine in occupational dermatology—Current status and perspectives. *J. Dtsch. Dermatol. Ges.* **2018**, *16*, 969–974. [CrossRef]
55. Alipour, J.; Hayavi-Haghighi, M.H. Opportunities and Challenges of Telehealth in Disease Management during COVID-19 Pandemic: A Scoping Review. *Appl. Clin. Inform.* **2021**, *12*, 864–876. [CrossRef]
56. Giansanti, D.; Morone, G.; Loreti, A.; Germanotta, M.; Aprile, I. A Narrative Review of the Launch and the Deployment of Telemedicine in Italy during the COVID-19 Pandemic. *Healthcare* **2022**, *10*, 415. [CrossRef] [PubMed]
57. Damiani, G.; Conic, R.R.Z.; Pigatto, P.D.M.; Carrera, C.G.; Franchi, C.; Cattaneo, A.; Malagoli, P.; Uppala, R.; Linder, D.; Bragazzi, N.L.; et al. Predicting Secukinumab Fast-Responder Profile in Psoriatic Patients: Advanced Application of Artificial-Neural-Networks (ANNs). *J. Drugs Dermatol.* **2020**, *19*, 1241–1246. [CrossRef] [PubMed]
58. Damiani, G.; Buja, A.; Grossi, E.; Rivera, M.; De Polo, A.; De Luca, G.; Zorzi, M.; Vecchiato, A.; Del Fiore, P.; Saia, M.; et al. Use of an Artificial Neural Network to Identify Patient Clusters in a Large Cohort of Patients with Melanoma by Simultaneous Analysis of Costs and Clinical Characteristics. *Acta Derm. Venereol.* **2020**, *100*, adv00323. [CrossRef]
59. Damiani, G.; Grossi, E.; Berti, E.; Conic, R.R.Z.; Radhakrishna, U.; Pacifico, A.; Bragazzi, N.L.; Piccinno, R.; Linder, D. Artificial neural networks allow response prediction in squamous cell carcinoma of the scalp treated with radiotherapy. *J. Eur. Acad. Dermatol. Venereol.* **2020**, *34*, 1369–1373. [CrossRef]
60. Grossi, E.; Cazzaniga, S.; Crotti, S.; Naldi, L.; Di Landro, A.; Ingordo, V.; Cusano, F.; Atzori, L.; Tripodi Cutrì, F.; Musumeci, M.L.; et al. The constellation of dietary factors in adolescent acne: A semantic connectivity map approach. *J. Eur. Acad. Dermatol. Venereol.* **2016**, *30*, 96–100. [CrossRef]

61. Giansanti, D.; Di Basilio, F. The Artificial Intelligence in Digital Radiology: Part 1: The Challenges, Acceptance and Consensus. *Healthcare* **2022**, *10*, 509. [CrossRef]
62. Giovagnoli, M.R.; Ciucciarelli, S.; Castrichella, L.; Giansanti, D. Artificial Intelligence in Digital Pathology: What Is the Future? Part 2: An Investigation on the Insiders. *Healthcare* **2021**, *9*, 1347. [CrossRef] [PubMed]

International Journal of
Environmental Research and Public Health

MDPI

Review

Harnessing Machine Learning in Tackling Domestic Violence—An Integrative Review

Vivian Hui [1,*], Rose E. Constantino [2] and Young Ji Lee [2,3]

[1] Center for Smart Health, School of Nursing, The Hong Kong Polytechnic University, Hong Kong
[2] Health and Community Systems, School of Nursing, University of Pittsburgh, Pittsburgh, PA 15260, USA
[3] Department of Biomedical Informatics, School of Medicine, University of Pittsburgh, Pittsburgh, PA 15260, USA
* Correspondence: vivianc.hui@polyu.edu.hk

Abstract: Domestic violence (DV) is a public health crisis that threatens both the mental and physical health of people. With the unprecedented surge in data available on the internet and electronic health record systems, leveraging machine learning (ML) to detect obscure changes and predict the likelihood of DV from digital text data is a promising area health science research. However, there is a paucity of research discussing and reviewing ML applications in DV research. Methods: We extracted 3588 articles from four databases. Twenty-two articles met the inclusion criteria. Results: Twelve articles used the supervised ML method, seven articles used the unsupervised ML method, and three articles applied both. Most studies were published in Australia (n = 6) and the United States (n = 4). Data sources included social media, professional notes, national databases, surveys, and newspapers. Random forest (n = 9), support vector machine (n = 8), and naïve Bayes (n = 7) were the top three algorithms, while the most used automatic algorithm for unsupervised ML in DV research was latent Dirichlet allocation (LDA) for topic modeling (n = 2). Eight types of outcomes were identified, while three purposes of ML and challenges were delineated and are discussed. Conclusions: Leveraging the ML method to tackle DV holds unprecedented potential, especially in classification, prediction, and exploration tasks, and particularly when using social media data. However, adoption challenges, data source issues, and lengthy data preparation times are the main bottlenecks in this context. To overcome those challenges, early ML algorithms have been developed and evaluated on DV clinical data.

Keywords: domestic violence; intimate partner violence; machine learning; big data; abuse

1. Introduction

Domestic violence (DV) is a significant public health issue that threatens the physical and mental well-being of people around the world. According to the World Health Organization (WHO), strategies and advocacy campaigns to reduce DV have raised public awareness of the issue through media, including online platforms [1]. For example, the widespread use on social media of hashtags (i.e., a word or phrase denoted by a hash sign (#) to identify digital content on the same topic) such as #metoo, #notokay, #whyistayed, and #whyileft has aroused a whirlwind of online disclosure by victims and survivors, who have received emotional, informational, financial, and community support on various platforms such as Twitter, Facebook, and Reddit [2,3]. The DV experience is a sensitive and private topic, normally reserved to face-to-face conversations with healthcare providers and peers, but social media valuably serves as an anonymous platform for people to express their needs and feelings without the guilt or shame associated with traditional in-person interviews [4].

During the COVID-19 pandemic, in particular, the enormity of DV gained broad attention as victims were forced to isolate with their abusers under stay-at-home orders [5,6].

Traditional community centers, shelters, governmental buildings, or even social work services were paused or shut down during the pandemic. Victims turned to social media and other online platforms to express their emotions and concerns and seek help from others [7,8]. Interpreting digital content may offer a viable approach to identify potential victims, who can then be provided with social support. Analysis of social media content has been adopted in various fields to understand the patient population, such as in breast cancer, depression, and people with high suicide risk [9–11]. Extending that, social media could offer an important resource for clinicians, nurses, and researchers to understand the concerns and needs of DV victims and to guide further interventions.

Due to the large volume of text available from social media platforms, machine learning (ML) techniques have been widely adopted to process this wealth of data and analyze them systematically, thereby revealing patterns. ML is a method to learn and predict outcomes from patterns in data [12]. Over the past decade, ML studies have gained momentum in oncology, cardiology, and radiology. ML algorithms have been used in healthcare research across the continuum of early detection, diagnosis prediction, prognosis evaluation, and treatment [13–16]. They have been applied to various health data such as clinical notes, patient narratives, social media data, and patients' free-text answers to questionnaires, with the goals of improving patient outcomes, deepening understanding of patients' psychological conditions, and devising supportive management [17,18].

In this era of rapid technology advancement, there is a need to ground novel work in evidence-based research when advancing the field of ML in DV. However, to the best of our knowledge, current reviews have only examined technology-based interventions for violence against children [19], mental health detection [20], and concerning the challenges and opportunities of ML in general healthcare [21]. Although the application of ML to the DV population has increased over the past decade, no evidence summarizes the current state of science in ML applications in the DV field. Hence, the research questions were formulated as follows: 1. What types of ML have been applied in the DV field? 2. What data sources have been used for ML development and for what purposes in DV research? 3. What ML algorithms have been used? 4. What outcome variable has been assessed by ML? 5. What are the implementation challenges? An integrative review of ML applications in the DV arena will help clinicians and researchers understand how ML can be applied in the field, what data sources there are, what outcomes have been evaluated, and what challenges have commonly been encountered. This study will help clinicians and researchers design future ML applications by improving their understanding of the existing data sources and challenges facing ML applications, as well as generate clinical and policy implications. To those ends, this integrative review paper (1) reviews the current use of ML in DV research, and (2) identifies the challenges in implementing ML in DV research.

2. Materials and Methods

2.1. Research Design

In this study, domestic violence is defined as any type of violence that can happen in a household, including intimate partner violence (IPV), child abuse, and elder abuse. An integrative review is conducted from peer-reviewed scholarly articles on ML in DV research based on the framework from [22]. This review style is the broadest kind of method, covering different research designs, which enables us to fully understand the current state of the science of ML in DV.

2.2. Search Methods

We collected literature from PubMed, PsycINFO, CINAHL, Scopus, and Google Scholar on the application of machine learning in domestic violence research since this review paper is situated at the intersection of DV and machine learning. The rationale behind choosing Scopus and Google Scholar was to extract multidisciplinary research in the field via a natural language keyword search. Since we wanted to examine DV from social, psychological, and health-related perspectives, we decided to include PubMed, PsycINFO, and CINAHL as further search databases, for which we used controlled taxonomies. The key search terms were ("machine learning" OR "deep learning" OR "artificial intelligence" OR "AI" OR "supervised learning" OR "unsupervised learning") AND ("domestic violence" OR "family violence" OR "intimate partner violence" OR "gender-based violence" OR "elder abuse" OR "child abuse") (Table 1).

Table 1. Search strings for different search engines.

Search Engine	Search Strings
PubMed	(("machine learning"[Mesh] OR "supervised machine learning"[Mesh] OR "deep learning"[Mesh] OR "unsupervised machine learning"[Mesh] OR artificial intelligence[tiab] OR Twitter[tiab] OR social media[tiab]) AND ("intimate partner violence"[Mesh] OR "gender-based violence"[Mesh] OR "domestic violence"[Mesh] OR intimate partner violence[tiab] OR domestic violence[tiab] OR child abuse[tiab] OR spouse abuse[tiab]))
PsycINFO	((machine learning/OR supervised machine learning/OR unsupervised learning/OR artificial intelligence*.ti,ab. OR (Reddit or Facebook or Twitter or social media). ti,ab.) AND (domestic violence/OR intimate partner violence/OR child abuse/OR elder abuse))
CINAHL	(TI machine learning* OR AB machine learning* OR TI supervised learning OR AB supervised learning OR TI unsupervised learning* OR AB unsupervised learning OR MH "social media") AND (TI domestic violence OR AB domestic violence OR TI domestic abuse OR AB domestic abuse OR TI intimate partner violence OR AB intimate partner violence OR TI spouse abuse OR AB spouse abuse OR TI child abuse OR AB child abuse OR MH "domestic violence+")) NOT PT dissertation
Scopus	("domestic violence" OR "domestic abuse" OR "intimate partner violence" OR "spouse abuse" OR "child abuse" OR "partner abuse" OR "gender-based violence") ("mobile application*" OR app OR smartphone* OR Facebook OR Twitter OR "social media" OR "cell*phone*" OR "text message*" OR "smartphone*" OR "crowdsourcing" OR "online service*" OR "social media")
Google Scholar	"machine learning" OR "deep learning" AND "domestic violence" OR "intimate partner violence" OR "elder abuse" OR "child abuse" OR "gender-based violence" AND "classification" AND "prediction"

All types of supervised and unsupervised machine learning that are applied to DV were included. Supervised ML refers to building a model with a known goal of prediction or classification, while unsupervised ML works on feature extraction such as themes, topics, or sentiment [23]. This review was carried out in accordance with the Preferred Reporting Items for Systematic Review and Meta-Analysis (PRISMA) framework [24]. The inclusion criteria were use of the ML method to prevent, predict, assess, or explore DV, with the work published between 1 January 2010 and 1 January 2022. This study excluded any articles published before 2010, those neither applying the ML method nor applicable to the DV field, full texts other than in English, and review articles (Figure 1). The initial database of literature was collected and stored in Mendeley, a referencing software manager, to build a collection of scholarly articles. After data collection, we removed duplicates in the Mendeley software using its "duplicates removal" function, and subsequently performed manual screening to confirm the de-duplication results [25]. Abstract screening and full-text extraction were performed manually.

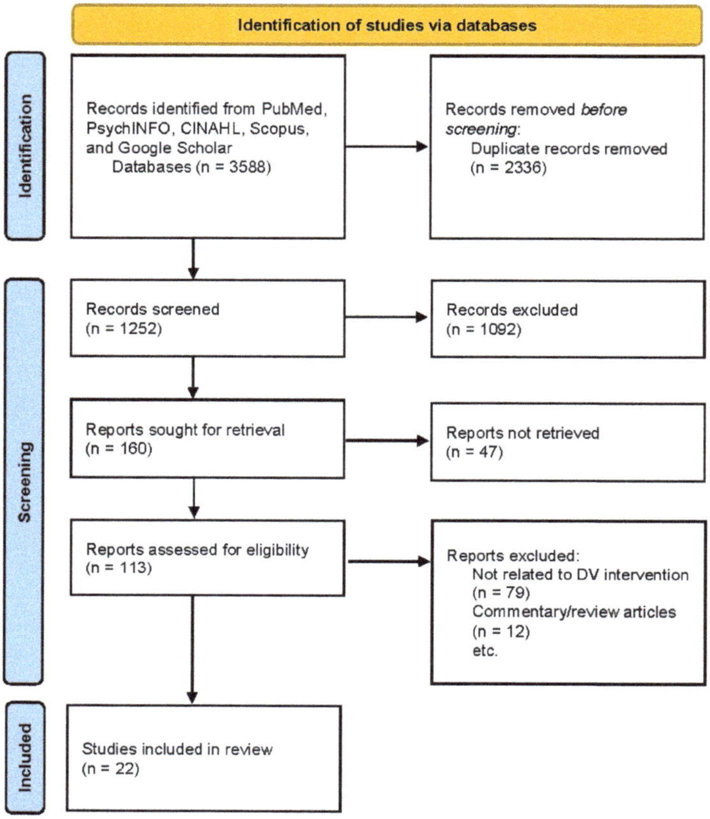

Figure 1. PRISMA Flow chart—integrative review of machine learning in domestic violence.

2.3. *Quality Appraisal*

To maintain internal validity and quality, two authors counterchecked the analysis and results of this study. The first author performed the initial screening based on the abstracts, created the tables and search strings, and synthesized the articles. The third author verified the screening process and counterchecked the result for each variable. Any disagreement was settled iteratively through discussion until the two researchers reached a consensus.

2.4. *Data Abstraction and Synthesis*

Data were evaluated and extracted from online databases with the full text available in English. Data retrieved from the articles included the ML method (i.e., supervised or unsupervised), study group, data source, use of ML, function, algorithm selection, outcome variable, and challenges, as shown in Tables 2 and 3.

Table 2. An integrative review of the included studies (results shown in alphabetical order).

Author (Year)	ML Method	Study Group	Country [1]	Data Source	Use of ML	ML Function	Algorithm Selection		Outcome Variable
							Training	Evaluation	
Amrit et al. (2017) [26]	S and US	Child abuse	Netherlands	Consultation notes	To predict whether a child suffers from abuse using classification models; To implement decision-support API.	Classification	Naïve Bayes RF, SVM	Precision, Accuracy, Recall, F1, ROC Curve	Child abuse case
Amusa et al. (2020) [27]	S	IPV	South Africa	Survey	To classify women based on their likelihood of experiencing IPV.	Classification	Decision Tree, RF, Gradient Boosting, LR Model	Precision, Accuracy, Recall, F1, ROC Curve	The likelihood of women experiencing IPV
Berk et al. (2016) [28]	S	DV	U.S.	Electronic records of arraignments	To forecast the future dangerousness of offenders in over 18,000 arraignment cases from a metropolitan area in which the offender faces DV charges.	Prediction	RF	Confusion Matrix	The likelihood of DV offenders
Chu et al. (2020) [29]	S and US	IPV	China	*Baidu Tieba's* IPV Group	To understand themes for emotional and informational support from IPV by analyzing with automatic content analytics.	Exploration	k-NN, Naïve Bayes, LR, LDA	Accuracy, F1	Themes for emotional and information support of IPV
Guerrero (2020) [30]	S	IPV	Peru	Registered denouncements	To compare the classifier models in order to predict IPV.	Classification	LR, RF, SVM, Naïve Bayes	Precision, Accuracy, Recall, F1	The likelihood of IPV cases
Hsieh et al. (2018) [31]	S	IPV	Taiwan	IPV report form and danger assessment form	To build a repeat victimization risk prediction model.	Prediction	RF	Accuracy, F1	The likelihood of re-victimization
Homan et al. (2020) [32]	S	IPV	U.S.	Twitter	To analyze social media data for the reasons victims give for staying in or leaving abusive relationships.	Exploration	Naïve Bayes, Linear SVM, Radial Basis Function	Accuracy, Confidence Score	IPV victim's reasons to stay or leave the relationship
Karystianis et al. (2020) [33]	US	DV	Australia	Electronic police records	To present the prevalence of extracted mental illness mentions for persons of interest (POIs) and victims in police-recorded DV events.	Exploration	GATE Text Engineering, International Classification of Diseases (ICD-10)	Precision	DV victims' mental illness
Liu et al. (2021) [34]	US	DV	China	Weibo	To explore the short-term outcomes of DV for individuals' mental health.	Exploration	Linguistic Inquiry and Word Count	Pearson's Correlation Coefficient	DV mental health short-term outcome

Table 2. *Cont.*

Author (Year)	ML Method	Study Group	Country [1]	Data Source	Use of ML	ML Function	Algorithm Selection		Outcome Variable
							Training	Evaluation	
Majumdar et al. (2018) [35]	S	DV	India	News (or social media)	To develop a DV face database and a deep learning framework for detecting injuries.	Classification	SVM, k-NN, Naïve Bayes, Random Decision Forest (RDF)	Accuracy	DV face injuries
Özyirmidokuz et al. (2014) [36]	S	DV	Turkey	(TURKSTAT) website	To extract meaningful knowledge from the "emotional violence against women" dataset.	Exploration	Decision Tree	Accuracy, Cross-Validation	Knowledge about emotional violence in DV
Perron et al. (2019) [37]	S and US	Child abuse	U.S.	Child welfare agencies wrote summaries	To better understand and detect substance-related problems among families investigated for abuse or neglect.	Prediction	Rule-Based Model, LR, RF	Global Accuracy, Sensitivity, Specificity	The likelihood of substance-related problems in child abuse
Rodríguez-Rodríguez et al. (2020) [38]	S	GBV	Spain	Spanish national database	To forecast the reports and complaints of GBV.	Prediction	LR, RF, k-NN, Gaussian Process	Accuracy from Root Mean Squared Error and Standard Deviation	The likelihood of GBV reports
Schrading et al. (2015) [39]	S	DV	U.S.	Reddit	To develop classifiers to detect submissions discussing domestic abuse.	Classification	Perceptron, Naïve Bayes, LR, RF, Radial Basis Function SVM, linear SVM	Confusion Matrix, 10-Fold Cross-Validation	Building a classifier of DV content in the post
Subramani et al. (2018) [40]	US	DV	Australia	Twitter	To discover the various themes related to DV.	Exploration	MapReduce, Frequency, Tag Cloud	Precision, Recall, F1	Themes related to DV
Subramani et al. (2018) [41]	S	CA and DV	Australia	Facebook	To develop a framework to identify CA and DV posts from social media automatically.	Classification	Linguistic Inquiry and Word Count, Bag of Words, SVM, Decision Tree, k-NN	Precision, Recall, F1, Accuracy	Building framework of CA and DV content in the post
Subramani et al. (2019) [42]	S	DV	Australia	Twitter	To classify DV online posts on Twitter.	Classification	CNNs, RNNs, LSTMs, GRUs, BLSTMs, RF, SVM, LR, Decision Tree	Precision, Recall, F1, Accuracy	Building a classifier of DV content in the post

Table 2. *Cont.*

Author (Year)	ML Method	Study Group	Country [1]	Data Source	Use of ML	ML Function	Algorithm Selection		Outcome Variable
							Training	Evaluation	
Subramani et al. (2017) [43]	S	DV	Australia	Facebook	To predict the accuracy of the classifiers between abuse or advice discourse.	Prediction	SVM, Naïve Bayes, Decision Tree, k-NN	Precision, Recall, F1, Accuracy	The likelihood of abuse or advice based on the post
Subramani et al. (2018) [44]	S	DV	Australia	Facebook	To identify DV victims in critical need automatically.	Classification	CNNs, RNNs, LSTMs, GRUs, BLSTMs	Precision, Recall, F1, Accuracy	Building a classifier for DV critical cases
Wijenayake et al. (2018) [45]	S	DV	Sri Lanka	Re-offending database	To predict recidivism in DV.	Prediction	Decision Tree	ROC Curve	The likelihood of recidivism in DV
Xue et al. (2019) [46]	US	DV	Canada	Twitter	To examine DV topics on Twitter.	Exploration	LDA		DV-related topics
Xue et al. (2020) [8]	US	DV	Canada	Twitter	To examine the hidden pattern of DV during COVID-19.	Exploration	LDA		DV-related topics

Note: Literature is shown in alphabetical order. S: Supervised, US: Unsupervised, NLP: Natural language processing, C: Classification, IPV: Intimate partner violence, GBV: Gender-based violence, CA: Child abuse, SVM: Supper vector machine, RF: Random forest, LR: Linear regression, LDA: Latent Dirichlet allocation, ROC: Receiver operating characteristic, CNNs: Convolutional neural network, RNNs: Recurrent neural network, LSTMs: Long short-term memory neural networks, GRUs: Gated recurrent units, BLSTMs: Bidirectional long short-term memory networks, k-NN: k-nearest neighbors. Note. [1]. Country was determined by affiliated institutions of the first author in each article.

Table 3. Challenges in implementing machine learning in domestic violence.

Author (Year)	Challenges Mentioned
Amrit et al. (2017) [26]	▪ Moral and ethical challenges ▪ Limited understandability of the model for the end users ▪ Having a prototype based on the prediction model accepted by the end users ▪ Suggestion: option for a professional to provide the model with feedback
Amusa et al. (2020) [27]	▪ Data sources from a cross-sectional survey cannot guarantee accurate predictions due to self-reported responses, recall bias, etc. ▪ The decision tree model is not robust to bias resulting from other essential risk factors that were not included in the model

Table 3. *Cont.*

Author (Year)	Challenges Mentioned
Berk et al. (2016) [28]	▪ The leniency of the magistrates may potentially lead to more unreported DV cases that are difficult to manage without a court order during the post-arraignment period ▪ Limited electronic data availability for DV cases and court documents ▪ The difficulties of obtaining information from jurisdictions in electronic form
Hsieh et al. (2018) [31]	▪ Using a survey may have a lapse of time, and the victim's negative perception toward the violent experience may be reduced over time, which may affect the accuracy of the machine learning model prediction
Chu et al. (2020) [29]	▪ Frequent appearance of words such as "mother", "abuse", and "perpetrator" makes it hard to differentiate between topics (too much noise for topic modeling) ▪ Generalizability
Guerrero (2020) [30]	N/A
Homan et al. (2020) [32]	▪ Bias toward female victims and male abusers ▪ Unique or rare forms of abuse missing ▪ Noise (spam bots, lies by the users, jokes that were missed by filters)
Karystianis et al. (2020) [33]	▪ The police officer's training on mental health and DV is limited ▪ The compliance from the police officers with taking records
Liu et al. (2021) [34]	▪ User information on posts can be inaccurate (fake profile and reports) ▪ Unavoidable subjectivity when judging the posts even with multiple judges ▪ Demographic information is incomplete on social media
Majumdar et al. (2018) [35]	N/A
Özyirmidokuz et al. (2014) [36]	N/A
Perron et al. (2019) [37]	▪ The number of documents that were manually coded was determined almost exclusively by available financial resources ▪ The core training curriculum in the applied social sciences needs to consider the variety of skills and knowledge needed to maximize the value of different types of data (scientific training is important)

Table 3. *Cont.*

Author (Year)	Challenges Mentioned
Rodríguez-Rodríguez et al. (2020) [38]	N/A
Schrading et al. (2015) [39]	■ Annotators had a hard time differentiating the categories
Subramani et al. (2018) [40]	■ Domain experts from DV are needed to analyze the various health problems that were extracted
Subramani et al. (2018) [41]	N/A
Subramani et al. (2019) [42]	■ The annotated corpora in the DV domain are important for ML ■ The annotation process is tedious and laborious
Subramani et al. (2017) [43]	■ Informal language use in short-text messages creates ambiguity ■ The sparsity of instances of specific intent classes creates data imbalance
Subramani et al. (2018) [44]	■ Laborious annotation process
Wijenayake et al. (2018) [45]	N/A
Xue et al. (2019) [46]	■ No information about the gender or demographic information on Twitter users, which limits the generalization of the study findings to the general population
Xue et al. (2020) [8]	■ Twitter data cannot represent the entire population's opinions ■ The search terms used in the study mostly reflect the terminology used by professionals rather than victims when discussing DV

Supervised learning refers to the use of labeled datasets for classification or prediction of outcomes, while unsupervised learning refers to the use of unlabeled datasets for uncovering hidden patterns [47]. The form of learning was determined by the algorithm selected for training and evaluation in the literature. For the ML method, any studies that used supervised learning algorithms such as linear regression, logistic regression, decision trees, and support vector machine (SVM) were classified as supervised learning, whereas studies that used techniques such as natural language processing (NLP), clustering, and principal component analysis (PCA) were classified as unsupervised learning. The challenges in conducting and implementing ML in domestic violence studies are presented in Table 3.

3. Results

3.1. Overview

A total of 3588 articles were identified by the search strings used in Table 1. After the removal of duplicates (n = 2336), the remaining 1252 unique articles were screened based on the title and abstract; of those, 1092 articles were excluded as they were not about machine learning or domestic violence. The remaining 113 articles were assessed for eligibility, and 91 of the articles were removed after screening the full text, while 22 articles met the inclusion criteria (Figure 1).

Twelve articles used the supervised ML method, seven articles used the unsupervised ML method, and three articles applied a mixture of supervised and unsupervised techniques. There was often a DV population (n = 13) in the studies, followed by IPV (n = 5), gender-based violence (n = 1), child abuse (n = 2), mixed DV, and child abuse (n = 1). In terms of location, Australia (n = 6) and the United States (n = 4) were the main contributors of ML research in the DV research field, while the rest of the studies were conducted in the Netherlands, South Africa, Turkey, Sri Lanka, Peru, Taiwan, Spain, and China. Data sources for the articles ranged from social media (n = 12) to professional notes (n = 5), national databases (n = 3), a survey (n = 1), and the news (n = 1). Three types of ML usage among DV studies were identified, and illustrated in Figure 2: classification of the likelihood of DV (n = 8), prediction of future crime or DV (n = 7), and an exploration of themes or hidden topics (n = 8). The top three algorithms used for supervised ML training were random forest (n = 10), support vector machine (n = 8), and naïve Bayes (n = 7), while the most commonly used algorithm for unsupervised ML was latent Dirichlet allocation (LDA) for topic modeling (n = 2). Precision, recall, and the F1 measure were the most popular evaluation matrices for supervised learning studies (n = 13). There were eight types of outcomes assessed among the 22 articles: mental and emotional health (n = 3), substance-related problems in child abuse (n = 2), offenders and recidivism-related (n = 2), victimization or revictimization (n = 5), facial injuries (n = 1), reasons for staying/leaving relationship (n = 1), building a classifier/framework for DV and CA cases (n = 4), and themes and topics (n = 4). Of the 22 articles, 16 were found to be relevant to the challenges of conducting and implementing ML in DV research.

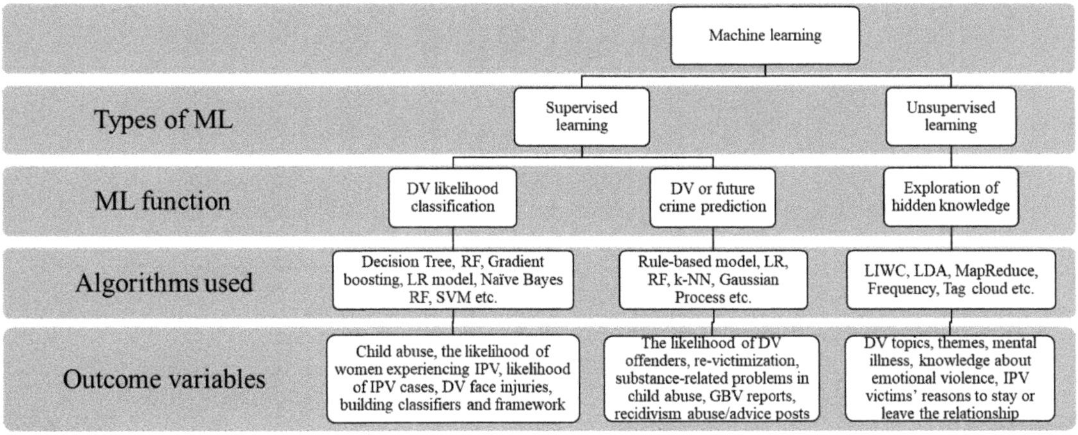

Figure 2. Technicalities of ML application in DV research. Note: SVM: Supper vector machine, RF: Random forest, LR: Linear regression, LDA: Latent Dirichlet Allocation, CNNs: Convolutional neural network, RNNs: Recurrent neural network, LIWC: Linguistic Inquiry Work Count, k-NN: k-nearest neighbors.

3.2. The Current Use of ML in DV Research and the Outcome of the Study

In terms of the current use of ML in DV research, three purposes were identified: classification ($n = 8$), prediction ($n = 7$), and exploration ($n = 8$). As DV crisis support groups have thrived on social media and formed online communities recently, identification of critical posts requires manual browsing to classify people at high risk of DV, which is time-consuming and ineffective with such a large amount of data. Recent research published by Subramani et al. (2018) [44] delineated the steps needed to apply supervised ML to classify critical posts (i.e., posts with emergency needs or red flags on DV) from a Facebook DV support group. Subramani et al. (2019) [42] also published another study on multi-class identification (i.e., identifying multiple classes of terms with the most common words) from domestic violence online posts on Twitter. They constructed the novel "gold standard" dataset from the social media DV crisis support group with multi-class annotation (i.e., manually annotate postings and train the ML model) using supervised ML techniques.

In terms of prediction, Berk et al. (2016) applied supervised ML to forecast the future dangerousness of offenders in over 18,000 arraignment cases from a metropolitan area in which the offender faced DV charges [28]. Another crime prediction study on DV was conducted by Wijenayake et al. (2018) [45]. Their team employed the decision tree approach to predict recidivism among DV offenders. Their results achieved a good prediction under the ROC area with only three features and four leaf nodes, which supported an effective prediction model of recidivism among DV cases.

Apart from crime detection and forecasting, exploratory research is abundant on DV in online forums such as Sina Weibo, Reddit, and Twitter. Liu et al. (2021) [34] explored the short-term outcomes of DV on mental health by collecting data from Sina Weibo. They utilized unsupervised ML to identify an individual's mental health status. Similar approaches have been applied on Reddit to understand the online disclosure of DV and develop classifiers for "abuse" and "non-abuse" posts [39]. Moreover, Xue et al. (2019) [46] used topic modeling techniques on Twitter to understand the DV topics among Twitter users. They used unsupervised ML techniques to identify topics that appear most frequently. Overall, the social media online disclosure of DV has been examined, covering general topics, emergency classification, and mental health state classification.

3.3. Challenges in Conducting and Implementing ML in DV Research

3.3.1. Limited Availability of Data Sources

One of the main challenges to implementing ML in DV has been the data source issue ($n = 9$), including generalizability, reliability, and availability. Studies using a national database ($n = 3$) are mostly cross-sectional surveys, and self-reported responses lead to recall bias or lapse of time issues, which may affect the accuracy of the prediction. As discussed by Berk et al. (2016) [28], limited electronic data and court documents for DV cases can be extracted for ML algorithms' development. Some jurisdictions' records are still in written form instead of electronic. In terms of social media data, Liu et al. (2021) [34] illustrated that the user's information on posts can be inaccurate, and that only incomplete demographic data can be captured from online posts (Table 3).

3.3.2. Excessive Data Collection, Annotation, and Model Interpretation Time

Eight studies reported that the excessive time spent on collecting, annotating, and interpreting data is another critical challenge to conducting an ML study in DV research. Subramani and colleagues highlighted the difficulties for annotators in differentiating the categories [40–44], including the laborious annotation process and agreement between annotators. Similar comments were also made by Liu et al. (2021) [34] regarding unavoidable subjectivity when different judges were judging the data. Social media data contain many daily conversations, which generate much noise. For example, Chu et al. (2020) [29] reported that frequent use of words such as "mother" and "abuse" can confuse researchers, making it hard for them to differentiate between topics, while Homan et al. (2020) [32] also mentioned that noise from spam bots, along with jokes or mistruths from users, are not easily filtered by the text-mining method.

3.3.3. Difficulties in Technology Adoption

In terms of the implementation, four articles ($n = 4$) were included [26,28,33,37], and three issues were identified: end users' acceptance ($n = 1$) [26], professional compliance ($n = 2$) [28,33], and professional training ($n = 1$) [37]. As discussed by Amrit et al. (2017) [26], end users (i.e., nurses and physicians) have limited understanding of the model development or how to apply a prototype (i.e., early product sample) in their work; providing further information in these regards is important to increase the acceptance by end users.

Apart from end users' acceptance, compliance from professionals such as police officers and magistrates was discussed by Karystianis et al. (2020) [33] and Berk et al. (2016) [28], respectively. The leniency of magistrates and non-systematic guidelines for how police officers should take records contributed to the unreported DV cases. Therefore, professional training is critically important to implement ML in DV research. In that spirit, Perron et al. (2019) [37] highlighted the importance of adding scientific training and data science skillsets to the curriculum for social science and healthcare professionals.

4. Discussion

Over the past decade, ML has been used to classify high-risk victims, predict future violent episodes, and explore the hidden themes from victims and survivors among different types of data sources through both supervised learning and unsupervised learning. Given that this is the first wave of ML research in DV, several challenges have been identified, overcoming which may facilitate future research.

4.1. Current Use of ML in DV

4.1.1. Supervised Method

Leveraging ML to predict the likelihood of DV and uncover the hidden themes or patterns from DV are the main goals identified in our review. We found that supervised ML dominates in the development of classification models to predict the future occurrence of DV, re-victimization, and recidivism. This trend can be explained by the difficulties in detecting DV in advance [48,49]. Traditionally, detecting victims has relied heavily on self-reports from victims or reports from healthcare providers after assessing injuries in the emergency room [48,50]. Early detection and screening of DV are time-consuming because those methods involve long-term observation through home visits by social workers, wound nurses, or community nurses. Usually, it is too late to intervene when healthcare professionals identify a suspected DV case from their work. Leveraging ML for DV interventions is not just limited to early crisis identification and classification from digital documents, but can also be extended to legal arraignments and decisions. Apart from assisting healthcare professionals to make clinical decisions, the use of ML in DV research has also improved legal judgment-making from the judicial perspective. Therefore, using ML to classify the level of danger of DV can potentially improve screening efficiency and increase the early detection rate to avoid severe physical injuries or further victimization from DV exposure.

4.1.2. Unsupervised Method

Exploring the themes and topic patterns from DV survivors using unsupervised ML ($n = 5$) was another trend found in our study. Over the past decade, social media has become a mainstream source of news delivery, promotion, and information exchange, where DV survivors can express their feelings and stories to draw public attention to DV anonymously [3]. It has also provided a dynamic source of support for victims, who can seek help and support from each other. Simultaneously, many non-governmental organizations and activists have launched online health promotion campaigns on DV prevention by using hashtags such as #metoo, #notokay, and #maybehedoesnthurtyou [51–53]. Accompanying these trends, many DV stories have been shared and forwarded globally over social media, allowing researchers to explore firsthand stories through text-mining techniques such as topic modeling and sentiment analysis. Since DV cases are underreported, social media sheds light on the need to create more sources of DV information that are beneficial to early detection, prevention, and intervention.

Our study also found that digital professional notes were used as resources for unsupervised ML. With the popularity of digitizing documents for efficient management, different professions are now transforming their written notes into digital notes [54]. In our review, the digital notes included consultation notes [26], electronic records of arraignments [28], police records [33], child welfare agency written summaries [37], and reoffending records [45]. Most of the data sources were from professions that commonly deal with DV such as law, disciplinary forces, social work, and counseling. Surprisingly, our review did not find any data sources from electronic health records (I) or DV shelter databases. One of the plausible reasons is they may contain too much information or they may be restricted by privacy considerations and hospital security policies. The data preprocessing time for clinical EHR data is relatively long and the procedure to request data that contain DV information is complicated due to restricted data availability across institutions. Some records, however, such as wound assessments from emergency rooms, or outpatient clinic social worker assessments that specifically capture the recent injury and family functioning, may arise as sources of data for future data-mining studies. Additionally, traditional qualitative studies in DV mainly recruited survivors from shelters for convenience and privacy protection, which may have limited the number of participants. We expect that more online narratives will become available from shelter websites or support group forums under the trend of self-disclosure encouraged by social media.

4.1.3. Current Outcomes Evaluated by ML in DV Research

In terms of the outcome variables evaluated, our review identified eight types of variables. Building an ML classifier to predict DV cases is the dominant outcome variable. One of the reasons is that screening and early detection of DV have posed a challenging task for decades, and leveraging ML techniques could potentially identify more victims at risk with minimal manpower and time. As DV victims have higher odds of mental health disorders [55], extracting wordings and features for mental or emotional health prediction is reasonable because ML allows researchers to cluster the patterns and identify possible features of multidimensional data. Our review has shown that current outcome variables also focus on a psychosocial aspect, such as the reasons for staying in or leaving a relationship, and legal aspect, such as offenders and recidivism-related issues. This finding is consistent with previous literature regarding the needs and safety concerns of DV victims, where legal help is of the highest priority [56].

4.2. Challenges in Conducting and Implementing ML in DV

An essential issue reported around conducting ML in DV research is the lack of data sources. The availability of electronic records for ML building is a critical component. As reported by Berk et al. (2016) [28], some records are still in a paper format. In certain rural areas, some clinicians and consultants still use a paper format for filing storage [57]. The scanning of documents is labor-intensive, and text identified from handwriting can be inaccurate, which can impede the use of text-mining techniques to retrieve the data. This result aligns with a recent review illustrating how to standardize clinical processes and integrate fragmented records for ML training in healthcare [21]. Furthermore, there are noises and response biases in patient-reported data, especially on social media [58]. Social media research mainly relies on users' posts, and self-reported DV experiences may undermine the reliability and accuracy of real situations. Social media research data should only comprise those that are public, all the posts should be anonymized, and personal identifiers such as specific geographic locations should be removed from the dataset.

We also observed that current study populations were largely limited to DV and IPV, while child abuse and elder abuse were rarely selected for ML. This may be explained by the lack of self-reported child abuse and elder abuse cases on the internet or in digitized notes. Besides the fact that DV and IPV are more commonly reported by healthcare professionals when compared to elder abuse [59], there is also the fact to consider that children and the elderly have not traditionally been likely to share their abuse experiences in person or through online disclosure. However, with increasing computer literacy and the prevalence of technology use, Haris (2014) [60] and Dilci (2019) [61] suggested that the elderly and teenagers may increasingly use social media or online chat box systems to disclose their experiences. The rise of social media influencers or key opinion leaders can contribute to self-disclosure behavior among teenagers [62]. A recent study showed that there was a significant increase in child abuse and DV content generated on Twitter by children during the COVID-19 pandemic [63]. Moreover, since working from home became widely accepted and adopted, violence against family members appeared as an escalating threat to public health [64]. Although the COVID-19 pandemic is thought to have passed its peak, it is expected that online platforms will continue to grow and become the main source of self-disclosure.

Currently, ML is mainly focused on predicting future abuse and uncovering underlying risks, meaning, information needs, and mental health consequences from DV survivors. Attention to the psychological status of DV survivors has only examined short-term mental health outcomes such as stress and depression [34], and future research efforts can be devoted to promoting positive mental change following the traumatic experience of DV. Across the variables covered in our review, few ML studies identified positive mental health outcomes (e.g., resilience and personal growth). One of the reasons for this could be the challenges of measuring the psychological status from big data, which requires a systematic way to interpret the findings, such as an ontology or a dictionary. Similar to the findings from Lee et al. (2020), we note that utilizing social media data to extract emotional needs via ML techniques is challenging [65]. Compared to negative outcomes, positive mental health concepts usually have obscure and inconsistent linguistic features that are not yet standardized. Further studies are required to develop a pipeline to structure and extract this psychological information from the various available data resources. Additionally, using ML models to examine psychological traits, states, and changes can be beneficial for advancing health science research and monitoring the mental health status of patients.

However, it is commonly warned that improper use of predicted results may constitute a threat to the well-being of people.

In addition to the challenges of psychological prediction, leveraging ML techniques in DV research also suffers from limitations. Only two studies found that ML techniques were useful and practical when applied to real-world settings [29,32]. While a model may appear successful in classifying the correct groups and needs, deployment in real-world settings throws up different challenges. For example, computer systems and formats differ between medical institutions and clinics. Aggregation of clinical data across institutions to address semantic interoperability but without clear guidelines and consent from the concerned parties may trigger privacy issues and ethical concerns, as well as posing a risk of data leakage [66]. In addition, the ethics of collecting, storing, and sharing mental health data present another significant obstacle in ML research, as do the degrees of privacy and autonomy afforded to ML systems.

5. Implications

Our study revealed the discrepancies between law enforcement and unsystematic reporting of DV cases. Training among magistrates on how to standardize the reporting procedure in a digital format could offer a chance to remove any leniency and improve the accuracy of ML prediction. In addition, our study showed that there is acceptance by end users in different professions, ranging from police officers to legal magistrates and healthcare professionals. However, we are uncertain whether ML techniques are clinically meaningful and practically useful in reality. It is suggested that including DV domain experts from in the multidisciplinary team, to provide feedback and monitor ML implementation, could be helpful to improve the adoption rate of this technology in clinical settings. For example, the prediction results from ML models can be reviewed by DV domain experts (i.e., medical social workers, nurses in emergency room, community nurses, and lawyers), who compare the results with manual screening to check for sensitivity and specificity qualitatively. In addition, future research could examine the level of technology adoption after implementation and validate the accuracy of ML models in different settings.

Using ML as a method to curate data from digital text is promising in DV research. Most of the current reviewed publications were produced by researchers from the computer science and social sciences fields. Increased training for DV researchers regarding the use of ML and what algorithms are available for them to analyze their data could facilitate greater ML research from healthcare perspectives. For practitioners, ML techniques are impactful for real-life applications in clinics or community centers to identify DV victims from a digital database. The development of cross-reporting systems between multiple community centers or clinics, with ML functions to screen victims who are seeking help online, could better identify DV perpetrators and potential victims in the community. However, the results generated from ML should be interpreted with caution as the current state of the science in ML research uses diverse datasets, which limit the applicability of the outcomes. In addition, considering that the prediction accuracy of ML algorithms is not compared against the usual traditional screening methods, practitioners working with DV populations are advised to interpret ML results with critical judgment based on their clinical experience.

6. Limitations

There are several limitations to this study. First, the scope of this review covers the broad spectrum of ML applications in DV for any country. In the field of nursing and public health, healthcare settings differ, the practices and systems for supporting DV survivors vary tremendously, and so do the characteristics of DV. Accordingly, the use of ML in DV research may not be the same internationally. Therefore, it may not be possible to generalize the conclusions of our study to all countries. While we summarized the challenges of ML application in DV based on the limitations mentioned in each included study, other variables such as the setting, target population, data source, and use of ML were not compared. Hence, future studies considering the challenges of ML in DV research should regard our findings with caution.

7. Conclusions

ML research in DV has advanced exponentially in the past decade. This review provides direction for researchers and clinicians on how ML has been deployed in the field of DV for the classification, prediction, and exploration of DV topics, and identifies the challenges of technology adoption, data source availability, and lengthy data preparation, which were highlighted in previous literature. The development of ML algorithms is still in its infancy within clinical settings due to restricted interoperability between institutions. With ML tools and research funding becoming more accessible, it is expected that ML in DV research will keep expanding, and more innovative strategies will be explored shortly.

Author Contributions: V.H.: conceptualization, methodology, writing—original draft preparation, data curation; R.E.C.: validation, writing—review and editing, supervision; Y.J.L.: conceptualization, methodology, writing—review and editing, supervision. All authors have read and agreed to the published version of the manuscript.

Funding: This research received no external funding.

Institutional Review Board Statement: Not applicable.

Informed Consent Statement: Not applicable.

Data Availability Statement: Data supporting reported results can be obtained on request.

Conflicts of Interest: The authors declare no conflict of interest.

References

1. World Health Organization. Global and Regional Estimates of Violence Against Women: Prevalence and Health Effects of Intimate Partner Violence and Non-Partner Sexual Violence. Italy. 2013. Available online: http://app.who.int/iris/bitstream/10665/85239/1/9789241564625_eng.pdf (accessed on 6 January 2023).
2. Alaggia, R.; Wang, S. "I never told anyone until the #metoo movement": What can we learn from sexual abuse and sexual assault disclosures made through social media? *Child Abus. Negl.* **2020**, *103*, 104312. [CrossRef]
3. Cravens, J.D.; Whiting, J.B.; Aamar, R.O. Why I Stayed/Left: An Analysis of Voices of Intimate Partner Violence on Social Media. *Contemp. Fam. Ther.* **2015**, *37*, 372–385. [CrossRef]
4. Suler, J. The Online Disinhibition Effect. *CyberPsychol. Behav.* **2004**, *7*, 321–326. [CrossRef]
5. Kofman, Y.B.; Garfin, D.R. Home is not always a haven: The domestic violence crisis amid the COVID-19 pandemic. *Psychol. Trauma Theory Res. Pract. Policy* **2020**, *12*, S199–S201. [CrossRef] [PubMed]
6. Hartmann, J. Several Police Departments Say They've Seenan Uptick in Domestic Violence Calls Since Start of COVID-19 Pandemic. WPXI. Available online: https://www.wpxi.com/news/top-stories/several-police-departments-say-theyve-seen-an-uptick-domestic-violence-calls-since-start-covid-19-pandemic/JJLDGXYPJVH3DALTQ3LOFVIODY/ (accessed on 21 April 2020).
7. Lyons, M.; Brewer, G. Experiences of Intimate Partner Violence during Lockdown and the COVID-19 Pandemic. *J. Fam. Violence* **2021**, *37*, 969–977. [CrossRef] [PubMed]
8. Xue, J.; Chen, J.; Chen, C.; Hu, R.; Zhu, T. The Hidden Pandemic of Family Violence During COVID-19: Unsupervised Learning of Tweets. *J. Med. Internet Res.* **2020**, *22*, e24361. [CrossRef] [PubMed]
9. De Choudhury, M.; Gamon, M.; Counts, S.; Horvitz, E. Predicting depression via social media. In Proceedings of the Seventh International AAAI Conference on Weblogs and Social Media, Cambridge, MA, USA, 8–11 July 2013.
10. Kumar, E.R.; Rao, K.R.; Nayak, S.R.; Chandra, R. Suicidal ideation prediction in twitter data using machine learning techniques. *J. Interdiscip. Math.* **2020**, *23*, 117–125. [CrossRef]
11. Nzali, M.D.T.; Bringay, S.; Lavergne, C.; Mollevi, C.; Opitz, T. What Patients Can Tell Us: Topic Analysis for Social Media on Breast Cancer. *JMIR Public Health Surveill.* **2017**, *5*, e23. [CrossRef]
12. Abu-Mostafa, Y.S.; Magdon-Ismail, M.; Lin, H.T. *Learning from Data*; AMLBook: New York, NY, USA, 2012; Volume 4.
13. Kourou, K.; Exarchos, T.P.; Exarchos, K.P.; Karamouzis, M.V.; Fotiadis, D.I. Machine learning applications in cancer prognosis and prediction. *Comput. Struct. Biotechnol. J.* **2015**, *13*, 8–17. [CrossRef]
14. Doucette, J.A.; Khan, A.; Cohen, R.; Lizotte, D.; Moghaddam, H.M. A framework for AI-based clinical decision support that is patient-centric and evidence-based. In Proceedings of the International Workshop on Artificial Intelligence and NetMedicine, Montpellier, France, 27 August 2012; p. 26.
15. Phillips-Wren, G.E. AI tools in decision making support systems: A review. *Int. J. Artif. Intell. Tools* **2012**, *21*, 52. [CrossRef]

16. Hosseinzadeh, A.; Izadi, M.; Verma, A.; Precup, D.; Buckeridge, D. Assessing the Predictability of Hospital Readmission Using Machine Learning. In Proceedings of the Twenty-Fifth Conference on Innovative Applications of Artificial Intelligence, Bellevue, WA, USA, 14–18 July 2013; Volume 27, pp. 1532–1538. [CrossRef]
17. Gorrell, G.; Roberts, A.; Jackson, R.; Stewart, R. Finding negative symptoms of schizophrenia inpatient records. In Proceedings of the Workshop on NLP for Medicine and Biology associated with RANLP 2013, Hissar, Bulgaria, 13 September 2013; pp. 9–17.
18. Wagholikar, A. Automated classification of limb fractures from free-text radiology reports using a clinician-informed gazetteer methodology. *Australas. Med. J.* **2013**, *6*, 301–307. [CrossRef]
19. Hunt, X.; Tomlinson, M.; Sikander, S.; Skeen, S.; Marlow, M.; Du Toit, S.; Eisner, M. Artificial Intelligence, Big Data, and mHealth: The Frontiers of the Prevention of Violence Against Children. *Front. Artif. Intell.* **2020**, *3*, 543305. [CrossRef] [PubMed]
20. Shatte, A.B.R.; Hutchinson, D.M.; Teague, S.J. Machine learning in mental health: A scoping review of methods and applications. *Psychol. Med.* **2019**, *49*, 1426–1448. [CrossRef] [PubMed]
21. Ghassemi, M.; Naumann, T.; Schulam, P.; Beam, A.L.; Chen, I.Y.; Ranganath, R. A review of challenges and opportunities in machine learning for health. *AMIA Summits Transl. Sci. Proc.* **2020**, *2020*, 191–200.
22. De Souza, M.T.; Da Silva, M.D.; De Carvalho, R. Integrative review: What is it? How to do it? *Einstein* **2010**, *8*, 102–106. [CrossRef]
23. Deo, R.C. Machine Learning in Medicine. *Circulation* **2015**, *132*, 1920–1930. [CrossRef] [PubMed]
24. Page, M.J.; E McKenzie, J.; Bossuyt, P.M.; Boutron, I.; Hoffmann, T.C.; Mulrow, C.D.; Shamseer, L.; Tetzlaff, J.M.; Moher, D. Updating guidance for reporting systematic reviews: Development of the PRISMA 2020 statement. *J. Clin. Epidemiol.* **2021**, *134*, 103–112. [CrossRef] [PubMed]
25. Kwon, Y.; Lemieux, M.; McTavish, J.; Wathen, N. Identifying and removing duplicate records from systematic review searches. *J. Med. Libr. Assoc.* **2015**, *103*, 184–188. [CrossRef]
26. Amrit, C.; Paauw, T.; Aly, R.; Lavric, M. Identifying child abuse through text mining and machine learning. *Expert Syst. Appl.* **2017**, *88*, 402–418. [CrossRef]
27. Amusa, L.B.; Bengesai, A.V.; Khan, H.T.A. Predicting the Vulnerability of Women to Intimate Partner Violence in South Africa: Evidence from Tree-based Machine Learning Techniques. *J. Interpers. Violence* **2020**, *37*, NP5228–NP5245. [CrossRef] [PubMed]
28. Berk, R.A.; Sorenson, S.B.; Barnes, G. Forecasting Domestic Violence: A Machine Learning Approach to Help Inform Arraignment Decisions. *J. Empir. Leg. Stud.* **2016**, *13*, 94–115. [CrossRef]
29. Chu, T.H.; Su, Y.; Kong, H.; Shi, J.; Wang, X. Online Social Support for Intimate Partner Violence Victims in China: Quantitative and Automatic Content Analysis. *Violence Against Women* **2020**, *27*, 339–358. [CrossRef]
30. Guerrero, A.; Cárdenas, J.G.; Romero, V.; Ayma, V.H. Comparison of Classifiers Models for Prediction of Intimate Partner Violence. In Proceedings of the Future Technologies Conference, Online Conference, 5–6 November 2020; Springer: Cham, Switzerland, 2020; pp. 469–488. [CrossRef]
31. Hsieh, T.C.; Wang, Y.-H.; Hsieh, Y.-S.; Ke, J.-T.; Liu, C.-K.; Chen, S.-C. Measuring the Unmeasurable—A Study of Domestic Violence Risk Prediction and Management. *J. Technol. Hum. Serv.* **2018**, *36*, 56–68. [CrossRef]
32. Homan, C.M.; Schrading, J.N.; Ptucha, R.W.; Cerulli, C.; Alm, C.O. Quantitative Methods for Analyzing Intimate Partner Violence in Microblogs: Observational Study. *J. Med. Internet Res.* **2020**, *22*, e15347. [CrossRef] [PubMed]
33. Karystianis, G.; Simpson, A.; Adily, A.; Schofield, P.; Greenberg, D.; Wand, H.; Nenadic, G.; Butler, T. Prevalence of Mental Illnesses in Domestic Violence Police Records: Text Mining Study. *J. Med. Internet Res.* **2020**, *22*, e23725. [CrossRef]
34. Liu, M.; Xue, J.; Zhao, N.; Wang, X.; Jiao, D.; Zhu, T. Using Social Media to Explore the Consequences of Domestic Violence on Mental Health. *J. Interpers. Violence* **2018**, *36*, NP1965–1985NP. [CrossRef]
35. Majumdar, P.; Chhabra, S.; Singh, R.; Vatsa, M. On detecting domestic abuse via faces. In Proceedings of the IEEE Conference on Computer Vision and Pattern Recognition Workshops, Salt Lake City, UT, USA, 18–23 June 2018; pp. 2173–2179.
36. Zyirmidokuz, E.K.; Kaya, Y. Decision Tree Induction of Emotional Violence against Women. In Proceedings of the INTCESS14-International Conference on Education and Social Sciences, Istanbul, Turkey, 3–5 February 2014; pp. 847–856.
37. Perron, B.E.; Victor, B.G.; Bushman, G.; Moore, A.; Ryan, J.P.; Lu, A.J.; Piellusch, E.K. Detecting substance-related problems in narrative investigation summaries of child abuse and neglect using text mining and machine learning. *Child Abus. Negl.* **2019**, *98*, 104180. [CrossRef] [PubMed]
38. Rodríguez-Rodríguez, I.; Rodríguez, J.-V.; Pardo-Quiles, D.-J.; Heras-González, P.; Chatzigiannakis, I. Modeling and Forecasting Gender-Based Violence through Machine Learning Techniques. *Appl. Sci.* **2020**, *10*, 8244. [CrossRef]
39. Schrading, N.; Alm, C.O.; Ptucha, R.; Homan, C. An analysis of domestic abuse discourse on Reddit. In Proceedings of the 2015 Conference on Empirical Methods in Natural Language Processing, Lisbon, Portugal, 17–21 September 2015; pp. 2577–2583.
40. Subramani, S.; O'Connor, M. Extracting Actionable Knowledge from Domestic Violence Discourses on Social Media. *ICST Trans. Scalable Inf. Syst.* **2018**, *5*, 807. [CrossRef]
41. Subramani, S.; Wang, H.; Islam, R.; Ulhaq, A.; O'Connor, M. Child Abuse and Domestic Abuse: Content and Feature Analysis from Social Media Disclosures. In Proceedings of the Australasian Database Conference, Gold Coast, Australia, 24–27 May 2018; Springer: Cham, Switzerland, 2018; pp. 174–185.
42. Subramani, S.; Michalska, S.; Wang, H.; Du, J.; Zhang, Y.; Shakeel, H. Deep Learning for Multi-Class Identification from Domestic Violence Online Posts. *IEEE Access* **2019**, *7*, 46210–46224. [CrossRef]

43. Subramani, S.; Vu, H.Q.; Wang, H. Intent classification using feature sets for domestic violence discourse on social media. In Proceedings of the 2017 4th Asia-Pacific World Congress on Computer Science and Engineering (APWC on CSE), Mana Island, Fiji, 11–13 December 2017; IEEE: Manhattan, NY, USA, 2017; pp. 129–136.
44. Subramani, S.; Wang, H.; Vu, H.Q.; Li, G. Domestic Violence Crisis Identification from Facebook Posts Based on Deep Learning. *IEEE Access* **2018**, *6*, 54075–54085. [CrossRef]
45. Wijenayake, S.; Graham, T.; Christen, P. A Decision Tree Approach to Predicting Recidivism in Domestic Violence. In Proceedings of the Pacific-Asia Conference on Knowledge Discovery and Data Mining. Springer: Cham, Switzerland, Chengdu, China, 16–19 May 2018; pp. 3–15. [CrossRef]
46. Xue, J.; Chen, J.; Gelles, R. Using Data Mining Techniques to Examine Domestic Violence Topics on Twitter. *Violence Gend.* **2019**, *6*, 105–114. [CrossRef]
47. Beam, A.L.; Kohane, I.S. Big data and machine learning in health care. *JAMA* **2018**, *319*, 1317–1318. [CrossRef] [PubMed]
48. Perera, N.; Hanson, D.; Franklin, R. Breaking the cycle of violence: Detection of domestic violence in a regional emergency department. *Inj. Prev.* **2012**, *18*, A184. [CrossRef]
49. Elliott, L.; Nerney, M.; Jones, T.; Friedmann, P.D. Barriers to screening for domestic violence. *J. Gen. Intern. Med.* **2002**, *17*, 112–116. [CrossRef] [PubMed]
50. Voce, I.; Boxall, H. Who reports domestic violence to police? A review of the evidence. *Trends Issues Crime Crim. Justice* **2018**, *559*, 1–16.
51. Bogen, K.W.; Bleiweiss, K.K.; Leach, N.R.; Orchowski, L.M. #MeToo: Disclosure and Response to Sexual Victimization on Twitter. *J. Interpers. Violence* **2019**, *36*, 8257–8288. [CrossRef]
52. Bailey, M.; Jackson, S.; Welles, B.F. Women Tweet on Violence: From #YesAllWomen to #MeToo. *Ada A J. Gender New Media Technol.* **2019**, *2019*, 6. [CrossRef]
53. Weiss, S. "MaybeHeDoesntHitYou" Twitter Hashtag Reminds Us That Intimate Partner Violence Isn't Always Physical. Bustle. 2016. Available online: www.bustle.com/articles/159909-maybe-he-doesnt-hit-you-twitter-hashtag-reminds-us-that-intimate-partner-violence-isnt-always-physical (accessed on 16 November 2017).
54. Hsiao, C.-J.; Hing, E.; Ashman, J. *Trends in Electronic Health Record System Use among Office-Based Physicians: United States, 2007–2012*; National Health Statistics Reports No. 75; NCHS: Atlanta, GA, USA, 2014; pp. 1–18. Available online: http://www.cdc.gov/nchs/data/nhsr/nhsr075.pdf (accessed on 20 May 2014).
55. Hui, V.; Constantino, R.E. The association between life satisfaction, emotional support, and perceived health among women who experienced intimate Partner violence (IPV)–2007 behavioral risk factor surveillance system. *BMC Public Health* **2021**, *21*, 641. [CrossRef]
56. Lee, J.G.; Backes, B.L. Civil Legal Aid and Domestic Violence: A Review of the Literature and Promising Directions. *J. Fam. Violence* **2018**, *33*, 421–433. [CrossRef]
57. Kanade, P.; Kumar, A. Mapping of Disease Names to Standard Codes for Effective EHR System in India. In Proceedings of the International Conference on Computational and Bio Engineering, Virtual Conference, 26–28 October 2020; Springer: Cham, Switzerland, 2020; pp. 273–285. [CrossRef]
58. Yin, J.; Lampert, A.; Cameron, M.; Robinson, B.; Power, R. Using Social Media to Enhance Emergency Situation Awareness. *IEEE Intell. Syst.* **2012**, *27*, 52–59. [CrossRef]
59. Evans, C.S.; Hunold, K.M.; Rosen, T.; Platts-Mills, T.F. Diagnosis of Elder Abuse in U.S. Emergency Departments. *J. Am. Geriatr. Soc.* **2016**, *65*, 91–97. [CrossRef] [PubMed]
60. Haris, N.; Majid, R.A.; Abdullah, N.; Osman, R. The role of social media in supporting elderly quality daily life. In Proceedings of the 2014 3rd International Conference on User Science and Engineering (i-USEr), Shah Alam, Malaysia, 2–5 September 2014; IEEE: Manhattan, NY, USA, 2014; pp. 253–257. [CrossRef]
61. Dilci, T.; Eranıl, A.K. The Impact of Social Media on Children. In *Handbook of Research on Children's Consumption of Digital Media*; IGI Global: Hershey, PA, USA, 2019; pp. 1–10. [CrossRef]
62. Zahara, F.N.; Effendi, R.; Sukmayadi, V. The Effect of Instagram Influencers Content Exposure on The Motivation for Online Self-Disclosing. *J. Pendidik. ILMU Soc.* **2020**, *29*, 19. [CrossRef]
63. Babvey, P.; Capela, F.; Cappa, C.; Lipizzi, C.; Petrowski, N.; Ramirez-Marquez, J. Using social media data for assessing children's exposure to violence during the COVID-19 pandemic. *Child Abus. Negl.* **2020**, *116*, 104747. [CrossRef] [PubMed]
64. Bradbury-Jones, C.; Isham, L. The pandemic paradox: The consequences of COVID-19 on domestic violence. *J. Clin. Nurs.* **2020**, *29*, 2047–2049. [CrossRef] [PubMed]
65. Lee, Y.J.; Park, A.; Roberge, M.; Donovan, H. What Can Social Media Tell Us About Patient Symptoms: A text-mining approach to online ovarian cancer forum. *Cancer Nurs.* **2022**, *45*, E27–E35. [CrossRef]
66. Naveed, T.S.A. Addressing Semantic Interoperability, Privacy and Security Concerns in Electronic Health Records. *J. Eng. Sci. Res.* **2020**, *2*, 40. [CrossRef]

Journal of
Clinical Medicine

MDPI

Systematic Review

Generative Adversarial Networks (GANs) in the Field of Head and Neck Surgery: Current Evidence and Prospects for the Future—A Systematic Review

Luca Michelutti [1,†], Alessandro Tel [1,†], Marco Zeppieri [2,*], Tamara Ius [3], Edoardo Agosti [4], Salvatore Sembronio [1] and Massimo Robiony [1]

1 Clinic of Maxillofacial Surgery, Head-Neck and NeuroScience Department, University Hospital of Udine, p.le S. Maria della Misericordia 15, 33100 Udine, Italy; alessandro.tel@icloud.com (A.T.)
2 Department of Ophthalmology, University Hospital of Udine, Piazzale S. Maria della Misericordia 15, 33100 Udine, Italy
3 Neurosurgery Unit, Head-Neck and NeuroScience Department, University Hospital of Udine, p.le S. Maria della Misericordia 15, 33100 Udine, Italy
4 Division of Neurosurgery, Department of Medical and Surgical Specialties, Radiological Sciences and Public Health, University of Brescia, Piazza Spedali Civili 1, 25123 Brescia, Italy
* Correspondence: markzeppieri@hotmail.com
† These authors contributed equally to this work.

Abstract: Background: Generative Adversarial Networks (GANs) are a class of artificial neural networks capable of generating content such as images, text, and sound. For several years already, artificial intelligence algorithms have shown promise as tools in the medical field, particularly in oncology. Generative Adversarial Networks (GANs) represent a new frontier of innovation, as they are revolutionizing artificial content generation, opening opportunities in artificial intelligence and deep learning. **Purpose:** This systematic review aims to investigate what the stage of development of such technology is in the field of head and neck surgery, offering a general overview of the applications of such algorithms, how they work, and the potential limitations to be overcome in the future. **Methods:** The Preferred Reporting Items for Systematic Reviews and Meta-Analyses (PRISMA) guidelines were followed in conducting this study, and the PICOS framework was used to formulate the research question. The following databases were evaluated: MEDLINE, Embase, Cochrane Central Register of Controlled Trials (CENTRAL), Scopus, ClinicalTrials.gov, ScienceDirect, and CINAHL. **Results:** Out of 700 studies, only 9 were included. Eight applications of GANs in the head and neck region were summarized, including the classification of craniosynostosis, recognition of the presence of chronic sinusitis, diagnosis of radicular cysts in panoramic X-rays, segmentation of craniomaxillofacial bones, reconstruction of bone defects, removal of metal artifacts from CT scans, prediction of the postoperative face, and improvement of the resolution of panoramic X-rays. **Conclusions:** Generative Adversarial Networks may represent a new evolutionary step in the study of pathology, oncological and otherwise, making the approach to the disease much more precise and personalized.

Keywords: generative adversarial network (GAN); artificial generating content; maxillofacial surgery; otolaryngology surgery

1. Introduction

1.1. Background

For several years now, artificial intelligence (AI) algorithms have been a topic of strong interest. Scientific studies in the literature are showing how these algorithms are excellent and promising tools that can be applied in various fields, particularly in the medical field. Artificial intelligence models are gaining more and more importance especially in oncology. Indeed, through the analysis of histologic, radiomic, genomic, and clinical–epidemiological data, these algorithms are proving to be potential tools for the detection of precancerous lesions, for diagnosis, for staging, for predicting response to treatment, and for the prognostic evaluation of a tumor [1–5].

"Artificial intelligence", "machine learning", "deep learning", and "artificial neural network" are often used as synonyms, but they refer to different concepts. The widest semantic area includes AI, which includes machine learning, and, on a further subdivision level, there are other models, including deep learning and artificial neural networks. ML is a field of artificial intelligence that focuses on learning through data input, and there are four kinds of learning methods: reinforcement learning and supervised, semi-supervised, and unsupervised learning. DL models are inspired by neural networks present in human beings. They are artificial neural networks that allow multilevel computational models to learn data representations with different and various levels of abstraction. In fact, there is an analogy with the cell bodies of a neuron, i.e., the nodes of the neural network, and axons, i.e., the connections that are generated between different nodes. An ANN, called a feedforward neural network, consists of an input layer and an output layer, and in between these are several hidden layers (which, in deep ANNs, can be dozens or hundreds in number). Information passes from each node in one layer to the next, and during this step the information is processed and transformed. As the input proceeds through an ANN, it is transformed so that when it reaches the final layer, it is no longer the same as its initial state. A particular type of ANN is the convolutional neural network (CNN), which sees wide application in image processing [6–9]. Figure 1 graphically describes the hierarchical organization of artificial intelligence networks.

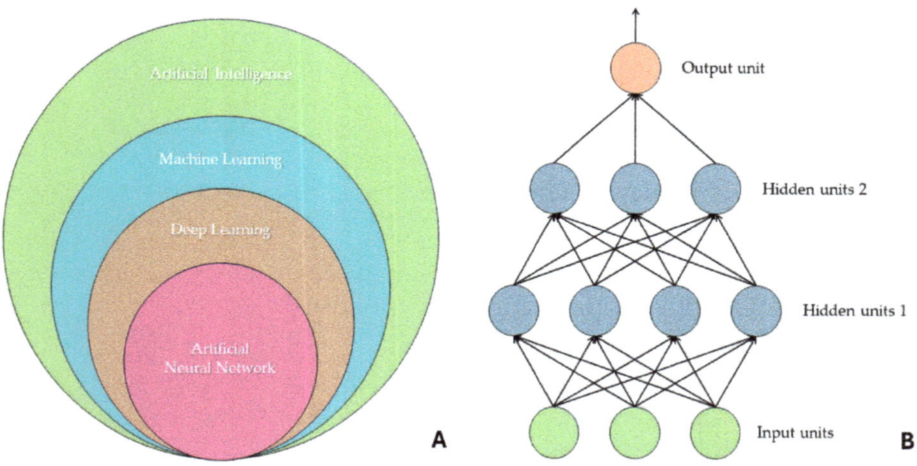

Figure 1. (**A**) Hierarchy between machine learning, deep learning, and artificial neural networks. (**B**) The composition of an artificial neural network consisting of an input layer (in green), two hidden layers (in blue), and an output layer (in orange) is shown. Each output within the ANN is used as input for the next layer. These artificial intelligence models, to perform the task for which they are trained, require a significant amount of data for the training set, particularly CNNs. In fact, there are studies in the literature that report the size of the data sample analyzed as a limitation. For example, the study conducted by Romeo et al. (2020) showed how the application of radiomic ML to primary tumor lesions has great potential in predicting the lymph node status of patients with oral cavity and oropharynx lesions, but they report how the small sample size is a problem. This is just one of many promising studies in the literature that report a similar impediment in evaluating the effectiveness and accuracy of such artificial intelligence models [10].

To overcome the problem related to limited sample size, especially when studying rare diseases for which clinical data are complex, researchers are investigating the capabilities of Generative Adversarial Networks (GANs) as a tool to generate synthetic data, i.e., created by the AI model, in order to use them to train deep learning algorithms [11].

1.2. Generative Adversarial Network (GAN)

Although GANs have become the subject of strong interest only in recent years, these models were first introduced in 2014 by Ian J. Goodfellow et al. [12] during their doctoral work at the University of Montréal.

Generative Adversarial Networks are a class of artificial neural network capable of creating artificial content such as images. Precisely, they consist of two networks: the generator and the discriminator (Figure 2). These have the task of competing with each other. Specifically, the generator must learn the data distribution and generate artificial data by receiving a random vector as input. The discriminator is trained to discriminate the difference between true data and synthetic data. Specifically, the discriminator receives synthetic and real data and calculates the probability that the generated data is real or false. The value of this probability represents a feedback signal that is sent to the discriminator itself and to the generator. This interactive process between the two networks (generator and discriminator) results in continuous mutual improvement, resulting in images similar to the real ones. The goal of a GAN is to generate synthetic images that are indistinguishable from real ones [11,13].

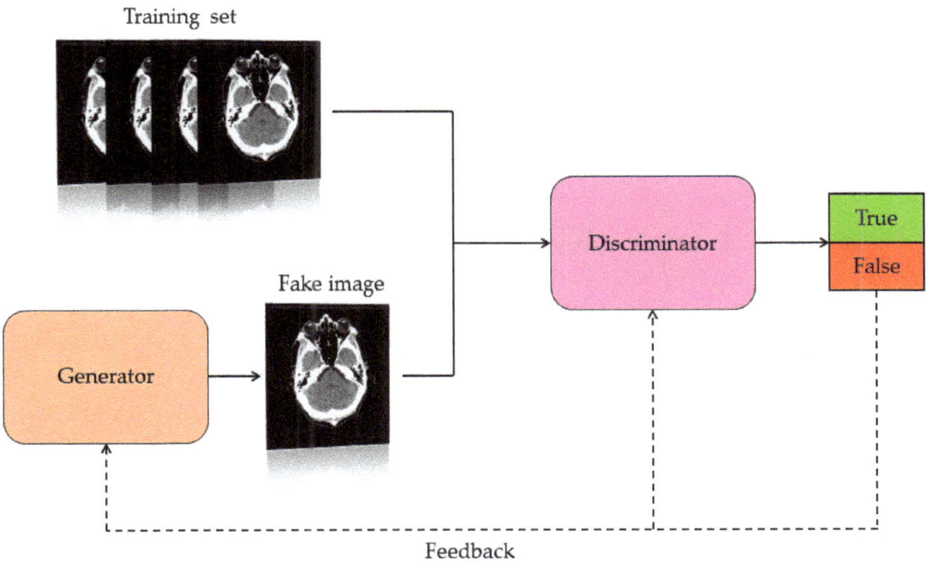

Figure 2. Basic architecture operation of a GAN.

From 2014, when GANs were born, to the present, these artificial neural networks have undergone continuous evolutions that have given birth to new and numerous architectures, some specific to certain functions (Table 1) [13,14].

Table 1. GAN functions found in the literature.

Classification	Model that can correctly classify input data by only emitting labels. In this model, the discriminator is a classification network.
Segmentation	It is used to classify voxels in order to identify objects using two GANs: the first produces synthetic scans, while the second has a segmentation network (using synthetic and real data) and a discriminator.
Reconstruction	GANs trained to reconstruct incomplete objects through a process with the purpose of acquiring the form and appearance of real objects.
Denoising	GANs trained to rebuild the true appearance of the object by removal of noise, artifacts, and causal data.
Image translation	GAN capable of converting an input image into another artificial version of that image, for example, transforming a CT scan into an MRI image.
General activities	GAN capable of generating synthetic data without applying it in a specific activity.

1.3. *Objective of the Study*

Already, several studies have shown how GANs are promising tools, especially to overcome the problem of the scarcity of clinical data for given diseases. For example, the study conducted by Loey et al. (2020) presented a GAN capable of generating synthetic data for coronavirus detection in chest X-rays [15], or the study conducted by Fujioka et al. (2020) reported the use of a GAN to create a computational model capable of detecting abnormal lesions in breast ultrasound images [16].

These models can represent a useful tool for the work of doctors and healthcare professionals. For example, the study conducted by Maniaci et al. (2024) [17] reported how the use of ChatGPT can be a tool capable of providing support in the diagnostic process in imaging for pathologies of the head and neck region. Furthermore, ChatGPT is proving to be a potential means to strengthen the relationship between doctor and patient, helping the latter to better understand their health status.

Considering that GANs have already been applied in different areas of medicine and in different pathologies, oncological and otherwise, the aim of this study is to propose an overview of what the applications of generative adversarial networks in pathologies affecting the head and neck region are, to report the reasons why researchers have been studying these particular artificial neural networks, to describe the types of GAN architectures used, and to analyze the results obtained from the studies included in this paper. Given that this is a technology that is gaining ground recently and considering that it is demonstrating promising applications in the management and study of many pathologies, we believe that it is interesting to investigate what the current applications and the possible prospects of such artificial intelligence models are.

2. Materials and Methods

This study was performed according to the Preferred Reporting Items for Systematic Review and Meta-Analyses (PRISMA) statement [18]. The PRISMA checklist is inserted in the Supplementary Materials. This review was recorded in the PROSPERO database (International Prospective Register of Systematic Review), and the ID number is 523954. The research question of this systematic review was constructed according to the PICOS framework (Table 2) and can be explained as follows: "Which are the applications of Generative Adversarial Networks for pathologies affecting the head and neck region?".

Table 2. PICOS framework.

Participant	Patients with diseases, oncological and otherwise, of the head-neck region
Interventions	Evaluation of the effects of the application of GANs
Comparators	N/A
Outcomes	AUC, sensibility, specificity
Study design	Research articles, original articles, cohort studies, clinical trials, randomized clinical trials

2.1. Literature Search

The query used is: ((GAN) OR (generative adversarial network)) AND ((maxillofacial surgery) OR (otolaryngology surgery) OR (head neck surgery)). The MeSH query used to improve and extend the search is the following: ((“Artificial Intelligence” [Mesh]) OR “Neural Networks, Computer” [Mesh]) AND “Orthognathic Surgical Procedures” [Mesh]. Using keyword combinations, the literature search was conducted until 13 March 2024, searching for studies included in the following databases: MEDLINE, Cochrane Central Register of Controlled Trials (CENTRAL), ClinicalTrials.gov (accessed on 29 April 2024), ScienceDirect, Embase, Scopus, CINAHL. The types of included articles are clinical trials, randomized clinical trials, cohort studies, original articles, research articles, and also reviews, systematic reviews, and meta-analysis since there are few papers in the literature concerning this topic.

The articles found in the databases consulted were imported into EndNote21 (Clarivate, Analytics, Philadelphia, PA, USA). All articles exported to EndNote21 were screened by two separate investigators (L.M. and A.T.). The primary screening consists of evaluating first the titles and then the abstracts of the included studies, as reported in the PRISMA flowchart (Figure 3), and in case of doubt, a third investigator (M.R.) was included in the evaluation.

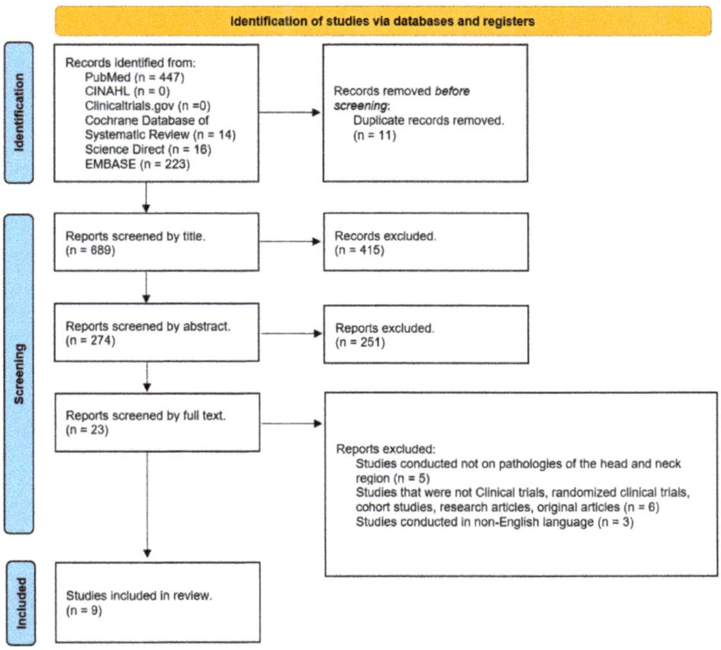

Figure 3. PRISMA flowchart of the systematic review process.

2.2. Data Collection

The data extracted from the studies included in this systematic review are study topic, reasons that motivated the researchers to study the application of GANs, architecture of GAN used, type of data used, parameters adopted to measure the functioning of the GANs, and the results obtained from the individual studies included. The data were manually exported by the two independent researchers (L.M and A.T.) and collected in a Microsoft Excel 2019 spreadsheet. These data are displayed in Table 3 of Section 3.

2.3. Inclusion and Exclusion Criteria Applied in the Collected Studies

The two researchers independently (L.M. and A.T.) applied the inclusion and exclusion criteria below on the collected articles through an initial evaluation on the title and abstract and then through a thorough analysis of the full text of the articles.

Articles analyzing the application of GANs in any pathology, oncologic or otherwise, of the head–neck region were considered. Articles dealing with GANs applied in pathologies not of the head–neck region, articles without the abstract, and systematic reviews and meta-analyses were excluded. Only studies conducted on the human species and published in English were included. The articles considered in this study are all papers that have a publication date between 2014 and 2024, and the types of studies included are clinical trials, original articles, cohort studies, and research articles.

2.4. Bias Assessment

Five types of bias were assessed: bias arising from the randomization process, bias due to deviations from the intended interventions, bias due to missing outcome data, bias in outcome measurement, and bias in reported outcome selection (Figure 4). The Robvis tool [19] was used to analyze the presence of these biases, and two investigators (L.M. and A.T.) were involved, who worked independently.

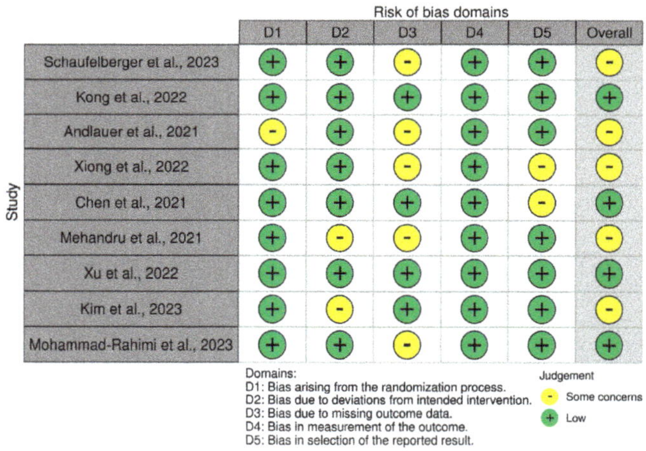

Figure 4. Robvis tool for assessing the risk of bias.

3. Results

PRISMA guidelines were followed in the search for scientific evidence to be included in this study. Figure 3 shows the PRISMA flowchart that illustrates the entire process of article selection. The total number of articles collected from the databases consulted and exported to EndNote is 700. Of these, 11 were removed because they were dubbed. Of the 689 remaining, 415 were excluded by analyzing the titles of the studies (although some collected studies did not have the word "GAN" in the title, the abstracts were carefully analyzed before deciding whether or not to exclude these studies). Screening based on abstract analysis resulted in the elimination of 251 reports. Of the remaining 23 studies, after careful and attentive analysis of the complete texts, 9 studies remained.

Through the use of the Robvis tool [19], the biases of the nine included studies were analyzed. Figure 4 illustrates the results obtained from this assessment.

3.1. Topics

Eight different types of topics were covered in the studies included in this paper (Figure 5): classification of craniosynostosis, chronic sinusitis, temporomandibular disorders and malocclusion, reconstruction of bone defects, craniomaxillofacial (CMF) bone segmentation, radicular cysts, correction of metal artifacts in CT scans, and improvement of panoramic X-ray resolution.

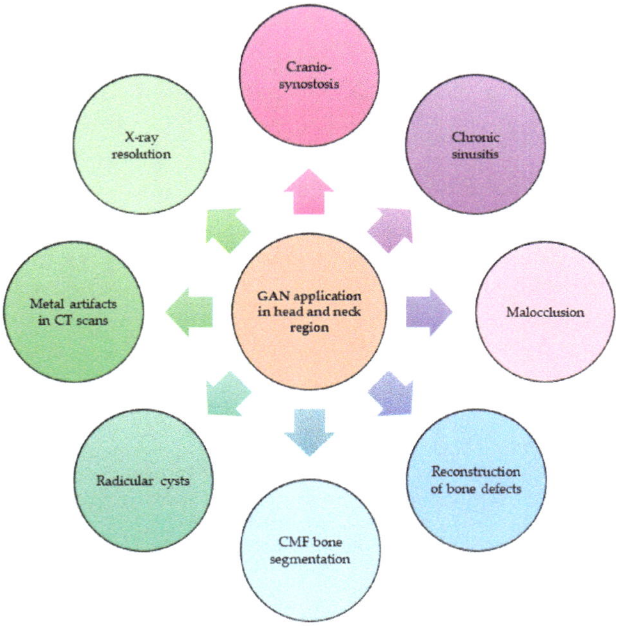

Figure 5. Different applications of GANs for the head and neck region.

3.2. Reasons Why GANs Have Been Applied

One of the most common reasons for researchers to study and apply GANs is the scarcity of clinical data. As repeated many times, artificial intelligence algorithms, especially artificial neural networks, need a large amount of data to be trained in order to perform the task for which they were created. The difficulty in finding clinical data is attributed to multiple factors that make obtaining such data complex: the presence of a rare disease for which little information and data are available; the need for experienced radiologists; the use of scans and images with specific characteristics in terms of format and source; and privacy issues.

In addition to obviating the problem of clinical data retrieval by generating synthetic data identical to real data, GANs have also been applied for other reasons, including the ability to overcome the limitations of current methods of reconstructing midfacial bone defects, translation of a CT scan into an MRI image, removal of metal artifacts, and improvement of the resolution of panoramic X-rays by exploiting the denoising function.

3.3. GAN Architectures Used

In the included studies, we have reported several types of GAN architectures, including cDC-WGAN-GP (Conditional Deep Convolutional Wasserstein GAN with Gradient Penalty), AC-GAN (Auxiliary Classifier GAN), Cycle-GAN, DDA-GAN (Diverse Data Augmentation Generative Adversarial Network), CD-GAN (Cyclic Discriminative GAN), MAR-GAN (metal artifact reduction GAN), Pix2pix-GAN, and SR-GAN (Super-Resolution GAN). Their functioning is briefly illustrated in Table 3.

Table 3. Functioning of the GAN architectures of the included studies.

cDC-WGAN-GP	It is a model that combines the Wasserstein GAN (WGAN) and the Gradient Penalty (GP). The former can produce better quality samples, the latter introduces a penalty on gradients preventing them from vanishing or exploding further enhancing stability. In addition, being a conditional model, it can generate specific images, resulting in an advanced model for synthetic image generation.
AC-GAN [20]	It is an extension of conditional GAN (cGAN), which in turn is an extension of the GAN architecture. The cGAN can predict the class label of an image received as input. The AC-GAN has a discriminator that predicts the class label of an image.
Cycle-GAN [21]	It is an image–image translation model without the need to have paired examples. By image–image translation, we mean the creation of a new artificial version of an image with specific modifications.
DDA-GAN [22]	It is a model that can segment bone structures and exploit synthetic data generated from an annotated domain to improve the quality of segmentation of images from an unannotated domain.
CD-GAN [23]	It is a model for image-to-image transformation, transforming an image from one domain to another. It is based on a Cycle-GAN architecture, but unlike the latter, it evaluates the quality of synthetic images by additional cyclic discriminators, making them more realistic.
MAR-GAN	GAN model capable of removing metal artifacts present in CT scans.
Pix2pix-GAN [24]	It is a model of cGAN (conditional generative adversarial network) used for image-to-image translation. It features a generator that is based on the U-Net architecture and a discriminator represented by a PatchGAN classifier.
SR-GAN [25]	It is a model used for super-resolution imaging. It has the function of generating high-definition images from low-resolution images.

3.4. Type of Data Analyzed

The data that were used were exclusively imaging data. In terms of percentages, in 44.4% of the included studies panoramic X-rays were used, 55.5% used CT scans, and 11.1% used MRI images.

Some studies are not limited in using only one type of imaging data. The study conducted by Kong et al., 2022 [26] exploits both CT and paranasal RX scans, the study conducted by Andlauer et al., 2021 [27] crosses both 2D images and postoperative 3D simulated images obtained from processing CT scans, and the study conducted by Chen et al. [28] analyzes both CT and MRI scans.

3.5. Parameters Adopted to Evaluate GANs

In the included studies, the parameters used to evaluate the results obtained are F1 score, AUC (area under the curve), sensibility, specificity, PSNR (peak signal-to-noise ratio), Euclidean distance, DSC (coefficient of symmetry), average symmetric superficial distance, SSIM (structural similarity index measurements), MSE (mean square error), PPV (positive predictive value), NPV (negative predictive value), and MOS (mean for expert opinion score).

3.6. Results Obtained for the Single Studies Included

In the study conducted by Schaufelberger et al., 2023 [29] a CNN (convolutional neural network) was trained to classify the different types of craniosynostosis using only synthetic data generated by different generative models, including GANs. The CNN was able to grade four different types of deformity.

The study conducted by Kong et al., 2022 [26] also demonstrated how GANs are an effective source of data that can be exploited to train artificial intelligence models to perform the job for which they were created. Through a particular type of GAN, synthetic data were generated to train a deep learning model created to diagnose the presence of sinus pathology by studying panoramic RX images and CT scans. It was shown that the deep learning model had better diagnostic performance when trained with original data and synthetic data generated GAN data.

The study conducted by Mehandru et al., 2021 [30] also demonstrated how GANs can generate useful data to train a CNN to recognize the presence of root cysts by studying panoramic X-rays. Analyzing the ROC curve, the CNN trained without synthetic images had lower accuracy than the CNN trained with synthetic images created by GANs (89.3% vs. 95.1%, respectively). The study conducted by Andlauer et al., 2022 [27] used a Cycle-GAN to predict the postoperative face of a patient with class II and III malocclusion to undergo bimaxillary surgery. Using 2D images and a 3D simulation of the surgery, the GAN was able to predict the outcome of the surgery. The Cycle-GAN was shown to predict realistic chin and nose changes on selected examples.

The study conducted by Xiong et al., 2022 [31] used a GAN to reconstruct midfacial bone defects. On the real and normal CT scans, spherical, cuboid, and semi-cylindrical artificial defects were manually inserted in five structural regions to simulate the bone defects. To train GANs, scans with corresponding artificially created defects were important. By analyzing the cosine similarity, this was about 0.97 in the reconstruction of artificially created defects and 0.96 in the reconstruction of unilateral clinical defects.

GANs also show promise for segmentation of craniomaxillofacial bones, as shown in the study conducted by Chen et al., 2021. [28] The GAN architecture used in the study is the DDA-GAN, which was compared to other segmentation tools, including PnP-AdaNet, SIFA, and SynSeg-Net. The DDA-GAN outperformed SynSeg-Net by 2.68 in terms of Dice symmetry coefficient (DCS) and 0.13 in terms of average surface symmetric distance (ASSD).

The study conducted by Xu et al., 2022 [32] applied a particular type of GAN, a MAR-GAN, to eliminate metal artifacts present in CT scans. The MAR-GAN performed better, demonstrating excellent abilities in restoring the original structures near metals and removing metal artifacts.

The two included studies that applied GANs to improve the resolution of panoramic X-rays, Kim et al., 2023 and Mohammad-Rahimi et al., 2023 [33,34] showed promising performance. The first study used a Pix2Pix-GAN model, demonstrating good performance on images with blurring in the anterior tooth region, while the second study used an SR-GAN model, demonstrating in terms of MOS (mean opinion score) significant improvements in resolution compared to the other tools used and compared.

Table 4 provides a comprehensive overview of papers selected for this systematic review.

Table 4. Data extracted by the included studies.

	Topics	Reason for Applying GANs	Architecture GAN Used	Data Used	Method	Results
Schaufelberger et al., 2023 [29]	Craniosynostosis classification	Generation of synthetic data to train a CNN to classify craniosynostosis, given the paucity of clinical data	cDC-WGAN-GP	75% of the clinical data were used to train GANs to generate synthetic data on which CNN was trained, while the remaining 25% was used for the test set for CNN.	A CNN was trained with purely synthetic data to classify craniosynostosis. The synthetic data were generated from three different generative models: GAN, SSM, and PCA.	Classification of craniosynostosis with a synthetic data set has been shown to have similar performance to that of a classifier trained on clinical data.
Kong et al., 2022 [26]	Imaging data generation for paranasal pathology (chronic sinusitis)	Synthetic data generation to improve the diagnostic performance of a DL model given the presence of possible problems in procuring clinical data, including: poor availability, need for experienced radiologists, and privacy issues	AC-GAN	Patients diagnosed with chronic sinusitis and undergoing X-ray examination were included. Included only patients who underwent both RX and CT with time distance of less than 14 days. The 389 paranasal RXs of the internal data set (212 images with sinusitis and 177 normal) were divided: 80% training set, 10% validation set, 20% test set).	All conventional radiographs were labeled as "sinusitis" or "normal" by experienced rhinologists by studying CT scans. One DL model, ChexNet, was trained in several ways, among them only with the original training data and with data obtained through GANs.	Of the various models analyzed in this study, the GBC + OMGDA model performed better in terms of AUC, accuracy, sensitivity, specificity, F1 score, PPV, and NPV. It was shown that the DL model had better diagnostic performance when trained with original data and synthetic data generated GAN data.

Table 4. *Cont.*

	Topics	Reason for Applying GANs	Architecture GAN Used	Data Used	Method	Results
Andlauer et al., 2021 [27]	Postoperative prediction for temporomandibular disorders and malocclusion	Predicting the postoperative face using preoperative 2D images and 3D simulation of postoperative soft tissue, without the need for difficult-to-acquire preoperative 3D images, for patients to undergo bimaxillary surgery for class II and class III malocclusion	Cycle-GAN	Used preoperative 2D images and a postoperative 3D simulation using preoperative facial CT images of four patients with malocclusion	CT scans were used to simulate bimaxillary surgery, and bone and soft tissue segmentations were applied on being. These 3D simulations, along with preoperative 2D images, were used to train the GAN.	Cycle-GAN was shown to predict realistic chin and nose changes on selected examples. The accuracy of the predictions was evaluated by the Euclidean distance of the facial landmarks. Unfortunately, some prediction errors were found concerning the nose region, while there appeared to be no errors for the chin region. According to the authors, this is probably due to the need for more detailed plots for the study of the nose that change based on different head poses. Nevertheless, it seems to be a promising tool for predicting postoperative outcome.
Xiong et al., 2022 [31]	Reconstruction of midfacial bone defects	Training a GAN to reconstruct midfacial defects. There are reconstruction methods such as mirror technology, but it cannot be used for I midspan and bilateral defects. In addition, training the DL model requires a large amount of data, which is not always achievable with clinical data alone.	GAN	CT scans with different defects: median and unilateral were used in this study	For GAN training, spherical, cuboid and half-cylindrical artificial defects were manually inserted on the real and normal CT scans in 5 structural regions to simulate bone defects. To evaluate the performance of GAN, cosine similarity (an indicator to assess the similarity of two objects) was calculated. The reconstructed images were compared with the real ones, and the obtained effect of the rebuilt area was evaluated by surgeons.	To evaluate the performance of the GAN used, cosine similarity was assessed. The study obtained a result of 0.97 in terms of reconstruction of artificial defects and 0.96 in terms of reconstruction of unilateral defects.

Table 4. *Cont.*

	Topics	Reason for Applying GANs	Architecture GAN Used	Data Used	Method	Results
Chen et al., 2021 [28]	Craniomaxillofacial bone segmentation	Synthetic data generation to train DL model to segment craniomaxillofacial CT scan. The paucity of available clinical data is a problem for having reliable segmentation models. In addition, we want to investigate whether from CT scans can be used to train segmentation models for MRI.	DDA-GAN	Use 50 CT scans as a training set and 50 MRI scans.	MRI-CT data were used to train the GAN to perform segmentations, and MRI scans were used for validation. The performance of the GAN was evaluated using DSC and ASSD, compared with different image segmentation methods, including PnP-AdaNet, SIFA, and SynSeg-Net.	The GAN analyzed by the study (DDA-GAN), outperforms SynSeg-Net, a Cycle-GAN used to train segmentation models. The DDA-GAN was shown to be superior because it avoids geometric distortions and improves segmentation performance.
Mehandru et al. 2021 [30]	Pathology detection in panoramic RX (root cysts)	Synthetic data generation to train a CNN to recognize root cysts in panoramic X-rays	CD-GAN	34 panoramic RXs of root cysts and 34 normal ones were divided into training and test sets (75% and 25% respectively). In addition to these, synthetic images generated by GAN were added.	Two CNNs were compared for the purpose of recognizing root cysts from panoramic X-rays: the first uses non-GAN-generated data, while the second also takes advantage of synthetic images. Both CNNs were then evaluated in terms of AUC.	The proposed model has demonstrated better performance in terms of area under the curve (AUC), sensitivity, and specificity. Comparing the receiver operating characteristic (ROC) curves, the performance of the convolutional neural network (CNN) trained with synthetic images was superior to that of the CNN trained with non-artificial images (95.1% vs. 89.3%).
Xu et al., 2022 [32]	Reduction of metal artifacts in oral maxillofacial CT	Build a GAN-based model to reduce artifacts and improve image quality	MAR-GAN	For this study, CT scans were used on which metal artifacts were artificially simulated.	The parameters used to evaluate the performance of the studied GAN are RMSE and SSIM.	The used GAN in this study has high performance, demonstrainting its ability to effictibely reduce the metallic artifacts that were artificially inserted.

Table 4. *Cont.*

	Topics	Reason for Applying GANs	Architecture GAN Used	Data Used	Method	Results
Kim et al., 2023 [33]	Image resolution refinement of panoramic RX	Create a GAN model that can improve image quality	Pix2Pix-GAN	In this study, panoramic X-rays were used. From these, images with poor quality were obtained to test the Pix2Pix-GAN's ability to improve image quality.	The quality of the generated images was evaluated by radiologist experienced in maxillofacial pathology.	The proposed model performed very well on images with blur in the anterior tooth region, while it was less effective in improving image quality with blur and noise.
Mohammad-Rahimi et al., 2023 [34]	Image resolution refinement of panoramic RX	Compare different DL-based super resolution (SR) models to improve the resolution of panoramic RXs	SR-GAN	888 Dental panoramic X-rays	Five super-resolution models were compared, including SRCNN, SRGAN, U-Net, Swinlr, and LTE. The results were compared with each other by conventional bicubic interpolation. The parameters of MSE, PNSR, SSIM, and MOS were evaluated.	The GAN included in this study (SR-GAN) has demonstrated significant performance in improving the resolution of panoramic X-rays in termins of mean opinion score (MOS).

Legends: AC-GAN—auxiliary classifier; ASSD—average symmetric superficial distance; AUC—area under the curve; CD-GAN—Cyclic Discriminative GAN; cDC-WGAN-GP—Wasserstein GAN and the Gradient Penalty; CNN—convolutional neural network; CT—computed tomography; DDA-GAN—Diverse Data Augmentation Generative Adversarial Network); DSC—Dice's coefficient of symmetry; DL—deep learning; GAN—Generative Adversarial Network; LTE—local texture estimator; MAR-GAN—metal artifact reduction GAN; ML—machine learning; MOS—mean opinion score; MRI: magnetic resonance imaging; MSE: mean square error; NPV—negative predictive value; PCA—principal component analysis; PPV—positive predictive value; PSNR—peak signal-to-noise ratio; ROC—receiver operating characteristic; RMSE—root mean square error; RX—X-rays; SR—super-resolution; SRCNN—SR convolutional neural network; SSIM—structural similarity index measure; SSM—Statistical Shape Model; Swinlr—Swin for image restoration.

4. Discussion

As announced earlier in the introduction, this systematic review aims to present what the applications of GANs (Generative Adversarial Networks) in pathologies are, oncological and otherwise, affecting the head and neck region. GANs are proving to be very promising tools in the field of medicine and with multiple functions. One of the most important functions is the generation of synthetic images. In fact, the creation of artificial data is solving a problem that many studies have raised, namely the scarcity of clinical data to be used to train deep learning models developed to perform the different functions for which they were created. As we have also seen in this paper, to train a deep learning model requires a significant amount of clinical data, and often this is not always possible, for various reasons, including the need for experienced radiologists, issues related to patient privacy, and use of data with particular properties that are often not always the same, especially in multicenter studies that analyze data from multiple different centers using different modalities to obtain CT or MRI scans.

In this paper, we have reported eight applications of GANs for pathologies affecting the head and neck region: classification of craniosynostosis, recognition of the presence of chronic sinusitis, diagnosis of radicular cysts in panoramic X-rays, segmentation of craniomaxillofacial bones, reconstruction of bone defects, removal of metal artifacts from CT scans, prediction of the postoperative face, and improvement of the resolution of panoramic X-rays. In these areas, GANs have proven essential for their ability to generate large amounts of synthetic data and more. In fact, depending on the type of architecture, GANs can acquire multiple functions, including denoising, image translation, reconstruction, segmentation, and classification.

Unfortunately, we did not find any studies dealing with GANs applied in the field of head and neck cancers, although there are several papers in the literature analyzing the application of GANs for functions that are certainly useful in oncology, such as gene expression analysis, segmentation, tumor detection, and diagnosis. There are several examples of how GANs can be implemented in the study of cancer pathology. A recent study by Waters et al., 2024 [11] investigated the use of GANs for augmented gene expression analysis and demonstrated how this technology can reliably discover gene expression in a limited number of samples, proving to be extremely useful, especially for rare diseases for which little clinical data are available. Also, in the field of oncology, the study conducted by Park et al., 2021 [35] applied a GAN to generate synthetic images in order to observe morphological changes in glioblastomas to improve the diagnostic performance of this pathology.

Since there are already several studies applying such technology in the oncological setting, we invite future research to investigate what the potential of GANs might be in head and neck cancer, particularly in oral cancer. Artificial intelligence applied to head-neck cancer pathology has been a subject of strong interest for several years already. It has been successful in demonstrating how machine learning and deep learning models are promising tools in various areas of oncology, including diagnosis, segmentation, staging, and even prognostic evaluation of cancer, as also shown by the systematic review conducted by Michelutti et al., 2023 [36] and the study by Chinnery et al., 2021 [37].

Although GANs are proving to be innovative tools, some limitations may exist, as the study conducted by Chen et al., 2021 [38] points out. Some of the problems concern mode collapse, i.e., when the generator is no longer capable of producing a large amount of artificial data; nonconvergence, i.e., when the generator produces more and more realistic data and the discriminator is no longer able to follow this evolution as the latter's feedback becomes increasingly meaningless; diminished gradient, which is when the generator cannot improve its performance as fast as the discriminator; overfitting, which is when the amount of data is very limited; and imperfection, which is when no evaluation function can mimic human judgment.

These tools are showing great promise, but one must also consider that these tools, particularly ChatGPT, need to be evaluated and it is necessary to understand whether the performance is reliable. In this regard, the study conducted by Lechien et al. (2024) [39]

applied an instrument, the Artificial Intelligence Performance Instrument (AIPI), to evaluate the performance of ChatGPT in the management of ENT patients. Although it has demonstrated good performance, which has also been validated by ENT surgeons, the authors highlight the need for further future studies to investigate the usefulness of such an instrument in medicine and surgery.

While we are aware that GANs applied in the medical field are an innovative and recently popularized topic, we must reiterate the absence of articles related to the study of this technology applied to head and neck oncology. We understand the reason why there are few reports on this subject in the literature, and precisely because the study of these artificial intelligence models is recent, we urge future research to conduct multicenter studies and protocols to standardize the application of GANs. We urge the study of such technology applied in the context of head and neck cancers. As mentioned above, many studies applying deep learning models in radiomics unfortunately have small patient samples and insufficiently large data sets. This technology could solve these limitations encountered. It is essential to investigate the impact that GANs can have in radiomics and in the study of CT and MRI scans of head and neck cancers so that we can have a useful tool in the study of oncological pathology through artificial intelligence algorithms. We believe that GANs can represent an important evolutionary step in the study of cancer, succeeding in overcoming the obstacles presented by deep learning models and making the transition to increasingly cutting-edge precision medicine faster and faster.

5. Conclusions

Generative Adversarial Networks (GANs) are artificial neural networks capable of performing many functions, particularly the generation of synthetic data. These artificial data are proving to be useful and essential for training deep learning algorithms, especially when dealing with a rare disease for which little clinical data are available. With regard to the application of GANs in the head and neck district, we found several areas where they are proving to be useful and promising tools, including classification of craniosynostosis, recognition of the presence of chronic sinusitis, diagnosis of radicular cysts in panoramic X-rays, segmentation of craniomaxillofacial bones, reconstruction of bone defects, removal of metal artifacts from CT scans, prediction of the postoperative face, and improvement of the resolution of panoramic X-rays. Unfortunately, no articles were found dealing with GAN applied in the specific study of head and neck cancer, although we believe that future research will be able to fill this hole. In conclusion, we believe that Generative Adversarial Networks may represent a new evolutionary step in the study of pathology, oncological and otherwise, making the approach to the disease much more precise and personalized.

Supplementary Materials: The following supporting information can be downloaded at: https://www.mdpi.com/article/10.3390/jcm13123556/s1, PRISMA 2020 Checklist.

Author Contributions: Conceptualization L.M., A.T., M.Z., T.I., E.A., S.S. and M.R.; methodology, L.M., A.T. and M.R.; validation, L.M., A.T., M.Z., T.I., E.A., S.S. and M.R.; formal analysis, L.M. and A.T.; investigation, L.M. and A.T.; resources, L.M., A.T., M.Z., T.I., E.A., S.S. and M.R.; data curation, L.M., A.T., M.Z., T.I., E.A., S.S. and M.R.; writing—original draft preparation, L.M. and A.T.; writing—review and editing, L.M. and A.T. visualization, L.M., A.T., M.Z., T.I., E.A., S.S. and M.R.; supervision, A.T., M.Z. and M.R.; project administration, A.T., M.Z. and M.R. All authors have read and agreed to the published version of the manuscript.

Funding: This research received no external funding.

Institutional Review Board Statement: Not applicable.

Informed Consent Statement: Not applicable.

Data Availability Statement: Data are available in a publicly accessible repository.

Conflicts of Interest: The authors declare no conflicts of interest.

References

1. Mahmood, H.; Shaban, M.; Indave, B.I.; Santos-Silva, A.R.; Rajpoot, N.; Khurram, S.A. Use of Artificial Intelligence in Diagnosis of Head and Neck Precancerous and Cancerous Lesions: A Systematic Review. *Oral Oncol.* **2020**, *110*, 104885. [CrossRef]
2. Resteghini, C.; Trama, A.; Borgonovi, E.; Hosni, H.; Corrao, G.; Orlandi, E.; Calareso, G.; De Cecco, L.; Piazza, C.; Mainardi, L.; et al. Big Data in Head and Neck Cancer. *Curr. Treat. Options Oncol.* **2018**, *19*, 62. [CrossRef]
3. Mäkitie, A.A.; Alabi, R.O.; Ng, S.P.; Takes, R.P.; Robbins, K.T.; Ronen, O.; Shaha, A.R.; Bradley, P.J.; Saba, N.F.; Nuyts, S.; et al. Artificial Intelligence in Head and Neck Cancer: A Systematic Review of Systematic Reviews. *Adv. Ther.* **2023**, *40*, 3360–3380. [CrossRef]
4. Abdel Razek, A.A.K.; Khaled, R.; Helmy, E.; Naglah, A.; AbdelKhalek, A.; El-Baz, A. Artificial Intelligence and Deep Learning of Head and Neck Cancer. *Magn. Reson. Imaging Clin. N. Am.* **2022**, *30*, 81–94. [CrossRef] [PubMed]
5. Peng, Z.; Wang, Y.; Wang, Y.; Jiang, S.; Fan, R.; Zhang, H.; Jiang, W. Application of Radiomics and Machine Learning in Head and Neck Cancers. *Int. J. Biol. Sci.* **2021**, *17*, 475–486. [CrossRef] [PubMed]
6. Chen, M.M.; Terzic, A.; Becker, A.S.; Johnson, J.M.; Wu, C.C.; Wintermark, M.; Wald, C.; Wu, J. Artificial Intelligence in Oncologic Imaging. *Eur. J. Radiol. Open* **2022**, *9*, 100441. [CrossRef] [PubMed]
7. Choi, R.Y.; Coyner, A.S.; Kalpathy-Cramer, J.; Chiang, M.F.; Campbell, J.P. Introduction to Machine Learning, Neural Networks, and Deep Learning. *Transl. Vis. Sci. Technol.* **2020**, *9*, 14. [CrossRef]
8. LeCun, Y.; Bengio, Y.; Hinton, G. Deep Learning. *Nature* **2015**, *521*, 436–444. [CrossRef] [PubMed]
9. Shen, D.; Wu, G.; Suk, H.-I. Deep Learning in Medical Image Analysis. *Annu. Rev. Biomed. Eng.* **2017**, *19*, 221–248. [CrossRef]
10. Romeo, V.; Cuocolo, R.; Ricciardi, C.; Ugga, L.; Cocozza, S.; Verde, F.; Stanzione, A.; Napolitano, V.; Russo, D.; Improta, G.; et al. Prediction of Tumor Grade and Nodal Status in Oropharyngeal and Oral Cavity Squamous-Cell Carcinoma Using a Radiomic Approach. *Anticancer Res.* **2020**, *40*, 271–280. [CrossRef]
11. Waters, M.R.; Inkman, M.; Jayachandran, K.; Kowalchuk, R.M.; Robinson, C.; Schwarz, J.K.; Swamidass, S.J.; Griffith, O.L.; Szymanski, J.J.; Zhang, J. GAiN: An Integrative Tool Utilizing Generative Adversarial Neural Networks for Augmented Gene Expression Analysis. *Patterns* **2024**, *5*, 100910. [CrossRef] [PubMed]
12. Goodfellow, I.; Pouget-Abadie, J.; Mirza, M.; Xu, B.; Warde-Farley, D.; Ozair, S.; Courville, A.; Bengio, Y. Generative Adversarial Nets. In Proceedings of the 27th International Conference on Neural Information Processing Systems, Montreal, QC, Canada, 8–13 December 2014; Curran Associates, Inc.: New York, NY, USA, 2014; Volume 27.
13. Ferreira, A.; Li, J.; Pomykala, K.L.; Kleesiek, J.; Alves, V.; Egger, J. GAN-Based Generation of Realistic 3D Volumetric Data: A Systematic Review and Taxonomy. *Med. Image Anal.* **2024**, *93*, 103100. [CrossRef] [PubMed]
14. Osuala, R.; Kushibar, K.; Garrucho, L.; Linardos, A.; Szafranowska, Z.; Klein, S.; Glocker, B.; Diaz, O.; Lekadir, K. Data Synthesis and Adversarial Networks: A Review and Meta-Analysis in Cancer Imaging. *Med. Image Anal.* **2023**, *84*, 102704. [CrossRef] [PubMed]
15. Loey, M.; Smarandache, F.; M. Khalifa, N.E. Within the Lack of Chest COVID-19 X-Ray Dataset: A Novel Detection Model Based on GAN and Deep Transfer Learning. *Symmetry* **2020**, *12*, 651. [CrossRef]
16. Fujioka, T.; Kubota, K.; Mori, M.; Kikuchi, Y.; Katsuta, L.; Kimura, M.; Yamaga, E.; Adachi, M.; Oda, G.; Nakagawa, T.; et al. Efficient Anomaly Detection with Generative Adversarial Network for Breast Ultrasound Imaging. *Diagnostics* **2020**, *10*, 456. [CrossRef] [PubMed]
17. Maniaci, A.; Fakhry, N.; Chiesa-Estomba, C.; Lechien, J.R.; Lavalle, S. Synergizing ChatGPT and General AI for Enhanced Medical Diagnostic Processes in Head and Neck Imaging. *Eur. Arch. Otorhinolaryngol.* **2024**, *281*, 3297–3298. [CrossRef] [PubMed]
18. Page, M.J.; McKenzie, J.E.; Bossuyt, P.M.; Boutron, I.; Hoffmann, T.C.; Mulrow, C.D.; Shamseer, L.; Tetzlaff, J.M.; Akl, E.A.; Brennan, S.E.; et al. The PRISMA 2020 Statement: An Updated Guideline for Reporting Systematic Reviews. *BMJ* **2021**, *372*, n71. [CrossRef] [PubMed]
19. McGuinness, L.A.; Higgins, J.P.T. Risk-of-bias VISualization (Robvis): An R Package and Shiny Web App for Visualizing Risk-of-bias Assessments. *Res. Synth. Methods* **2021**, *12*, 55–61. [CrossRef] [PubMed]
20. GitHub. ChenKaiXuSan/ACGAN-PyTorch: PyTorch Implements of Auxiliary Classifier GAN. Available online: https://github.com/ChenKaiXuSan/ACGAN-PyTorch (accessed on 1 April 2024).
21. GitHub. Junyanz/CycleGAN: Software That Can Generate Photos from Paintings, Turn Horses into Zebras, Perform Style Transfer, and More. Available online: https://github.com/junyanz/CycleGAN (accessed on 1 April 2024).
22. Huang, C.-E.; Li, Y.-H.; Aslam, M.S.; Chang, C.-C. Super-Resolution Generative Adversarial Network Based on the Dual Dimension Attention Mechanism for Biometric Image Super-Resolution. *Sensors* **2021**, *21*, 7817. [CrossRef] [PubMed]
23. GitHub. KishanKancharagunta/CDGAN: CDGAN: Cyclic Discriminative Generative Adversarial Networks for Image-to-Image Transformation. Available online: https://github.com/KishanKancharagunta/CDGAN (accessed on 1 April 2024).
24. GitHub. 4vedi/Pix2Pix_GAN: Image-to-Image Translation with Conditional Adversarial Nets. Available online: https://github.com/4vedi/Pix2Pix_GAN (accessed on 1 April 2024).
25. GitHub. Tensorlayer/SRGAN: Photo-Realistic Single Image Super-Resolution Using a Generative Adversarial Network. Available online: https://github.com/tensorlayer/srgan (accessed on 1 April 2024).
26. Kong, H.-J.; Kim, J.Y.; Moon, H.-M.; Park, H.C.; Kim, J.-W.; Lim, R.; Woo, J.; Fakhri, G.E.; Kim, D.W.; Kim, S. Automation of Generative Adversarial Network-Based Synthetic Data-Augmentation for Maximizing the Diagnostic Performance with Paranasal Imaging. *Sci. Rep.* **2022**, *12*, 18118. [CrossRef]

27. Andlauer, R.; Wachter, A.; Schaufelberger, M.; Weichel, F.; Kuhle, R.; Freudlsperger, C.; Nahm, W. 3D-Guided Face Manipulation of 2D Images for the Prediction of Post-Operative Outcome after Cranio-Maxillofacial Surgery. *IEEE Trans. Image Process.* **2021**, *30*, 7349–7363. [CrossRef] [PubMed]
28. Chen, X.; Lian, C.; Wang, L.; Deng, H.; Kuang, T.; Fung, S.H.; Gateno, J.; Shen, D.; Xia, J.J.; Yap, P.-T. Diverse Data Augmentation for Learning Image Segmentation with Cross-Modality Annotations. *Med. Image Anal.* **2021**, *71*, 102060. [CrossRef] [PubMed]
29. Schaufelberger, M.; Kühle, R.P.; Wachter, A.; Weichel, F.; Hagen, N.; Ringwald, F.; Eisenmann, U.; Hoffmann, J.; Engel, M.; Freudlsperger, C.; et al. Impact of Data Synthesis Strategies for the Classification of Craniosynostosis. *Front. Med. Technol.* **2023**, *5*, 1254690. [CrossRef] [PubMed]
30. Mehandru, N.; Hicks, W.L.; Singh, A.K.; Hsu, L.; Markiewicz, M.R.; Seshadri, M. Detection of Pathology in Panoramic Radiographs via Machine Learning Using Neural Networks for Dataset Size Augmentation. *J. Oral Maxillofac. Surg.* **2021**, *79*, e6–e7. [CrossRef]
31. Xiong, Y.-T.; Zeng, W.; Xu, L.; Guo, J.-X.; Liu, C.; Chen, J.-T.; Du, X.-Y.; Tang, W. Virtual Reconstruction of Midfacial Bone Defect Based on Generative Adversarial Network. *Head Face Med.* **2022**, *18*, 19. [CrossRef] [PubMed]
32. Xu, L.; Zhou, S.; Guo, J.; Tian, W.; Tang, W.; Yi, Z. Metal Artifact Reduction for Oral and Maxillofacial Computed Tomography Images by a Generative Adversarial Network. *Appl. Intell.* **2022**, *52*, 13184–13194. [CrossRef]
33. Kim, H.-S.; Ha, E.-G.; Lee, A.; Choi, Y.J.; Jeon, K.J.; Han, S.-S.; Lee, C. Refinement of Image Quality in Panoramic Radiography Using a Generative Adversarial Network. *Dentomaxillofac. Radiol.* **2023**, *52*, 20230007. [CrossRef] [PubMed]
34. Mohammad-Rahimi, H.; Vinayahalingam, S.; Mahmoudinia, E.; Soltani, P.; Bergé, S.J.; Krois, J.; Schwendicke, F. Super-Resolution of Dental Panoramic Radiographs Using Deep Learning: A Pilot Study. *Diagnostics* **2023**, *13*, 996. [CrossRef] [PubMed]
35. Park, J.E.; Eun, D.; Kim, H.S.; Lee, D.H.; Jang, R.W.; Kim, N. Generative Adversarial Network for Glioblastoma Ensures Morphologic Variations and Improves Diagnostic Model for Isocitrate Dehydrogenase Mutant Type. *Sci. Rep.* **2021**, *11*, 9912. [CrossRef]
36. Michelutti, L.; Tel, A.; Zeppieri, M.; Ius, T.; Sembronio, S.; Robiony, M. The Use of Artificial Intelligence Algorithms in the Prognosis and Detection of Lymph Node Involvement in Head and Neck Cancer and Possible Impact in the Development of Personalized Therapeutic Strategy: A Systematic Review. *J. Pers. Med.* **2023**, *13*, 1626. [CrossRef]
37. Chinnery, T.; Arifin, A.; Tay, K.Y.; Leung, A.; Nichols, A.C.; Palma, D.A.; Mattonen, S.A.; Lang, P. Utilizing Artificial Intelligence for Head and Neck Cancer Outcomes Prediction From Imaging. *Can. Assoc. Radiol. J.* **2021**, *72*, 73–85. [CrossRef] [PubMed]
38. Chen, H. Challenges and Corresponding Solutions of Generative Adversarial Networks (GANs): A Survey Study. *J. Phys. Conf. Ser.* **2021**, *1827*, 012066. [CrossRef]
39. Lechien, J.R.; Maniaci, A.; Gengler, I.; Hans, S.; Chiesa-Estomba, C.M.; Vaira, L.A. Validity and Reliability of an Instrument Evaluating the Performance of Intelligent Chatbot: The Artificial Intelligence Performance Instrument (AIPI). *Eur. Arch. Otorhinolaryngol.* **2024**, *281*, 2063–2079. [CrossRef] [PubMed]

applied sciences

MDPI

Technical Note

Machine Learning for Predicting Neutron Effective Dose

Ali A. A. Alghamdi

Department of Radiological Sciences, College of Applied Medical Science, Imam Abdulrahman Bin Faisal University, P.O. Box 2435, Dammam 31441, Saudi Arabia; alalghamdi@iau.edu.sa

Abstract: The calculation of effective doses is crucial in many medical and radiation fields in order to ensure safety and compliance with regulatory limits. Traditionally, Monte Carlo codes using detailed human body computational phantoms have been used for such calculations. Monte Carlo dose calculations can be time-consuming and require expertise in different processes when building the computational phantom and dose calculations. This study employs various machine learning (ML) algorithms to predict the organ doses and effective dose conversion coefficients (DCCs) from different anthropomorphic phantoms. A comprehensive data set comprising neutron energy bins, organ labels, masses, and densities is compiled from Monte Carlo studies, and it is used to train and evaluate the supervised ML models. This study includes a broad range of phantoms, including those from the International Commission on Radiation Protection (ICRP-110, ICRP-116 phantom), the Visible-Human Project (VIP-man phantom), and the Medical Internal Radiation Dose Committee (MIRD-Phantom), with row data prepared using numerical data and organ categorical labeled data. Extreme gradient boosting (XGB), gradient boosting (GB), and the random forest-based Extra Trees regressor are employed to assess the performance of the ML models against published ICRP neutron DCC values using the mean square error, mean absolute error, and R^2 metrics. The results demonstrate that the ML predictions significantly vary in lower energy ranges and vary less in higher neutron energy ranges while showing good agreement with ICRP values at mid-range energies. Moreover, the categorical data models align closely with the reference doses, suggesting the potential of ML in predicting effective doses for custom phantoms based on regional populations, such as the Saudi voxel-based model. This study paves the way for efficient dose prediction using ML, particularly in scenarios requiring rapid results without extensive computational resources or expertise. The findings also indicate potential improvements in data representation and the inclusion of larger data sets to refine model accuracy and prevent overfitting. Thus, ML methods can serve as valuable techniques for the continued development of personalized dosimetry.

Keywords: machine learning; Monte Carlo; neutron dosimetry; effective dose

1. Introduction

In the field of nuclear medicine, the use of radioisotopes for diagnostic and therapeutic purposes was introduced in the 1960s. Safety prerequisites and compliance with regulatory limits led to the need to pre-calculate the dose distributions in the target organ and surrounding tissues. To calculate the dose received by the internal organs, a detailed model was introduced to estimate the diagnostic or therapeutic dose for both the organ and the entire body. This work resulted in the creation of an MIRD phantom (Medical Internal Radiation Dose Committee) [1] in conjunction with the state-of-the-art Monte Carlo N-Particle Transport code (MCNP). This model considers the full body size and shape, as well as physical characteristics, such as the density and elemental composition of organs [2]; furthermore, it has the advantage of using less computational memory. During the 1980s and 1990s, a second type of anthropomorphic phantom—known as the voxel-based phantom—was developed. This phantom takes advantage of sectional tomographic images to better represent the shape and size of organs, and it can include smaller organs in more detail. Additionally, a third type of phantom—known as the mesh-based or boundary representation (BREP) deformable phantom—was developed, which is also based on medical images. This phantom has higher resolution than the earlier phantoms and also possesses the ability to deform. All types of anthropomorphic phantoms are currently employed for research and operations in many radiological fields. Furthermore, all types have multiple versions available in different Monte Carlo codes, covering both gender and different age groups, as well as organ-specific models [3–5].

The concept of effective dose was set out by the International Commission for Radiation Protection (ICRP) [6,7]. It considers weighting factors for the selected organ tissue (radiation sensitivity) multiplied by radiation weighting factors associated with the radiation damage quality factor. The definition of the effective dose has great application potential, as it sets the dose limits for patients, workers, and the public [8]. Therefore, effective dose conversion coefficients (DCCs) have been calculated by employing all types of anthropomorphic phantoms and utilizing different Monte Carlo codes. This was achieved to accommodate the fact that defining an average person is difficult. Different locations use different types of population-based anthropomorphic phantoms [5] with the same elemental composition reference values [9,10] and varying physical characteristics, in terms of total weight, height, organ size, and shape, against the ICRP reference model.

Machine learning (ML) algorithms have been effectively applied in radiotherapy treatment planning [11], including for the segmentation and building of higher-resolution anthropomorphic tomography-based phantoms [5]. These applications depend on large amounts of evaluated data, increased computer capacity, and the development of powerful ML algorithms. One of the main advantages of ML is that it provides fast and accurate results, enabling rapid predictions [12].

This pilot study attempted to predict organ doses using supervised ML methods through tabulating several published Monte Carlo calculations of neutron DCCs for different types of anthropomorphic phantoms. The construction of the used data set and the accuracy constraints of the ML models are presented, and the results regarding organ doses and effective doses for previously uncalculated anthropomorphic phantom data are compared to the neutron DCCs published by the International Commission for Radiation Protection (ICRP) [13,14].

2. Methodology

Raw data were collected from published studies [13–17], and Python programming language was employed for ML models fitting and analysis. Table 1 shows the different types of anthropomorphic phantoms, the organs included in the study, and the target organs for the uncalculated neutron DCC in the anthropomorphic voxel phantom based on the population of Saudi Arabia [17]. This study included ICRP-110 voxel-based male and female phantoms, ICRP-116 mesh-based (a type of BREP deformable) male and female phantoms, the Visible Human Project VIP-man voxel-based phantom, and an MIRD mathematical-based phantom. Different general-purpose Monte Carlo codes were used, including the MCNP series, Geometry and Tracking 4 (GEANT4), FLUktuierend KAskade (FLUKA), and the Particle and Heavy Ion Transport Code System (PHITS). The inclusion criterion for selecting the data required for the anthropomorphic models was consistency in the calculated neutron energy bins. The data were organized vertically, with the neutron energy bins listed along with the corresponding organ labels, which were repeated for each of the 48 energy bin ranges (from 10^{-9} to 20 MeV). In addition, the associated data features, such as the weight of each organ in grams, the density in grams per cubic centimeters, and the calculated doses for anterior posterior (AP), posterior anterior (PA), and lateral (LAT) irradiation conditions were considered.

Table 1. Different types of anthropomorphic phantoms, the organs included in the study, and the target organs for uncalculated neutron effective dose conversion coefficients.

	ICRP-110-Male	ICRP-110-Female	ICRP-116-Female	ICRP-116-Male	VIP-Man	MIRD-Male	Saudi Voxel_Male
1	RBM	RBM	RBM	RBM	Adrenals	Bladder	* RBM
2	Colon	Colon	Colon	Colon	Bladder	Bone	* Colon
3	Stomach	Stomach	Stomach	Stomach	Esophagus	Colon	* Stomach
4	Gonad	Breast	Breast	Bone	Bone	Gonad	* Gonad
5	Bladder	Bladder	Bladder	Gonad	Brain	Lung	* Lung
6	Esophagus	Esophagus	Esophagus	Bladder	Liver	Liver	* Bladder
7	Liver	Liver	Liver	Esophagus	Heart	Esophagus	* Bone
8	Thyroid	Thyroid	Thyroid	Liver	RBM	RBM	* Esophagus
9	Brain	Brain	Brain	Thyroid	Kidneys	Skin	* Liver
10	Skin	Skin	Skin	Brain	Lung	Stomach	* Thyroid
11	Adrenals	Adrenals	Adrenals	Skin	Thyroid		* Brain
12	Salivary	Salivary	Salivary	Adrenals	Muscle		* Skin
13	Heart	Heart	Heart	Salivary	Skin		* Breast
14	Kidneys	Kidneys	Kidneys	Heart	Stomach		* Salivary
18	Lymph	Lymph	Lymph	Kidneys	Gonad		† Adrenal
19	Muscle	Muscle	Muscle	Lymph			† Heart
20	Pancreas	Pancreas	Pancreas	Muscle			† Kidneys
21	Prostate	Ovaries	Ovaries	Pancreas			† Lymph
22	Intestine	Intestine	Intestine	Prostate			† Muscle
23	Spleen	Spleen	Spleen	Intestine			† Pancreas
24	Thymus	Thymus	Thymus	Spleen			† Prostate
26	Eye lens	Eye lens	Eye lens	Thymus			† Intestine
27	Gall Bladder	Uterus	Uterus	Eye lens			† Spleen
28	Endothoracic	Gall bladder					† Thymus
29	Mucosa	Endothoracic					† Gall Bladder
30	Breast	Mucosa					

* ICRP 103 recommended organs assigned radiation tissues weighting factor. † Remainder tissues included in this study.

Overall, the data included 5618 rows of vertically repeated neutron energy bins for all organs from all anthropomorphic models in the energy range from 10^{-9} to 20 MeV and 6 columns representing 6 features: organ label, organ mass, organ density, AP DCC, PA DCC, and LAT DCC. Data for the final shape are provided in an Excel file (Supplementary Material Table S1). The steps and processes (known as pipelines) in ML are well documented, and further details can be found in the study of Raschka and Mirjalili [18]. The most important steps are described as follows.

2.1. Data Preparation

The number of group labels investigated included 32 labeled organs generated from the 6 anthropomorphic phantoms. These data can be used in two ways: (1) employing only numerical data for prediction and (2) converting the labeled categorical data to encode false and true tables using the "one-hot-encoder" Python function to distinguish each group of labeled organs. The results from this step were added back into the original data file, and the organ column was replaced with 32 columns.

2.2. ML Model Selection

Extreme gradient boosting (XGB) and random forest models for tabulated data are preferred over artificial neural networks (ANNs) [19–21]. Three models were selected for fitting the pilot data: XGB, gradient boosting (GB), and the random forest-based Extra Trees regressor (EXTR). The detailed parameter options can be found in [22]. Default parameters were used, with a fixed number of estimators (n-estimator = 100), and the data (5168 × 38 after dropping the desired fitting target) were divided into a 75% sample for training and a 25% sample for testing.

2.3. Evaluation and Cross Validation

Table 2 shows a sample of the cross-validation scores of the ML models for the mean square error, mean absolute error, and R^2, employing categorical labeled data for the EXTR-C, XGB-C, and GB-C ML models and numerical data for the EXTR, XGB, and GB ML models.

Table 2. Cross-validation scores (fractional unit) of the ML models for mean square error, mean absolute error, and R^2, employing categorical labeled data (for the EXTR-C, XGB-C, and GB-C ML models) and numerical data (for the EXTR, XGB, and GB ML models).

ML Model	Mean Square Error	Mean Absolute Error	R^2
EXTR-C	3.42	0.88	0.992
XGB-C	1.57	0.01	0.996
GB-C	5.41	1.32	0.987
EXTR	6.54	1.24	0.984
XGB	2.30	0.65	0.994
GB	3.82	1.14	0.990

Figure 1 illustrates a sample of R^2 values for the categorically labeled data models. In addition, the three models were compared in terms of k-fold accuracy for both the training and testing sets. The box plot in Figure 1 displays the results of the k-fold accuracy analysis with five cross-validations, showing the performance of all models for both types of data fitting, including the training and testing sets. In general, all three models performed well and demonstrated better results when fitting the categorical data. K-fold analysis can be used with large or small size data. However, while the hyperparameter tuning of any of the three models may lead to improved results, hyperparameters tuning except for k-fold analysis were avoided in this study, as it was found to potentially cause overfitting of the results. Future studies involving larger data sets should consider the use of hyperparameter tuning techniques.

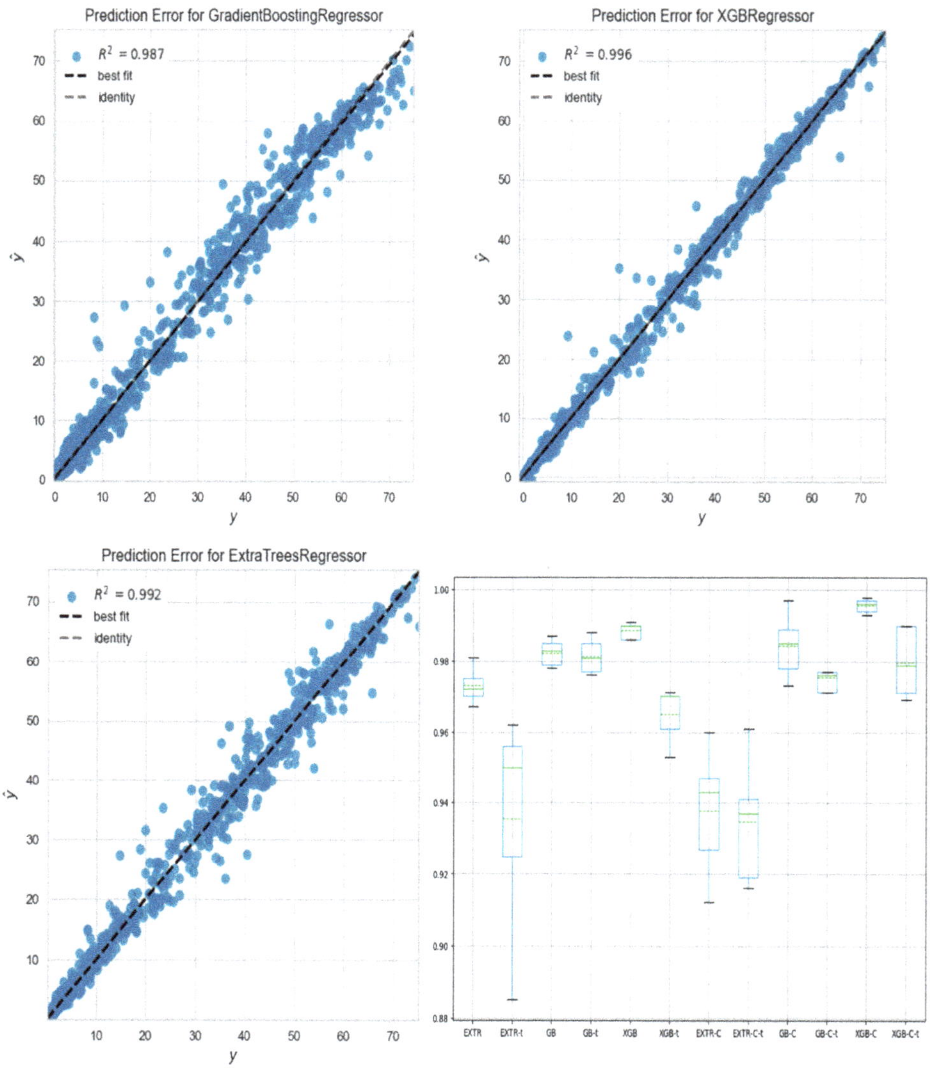

Figure 1. R^2 values for the categorical labeled data training set for the EXTR-C, XGB-C, and GB-C models, both actual (y) and predicted ($\hat{y}$) units in pSv. The box plot in the lower right corner of the figure shows the results for the k-fold accuracy analysis with five cross-validations for all models on the training set for numerical data (EXTR, GB, XGB), categorical data (EXTR-C, GB-C, XGB-C), testing set for numerical data (EXTR-t, GB-t, XGB-t) and categorical data (EXTR-C-t, GB-C-t, XGB-C-t).

3. Results and Discussion

Figure 2 shows a comparison of the XGB, GB, and EXTR models. These models used both numerical and categorical data (XGB-C, GB-C, and EXTR-C) to predict doses for the target voxel-based anthropomorphic phantom. Selected organ doses for the colon and red bone marrow (RBM) at different irradiation positions (AP, PA, and LAT) were compared with the ICRP-116 mesh-based and ICRP-110 voxel-based anthropomorphic reference calculated the organ doses. The results obtained when using predictive ML models (numerical and categorical) overlapped with each other; however, a deviation in the results of some models was observed. For red bone marrow (RBM) AP irradiation conditions, the values for neutron energies lower than 1 eV had percentile differences that varied between 40% (for the EXTR, EXTR-C, and XGB-C models) and 87% (for GB, GB-C, and XGB). For higher neutron energies, the values varied between 3% and 27% for all of the models.

The ML model predictions varied, and the EXTR-C and XGB-C models generally performed better than the other models; for example, for the colon LAT DCCs in Figure 2, the XGB model using numerical data presented signs of underestimation and overfitting. All ML models scored an average percentile difference of less than 9% with respect to ICRP-116 LAT DCCs.

The models employed for fitting categorical data (XGB-C, GB-C, and EXTR-C) showed reasonable agreement with the reference values of ICRP-116 and ICRP-110, considering the variation in the physical characteristics of the organ (assigned features weight and density) for the target voxel phantom. Notably, the results of ICRP-116 and ICRP-110 represented the average of several Monte Carlo codes calculations with a variation of 15% [13,14].

For effective dose calculations, categorical data for organ dose prediction were considered using three linear ML models (XGB-C, GB-C, and EXTR-C). The calculation methods described in ICRP-103 and ICRP-116 using a function for the neutron energy radiation weighting factor dependency were adopted. ICRP-103 recommends a radiation-sensitive assigned weighting factor for 14 organs (Table 1) with the remaining tissues segmented in the Saudi voxel anthropomorphic phantom.

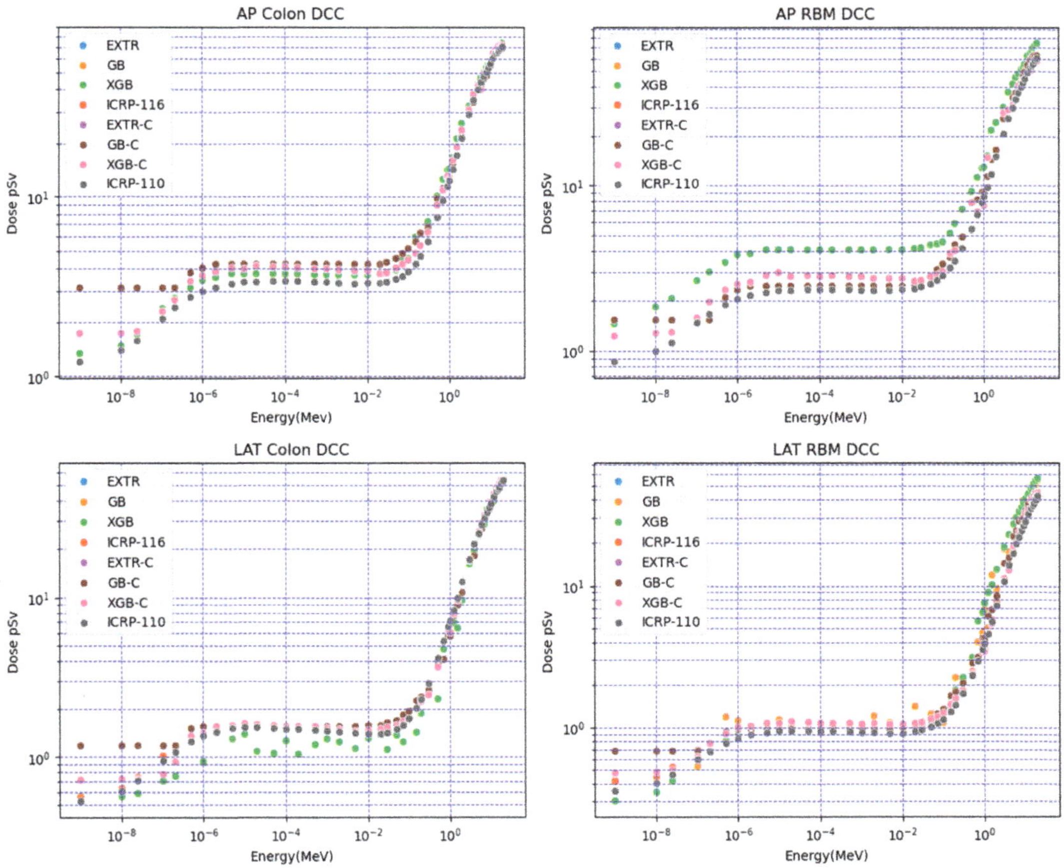

Figure 2. *Cont.*

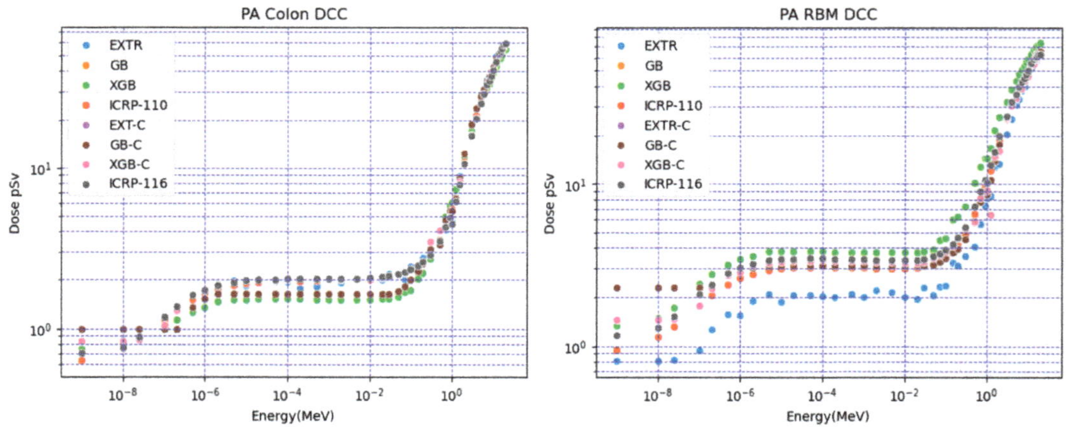

Figure 2. Comparison of predicted doses for colon and red bone marrow (RBM) in different irradiation positions (AP, PA, and LAT) using the ICRP (116 mesh-based and 110 voxel-based) anthropomorphic reference.

Figure 3 shows the results of the neutron effective dose CC for the AP, PA, and LAT irradiation conditions compared with ICRP-116. The comparison results, obtained through dividing the ML model-predicted value by the ICRP-116 values, are shown in Figure 3 (right lower corner graph). The PA had the largest deviation, which was followed by the AP and LAT. The major contributors to the received dose in organs depend primarily on the position of the organ relative to the irradiation source and the mean position volume of the organ within the phantom. Therefore, differences can be expected when comparing with the agreed reference anthropomorphic phantom provided by the ICRP. Figure 3 shows the PA effective dose calculations for the FAX voxel-based phantom using the ICRP-103 radiation weighting factors [23] and the Zubal voxel-based phantom [24]. The deviation was larger than the Saudi voxel-based ML model-predicted neutron effective dose CC versus the ICRP reference values. The use of different neutron radiation weighting factors and different numbers of organs in the calculations may explain the larger deviation for the FAX voxel phantom and, to a lesser extent, Zubal voxel-based phantoms, compared to that in the current study. Despite the possible sources of variation, the present results indicate that the ML model predictions were within the range of expected differences given the large variations between neutron effective doses from different anthropomorphic phantoms [13–17,23,24].

The prediction of the categorical data models for the neutron effective dose exhibited reasonable results, considering the differences in the voxel phantom based on the Saudi population for organ sizes and assigned physical characteristics for weights and densities.

Finally, the size of the row data used in this study (5618 rows $\times$ 6 columns) was within the medium range. Therefore, while the interpretations of the current results show reasonable agreement with the expected neutron DCC trend, the results may be improved further through increasing the size of the sample.

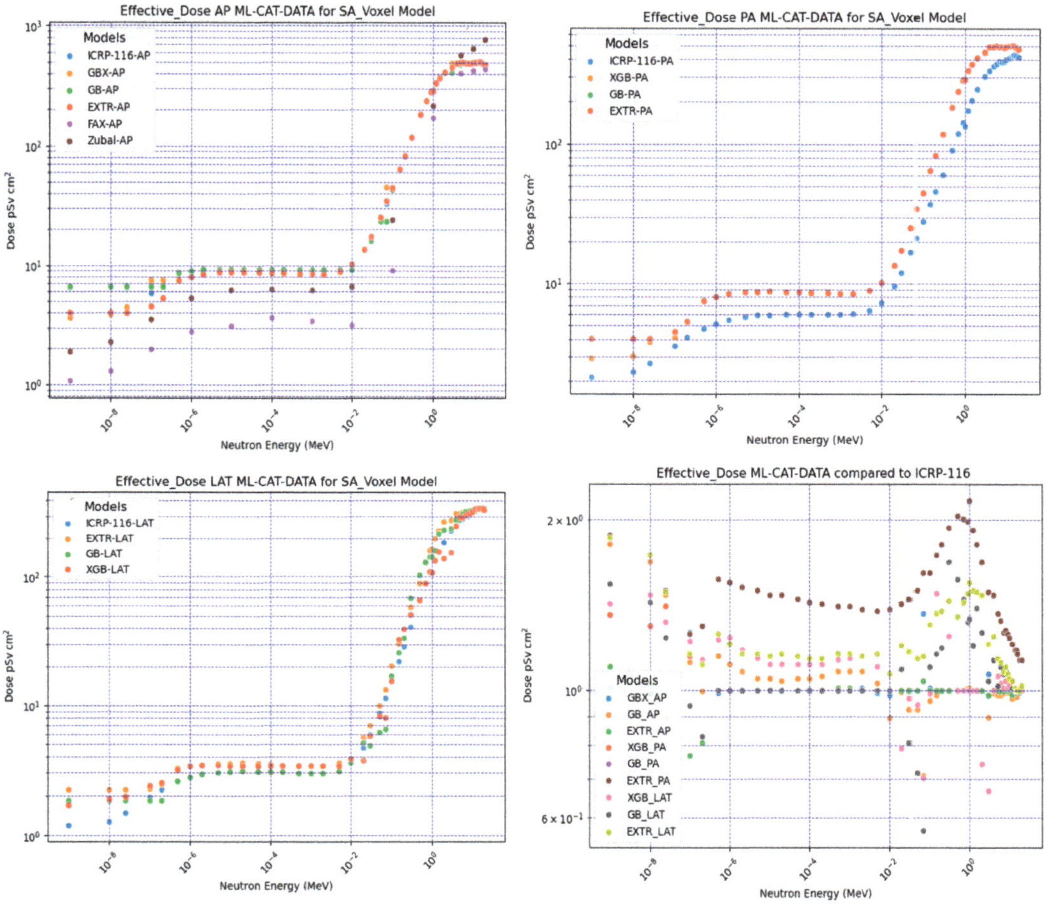

Figure 3. ML prediction using categorical data (ML-CAT-DATA) for the Saudi voxel phantom (SA-Voxel model) neutron effective dose CC for AP, PA, and LAT irradiation conditions compared with ICRP-116.

4. Conclusions

In this study, we presented a method for constructing a data set which enables ML-based prediction from previously calculated Monte Carlo neutron DCCs from different types of anthropomorphic phantoms. The results of the ML models were in agreement with the ICRP values at medium neutron energies but presented large deviations at lower energies and relatively acceptable deviation at higher energy ranges; however, these observed differences were expected and fell within a reasonable range. Although the current study covered more than 75% of the published calculated neutron effective DCCs, the overall number of such studies remains low. Therefore, to eliminate the possibility of overfitting, the size of the data set could be increased in future investigations through including more simulation studies or applying ML models to photon DCCs, for which more investigations of anthropomorphic phantoms have been conducted on a larger scale.

Better fitting results were obtained with categorical arranged data than when using numerical data; however, numerical data offer the possibility to predict one or multiple organs and one or multiple energy bins.

This study demonstrated that ML can be an efficient tool for dose prediction, depending on the number of available Monte Carlo studies covering different anthropomorphic phantoms. In many cases, such Monte Carlo dose calculations are time-consuming, require expertise, and require the computational capacity to incorporate a large number of voxels. Therefore, ML methods offer the possibility of dose prediction when rapid results are required. ML has some additional advantages in terms of flexibility in accommodating different data; however, it should be considered that ML models are very sensitive to irregularities in the data, such as the number of energy bins considered in the Monte Carlo calculations.

Supplementary Materials: The following supporting information can be downloaded at: https://www.mdpi.com/article/10.3390/app14135740/s1, Table S1: Anthropomorphic Phantom's Data.

Funding: This research received no external funding.

Conflicts of Interest: The author declares no conflicts of interest.

References

1. Snyder, W.S.; Ford, M.R.; Warner, G.G.; Fisher, H.L., Jr. *Estimates of Absorbed Fractions for Monoenergetic Photon Sources Uniformly Distributed in Various Organs of a Heterogeneous Phantom*; Oak Ridge National Lab: Oak Ridge, TN, USA, 1969.
2. Howell, R.W.; Wessels, B.W.; Loevinger, R.; MIRD Committee. The MIRD perspective 1999. *J. Nucl. Med.* **1999**, *40*, 3S–10S. [PubMed]
3. Abadi, E.; Segars, W.P.; Tsui, B.M.; Kinahan, P.E.; Bottenus, N.; Frangi, A.F.; Maidment, A.; Lo, J.; Samei, E. Virtual clinical trials in medical imaging: A review. *J. Med. Imaging* **2020**, *7*, 042805–042845. [CrossRef] [PubMed]
4. Kim, C.H.; Yeom, Y.S.; Petoussi-Hen, N.; Zankl, M.; Bolch, W.E.; Lee, C.; Choi, C.; Nguyen, T.T.; Eckerman, K.; Kim, H.S.; et al. ICRP publication 145: Adult mesh-type reference computational phantoms. *Ann. ICRP* **2020**, *49*, 13–201. [CrossRef]
5. Peng, Z.; Gao, N.; Wu, B.; Chen, Z.; Xu, X.G. A review of computational phantoms for quality assurance in radiology and radiotherapy in the deep-learning era. *J. Radiat. Prot. Res.* **2022**, *47*, 111–133. [CrossRef]
6. International Commission on Radiological Protection. *Recommendations of the International Commission on Radiological Protection*; ICRP Publication 26; ICRP Publication: Oxford, UK, 1977.
7. International Commission on Radiological Protection. *1990 Recommendations of the International Commission on Radiological Protection*; ICRP Publication 60; The International Commission on Radiological Protection: New York, NY, USA, 1991.
8. McCollough, C.H.; Schueler, B.A. Calculation of effective dose. *Med. Phys.* **2000**, *27*, 828–837. [CrossRef] [PubMed]
9. Scott, J.A. *Photon, Electron, Proton and Neutron Interaction Data for Body Tissues: ICRU Report 46*; International Commission on Radiation Units and Measurements: Bethesda, MD, USA, 1992.
10. Zankl, M.; Schlattl, H.; Petoussi-Henss, N.; Hoeschen, C. Electron specific absorbed fractions for the adult male and female ICRP/ICRU reference computational phantoms. *Phys. Med. Biol.* **2012**, *57*, 4501. [CrossRef] [PubMed]
11. Wang, M.; Zhang, Q.; Lam, S.; Cai, J.; Yang, R. A review on application of deep learning algorithms in external beam radiotherapy automated treatment planning. *Front. Oncol.* **2020**, *10*, 580919. [CrossRef] [PubMed]
12. Shao, W.; Lin, X.; Yi, Y.; Huang, Y.; Qu, L.; Zhuo, W.; Liu, H. Fast prediction of patient-specific organ doses in brain CT scans using support vector regression algorithm. *Phys. Med. Biol.* **2024**, *69*, 025010. [CrossRef]
13. ICRPP. Adult reference computational phantoms. ICRP Publication 110. *Ann. ICRP.* **2009**, *39*, 1.
14. ICRP. Conversion Coefficients for Radiological Protection Quantities for External Radiation Exposures. ICRP Publication 116. *Ann. ICRP* **2010**, *40*, 2–5.
15. Bozkurt, A.; Chao, T.C.; Xu, X.G. Fluence-to-dose conversion coefficients from monoenergetic neutrons below 20 MeV based on the VIP-man anatomical model. *Phys. Med. Biol.* **2000**, *45*, 3059. [CrossRef] [PubMed]
16. Hakimabad, H.M.; Motavalli, L.R.; Shahri, K.K. Assessment of neutron fluence to organ dose conversion coefficients in the ORNL analytical adult phantom. *J. Radiol. Prot.* **2009**, *29*, 51. [CrossRef] [PubMed]
17. Ma, A.K.; Hussein, M.A.; Altaher, K.M.; Farid, K.Y.; Amer, M.; Aldhafery, B.F.; Alghamdi, A.A. Fluence-to-effective dose conversion coefficients from a Saudi population based phantom for monoenergetic photon beams from 10 keV to 20 MeV. *J. Radiol. Prot.* **2014**, *35*, 75. [CrossRef] [PubMed]
18. Raschka, S.; Mirjalili, V. *Python Machine Learning: Machine Learning and Deep Learning with Python, Scikit-Learn, and TensorFlow 2*; Packt Publishing Ltd.: Birmingham, UK, 2019.
19. Deka, B.; Maji, P.; Mitra, S.; Bhattacharyya, D.; Bora, P.; Pal, S. Pattern Recognition and Machine Intelligence. In Proceedings of the 8th International Conference, PReMI 2019, Tezpur, India, 17–20 December 2019.
20. Geurts, P.; Ernst, D.; Wehenkel, L. Extremely randomized trees. *Mach. Learn.* **2006**, *63*, 3–42. [CrossRef]
21. Luo, Y.; Chen, S.; Valdes, G. Machine learning for radiation outcome modeling and prediction. *Med. Phys.* **2020**, *47*, e178–e184. [CrossRef]
22. Pedregosa, F.; Varoquaux, G.; Gramfort, A.; Michel, V.; Thirion, B.; Grisel, O.; Blondel, M.; Prettenhofer, P.; Weiss, R.; Dubourg, V.; et al. Scikit-learn: Machine learning in Python. *JMLR* **2011**, *12*, 2825–2830.

23. Cordeiro, T.P.V.; Silva, A.X.; Crispim, V.R. Calculation of conversion coefficients for effective dose for neutrons using a female voxel anthropomorphic model and the MCNPX code. In Proceedings of the INAC 2009: International Nuclear Atlantic Conference. Innovations in Nuclear Technology for a Sustainable Future, Rio de Janeiro, Brazil, 27 September–2 October 2009.
24. Alghamdi, A.A.; Ma, A.; Tzortzis, M.; Spyrou, N.M. Neutron-fluence-to-dose conversion coefficients in an anthropomorphic phantom. *Radiat. Prot. Dosim.* **2005**, *115*, 606–611. [CrossRef]

MDPI AG
Grosspeteranlage 5
4052 Basel
Switzerland
Tel.: +41 61 683 77 34

MDPI Books Editorial Office
E-mail: books@mdpi.com
www.mdpi.com/books

www.ingramcontent.com/pod-product-compliance
Lightning Source LLC
LaVergne TN
LVHW070054160926
848129LV00013B/623
* 9 7 8 3 7 2 5 8 5 4 7 1 4 *